Biosurfactants

ADVANCES IN EXPERIMENTAL MEDICINE AND BIOLOGY

Biosurfactants

Edited by

Ramkrishna Sen, MTech, PhD
*Bioprocess and Bioproduct Development Laboratory, Department of Biotechnology,
Indian Institute of Technology Kharagpur, West Bengal, India*

Springer Science+Business Media, LLC

Landes Bioscience

Springer Science+Business Media, LLC
Landes Bioscience

Printed in the USA.

Springer Science+Business Media, LLC, 233 Spring Street, New York, New York 10013, USA
http://www.springer.com

Please address all inquiries to the publishers:
Landes Bioscience, 1002 West Avenue, Austin, Texas 78701, USA
Phone: 512/ 637 6050; FAX: 512/ 637 6079
http://www.landesbioscience.com

The chapters in this book are available in the Madame Curie Bioscience Database.
http://www.landesbioscience.com/curie

Biosurfactants, edited by Ramkrishna Sen. Landes Bioscience / Springer Science+Business Media, LLC
dual imprint / Springer series: Advances in Experimental Medicine and Biology.

ISBN: 978-1-4419-5978-2

Library of Congress Cataloging-in-Publication Data

Library of Congress Cataloging-in-Publication Data

Biosurfactants / edited by Ramkrishna Sen.
    p. cm.
ISBN 978-1-4419-5978-2
1. Biosurfactants. I. Sen, Ramkrishna, 1966-
TP248.B57B558 2010
668'.1--dc22
                        2009052185

DEDICATION

To my parents—my Maa, Manjushree Sen and Baba, Gouranga Prasad Sen

FOREWORD

The microbial world has given us many surprises including microbes that grow under extremely harsh conditions (122°C at 40 MPa), novel metabolisms such as the uranium and perchlorate reduction, and novel chemicals that can be used to control diseases. We continually face new and difficult problems such as the need to transition to more carbon-neutral energy sources and to find eco-friendly chemicals and to find new drugs to treat disease. Will it be possible to tap into the seemingly limitless potential of microbial activity to solve our current and future problems? The answer to this question is probably yes. We are already looking to the microbial world to provide new energy sources, green chemicals to replace those made from petroleum, and new drugs to fight disease. To help us along these paths, we are deciphering how microorganisms interact with each other. We know that microbial populations interact and communicate with each other. The language that microbes use is chemical where small molecules are exchanged among different microbial cells. Sometimes, these chemicals suppress activities of competitors and could be used as antibiotics or may have other therapeutic uses. Other times, the chemicals stimulate complex responses in microbial populations such as fruiting body or biofilm formation. By understanding the conversation that microbes are having among themselves, e.g., what chemicals are made and why these chemicals are made, we should be able to discover new chemicals that control microbial growth and activity; some of these will have other applications. One class of chemicals made by microorganisms that is finding more and more practical use is biosurfactants.

Biosurfactants are low molecular weight, amphiphilic compounds produced by a wide variety of microorganisms. Due to their amphiphilic nature, biosurfactants have hydrophilic and lipophilic moieties that allow the biosurfactants to partition at water/air, oil/air, or the oil/ water interfaces where it lowers surface and/or interfacial tension. We have known for many years that hydrocarbon-degrading microorganisms make biosurfactants to increase the apparent aqueous solubility of the hydrocarbon by forming micelles or to alter surface properties of the cell to bring the microbe to the hydrocarbon. However, it was unclear until recently why non-hydrocarbon-degrading bacteria make biosurfactants. Recent research indicates that there are a number of reasons why microorganisms make biosurfactants; mainly these reasons relate to the need to change surface or interfacial properties of the cell or local environment. Surface or interfacial tension changes are needed for the erection of fruiting bodies, swarming of cells, gliding motility, and biofilm formation and development. Because biosurfactants are involved in the complex social responses that control cell development, they also have a number of therapeutic functions including anti-microbial and anti-tumor activities.

One important feature of biosurfactants is that they have very low critical micelle concentrations (CMC), much lower than chemically made surfactants. The low CMC of biosurfactants means that biosurfactants are effective at low concentrations, lower than many chemically made surfactants, so only small amounts of biosurfactants are needed to reduce surface and interfacial tension. The fact that only small amounts of biosurfactants coupled with their known biodegradability make them excellent candidates for "green" detergents and surfactants. More productive strains, better fermentation conditions and cheaper substrates are needed to reduce costs and expand the applications of biosurfactants. This book presents a number of outlooks on the production and use of biosurfactants. Dr. Cameotra et al reviews the synthesis and advantages of biosurfactants. Dr. Nerurkar and Dr. Sen each discuss the structural and functional features of the well-studied lipopeptide biosurfactants, lichenysin and surfactin, respectively. Methods to screen for biosurfactant producers are discussed by Walter et al, which should assist those interested in obtaining new biosurfactant producers. Das et al discuss the potential to obtain new biosurfactant producers from marine environments. Two chapters discuss biosurfactant production by yeasts. Campos-Takaki et al reviews environmentally friendly biosurfactants made by yeast while Amaral et al discusses the characteristics, production and applications of biosurfactants made by yeasts.

One problem with commercial applications of biosurfactants is that they are made in low concentrations, which make product recovery difficult and expensive. A major theme of the book is the use of alternative substrates and fermentation approaches to reduce cost and optimize biosurfactant production. Chapters by Benincasa et al and Pornsunthorntawee et al discuss new or alternate strategies for the production and use of rhamnolipids. Solid-state cultivation for biosurfactant production (chapter by Krieger et al) is a logical outcome of role of biosurfactants in biofilm formation. Non-aqueous phase production may also be an economic way to make biosurfactants as discussed by Zinjarde and Ghosh. Finally, Baker and Chen discuss how one can take advantage of the ability of biosurfactants to form micelles to facilitate recovery.

An important factor limiting the application of biosurfactants is that chemically made surfactants have better interfacial properties with diverse hydrophobic compounds than biosurfactants do. New structures with better properties are needed. The chapter by Koglin et al discusses strategies to redesign biosurfactant structure to optimize activity for specific applications. Palme et al discuss the properties, production and chemoenzymatic modification of glycoglycerolipids and oligosaccharide lipids. Mehta et al discuss the structural features that govern surface activity and biological function. The interaction of di-rhamnolipids with phospholipids membranes and the mechanism of how these molecules disrupt membranes are discussed by Ortiz et al.

Another important theme of the book is the diverse applications of biosurfactants for environmental clean-up, oil recovery, and medicine. Mukherjee and Das provide an overview of these applications. Prof. Ward lends his considerable expertise to review the use of biosurfactants to stimulate biodegradation. Joshi and Desai review the use of biosurfactants in bioremediation of non-aqueous phase liquids while Franzetti et al review the use of biosurfactants in bioremediation. Two chapters, one by Perfumo et al and the other by Khire, discuss the use of biosurfactants for oil recovery. Rodrigues and Teixeira discuss the growing biomedical and therapeutic applications of biosurfactants.

With a greater understanding of how and why microorganisms make biosurfactants with an insight into the molecular genetics of their biosynthesis (chapter by Shete et al), we can better manipulate the physiology of biosurfactant producers to enhance productivity and to identify more active compounds. The book provides comprehensive overviews on the diversity of biosurfactant-producing microorganisms and types of biosurfactant molecules that are made. Also, the book includes a state-of-the-art discussion on the use of alternative substrates and fermentation approaches for biosurfactant production.

Prof. Michael J. McInerney
Department of Botany and Microbiology
University of Oklahoma
Norman, Oklahoma
USA

PREFACE

The idea of writing or editing a book on 'Biosurfactants' struck me immediately after we published a review in *Trends in Biotechnology* [2006; 24(11):509-515], which received very good feedback from the world biosurfactant research community. In one fine morning, when I received an email from Ron Landes of Landes Bioscience, USA, requesting me to edit a book on biosurfactants, I spared no time to grab the opportunity and contacted all those who are international experts in the area of biosurfactant research and development. It is the prompt and positive responses from my dear colleagues who through their valuable contributions made my wish and endeavor of bringing out the book on comprehensive review of the background and recent advances in the field of biosurfactants a reality. Their timely efforts and contributions are thus gratefully appreciated. The book, which deserves to be an excellent reference book on various facets of the fascinating world of biosurfactants, would surely live up to the expectations of the researchers actively involved and keenly interested in biosurfactant R&D, both in academia and industry. The book consists of 24 chapters from different research groups—each one represents the progress, prospect and challenges in biosurfactant research.

This is supposed to be the most up-to-date book on 'biosurfactants'. Moreover, the enormous commercial and healthcare potentials of biosurfactants and the current market demand for cost competitive and environment friendly alternatives to synthetic surfactants, particularly when an impending petroleum crisis is looming large all over the world, have encouraged me to undertake the challenge of editing this book on 'Biosurfactants'. We endeavor not only to highlight the tremendous progress made by the scientific community in this field of research, but also to critically analyze the lacuna to improve the commercial prospects of these wonder biomolecules by resorting to novel screening methods, metabolic pathway engineering, and innovative process development and application strategies. I do fervently hope that the book will be able to cater to the needs of the research scientists and technologists at large. We will be very happy if our sincere efforts enhance the reader's understanding of the new developments in this subject area.

I thankfully acknowledge all the authors and co-authors of each chapter of the book for their valuable and inspiring contributions. I do highly appreciate the help that I have constantly received from my colleagues at Landes Bioscience; particularly from Cynthia, Celeste, Erin and Scott. I also thank my research students, particularly Soumen; my wife, Anamika and my little son, Adi for their support, understanding and forbearance.

Ramkrishna Sen, MTech, PhD
Bioprocess and Bioproduct Development Laboratory
Department of Biotechnology
Indian Institute of Technology Kharagpur
West Bengal, India

ABOUT THE EDITOR...

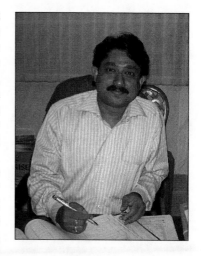

RAMKRISHNA SEN is an Assistant Professor (Bioprocess Engineering) in the Department of Biotechnology, Indian Institute of Technology (IIT) Kharagpur, India. Before joining IIT Kharagpur, Dr. Sen served BITS, Pilani as an Assistant Professor and Cadila Pharmaceuticals Ltd., Ahmedabad as the Manager (R&D–Biotech). He successfully completed some industrial projects and launched modern biotechnology products. At the IIT Kharagpur, he currently heads the 'Bioprocess and Bioproduct Development' group, consisting of 11 research scholars, 2 MTech and 2 BTech project students, who are actively involved in developing, optimizing, modeling and scaling up bioprocesses for the production and applications of marine biosurfactants, probiotics based nutraceuticals, water-repellant durable jute geotextiles and biofuels. Dr. Sen, being a biochemical engineer with industrial R&D experience had set his research priorities in broader areas of biotherapy and bioenergy. His Biosurfactant group is engaged in characterizing marine microbial surfactants for their potential commercial, healthcare (antimicrobial and anticancer) and environmental (including bioremediation and MEOR) applications. His Nutraceutical group is developing probiotic based nutraceuticals and also working on probioactive molecules like bacteriocin and antihyperglycemic EPS molecule with significant antioxidant activities (Patent Application No.: 594/KOL/2009) and industrial enzymes. Dr. Sen was also involved in developing a biofuel additive for diesel engine, which showed superior fuel properties and pollution characteristics (Patent Appl. No.: KOL/1373/2006). His group is recently involved in developing hydrophobic geotextiles, continuous processes for biodiesel production (sponsored by PfP Technology LLC., Houston, USA) and process integration for bio-ethanol (in collaboration with NEERI, Nagpur) production. Dr. Sen has international research collaborations with some foreign universities and has visited many foreign countries including USA, UK, Brazil, Portugal, Czech Republic, Malaysia, Australia, etc. He has a number of sponsored research and consultancy projects and several research/review articles and book chapters in high impact international journals and highly rated books in the field of biotechnology and biochemical engineering. He serves as a reviewer of 17 peer reviewed international journals and has edited this book being published by Landes Bioscience and Springer Science+Business Media, LLC. Dr. Sen was recently invited as one of the founding members of the recently launched Global Biorenewables (BioEnergy) Research Society (GBR Society) in Lisbon. His biography has been published in Who's Who in Science & Engineering (2007) and Who's Who in the World (2008).

PARTICIPANTS

Clarissa Daisy C. Albuquerque
Nucleus of Research in Environmental
  Sciences
Center of Sciences and Technology
Catholic University of Pernambuco
Pernambuco
Brazil

Priscilla F.F. Amaral
Department of Biochemistry
  Engineering
Escola de Química/Universidade Federal
  do Rio de Janeiro
Rio de Janeiro
Brazil

Francisco J. Aranda
Departamento de Bioquímica y Biología
  Molecular-A
Universidad de Múrcia
Múrcia
Spain

Simon C. Baker
School of Life Sciences
Oxford Brookes University
Oxford
UK

Ibrahim M. Banat
School of Biomedical Sciences
University of Ulster, Coleraine
Northern Ireland
UK

Maria Benincasa
Departamento Biologia Aplicada
  Agropecuária
Universidade Estadual Paulista
Jaboticabal
Brazil

Frank Bernhard
Center for Biomolecular Magnetic
  Resonance
Goethe-University of Frankfurt/Main
Institute for Biophysical Chemistry
Frankfurt/Main
Germany

Smita S. Bhuyan
Department of Microbiology
University of Pune
Maharashtra
India

Swaranjit Singh Cameotra
Institute of Microbial Technology
and
Microbial Type Culture Collection
  and Gene Bank
International Development Association
Chandigarh
India

Galba M. Campos-Takaki
Nucleus of Research in Environmental
   Sciences
Center of Sciences and Technology
Catholic University of Pernambuco
Pernambuco
Brazil

Chien-Yen Chen
Department of Earth and Environmental
   Sciences
National Chung Cheng University
Chia-Yi
Taiwan

Balu A. Chopade
Institute of Bioinformatics
   & Biotechnology
and
Department of Microbiology
University of Pune
Maharashtra
India

Maria Alice Z. Coelho
Department of Biochemistry
   Engineering
Escola de Química/Universidade Federal
   do Rio de Janeiro
Centro de Tecnologia
Rio de Janeiro
Brazil

João A.P. Coutinho
CICECO, Department of Chemistry
University of Aveiro
Aveiro
Portugal

Kishore Das
Department of Diagnostic Medicine and
   Pathobiology
Kansas State University
Manhattan, Kansas
USA

Palashpriya Das
Bioprocess and Bioproduct
   Development Laboratory
Department of Biotechnology
Indian Institute of Technology
   Kharagpur
West Bengal
India

Anjana J. Desai
Department of Microbiology
   and Biotechnology Center
The M.S. University of Baroda
Vadodara
India

Prashant K. Dhakephalkar
Division of Microbial Sciences
Agharkar Research Institute
Maharashtra
India

Volker Doetsch
Center for Biomolecular Magnetic
   Resonance
Goethe-University of Frankfurt/Main
Institute for Biophysical Chemistry
Frankfurt/Main
Germany

Andrea Franzetti
Department of Environmental Sciences
University of Milano-Bicocca
Milano
Italy

Mahua Ghosh
Department of Chemical Technology
University of Calcutta
Calcutta
India

Rudolf Hausmann
Institute of Engineering in Life Sciences
Department Technical Biology
University of Karlsruhe
Karlsruhe
Germany

Dimitri Iphöfer
Biotechnology Group
Institute of Biochemistry
   and Biotechnology
Technical University of Braunschweig
Braunschweig
Germany

Sanket J. Joshi
N.V. Patel College of Basic and Applied
   Sciences
Vallabh Vidyanagar
Gujarat
India

Jasminder Kaur
Home Science
Chandigarh Admn.
Chandigarh
India

J.M. Khire
NCIM Resource Center
Division of Biochemical Sciences
National Chemical Laboratory
Pune
India

Alexander Koglin
Department of Biological Chemistry
   and Molecular Pharmacology
Harvard Medical School
Boston, Massachusetts
USA

Nadia Krieger
Chemistry Department
Federal University of Parana
Curitiba
Brazil

Siegmund Lang
Biotechnology Group
Institute of Biochemistry
   and Biotechnology
Technical University of Braunschweig
Braunschweig
Germany

Randhir S. Makkar
Department of Developmental
   Neurogenetics
Children Research Institute
Medical University of South Carolina
Charleston, South Carolina
USA

Angels Manresa
Laboratori de Microbiologia
Universitat de Barcelona
Barcelona
Spain

Isabel M.J. Marrucho
CICECO, Department of Chemistry
Universidade de Aveiro
Aveiro
Portugal

AnaM^a Marqués
Laboratori de Microbiologia
Universitat de Barcelona
Barcelona
Spain

Michael J. McInerney
Department of Botany and Microbiology
University of Oklahoma
Norman, Oklahoma
USA

Neena Mehta
S.D.D. Dental College
Golpura
Barwala
India

S.K. Mehta
Center of Advanced Studies
   in Chemistry
Department of Chemistry
Panjab University
Chandigarh
India

David Alexander Mitchell
Departamento de Bioquímica e Biologia
   Molecular
Universidade Federal do Paraná
Curitiba
Brazil

Anja Moszyk
Biotechnology Group
Institute of Biochemistry
   and Biotechnology
Technical University of Braunschweig
Braunschweig
Germany

Shilpa S. Mujumdar
Department of Microbiology
Modern College of Arts, Science
   and Commerce
Maharashtra
Índia

Ashis K. Mukherjee
Department of Molecular Biology
   and Biotechnology
Tezpur University
Assam
India

Soumen Mukherjee
Bioprocess and Bioproduct
   Development Laboratory
Department of Biotechnology
Indian Institute of Technology
   Kharagpur
West Bengal
India

Anuradha S. Nerurkar
Department of Microbiology
   and Biotechnology Center
The Maharaja Sayajirao University
   of Baroda
Gujarat
India

Doumit Camilios Neto
Departamento de Bioquímica e Biologia
   Molecular
Universidade Federal do Paraná
Curitiba
Brazil

Antonio Ortiz
Departamento de Bioquímica y Biología
   Molecular-A
Universidad de Múrcia
Múrcia
Spain

Olof Palme
Biotechnology Group
Institute of Biochemistry
   and Biotechnology
Technical University of Braunschweig
Braunschweig
Germany

Karishma R. Pardesi
Department of Microbiology
University of Pune
Maharashtra
India

Amedea Perfumo
School of Biomedical Sciences
University of Ulster, Coleraine
Northern Ireland
UK

Aurora Pinazo
Departament de Tecnologia
   de Tensioactius
Consejo Superior de Investigaciones
   Científicas
Barcelona
Spain

Orathai Pornsunthorntawee
The Petroleum and Petrochemical
   College
Chulalongkorn University
Bangkok
Thailand

Ivo Rancich
Idrabel Italia S.r.L.
Genoa
Italy

Lígia R. Rodrigues
Institute for Biotechnology
    and Bioengineering
Center of Biological Engineering
Universidade do Minho
Braga
Portugal

Ratana Rujiravanit
The Petroleum and Petrochemical
    College
Chulalongkorn University
Bangkok
Thailand

Leonie Asfora Sarubbo
Nucleus of Research in Environmental
    Sciences
Center of Sciences and Technology
Catholic University of Pernambuco
Pernambuco
Brazil

Surekha K. Satpute
Department of Microbiology
University of Pune
Maharashtra
India

Ramkrishna Sen
Bioprocess and Bioproduct
    Development Laboratory
Department of Biotechnology
Indian Institute of Technology
    Kharagpur
West Bengal
India

Shweta Sharma
Center of Advanced Studies
    in Chemistry
Department of Chemistry
Panjab University
Chandigarh
India

Ashvini M. Shete
Praj Industries Limited
Maharashtra
Índia

C. Sivapathasekaran
Bioprocess and Bioproduct
    Development Laboratory
Department of Biotechnology
Indian Institute of Technology
    Kharagpur
West Bengal
India

Christoph Syldatk
Institute of Engineering in Life Sciences
Department Technical Biology
University of Karlsruhe
Karlsruhe
Germany

Elena Tamburini
Department of Biomedical Science
    and Technology
University of Cagliari
Monserrato
Italy

Jose A. Teruel
Departamento de Bioquímica y Biología
    Molecular-A
Universidad de Múrcia
Múrcia
Spain

José A. Teixeira
Institute for Biotechnology
    and Bioengineering
Center of Biological Engineering
Universidade do Minho
Braga
Portugal

Vanessa Walter
Institute of Engineering in Life Sciences
Department Technical Biology
University of Karlsruhe
Karlsruhe
Germany

Owen P. Ward
Department of Biology
University of Waterloo
Waterloo, Ontario
Canada

Panya Wongpanit
The Petroleum and Petrochemical
   College
Chulalongkorn University
Bangkok
Thailand

Smita Sachin Zinjarde
Institute of Bioinformatics and
   Biotechnology
University of Pune
Pune
India

CONTENTS

SECTION I. SCREENING, GENETICS AND BIOPHYSICS

SECTION II. PROPERTIES AND POTENTIAL APPLICATIONS

7. MICROBIAL SURFACTANTS OF MARINE ORIGIN: POTENTIALS AND PROSPECTS... 88

Palashpriya Das, Soumen Mukherjee, C. Sivapathasekaran and Ramkrishna Sen

8. BIOMIMETIC AMPHIPHILES: PROPERTIES AND POTENTIAL USE.. 102

S.K. Mehta, Shweta Sharma, Neena Mehta and Swaranjit Singh Cameotra

9. APPLICATIONS OF BIOLOGICAL SURFACE ACTIVE COMPOUNDS IN REMEDIATION TECHNOLOGIES................. 121

Andrea Franzetti, Elena Tamburini and Ibrahim M. Banat

10. POSSIBILITIES AND CHALLENGES FOR BIOSURFACTANTS USE IN PETROLEUM INDUSTRY 135

Amedea Perfumo, Ivo Rancich and Ibrahim M. Banat

11. BACTERIAL BIOSURFACTANTS, AND THEIR ROLE IN MICROBIAL ENHANCED OIL RECOVERY (MEOR)............ 146

J.M. Khire

SECTION III. BIOSURFACTANT PRODUCTION

12. MOLECULAR ENGINEERING ASPECTS FOR THE PRODUCTION OF NEW AND MODIFIED BIOSURFACTANTS 158

Alexander Koglin, Volker Doetsch and Frank Bernhard

20. SYNTHESIS OF BIOSURFACTANTS AND THEIR ADVANTAGES TO MICROORGANISMS AND MANKIND 261

Swaranjit Singh Cameotra, Randhir S. Makkar, Jasminder Kaur and S.K. Mehta

21. ENRICHMENT AND PURIFICATION OF LIPOPEPTIDE BIOSURFACTANTS 281

Simon C. Baker and Chien-Yen Chen

22. PRODUCTION OF SURFACE ACTIVE COMPOUNDS BY BIOCATALYST TECHNOLOGY 289

Smita Sachin Zinjarde and Mahua Ghosh

SECTION IV. THE MOST STUDIED
BIOSURFACTANTS

CHAPTER 1

Screening Concepts for the Isolation of Biosurfactant Producing Microorganisms

Vanessa Walter,* Christoph Syldatk and Rudolf Hausmann

Abstract

This chapter gives an overview of current methods for the isolation of biosurfactant producing microbes. The common screening methods for biosurfactants are presented.

Sampling and isolation of bacteria are the basis for screening of biosurfactant producing microbes. Hydrocarbon-contaminated sites are the most promising for the isolation of biosurfactant producing microbes, but many strains have also been isolated from undisturbed sites.

In subsequent steps the isolates have to be characterized in order to identify the strains which are interesting for a further investigation. Several techniques have been developed for identifying biosurfactant producing strains. Most of them are directly based on the surface or interfacial activity of the culture supernatant. Apart from that, some screening methods explore the hydrophobicity of the cell surface. This trait also gives an indication on biosurfactant production.

In recent years automation and miniaturization have led to the development of high throughput methods for screening. High throughput screening (HTS) for analyzing large amounts of potential candidates or whole culture collections is reflected in the end. However, no new principals have been introduced by HTS methods.

Introduction

The overall establishment of biosurfactants is well-known to be impeded by a lack of availability of economic and versatile products. Currently there is only a very limited offer of commercially available biosurfactants, e.g., surfactin, sophorolipids and rhamnolipids. A variety of new biosurfactants respectively producing strains are the key issue in overcoming the economic obstacles of the production of biosurfactants. Therefore, increased efforts in the discovery of new biosurfactant producing microbes must be made by applying a broad range of different screening methods, which is the focus of this chapter.

The principle aim in screening for new biosurfactants is finding new structures with strong interfacial activity, low critical micelle concentration (cmc), high emulsion capacity, good solubility and activity in a broad pH-range. Besides these physicochemical properties, commercial viable biosurfactants have to be economically competitive. Therefore, the second aim in screening is the discovery of good production strains with high yields.

*Corresponding Author: Vanessa Walter—Institute of Engineering in Life Sciences, Department of Technical Biology, University of Karlsruhe, Karlsruhe, Germany.
Email: vanessa.walter@tebi.uni-karlsruhe.de

Biosurfactants, edited by Ramkrishna Sen. ©2010 Landes Bioscience and Springer Science+Business Media.

Biosurfactants may be involved in pathogenesis due to their surface activity; however, for security and regulatory reasons, production strains should be nonpathogenic. In the above mentioned example of rhamnolipids this is not the case as *Pseudomonas aeruginosa*, the most common producing bacteria, is a pathogen.

A variety of methods for the screening of biosurfactant producing microbes has been developed and successfully applied. Since the 1970s there have been various trials in this field. These screenings have mostly been limited to a manageable number of samples. In recent years automation and miniaturization have led to the development of high throughput methods for screening of biosurfactant producing strains. A broad application of such methods could eventually lead to the desired upsurge of new commercially interesting strains.

An efficient screening strategy is the key to success in isolating new and interesting microbes or their variants, because a large number of strains needs to be characterized. A complete strategy for screening of new biosurfactants or production strains consists of three steps: sampling, isolation of strains and investigation of strains. Theses steps will be addressed in the next paragraphs. Bioinformatical approaches like homology search are not included herein.

Sampling

According to Ron and Rosenberg,[1] biosurfactants can fulfill various physiological roles and provide different advantages to their producing strains:

- increase the surface area of water-insoluble substrates by emulsification,
- increase the bioavailability of hydrophobic substrates,
- bind heavy metals,
- be involved in pathogenesis,
- possess antimicrobial activity,
- regulate the attachment/detachment of microorganisms to and from surfaces.

According to these physiological roles, biosurfactant producing microbes can be found in different environments. Many biosurfactant producing microbes were isolated from soils or water samples which are contaminated with hydrophobic organic compounds like e.g., refinery wastes.[2-13] One biosurfactant producing microbe, *Cladosporium resinae*, which is also called the "kerosene fungus", was even isolated from an aircraft fuel tank.[14] In contrast, also undisturbed environments have yielded several interesting isolates, e.g., natural soils.[9] Marine environments have also been reported as successful sampling sites.[6,16-19] However, Bodour and Miller-Maier[15] showed that contaminated soils are more yielding than uncontaminated soils. One exceptional example is the discovery of biosurfactant producing strains which were originally isolated when investigating the food hygiene of meat.[20,21]

Isolation

In natural environments, microbes occur almost always in a mixed population composed of a multitude of different strains and species. For analyzing the properties of a defined organism out of such a mixed population, a pure culture is required. Apart from direct isolation of strains by diluting and plating, enrichment cultures with hydrophobic substrates are very promising for the isolation of biosurfactant producing microbes. Additionally, hydrophobic interaction chromatography and the replica plate technique are also rewarding methods.

The principle of enrichment culture is to provide growth conditions that are very favorable for the organisms of interest and as unfavorable as possible for competing organisms. Hence, the microbes of interest are selected and enriched. For the screening of biosurfactant producing microbes, enrichment cultures utilizing hydrophobic compounds as the sole carbon source are applied.[3,5-7,11,12,22] This is an indirect screening method as the growth on hydrophobic compounds indicates the production of biosurfactants, but not always correlates with this trait.[3,5] Moreover, the applied screening medium and conditions will influence whether or not surfactants are produced.[9] Thus, it is possible that biosurfactant producing populations are present in the sample which are not enriched by the applied enrichment conditions.

Willumsen and Karlson[3] isolated biosurfactant producing bacteria from soil which was contaminated with polyaromatic hydrocarbons (PAHs). They used PAH-amended liquid minimal medium for enrichment culture. Furthermore, they used agar-plates coated with different PAHs and agar-plates with a PAH-soaked filter in the lid of the petri dish for the selection. The degradation of PAHs by the microorganisms then leads to a clearing zone agar around the colonies in the PAH coated agar. As result, they isolated 57 strains of which only 4 strains showed surface activity.

Mercadé et al.[5] isolated biosurfactant producing strains from petroleum-contaminated soil samples by using waste lubricating oil as the sole carbon source. They isolated 44 strains which were able to grow on hydrocarbons. Therefrom, five isolates produced biosurfactants.

Schulz and colleagues[6] isolated three bacterial strains of marine origin during a screening for biosurfactants among *n*-alkane degrading microorganisms. As enrichment medium, they used mineral media with C_{14}- and C_{15}-*n*-alkanes and also agar plates with an alkane-soaked filter in the lid. Yakimov and coworkers[17] isolated a biosurfactant producing bacterium of a new genus by using the same enrichment technique.

Rahman et al[7] isolated 130 oil-degrading isolates from hydrocarbon-polluted environments by enrichment techniques. A mineral salts medium containing crude oil as the sole carbon source was applied. Two of these strains were found to produce biosurfactants.

The degradation and consumption of hydrocarbons can also be visualized by the following colorimetric method developed by Hanson et al.[23] By adding a colored redox indicator, 2,6-dichlorophenol indophenol (DCPIP), to liquid cultures growing on hydrocarbons, a simple colorimetric assay results. The DCPIP is incorporated by bacteria that can degrade the hydrocarbons. It acts as electron acceptor and changes from blue (oxidized) to colorless (reduced). Thus, a decolorization of the culture shows degradation of hydrocarbons. However, the redox indicator DCPIP might be toxic to some organisms.

As a conclusion, sampling of contaminated sites combined with direct isolation or enrichment culture is an approved strategy for discovering new biosurfactant producing strains. However, as the proportion of positives is only in the range of a few percent, several dozen of isolates have to be tested for every hit.

Screening Methods

Biosurfactants are structurally a very diverse group of biomolecules, e.g., glycolipids, lipopeptides, lipoproteins, lipopolysaccharides or phospholipids. Therefore, most methods for a general screening of biosurfactant producing strains are based on the physical effects of surfactants. Alternatively, the ability of strains to interfere with hydrophobic interfaces can be explored. On the other hand, specific screening methods like the colorimetric CTAB agar assay are suitable only to a limited group of biosurfactants. The screening methods can give qualitative and/or quantitative results. For a first screening of isolates, qualitative methods are generally sufficient.

Surface/Interfacial Activity

The majority of screening methods for biosurfactant producing microbes are based on the interfacial or surface activity. Various methods have been developed for measuring this property. The methods which are applied for screening of biosurfactant producing microbes are reviewed in the next paragraph.

Direct Surface/Interfacial Tension Measurements

The direct measurement of the interfacial or surface activity of the culture supernatant is the most straightforward screening method and very appropriate for a preliminary screening of biosurfactant producing microbes.[24] This gives a strong indication on biosurfactant production. The interfacial or surface tension of a liquid can be measured by a variety of methods. However, there is a restriction in the range of measurement. The surface tension decreases with increasing surfactant concentration until the cmc is reached. If the concentration of biosurfactant is above the cmc, an increase in the concentration cannot be detected. Consequently, two cultures with very different concentrations of biosurfactant may display the same surface tension. This problem can be solved by serial diluting until a sharp increase in surface tension is observed.[2,20,25-29] The corresponding dilution of the supernatant is called critical micelle dilution (cmd) and correlates to the concentration of biosurfactant. Furthermore, the measurements are strongly affected by factors such as pH and ionic strength. In addition, the measurement can be affected by plant oils as carbon sources because of the resulting fatty acids or mono/di-glycerids interfacial activity.

For screening purposes, the following methods are established. They can all be used for measuring the surface and interfacial tension of a liquid. Especially the Du-Nouy-Ring method is quite easy and most frequently applied.

Du-Nouy-Ring Method

The Du-Nouy-Ring method is based on measuring the force required to detach a ring or loop of wire from an interface or surface.[30] The detachment force is proportional to the interfacial tension. It can be measured with an automated tensiometer which is available from many manufacturers. The ring must be free from contaminant, which is usually achieved by using a platinum ring that is flamed before use. Instead of a ring, a platinum plate, a so called Wilhelmy plate, can be applied in the same manner.[31-33]

The Du-Nouy-Ring assay is widely applied for screening of biosurfactant producing microbes.[3,5-7,15,20,27,34-36] Cooper considered a culture as promising if it reduces the surface tension of a liquid medium to 40 mN/m or less.[37] Willumsen and Karlson[3] give a similar definition: a good biosurfactant producer is defined as one being able to reduce the surface tension of the growth medium by ≥20 mN/m compared with distilled water.

The advantage of this method is the accuracy and the ease of use. However, it requires specialized equipment. A disadvantage is that measurements of different samples cannot be performed simultaneously. Other limitations of this assay include the volume of sample required for analysis, usually some milliliters and the restricted range of concentrations that can be analyzed without dilution.[15]

Stalagmometric Method

The surface tension of a liquid can alternatively be measured with a Traube stalagmometer.[38] This device is essentially a pipette with a broad flattened tip, which permits large drops of reproducible size to form and finally drop under the action of gravity. The surface tension can be determined on the basis of the number of drops which fall per volume, the density of the sample and the surface tension of a reference liquid, e.g., water. According to Dilmohamud et al,[38] the surface tension is given by:

$$\sigma_L = \frac{\sigma_W \cdot N_W \cdot \rho_L}{N_L \cdot \rho_W}$$

where as σ_L is the surface tension of the liquid under investigation, σ_W is the surface tension of water, N_L is the number of drops of the liquid, N_W is the number of drops of water, ρ_L is the density of the liquid and ρ_W is the density of water.

Again, a disadvantage of this assay is that only consecutive measurements can be performed. Also, the method seems to be variability prone. Plaza et al[36] applied this method and conclude that it is not recommendable due to the large variability they obtained in their results. The reason is probably that the process of drop formation is too fast to allow the complete adsorption of the surfactants to the newly generated drop surface.

Pendant Drop Shape Technique

The pendant drop shape technique is an optical method for measuring the interfacial tension. A drop of liquid is allowed to hang from the end of a capillary. It adopts an equilibrium profile that is a unique function of the tube radius, the interfacial tension, its density and the gravitational field.

According to Tadros,[30] the interfacial tension is given by the following equation:

$$\gamma = \frac{\Delta \rho \, g \, d_e^2}{H} \qquad H = f\left(\frac{d_s(t)}{d_e(t)}\right)$$

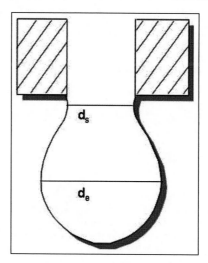

Figure 1. Shape of a pendant drop with the equatorial diameter d_e and the smallest diameter d_s.

in which $\Delta\rho$ is the density difference between the two phases, d_e is the equatorial diameter of the drop and d_s is the smallest diameter of the hanging drop (see Fig. 1). H is a function of d_s and d_e. Accurate values for H have been obtained by Nierderhauser and Bartell.[39]

A variant of this technique was applied by Chen et al[4] who measured in an inverse mode. A small volume of air was blown into a liquid and the shape of the air bubble in the liquid was measured. The disadvantage of the pendant drop shape technique is again that measurements cannot be performed simultaneously.

Axisymmetric Drop Shape Analysis by Profile

The drop shape analysis is another optical method for the determination of the surface tension. For screening purposes it was first applied by Van der Vegt et al[40] The underlying principle is that the shape of a liquid droplet depends greatly on the liquid surface tension. Droplets of liquids with a low surface tension are more apt to deviate from a perfectly spherical shape than droplets of liquids with a high surface tension.

According to Rotenberg et al,[41] the profile of a liquid droplet can be describes by the following equation:

$$\Delta p = \sigma \left(\frac{1}{r_1} + \frac{1}{r_2} \right)$$

in which Δp is the pressure difference across the interface, r_1 and r_2 are the principal radii of curvature and σ is the surface tension (see Fig. 2).

For the drop shape analysis, a 100 µl droplet of a bacterial suspension is put on a FEP-Teflon surface. The profile of the droplet is determined with a contour monitor as a function of time up to 2 hours. The surface tension of the suspension can then be calculated from the droplet profiles with a solution scheme developed by Rotenberg et al.[41] As shown by Van der Vegt et al,[40] the drop shape analysis can be used to monitor bacterial biosurfactant production. For this assay, just small amounts of sample are needed. But a special camera and software are required. The calculation of the surface tension is rather complex. Furthermore, different samples cannot be measured in parallel.

Measurements Based on Surface/Interfacial Tension

Many screening methods have been developed that rely on the interfacial activity of the biosurfactants but that do not measure it directly. They are presented in the following.

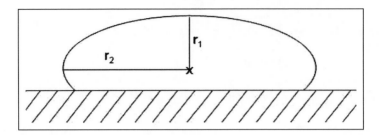

Figure 2. Shape of a sessile drop with the principal radii of curvature r_1 and r_2.

Drop Collapse Assay

Jain et al[29] developed the drop collapse assay. This assay relies on the destabilization of liquid droplets by surfactants. Therefore, drops of a cell suspension or of culture supernatant are placed on an oil coated, solid surface. If the liquid does not contain surfactants, the polar water molecules are repelled from the hydrophobic surface and the drops remain stable. If the liquid contains surfactants, the drops spread or even collapse because the force or interfacial tension between the liquid drop and the hydrophobic surface is reduced. The stability of drops is dependent on surfactant concentration and correlates with surface and interfacial tension.

Persson and Molin[20] described a similar assay using a glass surface instead of the oil coated surface. Furthermore, Bodour and Miller-Maier[15] showed that for pure surfactant, this assay can even be quantitative by measuring the drop size with a micrometer. An important distinction of this assay is that it can be transferred to an automated screening in microplates, as it has been reported by Maczek et al.[42] They stained the culture supernatant to enhance the visual effect.

The drop collapse assay is rapid and easy to carry out, requires no specialized equipment and just a small volume of sample.[36] In addition, it can be performed in microplates.[43] This assay has been applied several times for screening purposes.[2,9,36,44] But it displays a relative low sensitivity since a significant concentration of surface active compounds must be present in order to cause a collapse of the aqueous drops on the oil or glass surfaces.

Microplate Assay

The surface activity of individual strains can be determined qualitatively with the microplate assay developed and patented by Vaux and Cottingham.[45] This assay is based on the change in optical distortion that is caused by surfactants in an aqueous solution. Pure water in a hydrophobic well has a flat surface. The presence of surfactants causes some wetting at the edge of the well and the fluid surface becomes concave and takes the shape of a diverging lens. For this assay, a 100 µl sample of the supernatant of each strain is taken and put into a microwell of a 96-mircowell plate. The plate is viewed using a backing sheet of paper with a grid. If biosurfactant is present, the concave surface distorts the image of the grid below (see Fig. 3). The optical distortion of the grid provides a qualitative assay for the presence of surfactants.

The microplate assay is easy, rapid and sensitive and allows an instantaneous detection of surface-active compounds.[4] Just a small volume (100 µl) of sample is needed. Furthermore, the method is suitable for automated high throughput screening. Chen et al[4] demonstrated the efficiency of the microplate method for high throughput screening purposes.

Penetration Assay

Maczek et al[42] developed another assay suitable for high throughput screening, the penetration assay. This assay relies on the contacting of two unsoluble phases which leads to a color change.

For this assay, the cavities of a 96 well microplate are filled with 150 µl of a hydrophobic paste consisting of oil and silica gel. The paste is covered with 10 µl of oil. Then, the supernatant of the

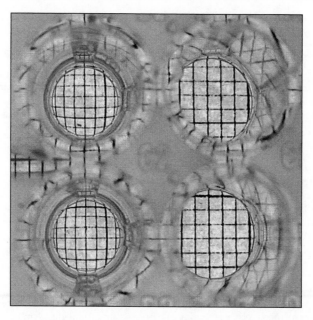

Figure 3. Microplate assay. Left) Biosurfactant rhamnolipid in water. Right) water.

culture is colored by adding 10 µl of a red staining solution to 90 µl of the supernatant. The colored supernatant is placed on the surface of the paste. If biosurfactant is present, the hydrophilic liquid will break through the oil film barrier into the paste. The silica is entering the hydrophilic phase and the upper phase will change from clear red to cloudy white within 15 minutes. The described effect relies on the phenomenon that silica gel is entering the hydrophilic phase from the hydrophobic paste much more quickly if biosurfactants are present. Biosurfactant free supernatant will turn cloudy but stay red.

The penetration assay is a simple, qualitative technique for screening large amounts of potential isolates. It can be applied in high throughput screening. The assay was described as recently as 2007 and to our knowledge there has been no further report of its application by now.

Oil Spreading Assay

The oil spreading assay was developed by Morikawa et al.[28] For this assay, 10 µl of crude oil is added to the surface of 40 ml of distilled water in a petri dish to form a thin oil layer. Then, 10 µl of culture or culture supernatant are gently placed on the centre of the oil layer. If biosurfactant is present in the supernatant, the oil is displaced and a clearing zone is formed. The diameter of this clearing zone on the oil surface correlates to surfactant activity, also called oil displacement activity. For pure biosurfactant a linear correlation between quantity of surfactant and clearing zone diameter is given.

The oil spreading method is rapid and easy to carry out, requires no specialized equipment and just a small volume of sample.[36] It can be applied when the activity and quantity of biosurfactant is low. Plaza et al[36] and Youssef et al[44] demonstrated that the oil spreading technique is a reliable method to detect biosurfactant production by diverse microorganisms. The assay was also applied for screening by Huy et al.[12]

Emulsification Capacity Assay

Another popular assay based on the emulsification capacity of biosurfactants was developed by Cooper and Goldenberg.[35] For measuring this trait, kerosene is added to an aqueous sample. The mixture is vortexed at high speed for 2 minutes. After 24 hours, the height of the stable emulsion layer is measured. The emulsion index E_{24} is calculated as the ratio of the height of the emulsion layer and the total height of liquid:[35]

$$E_{24} = \frac{h_{emulsion}}{h_{total}} \times 100\,\%$$

E_{24} correlates to the surfactant concentration. Evaluating the emulsification capacity is a simple screening method suitable for a first screening of biosurfactant producing microbes. It is applied in many screenings,[3,4,6,10,11,13,26,27,36,46,47] whereas the kerosene can be replaced with other hydrophobic compounds, e.g., hexadecane. But surface activity and emulsification capacity do not always correlate.[3,26,35,36,48] Consequently, this method gives just an indication on the presence of biosurfactants.

Solubilization of Crystalline Anthracene

Willumsen and Karlson[3] developed an assay based on the solubilization of crystalline anthracene. This screening method is based on the solubilization of a highly hydrophobic, crystalline compound, anthracene, by the biosurfactants. Therefore, crystalline anthracene is added to the culture supernatant and incubated on a shaker at 25°C for 24 h. The concentration of the dissolved hydrophobic anthracene is measured photometrically at 354 nm and correlates to the production of biosurfactant.

This is a simple and rapid screening method, but the anthracene might be toxic to some microbes. To our knowledge there have been no further reports on its application.

Cell Surface Hydrophobicity

The following screening methods are based on the hydrophobicity of the cell surface. Thus, they are indirect methods for the screening of biosurfactant producing microbes. Nevertheless, a rapid identification of biosurfactant producing strains can be achieved by assaying this trait.[46,49] A disadvantage is that the hydrophobicity of bacteria depends on physiological aspects like growth conditions or cellular age.[49]

Bacterial Adhesion to Hydrocarbons Assay (BATH)

Rosenberg et al[50] developed the bacterial adhesion to hydrocarbons method, a simple photometrical assay for measuring the hydrophobicity of bacteria. The method is based on the degree of adherence of cells to various liquid hydrocarbons. For measuring this trait, a turbid, aqueous suspension of washed microbial cells is mixed with a distinct volume of a hydrocarbon, e.g., hexadecane or octane. After mixing for 2 minutes, the two phases are allowed to separate. Hydrophobic cells become bound to hydrocarbon droplets and rise with the hydrocarbon. They are removed from the aqueous phase. The turbidity of the aqueous phase is measured. The decrease in the turbidity of the aqueous phase correlates to the hydrophobicity of the cells. The percentage of cells bound to the hydrophobic phase (H) is calculated by:[40]

$$H = \left(1 - \frac{A}{A_0}\right) \cdot 100\%$$

whereas A_0 is the absorbance of the bacterial suspension without hydrophobic phase added and A the absorbance after mixing with hydrophobic phase.

BATH is a simple but indirect screening method. Pruthi and Cameotra[49] showed that the ability of bacteria to adhere to hydrocarbons is a characteristic feature of biosurfactant producing microbes. This assay was applied several times for screening.[13,46,47] For example, Neu and Poralla[46] isolated 126 bacterial strains during screening for cell surface hydrophobicity. Forty-eight of the isolated strains produced an emulsifying agent.

Hydrophobic Interaction Chromatography (HIC)

A method which allows the simultaneous isolation and screening of microbes was developed by Smyth et al.[51] They used hydrophobic interaction chromatography (HIC) for this purpose. HIC is a chromatographic procedure based on hydrophobic interaction between the nonpolar groups on a hydrophobic chromatographic resin and the nonpolar regions of a particle.

A bacterial suspension is drained into a gel bed of hydrophobized sepharose. Hydrophobic microbes are retained by the gel and the degree of adsorption of the cells to the gel can be measured by the turbidity of the eluate or by bacteria counting. For desorption of the adherent microbes, the ionic strength of the buffer is decreased.

HIC is very convenient because screening and isolation of potential strains can be combined in one step. Pruthi and Cameotra[49] reported that HIC is a reliable screening method for biosurfactant production. The technique is also valid for comparative analysis of the hydrophobic properties of microorganisms.

Replica Plate Assay

A simple replica plate assay for the identification and isolation of hydrophobic microbes was developed by Rosenberg.[52] The principle of this assay is the adherence of bacterial strains to hydrophobic polystyrene which correlates to cell surface hydrophobicity. A flat, sterile disc of polystyrene is pressed on an agar containing the colonies to be screened. The replica of the colonies obtained on the polystyrene surface is washed under running water to remove all cells which are not firmly bound. To visualize the adherent colonies, they are fixed and stained. To isolate the hydrophobic strains the replica might be transferred to a new, sterile agar plate. Pruthi and Cameotra[49] demonstrated the strong correlation between cell surface hydrophobicity and affinity to polystyrene. They suggest that greater than 50% coverage of the disc by adherent cells can be scored as positive. This technique is an inexpensive way to identify an array of microbial strains for biosurfactant production simultaneously on readily available materials. Furthermore, the identification and isolation of potential strains might be combined in one step.

Salt Aggregation Assay

A salt aggregation assay for exploring the hydrophobic surface properties was first described by Lindahl et al.[53] It is similar to the "salting out" of proteins. The cells are precipitated by increasing salt concentrations. The more hydrophobic the surface of the cells, the lower the salt concentration required to aggregate the cells. So, the most hydrophobic cells precipitate first, at low salt concentrations.

For this assay, a dilution series of ammonium sulfate in sodium phosphate buffer is used, ranging from 4 M to 0.02 M ammonium sulfate. The bacterial suspension is then mixed with an equal volume of salt solution on glass depression slides. The suspension is mixed for 2 minutes at 20°C, then visual reading against black background is carried out. A positive aggregation reaction shows a clear solution and white aggregates with a diameter of appr. 0.1 mm. As positive control, all readings are compared to the reaction at the highest molarity. A bacterial suspension mixed with 0.002 M sodium phosphate without addition of salt is used as negative control.

The salt aggregation test provides a simple means for identifying bacteria associated with the production of biosurfactants. No special equipment is needed. Pruthi and Cameotra[49] showed that this technique gives a good estimation of the degree of cell surface hydrophobicity.

Specialities

This last section on screening methods deals with two special screening techniques: the CTAB agar plate assay and the hemolysis assay. They are exceptional because they are not suitable to a general screening for biosurfactant producing microbes.

CTAB Agar Plate

The CTAB agar plate method is a semi-quantitative assay for the detection of extracellular glycolipids or other anionic surfactants. It was developed by Siegmund and Wagner.[54] The microbes of interest are cultivated on a light blue mineral salts agar plate containing the cationic surfactant cetyltrimethylammonium bromide and the basic dye methylene blue. If anionic surfactants are secreted by the microbes growing on the plate, they form a dark blue, insoluble ion pair with cetyltrimethylammonium bromide and methylene blue. Thus, productive colonies are surrounded by dark blue halos (see Fig. 4).

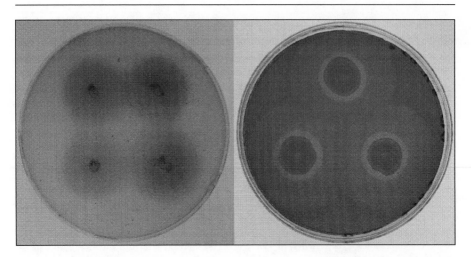

Figure 4. Left) *Pseudomonas sp.* grown on CTAB agar, dark blue halos around the 4 colonies indicate production of biosurfactant. Right) *Pseudomonas aeruginosa* grown on blood agar, lysis of erythrocytes is indicated by the lytic zones around the colonies. A color version of this image is available at www.landesbioscience.com/curie.

To strengthen the visual effect of this method, small wells can be melted into the agar surface with the heated point of a glass stick or pipette. The cultures are placed and incubated in the wells.

Even hydrophobic substrates like plant oils can be included in this test. Therefore, the oil droplets are stabilized with Gum Arabicum. Oil, agar and 1 g/L Gum Arabicum are mixed separately with ultrasound in a small volume of water. The homogenous mixture is added to the medium before sterilization.

The CTAB agar assay is a comfortable screening method, but it is specific for anionic biosurfactants. It has been applied in several screenings.[31,47,55-57] Different culture conditions can be applied directly on the agar plates, e.g., different substrates or temperature. Furthermore, it could be transferred to liquid culture conditions. The disadvantage is that CTAB is harmful and inhibits the growth of some microbes. But, as Siegmund et al[54] suggest, CTAB could be replaced by another cationic surfactant.

Hemolysis

Biosurfactants can cause lysis of erythrocytes. This principle is used for the hemolysis assay which was developed by Mulligan et al.[58] Cultures are inoculated on sheep blood agar plates and incubated for 2 days at 25°C. Positive strains will cause lysis of the blood cells and exhibit a colorless, transparent ring around the colonies (see Fig. 4). Hemolysis can also be shown with purified biosurfactant.

The blood agar method is often used for a preliminary screening of microorganisms for the ability to produce biosurfactants on hydrophilic media.[6,36,44] Blood agar is a rich growth medium for many organisms. But the method has some limitations.[29] First, the method is not specific, as lytic enzymes can also lead to clearing zones. Second, hydrophobic substrates cannot be included as sole carbon source in this assay. Third, diffusion restriction of the surfactant can inhibit the formation of clearing zones. In addition, Schulz et al[6] showed that some biosurfactants do not show any hemolytic activity at all. Youssef et al[44] and Plaza et al[36] also confirmed the poor specificity of this method. It can give a lot of false negative and false positive results. Mulligan et al[58] recommend the blood agar method as a preliminary screening method which should be supported by other techniques based on surface activity measurements.

Table 1. Comparison of the presented screening methods for biosurfactant production

Analytical Technique	Qualitative Analysis	Quantitative Analysis	Analysis Speed	Application in HTS
Direct surface/interfacial tension measurement	++	+	min	–
Drop collapse assay	++	–	min	+
Microplate assay	++	–	min	+
Penetration assay	++	–	min	+
Oil spreading assay	++	–	min	–
Emulsification capacity assay	+	–	d	–
Solubilization of crystalline anthracene	+	–	d	+/–
Bacterial adhesion to hydrocarbons assay	+	–	min	–
Hydrophobic interaction chromatography	+	–	h	–
Replica plate assay	+	–	d	–
Salt aggregation assay	+	–	min	+/–
CTAB agar assay	+	–	d	–
Hemolysis assay	+	–	d	–

Qualitative analysis: ++ = very efficient, + = efficient; quantitative analysis (of surface activity): + = Yes,– = No; Analysis speed: (required time per sample) min = analysis within minutes, h = within hours, d = within days; Application in HTS: + = Yes,– = No, +/– = not reported but principally applicable.

High Throughput Screening

The development of rapid and reliable methods for screening and selection of microbes from thousands of potentially active organisms and the subsequent evaluation of surface activity holds the key to the discovery of new biosurfactants or production strains. According to Chen et al,[4] a screening method for the isolation of biosurfactant producing microbes must fulfill three requirements:

- The ability to identify potential organisms
- The ability to assess quantitatively how effective the surfactant is
- The ability to screen many candidates quickly

The performance of the methods presented in this chapter according to these criteria is shown in Table 1.

The microplate assay, the penetration assay and the drop collapse assay can be performed in microplates. This is the basic requirement for high throughput screening. The solubilization of crystalline anthracene assay and the salt aggregation assay might as well be adopted for high throughput screening; however, this has not been reported yet. By now, there have been no other measurement principles adopted for high throughput screening.

Conclusion and Perspectives

Interest in biosurfactants has led to the development of a multitude of methods for the screening of biosurfactant producing strains. As every method has its advantages and disadvantages, a combination of different methods is appropriate for a successful screening.

Some screening methods can be automated and used for HTS. By using these rapid screening methods and by screening many isolates or large culture collections, in the near future various new production strains or new biosurfactants may be found. Accordingly, if new production strains become available, the economic obstacle of biosurfactants may eventually be overcome.

References

1. Ron E, Rosenberg E. Natural roles of biosurfactants. Environ Microbiol 2001; 3(4):229-236.
2. Batista S, Mounteer A, Amorim F et al. Isolation and characterization of biosurfactant/bioemulsifier-producing bacteria from petroleum contaminated sites. Bioresour Technol 2006; 97(6):868-875.
3. Willumsen P, Karlson U. Screening of bacteria, isolated from PAH-contaminated soils, for production of biosurfactants and bioemulsifiers. Biodegradation 1997; 7(5):415-423.
4. Chen C, Baker S, Darton R. The application of a high throughput analysis method for the screening of potential biosurfactants from natural sources. J Microbiol Methods 2007; 70:503-510.
5. Mercadé M, Monleón L, de Andrés C et al. Screening and selection of surfactant-producing bacteria from waste lubricating oil. J Appl Bacteriol 1996; 81(2):161-166.
6. Schulz D, Passeri A, Schmidt M et al. Marine biosurfactants.1. Screening for biosurfactants among crude-oil degrading marine microorganisms from the North-Sea. Z Naturforsch (C) 1991; 46(3-4):197-203.
7. Rahman K, Rahman T, McClean S et al. Rhamnolipid biosurfactant production by strains of Pseudomonas aeruginosa using low-cost raw materials. Biotechnol Prog 2002; 18:1277-1281.
8. Abalos A, Maximo F, Manresa M et al. Utilization of response surface methodology to optimize the culture media for the production of rhamnolipids by Pseudomonas aeruginosa AT10. J Chem Tech Biotech 2002; 77:777-784.
9. Bodour A, Drees K, Maier R. Distribution of biosurfactant-producing bacteria in undisturbed and contaminated arid southwestern soils. Appl Environ Microbiol 2003; 69(6):3280-3287.
10. Denger K, Schink B. New halo and thermotolerant fermenting bacteria producing surface-active compounds. Appl Microbiol Biotechnol 1995; 44(1-2):161-166.
11. Bento F, Camargo F, Okeke B et al. Diversity of biosurfactant producing microorganisms isolated from soils contaminated with diesel oil. Microbiol Res 2005; 160(3):249-255.
12. Huy N, Jin S, Amada K et al. Characterization of petroleum-degrading bacteria from oil-contaminated sites in Vietnam. J Biosci Bioeng 1999; 88(1):100-102.
13. Al-Mallah M, Goutx M, Mille G et al. Production of emulsifying agents during growth of a marine Alteromonas in sea water with eicosane as carbon source, a solid hydrocarbon. Oil Chem Pollut 1990; 6:289-305.
14. Muriel J, Bruque J, Olias J et al. Production of biosurfactants by Cladosporium resinae. Biotechnol Lett 1996; 18(3):235-240.
15. Bodour A, Miller-Maier R. Application of a modified drop-collapse technique for surfactant quantitation and screening of biosurfactant-producing microorganisms. J Microbiol Methods 1998; 32(3):273-280.
16. Lang S, Wagner F. Biosurfactants from marine microorganisms. In: Kosaric N, ed. Biosurfactants: Production, Properties, Applications. New York: Marcel Dekker, 1993:391-417.
17. Yakimov MM, Golyshin PN, Lang S et al. Alcanivorax borkumensis gen. nov., sp. nov., a new, hydrocarbon-degrading and surfactant-producing marine bacterium. Int J Syst Bacteriol 1998; 48:339-348.
18. Ramm W, Schatton W, Wagner-Dobler I et al. Diglucosyl-glycerolipids from the marine sponge-associated Bacillus pumilus strain AAS3: their production, enzymatic modification and properties. Appl Microbiol Biotechnol 2004; 64(4):497-504.
19. Yakimov M, Timmis K, Wray V et al. Characterization of a new lipopeptide surfactant produced by thermotolerant and halotolerant subsurface Bacillus licheniformis BAS50. Appl Environ Microbiol 1995; 61(5):1706-1713.
20. Persson A, Molin G. Capacity for biosurfactant production of environmental Pseudomonas and Vibrionaceae growing on carbohydrates. Appl Microbiol Biotechnol 1987; 26(5):439-442.
21. Enfors S, Molin G, Ternstrom A. Effect of packaging under carbon-dioxide, nitrogen or air on the microbial-flora of pork stored at 4°C. J Appl Bacteriol 1979; 47(2):197-208.
22. Giani C, Wullbrandt D, Rothert R et al. Hoechst Aktiengesellschaft, Frankfurt am Main. Pseudomonas aeruginosa and its use in a process for the biotechnological preparation of L-Rhamnose. US patent 1997; 5:658-793.
23. Hanson K, Desai J, Desai A. A rapid and simple screening technique for potential crude-oil degrading microorganisms. Biotechnol Techniques 1993; 7(10):745-748.
24. Lin S. Biosurfactants: Recent advances. J Chem Tech Biotech 1996; 66(2):109-120.
25. Duvnjak Z, Cooper D, Kosaric N. Production of Surfactant by Arthrobacter paraffineus ATCC 19558. Biotechnol Bioeng 1982; 24(1):165-175.
26. Bosch M, Robert M, Mercadé M et al. Surface-active compounds on microbial cultures. Tenside Surfactants Detergents 1988; 25:208-211.
27. Makkar R, Cameotra S. Biosurfactant production by a thermophilic Bacillus subtilis strain. J Ind Microbiol Biotechnol 1997; 18(1):37-42.
28. Morikawa M, Hirata Y, Imanaka T. A study on the structure-function relationship of lipopeptide biosurfactants. Biochim Biophys Acta 2000; 1488(3):211-218.

29. Jain D, Collins-Thompson D, Lee H et al. A drop-collapsing test for screening surfactant-producing microorganisms. J Microbiol Methods 1991; 13(4):271-279.
30. Tadros T. Adsorption of surfactants at the air/liquid and liquid/liquid interfaces. In: Applied Surfactants: Principles and Applications. Weinheim: Wiley VCH, 2005:81-82.
31. Tuleva B, Christova N, Jordanov B et al. Naphthalene degradation and biosurfactant activity by Bacillus cereus 28BN. Z Naturforsch (C) 2005; 60(7-8):577-582.
32. Wei Y, Chou C, Chang J. Rhamnolipid production by indigenous Pseudomonas aeruginosa J4 originating from petrochemical wastewater. Biochem Eng J. 2005; 27(2):146-154.
33. Chen S, Lu W, Wei Y et al. Improved production of biosurfactant with newly isolated Pseudomonas aeruginosa S2. Biotechnol Prog 2007; 23(3):661-666.
34. Das M, Das S, Mukherjee R. Surface active properties of the culture filtrates of a Micrococcus species grown on n-alkanes and sugars. Bioresour Technol 1998; 63(3):231-235.
35. Cooper D, Goldenberg B. Surface-active agents from 2 Bacillus species. Appl Environ Microbiol 1987; 53(2):224-229.
36. Plaza G, Zjawiony I, Banat I. Use of different methods for detection of thermophilic biosurfactant-producing bacteria from hydrocarbon-contaminated bioremediated soils. J Petro Science Eng 2006; 50(1):71-77.
37. Cooper D. Biosurfactants. Microbiol Sci 1986; 3(5):145-149.
38. Dilmohamud B, Seeneevassen J, Rughooputh S et al. Surface tension and related thermodynamic parameters of alcohols using the Traube stalagmometer. Euro J Physics 2005; 26(6):1079-1084.
39. Nierderhauser D, Bartell F. A corrected table for the calculation of boundary tensions by the pendent drop method. Baltimore: American Petroleum Institute, 1950.
40. Van der Vegt W, Van der Mei H, Noordmans J et al. Assessment of bacterial biosurfactant production through axisymmetrical drop shape-analysis by profile. Appl Microbiol Biotechnol 1991; 35(6):766-770.
41. Rotenberg Y, Boruvka L, Neumann A. Determination of surface-tension and contact-angle from the shapes of axisymmetric fluid interfaces. J Colloid Interface Science 1983; 93(1):169-183.
42. Maczek J, Junne S, Götz P. Examining biosurfactant producing bacteria—an example for an automated search for natural compounds. Application Note CyBio AG, 2007.
43. Tugrul T, Cansunar E. Detecting surfactant-producing microorganisms by the drop-collapse test. World J Microbiol Biotechnol 2005; 21(6-7):851-853.
44. Youssef N, Duncan K, Nagle D et al. Comparison of methods to detect biosurfactant production by diverse microorganisms. J Microbiol Methods 2004; 56(3):339-347.
45. Vaux D, Cottingham M. Method and apparatus for measuring surface configuration. patent number WO 2007/039729 A1, 2001.
46. Neu T, Poralla K. Emulsifying agents from bacteria isolated during screening for cells with hydrophobic surfaces. Appl Microbiol Biotechnol 1990; 32(5):521-525.
47. Christova N, Tuleva B, Lalchev Z et al. Rhamnolipid biosurfactants produced by Renibacterium salmoninarum 27BN during growth on n-hexadecane. Z Naturforsch [C] 2004; 59(1-2):70-74.
48. Van Dyke M, Gulley S, Lee H et al. Evaluation of microbial surfactants for recovery of hydrophobic pollutants from soil. J Ind Microbiol 1993; 11(3):163-170.
49. Pruthi V, Cameotra S. Rapid identification of biosurfactant-producing bacterial strains using a cell surface hydrophobicity technique. Biotechnol Techniques 1997; 11(9):671-674.
50. Rosenberg M, Gutnick D, Rosenberg E. Adherence of bacteria to hydrocarbons—a simple method for measuring cell-surface hydrophobicity. FEMS Microbiol Lett 1980; 9(1):29-33.
51. Smyth C, Jonsson P, Olsson E et al. Differences in hydrophobic surface characteristics of porcine enteropathogenic Escherichia coli with or without K88 antigen as revealed by hydrophobic interaction chromatography. Infect Immun 1978; 22(2):462-472.
52. Rosenberg M. Bacterial adherence to polystyrene—a replica method of screening for bacterial hydrophobicity. Appl Environ Microbiol 1981; 42(2):375-377.
53. Lindahl M, Faris A, Wadstrom T et al. A new test based on salting out to measure relative surface hydrophobicity of bacterial cells. Biochim Biophys Acta 1981; 677(3-4):471-476.
54. Siegmund I, Wagner F. New method for detecting rhamnolipids excreted by Pseudomonas species during growth on mineral agar. Biotechnol Techniques 1991; 5(4):265-268.
55. Gunther N, Nunez A, Fett W et al. Production of rhamnolipids by Pseudomonas chlororaphis, a nonpathogenic bacterium. Appl Environ Microbiol 2005; 71(5):2288-2293.
56. Tuleva BK, Ivanov GR, Christova NE. Biosurfactant production by a new Pseudomonas putida strain. Z Naturforsch [C]—Journal of Biosciences 2002; 57(3-4):356-360.
57. Tahzibi A, Kamal F, Assadi M. Improved production of rhamnolipids by a Pseudomonas aeruginosa mutant. Iran Biomed J 2004; 8(1):25-31.
58. Mulligan C, Cooper D, Neufeld R. Selection of microbes producing biosurfactants in media without hydrocarbons. J Fermentation Technol 1984; 62(4):311-314.

CHAPTER 2

Molecular Genetics of Biosurfactant Synthesis in Microorganisms

Surekha K. Satpute, Smita S. Bhuyan, Karishma R. Pardesi,
Shilpa S. Mujumdar, Prashant K. Dhakephalkar, Ashvini M. Shete
and Balu A. Chopade*

Abstract

Biosurfactant (BS)/bioemulsifier (BE) produced by varied microorganisms exemplify immense structural/functional diversity and consequently signify the involvement of particular molecular machinery in their biosynthesis. The present chapter aims to compile information on molecular genetics of BS/BE production in microorganisms. Polymer synthesis in *Acinetobacter* species is controlled by an intricate operon system and its further excretion being controlled by enzymes. Quorum sensing system (QSS) plays a fundamental role in rhamnolipid and surfactin synthesis. Depending upon the cell density, signal molecules (autoinducers) of regulatory pathways accomplish the biosynthesis of BS. The regulation of serrawettin production by *Serratia* is believed to be through non ribosomal peptide synthetases (NRPSs) and N-acylhomoserine lactones (AHLs) encoded by QSS located on mobile transposon. This regulation is under positive as well as negative control of QSS operon products. In case of yeast and fungi, glycolipid precursor production is catalyzed by genes that encode enzyme cytochrome P450 monooxygenase. BS/BE production is dictated by genes present on the chromosomes. This chapter also gives a glimpse of recent biotechnological developments which helped to realize molecular genetics of BS/BE production in microorganisms. Hyper-producing recombinants as well as mutant strains have been constructed successfully to improve the yield and quality of BS/BE. Thus promising biotechnological advances have expanded the applicability of BS/BE in therapeutics, cosmetics, agriculture, food, beverages and bioremediation etc. In brief, our knowledge on genetics of BS/BE production in prokaryotes is extensive as compared to yeast and fungi. Meticulous and concerted study will lead to an understanding of the molecular phenomena in unexplored microbes. In addition to this, recent promising advances will facilitate in broadening applications of BS/BE to diverse fields. Over the decades, valuable information on molecular genetics of BS/BE has been generated and this strong foundation would facilitate application oriented output of the surfactant industry and broaden its use in diverse fields. To accomplish our objectives, interaction among experts from diverse fields like microbiology, physiology, biochemistry, molecular biology and genetics is indispensable.

Introduction

Enormous structural and functional diversity are implicated in biosurfactant (BS)/bioemulsifiers (BE) produced by microorganisms. BS/BE possesses remarkable applications in diverse fields. With the need for green chemicals, their study is becoming imperative. Therefore, BS/BE

*Corresponding Author: Balu A. Chopade—Institute of Bioinformatics & Biotechnology, and Department of Microbiology, University of Pune, Pune 411007, Maharashtra, India.
Email: directoribb@unipune.ernet.in

Biosurfactants, edited by Ramkrishna Sen. ©2010 Landes Bioscience
and Springer Science+Business Media.

studies have been focused on by large number of researchers. However, commercial production of these compounds is quite expensive. Use of cheaper and renewable substrates is a necessity.[1-3] However, a great deal of monetary input is required in purification processes.[4] Thus, it represents two faces of a coin; so to overcome this dilemma and subsequently economize and commercialize BS production a better understanding at molecular level is mandatory.

Literature survey illustrates that detailed studies of BS/BE production have been carried out in *Acinetobacter, Pseudomonas, Bacillus, Serratia, Candida* spp. BS producing microbes from different resources, viz., fresh water, soil, marine, oil wells and industrial effluents have been studied extensively.[5,6] Among these natural resources, marine environment is attracting interest from many researchers due to its vastness and novelty with respect to products that can be obtained.[7-9] However, this survey clearly illustrates that the maximum reports are focused on rhamnolipid and surfactin production from *Pseudomonas* and *Bacillus* spp. respectively. Few researchers have reviewed the enormous data generated on BS/BE production in microorganisms, briefing molecular biological aspects.[5,6,10-18,19] However, it is important to note that, before and after Sullivan's review[20] on molecular genetics of BS not a single review is devoted exclusively to molecular biology of synthesis BS in microorganisms. A gap of ~10 years indicates that a compilation of molecular mechanisms involved in BS/BE production is essential. Enormous molecular and biotechnological developments have taken place in this decade and therefore, our understanding on the present topic has improved greatly. Therefore, present review is focused at compiling valuable developments in this area. To the best of our knowledge, this chapter would give comprehensive information on molecular genetics of BS/BE production in microorganisms.

Important Aspects Pertaining to Biosurfactant Production in Microorganisms

The mystery why microbes produce BS/BE is still unknown. Justifications include survival on various hydrophobic substrates[21] and desorption from the hydrophobic substrates allowing direct contact with cell, thereby increasing the bioavailability of insoluble substrates.[22] However, few microbes produce BS/BE on water soluble substrates.[23,24] Different biosynthetic pathways and specific enzymes are involved.[25] Synthesis takes place by de novo pathway and/or assembly from substrates.[26] Based on the four assumptions proposed by Syldatk and Wagner,[26] diagrammatic representations for biosurfactant synthesis in microorganisms is given in Figure 1. Induction/repression of BS/BE production are dependent on presence of carbon, nitrogen, phosphate, trace elements and multivalent cations.[27,28] BS/BE production is controlled by environmental parameters.[29,30] Literature survey suggests that complex pathways are involved in BS/BE production.[18] BS/BE producing microbes may harbour plasmids.[31,32] However, genes responsible for BS production are located on chromosomal DNA.[32] Interacellular communication and production of enzymes, pigments and BS occurs by QSS which depends on the production of diffusible signal molecules termed autoinducers.[33] The regulatory machinery is different for different BS/BE producers.

Molecular Genetics of Biosurfactant Production in Bacteria

Acinetobacter Species

Acinetobacter spp. are ubiquitous in nature, being isolated from various sources like soil, mud, marine water, fresh water, meat products etc.[34-38] and reported for production of BE.[34-36,39-40] *Acinetobacter* species are the most promising bacteria producing high molecular weight BS/BE. The first description of the best known marine BE, now exploited commercially as 'Emulsan' appeared in 1972. This emulsifier is produced by *A. calcoaceticus* RAG-1, isolated from the Mediterranean Sea. Emulsan produced by RAG-1 has a heteropolysaccharide backbone with a repeating trisaccharide of *N*-acetyl-D-galactosamine, *N*-acetylgalactosamine uronic acid and an unidentified *N*-acetyl amino sugar. Fatty acids (FA) are covalently linked to the polysaccharide through *o*-ester linkages.[42-45] Different species of *Acinetobacter* are known to produce protein polysaccharide complexes. Proteoglycan type bioemulsifier is produced by *Acinetobacter junii*

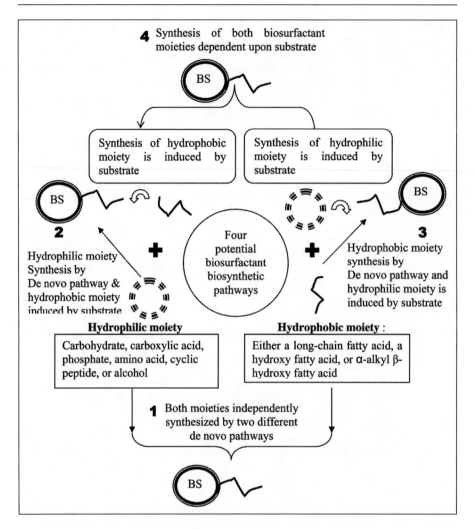

Figure 1. Potential biosurfactant biosynthetic pathways in microorganisms: BS: Biosurfactant molecule. Probable BS biosynthetic pathways operating in different microorganisms. Based on Syldatk and Wagner (1987)[26] four assumptions.

SC14. This bioemulsifier is made up of protein (50.5%), polysaccharide (43%) and lipid in a minor fraction (3.8%). 88.7% of the polysaccharide consisted of reducing sugars.[36,41] About 16% of patents on BS have been reported from *Acinetobacter* spp. alone,[38] which indicates the tremendous market potential of exopolysaccharide (EPS).

Emulsan

It is a complex polysaccharide (9.9×10^5) produced by *A. calcoaceticus* RAG-1 and stabilizes oil-water emulsions efficiently.[43,44] In spite of structural complexity, researchers have succeeded in identifying genes implicated in emulsan synthesis and emulsification phenomena. Polymer biosynthesis is accomplished by a single gene cluster of 27 kbp with 20 open reading frames (ORFs) called as *wee* regulon which contains *weeA* to *weeK* genes that accomplish polymer biosynthesis.[46,47] Putative proteins encoded by the *wee* cluster have been tabulated by Nakar and Gutnick[48] in detail.

These genes lead to the formation of polysaccharide containing amino sugars, with O-acyl- and N-acyl-bound side chain of FA. Further addition of intermediates takes place as follows: WeeA converts UDP-N-acetyl-D-glucosamine into UDP-N-acetylmannosamine. Consequently, WeeB oxidizes the UDP-N-acetylmannosamine into UDP-N-acetylmannosaminuronic acid. This regulon possess *wzb* and *wzc* genes which are responsible for biosynthesis of emulsan. Gene products Wzc and Wzb were over expressed, purified and a bulk of polysaccharide was produced successfully.[48,49] The *Wee*E or *Wee*F are possibly involved in formation of UDP-N-acetyl-L-galactosaminuronic acid. The gene *Wee*J further catalyses the formation of diamino 2, 4-diamino-6-deoxy-D-glucosamine, a component of the repeating unit, from UDP-4-keto-6-deoxy-D-glucosamine. The sequence of *Wee*K is similar to dTDP-glucose 4, 6-dehydratase and therefore could possibly be responsible for conversion of UDP-D-glucosamine into UDP-4-keto-6-deoxy-D-glucosamine. The overall process is summarized in detail by Nesper, et al.[50] The monomers gather on a lipid carrier on the cytoplasmic face of the inner membrane. Subsequently, they are transferred by Wzx protein to the periplasmic face of the membrane. Wzy polymerase further catalyzes the polymerization process. Finally, lipid intermediates lead to the formation of a protein-polysaccharide complex which is transported across the periplasm to the outer membrane. This assembly gets accumulated on cell surface and is further excreted as polymer complex in the exterior.[50]

Due to complex nature of exopolymers, genetic studies remained at a nascent level for a long period. However, with the advent of recent technologies and innovations, bioengineering of BE producing microorganisms has become possible. Complex polysaccharide backbone of emulsan was altered by modifying the culture conditions for *A. venetianus* RAG-1.[45,51-53] The emulsan structure was modified by transposon mutagenesis of FA moiety. Analysis of various factors viz., yield, FA content, molecular weight and emulsification behavior demonstrated that parent strain yielded high emulsan as compared to mutant strain. The factors are dependent on the type of FA supplemented during the production process. However, cloning and sequencing of mutants with enhanced emulsifying activity indicated that they were involved in biosynthesis of emulsan. The presence and composition of long chain FAs on the polysaccharide backbone influenced emulsification behaviour. Such studies are highly significant and open newer avenues for applications of amphiphiles in diverse fields.[54] Based on similar kind of studies, an interesting U.S. patent (20040265340) on "Emulsan adjuvant immunization formulations" was filed by Kaplan, et al.[55] The emulsan analog and mutants of *A. calcoaceticus* RAG-1 were produced in presence of different FA sources. Different molecular tools have been employed to modify and improve quality of emulsan produced by *Acinetobacter* spp. (Table 1).

Apoemulsan

It is an extracellular, polymeric lipoheteropolysaccharide produced by *A. venetianus* RAG-1. Purified deproteinized emulsan (apoemulsan, 103 kDa) consists of D-galactosamine, L-galactosamine uronic acid (pKa, 3.05) and a diamino, 2-desoxy *n*-acetylglucosamine.[44] It retained emulsifying activity towards certain hydrocarbon substrates but was unable to emulsify relatively nonpolar, hydrophobic, aliphatic materials.[63,64] It is now known that polymers are synthesized from Wzy pathway. However, there also appears a differing report which claims that the process is based on presence of polysaccharide-copolymerase (PCP).[65,66] However, recently Dams-Kozlowska and Kaplan[58] proved that synthesis of this polymer was dependant on Wzy pathway where, PCP protein controlled the length of the polymer. This was proved by inducing defined point mutations in the proline-glycine-rich region of apoemulsan PCP protein (Wzc). Five of the eight mutants produced higher weight BE than the wild type while four had modified biological properties. This study demonstrated the functional effect of Wzc modification on molecular weight of polymer and the genetic system controlling apoemulsan polymerization. It has been suggested that emulsifying activity and release of polymer is mediated via esterase gene *est* (34.5 kD). A study carried out by Leahy in 1993,[67] proved that lipase is responsible for enhanced emulsification properties. Lipase negative mutants exhibited less emulsification activity. The gene *est* has been cloned and over expressed in *E. coli* BL21 (DE3) behind the phage T7 promoter with His tag system.[68] Further Alon and Gutnick,[57] also showed that *est* gene encodes protein that is located on the outer membrane.

Table 1. *Employment of molecular tools for construction of recombinant/mutant strains of Acinetobacter and Pseudomonas spp.*

Organism	Mutation	Objective	Significant Feature	Reference
A. calcoaceticus RAG-1 (Emulsan)	CTAB (Cetyl trimethyl ammonium bromide)	Enhance the yield	High yield achieved	56,57
A. venetianus RAG-1 (Emulsan)	Recombinant point mutations in proline—glycine-rich region of the apoemulsan PCP protein (Wzc)	Alteration in Wzc gene	Molecular weight of polysaccharide was modified	58
A. calcoaceticus A2 (Biodispersan)	N-methyl-N-nitrosoguanidine (NTG)	Alteration of wild type strain	Mutant produced equal/higher polysaccharide; rich protein also secreted along with it.	59
A. calcoaceticus RAG-1	Transposon	Disruption of genes involved in biosynthetic pathways of biotin, histidine, cysteine or purines	Modification in fatty acid (FA) metabolism influenced level and types of FA incorporated into emulsan	54
A. venetianus RAG-1 (Emulsan)	M13 and Primers for parent esterase gene	The pET system for over expression of esterase in *E. coli* BL21 carrying pESTAL-14b/pESTAL-11c and plasmid constructed by ligation of the KpnI-NdeI-BamH1 fragment form parent est gene	Overproduction of His0 tagged recombinant esterase and affected protein confirmation that enhanced apoemulsan-mediated emulsifying activity.	
A. lwoffii RAG-1 (Emulsan)	Mini Tn10Km	One region, transcribed in the upstream direction, appears to encode for 3 complete ORFs, while the second region is transcribed in the opposite direction and encodes 17 complete ORFs	Identification of *wee* gene (27 kbp) containing 20-ORFs for polysaccharide synthesis; Defect in emulsan production with specific activities of 5–14% of parental emulsifying activity	48
P. aeruginosa (Rhamnolipid)	N-methyl-N-nitrosoguanidine (NTG)	Enhance yield of BS	Similar type of biosurfactant with 10 times more BS production	61
P. fluorescens	Tn5	Transposon integration into condensation domains of peptide synthetases	Rhamnolipid reduced surface tension effectively	62

The same gene was sequenced and expressed in *E. coli*. High amount of esterase was found to be associated when cell was grown in presence of nitrogen. Variants resistant to cetyl trimethyl ammonium bromide (CTAB) showed enhanced emulsan production.[56] Site directed mutagenesis revealed that esterase-defective mutants could not release emulsan. Mutant proteins defective were capable of enhancing apoemulsan-mediated emulsifying activity. Bach, et al[60] carried out studies on emulsan from *A. venetianus* RAG-1. It was seen that apoemulsan and esterase are essential for the formation of stable oil-water emulsions.[56,64]

Alasan

The polymer produced by *A. radioresistens* KA53 is designated as 'Alasan' and finds significant application in bioremediation.[69] Alasan is an alanine containing complex heteropolysaccharide and protein polymer that stabilizes oil in water emulsions in n-alkanes with chain length 10 or higher and alkyl aromatics, liquid paraffin, soyabean, coconut oil and crude oils.[70] The proteins of alasan have been identified as AlnA, AlnB and AlnC. One of the alasan protein (AlnA) of 45 kDa exhibiting highest emulsification activity was purified[71-74] and denoted high sequence homology to an OmpA-like protein from *Acinetobacter* spp.[75] Four hydrophobic regions in AlnA forming specific structure on the surface of hydrocarbon are responsible for surface activity.[73,74] The AlnB protein exhibited strong homology to perioxiredoxins (family of thiol—specific antioxidant enzymes). It was proposed that all three proteins may be released as a complex with AlnA entering the oil phase and Alnb forming a compact shell around the hydrocarbon, thereby forming stable emulsions.[71] *A. calcoaceticus* RA57 grown on crude oil sludge possesses three plasmids, one of which pSR4, a 20 kb fragment was found to be essential for growth and emulsification of crude oil in liquid culture.[76]

Biodispersan

It is an extracellular, anionic polysaccharide produced by *A. calcoaceticus* A2 which acts as a dispersing agent for water-insoluble solids.[77-79] It is nondialyzable, with an average molecular weight of 51,400 and contains four reducing sugars, namely, glucosamine, 6-methylaminohexose, galactosamine uronic acid and an unidentified amino sugar.[78] Rich protein was also secreted along with the extracellular polysaccharide. Protein defective mutants produced equal/enhanced biodispersion as compared to the parent strain.[59]

Exopolysaccharide (EPS)

A. calcoaceticus BD4, BD413 produces EPS with rhamnose and glucose.[80] EPS production is mediated by proteins like Ptk (protein tyrosine kinases) and was also found in *A. johnsonii*. These proteins encode for virulence factors and may serve as a target for the development of new antibiotics.[81]

Pseudomonas Species

Glycolipid BS production was first discovered by Jarvis and Johnson in 1949.[82] They reported production of an acidic, crystalline glycolipid L-rhamnose and ʟ- β-hydroxydecanoic acid from *P. aeruginosa*. This compound was found to be quite similar to a compound of polymer and higher rhamnose-hydroxyacid ratio which was isolated previously by Bergstrom, et al.[83] Later, Hauser and Karnovsky[84] demonstrated the biosynthetic pathway for rhamnolipid production in *Pseudomonas* spp. Burger, et al[85] and Lang and Wagner,[86] demonstrated that *P. aeruginosa* synthesizes mono as well as di-rhamnolipid. Similarly, *P. aeruginosa* synthesizes different rhamnolipid derivatives which include 3-(3-hydroxyalkanoyloxy-) alcanoic acid (HAA), mono-rhamnolipid (L-rhamnosyl-3-hydroxydecanoyl-3-hydroxydecanoate)[87-90] and di-rhamnolipid (L-rhamnosyl-L-rhamnosyl-3-hydroxydecanoyl-3-hydroxydecanoate).[91] Details of different intermediates have been accounted by Pamp and Tolker-Nielsen.[92]

However, studies on regulatory mechanisms came very late with the work of Ochnser, et al[88,89] and Latifi, et al[93] who proposed the involvement of quorum sensing system (QSS) for rhamnolipid biosynthesis in *Pseudomonas* spp. Various components involved in rhamnolipid biosynthesis are

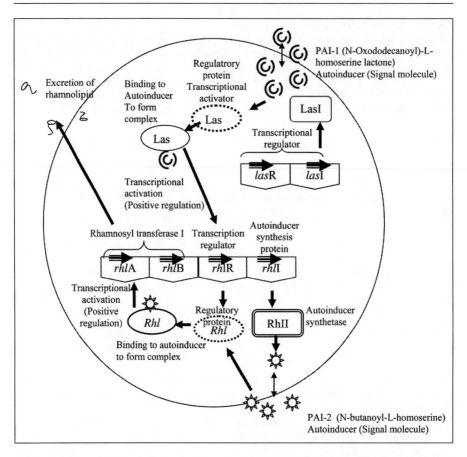

Figure 2. Rhamnolipid synthesis in *Pseudomonas* spp. by two quorum sensing system: Pictorial representation of two quorum sensing system (QSS) present at different regions of *Pseudomonas* spp. chromosome. Thick black bold arrows: Genes on chromosome of *Pseudomonas*; Black arrows: Protein synthesis from gene; Dotted oval indicates inactive regulatory protein; Continuous oval: Active complex of regulatory protein and autoinducer.[14,17,20]

represented diagrammatically in Figure 2. Two QSS regulating rhamnolipid synthesis are present on two different regions of chromosome.[94] Formation of mono and di-rhamnolipids is mediated through two different transferases viz., rhamnosyltransferase I and II. Rhamnolipid synthesis is coupled with nitrogen limitations to the cell.[95] Phosphate limiting conditions are found to enhance BS biosynthesis.[96] Detailed studies have been reported on rhamnosyltransferase I, which contains four genes viz., *rhl*A, *rhl*B, *rhl*R, *rhl*I. Plasmids encoding four genes are sufficient to produce rhamnolipid in heterologous hosts.[97] Genes *rhl*A, *rhl*B are located upstream while *rhl*R, *rhl*I are located downstream of the structural genes (Fig. 2). The *rhl*A and *rhl*B genes code for active rhamnosyltransferase I and are transcribed together as a bicistronic RNA.[88-89,97] Structural proteins are encoded by *rhl*B and present in the periplasm. Inner membrane proteins required for synthesis, transport or solubilization of rhamnosyltransferase are encoded on *rhl*A.[97] In first QSS, genes *rhl*A, *rhl*B are positively regulated by rhlR. Transcriptional activator and autoinducer are encoded by *rhl*R and *rhl*I respectively. Two signal molecules viz., N-butanoyl-Lhomoserine (PAI-2) and hexanoyl-L-homoserine lactone are produced by *rhl*I. Transcriptional activator produced by *rhl*R binds to autoinducer PAI-2 and this active complex causes transcriptional activation of *rhl*A and *rhl*B that encode rhamnosyltransferase I. The second QSS contains two genes namely *las*R and *las*I.[98,99] In this system autoinducer is encoded by *las*I namely N-(3-oxododecanoyl)-l-homoserine-Lactone (PAI-1) RhlR regulatory protein requires autoinducers N-butyryl-HSL and N-(3-oxohexanoyl)-HSL autoinducer for its activity.[100] Induction of second QSS occurs by cyclic AMP levels as indicated by the presence of *las*R promoter region of both lux-box and binding consensus sequence for cyclic AMP receptor protein.[101] The transcription of *rhl*R system is positively regulated by *las* system.[98,102] The *rhl* system is posttranslationally controlled by *las* system by hindrance of PAI-2 by PAI-1 from binding to RhlR. This situation is created till enough PAI-2 and/or PAI-1 are produced to create blockage effect.[98] Figure 2 illustrates the regulation of rhamnolipid synthesis in *Pseudomonas* spp. It is proved that rhlR expression is strongly influenced by environmental factors and is partially LasR-independent under certain culture conditions. Different regulatory proteins viz. Vfr sigma factor σ54 and RhlR itself regulates expression of rhlR.[103]

The *rhl*I negative mutant is unable to produce rhamnolipid on its own. However, addition of synthetic N-acylhomoserine lactone (signal molecule) initiates BS production by mutant. Holden, et al[104] carried out studies to find out whether the BS genes are expressed in unsaturated porous media contaminated with hexadecane and play role in biodegradation process. For this purpose, the *gfp* reporter gene was integrated with either the promoter region of *pra*, which encodes for the emulsifying PA protein and/or to the promoter of the transcriptional activator *rhl*R. It was found that GFP was produced in culture, which indicated that the *rhl*R and *pra* genes are both transcribed in unsaturated porous media. The *gfp* expression was localized at the hexadecane-water interface. Other interesting studies carried out by Pamp and Tolker-Nielsen[92] demonstrated the BS produced by *P. aeruginosa* has additional role in structural biofilm development. Genetic evidence showed that mutant deficient in *rhl*A lack the ability to synthesize BS and could not form microcolonies. This indicates significant role of *rhl*A in BS biosynthesis and biofilm development. The protein AlgR2 responsible for regulation of nucleoside diphosphate kinase also down regulates rhamnolipid production in *P. aeruginosa*.[105] Lequette and Greenberg[106] in 2005, worked on identifying the role of QSS responsible for rhamnolipid biosynthesis on biofilm architecture. They introduced a *rhl*A-*gfp* fusion into a neutral site in the *P. aeruginosa* genome and highlightened the activity of *rhl*AB promoter in rhamnolipid-producing biofilms. Campos-Garci´A, et al[107] identified a new *gene rhl*G which is a homologue of the *fabG* gene encoding NADPH-dependent β-ketoacyl acyl carrier protein (ACP) reductase. This is necessary for synthesis of FA. This gene *rhl*C is obligatory for synthesis of b-hydroxy acid moiety of rhamnolipids and partly contributes to production of poly-β-hydroxyalkanoate (PHA). This study proved that different pathways are involved in synthesis of FA moiety of rhamnolipids than those for general FA synthetic pathways.

Till the year 2001, it was obvious that, rhamnosyltransferase 1 (RhlAB) catalyses the synthesis of mono-rhamnolipid from dTDP-l-rhamnose and β-hydroxydecanoyl-β-hydroxydecanoate, whereas di-rhamnolipid is produced from mono-rhamnolipid and dTDP-l-rhamnose. For the first time, Rahim, et al[91] in 2001, reported dependance of di-rhamnolipid synthesis on rhamnosyltransferase gene. Gene *rhl*C encode for rhamnosyltransferase which catalyses di-rhamnolipid (l-rhamnose-l-rhamnose-β-hydroxydecanoyl-β-hydroxydecanoate) production in *P. aeruginosa*. RhlC is a protein consisting of 325 amino acids (35.9 kDa). The *rhl*C gene is located in an operon with an upstream gene (PA1131) of unknown function. A σ54-type promoter for the PA1131-*rhl*C operon was identified and a single transcriptional start site was mapped. Biological role of RhlC was confirmed by insertional mutagenesis studies and allelic replacement. Inhibition of QSS was demonstrated by work with mutants. Deletion mutants, complementation studies and northern blot analysis on *P. aeruginosa* strain PR1-E4: a *las*R deletion mutant revealed that overproduction of the *P. aeruginosa* DksA homologue down regulated transcription of the autoinducer synthase gene *rhl*I thereby inhibiting QSS.[108]

Pseudomonas species are known to produce different types of BS viz., rhamnolipids, cyclic lipopeptides- putisolvins, lipopolysaccharide. Two types of cyclic lipopeptides (putisolvins I and II) are produced by *P. putida* PCL1445, which possess surfactant activity and also plays

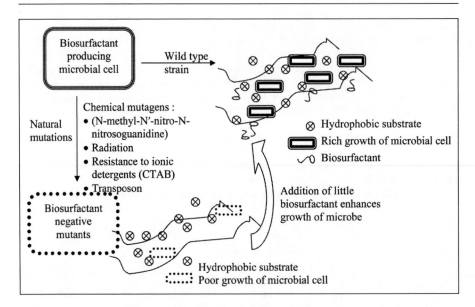

Figure 3. Effect of biosurfactant production on growth in presence of hydrophobic substrates.

significant role in biofilm formation and degradation. Mutants from Tn5*luxAB* library of strain PCL1627 defective in BS production contained transposon inserted in a *dnaK* homologue located downstream of *grpE* and upstream of *dnaJ* indicating positive regulation of these genes in BS synthesis. Two-component signaling system GacA/GacS was involved in BS synthesis.[109] Studies on co-existence of *Burkholderia cepacia* and *P. aeruginosa* in lungs of cystic fibrosis (CF) patients as mixed biofilms correlated the formation of biofilms to *cep*-regulated BS production.[110]

Generally hydrocarbon utilizing microbes produce BS. *P. aeruginosa* degrades hexadecane only if it can produce rhamnolipid.[10,111-113] Mutated *Pseudomonas* spp. produce low rhamnolipid BS.[114-116] Whereas, rhamnolipid defective mutants grow very poorly on hydrocarbons.[117] Pictorial representation is given in Figure 3. Ability of hydrocarbon uptake can be improved by addition of BS in the growth medium. This concept was proved by various studies viz., Koch, et al[118] constructed a transposon TN5-GM induced mutant of *P. aeruginosa* PG201 which could not grow on minimal medium with hexadecane. It was found that the same culture grew well with rhamnolipid supplementation. Al-Tahhan, et al[119] showed that emulsifier makes the cell surface more hydrophobic through release of lipopolysaccharide (LPS). *P. aeruginosa* grew well on paraffin in presence of emulsifier in the production medium. All these observations clearly suggest role of BS/BE in survival of microbes on hydrophobic substrates. Natural or chemical mutations are employed to improve quality and yield of BS/BE from microorganisms.[61] In the year 1995, Iqbal, et al[120] demonstrated hyper—production of BS, high biodegradation and emulsification of crude oil by an EBN-8 a gamma ray induced mutant of *P. aeruginosa*. The same mutant produced 4.1 and 6.3 of rhamnolipids (g/L) when grown on hexadecane and paraffin oil respectively.[113] Another gamma ray induced *P. putida* 300-B mutant gave high yield of rhamnolipid (4.1 g l^{-1}) on soybean waste frying oil as carbon source and glucose as growth initiator over the wild type strain.[121] A research team of Koch, et al[122] constructed a lactose utilizing strain of *P. aeruginosa* by insertion of *E. coli* lac Y genes. Two reporter systems, lacZY and lux4B, were incorporated into chromosome of *P. aeruginosa* UG2. This recombinant strain could utilize lactose and produced BS efficiently. Similar studies were also carried out by Flemming, et al.[123] Their work proved to be efficient in sensitive detection and quantitative enumeration of *P. aeruginosa* UG2Lr (spontaneous rifampin-resistant derivative) using supportive data from antibiotic resistance, bioluminescence and PCR analyses. Ochsner, et al[97] constructed recombinant strains of

P. putida and *P. fluorescence* by knocking down genes responsible for pathogenicity thereby produce harmless BS producing stains. This is the best example of application of molecular knowledge in producing biotechnologically improved stains.

Bacillus *Species*

Surfactin is a cyclic lipopeptide BS produced by *Bacillus* spp. The first report on surfactin production dates back almost to 4.5 decades. Arima, et al[124] were the pioneer researchers who reported production of surfactin from *Bacillus* species. Surfactin the most effective BS reducing surface tension efficiently (72-27 dynes/cm)[125,126] has low CMC (critical micelle concentration) value and finds potential applications in biotechnology and medicine. It is important to note that more than 70% of research on BS is accounted for *Bacillus* spp. alone. Surfactin production, structure, enzymes involved in biosynthesis, organization and genetics of production has been reviewed in great detail.[13] Due to great potential of surfactin and its diverse applications, it became necessary to study the underlying genetic mechanisms. However, the advent of these studies was not until 1988. Kluge, et al[127] laid the foundation for molecular studies by proposing a non ribosomal mechanism of surfactin synthetase. A brief summary of genetic machinery involved in surfactin synthesis is tabulated in Table 2.

Surfactin contains β-hydroxyl FA, usually β-hydroxytetradecanoic acid, synthesized by a 27 kb *srfA* operon. It is under regulation of QSS. First QSS involves nonribosomal peptide synthetases with four open reading frames (ORFs) in the *srf*A operon.[139,140] Operon *srf*A catalyses three multi-functional enzymes for surfactin synthesis.[141] (Cosmina, et al 1993). These modular building blocks are called as surfactin synthetases encoded by *srfA*, *srfB* and *srfC*. The *srf*A locus plays a key role in surfactin production; Nakano and coworkers[142] isolated *srf*A locus by cloning the DNA flanking srfA::Tn917 insertions followed by chromosome walking. This region was an operon (>25 kb) and the gene *srfA* codes for template enzymes while; another gene *Sfp* located downstream of the *srfA* operon encodes for 4'- phosphopantotheinyl transferase. This gene product modifies enzymes to their functional forms for their transcription.[143-146] Study on Tn9171ac mutations confirmed that surfactin production required both the intact 5' as well as 3' end of *srfA*. The 5' region was responsible for sporulation and competence for DNA uptake along with surfactin production and contains 20,535 bp. This region contains *srfA* promoter and two ORFs *srfAA* and *srfAB* encoding surfactin synthetase I and II. The *srfAA* contains three amino acid activating domains for Glu, Val and Leu, while *srfAB* peptide synthesizing domain contains domains for activating Val, Asp and D-Leu. Gene *srfC* contains activating regions for Leu[128-130] and encodes thioesterase Type I motif responsible for termination of peptide.[131]

A third locus within *srfA* operon, the *srfB* gene is required for surfactin production. *srfB* is also necessary for expression of *srfA-lacZ* and is identical to an early competence gene *comA*. Surfactin production is under *ComA* (*SrfB*)-dependent regulation operating at the transcriptional level. *srfA* is positively regulated by product of *srfB*.[147,148] Subsequently, SrfD stimulates the initiation process.[149] However, release of surfactin is still unknown. There is an assumption that passive diffusion releases surfactin across the cytoplasm membrane.[150] Once the cell density attains a maximum level, ComX get accumulated in the medium and interacts with membrane bound histidine kinase ComP and the response regulator ComA.[151] Further, after phosphorylation, by ComP; ComA binds to promoter *srf*A and transcription begins. Competence stimulating factor (CSF), a signal peptide influences *srf*A expression.[139,142,152] It is transported across the membrane and interacts with at least two different intracellular receptors depending upon its concentration. Mutation in ComA inhibits development of competence indicating that, *com*A gene is responsible for expression of *srf* and other com genes.[148] In addition to all these proteins, ComR and SinR also influence *srf*A expression.[138] ComA is regulated positively as well as negatively by ComP under the control of the ComX pheromone.[153] The authors also suggested that *srf* expression requires SpoOK and another, as yet unidentified, extracellular factor under variable pH conditions. The gene *spoOK* codes for an oligopeptide permease that functions in cell-density-dependent control of sporulation and competence.[154,155] Thus molecular machinery ensures appropriate surfactin synthesis.

Table 2. Genetic machinery involved in surfactin synthesis from Bacillus spp.

Operon/Genes/Operator/ Promoter/Protein	Function	Reference
Quorum sensing system I		
srfAA[†‡]	Amino acid activating domain for Glu, Leu, D-Leu	128,129
	Expression of *comS* gene[#]	
		130
SrfAC[†]	Encodes a thioesterase of a Type I motif responsible for peptide termination	131
sfp	Surfactin production	132
Sfp[†]	Activation of surfactin synthetase by post translational modification	132
Quorum sensing system II		
ComQ	Modification of *comX* to form signal peptide ComX	133,134
ComP (Membrane bound protein)	Gets autophosphorylated upon stimulation and transfers its phosphate group to ComA	
Phosphorylated ComA ComS (located within and out of frame srfA gene)	Binds comA-box and initiate transcription of surfactin peptide synthetase, *srf*AA-AD operon and *com*S Development of competence	135
ComX (Signal peptide)	Controls expression of *srf*A and interaction with	
	• Membrane bound histidine kinase ComP	
	• Response regulator ComA	
*Spo*OK (Oligopeptide permease) RapC	Transfer of Competence stimulating factor (CSF) through the cell membrane; Phosphotransferase activity	136
ComR (Polynucleotide phosphorylase)	Enhances *srf*A expression posttranscriptionally	137
SinR (Transcriptional regulator)	Negatively controls *srf*A possibility by regulating *com*R	138

‡: Multifunctional subunit of surfactin synthetase; †: Part of peptide synthetase; #: Embedded within but out of frame with *srf*B.

The sfp locus plays a significant regulatory role at the transcriptional level. The *sfp* locus from a producer strain *B. subtilis* ATCC 21332 was transferred to a standard *B. subtilis* 168 and further subjected to transposon mutagenesis. Studies suggested that, *B. subtilis with a sfp⁰* genotype contains some genes required for surfactin synthesis; *sfp* locus responsible for surfactin production alters the transcriptional regulation of *srf*.[128] A *gsp* gene with sequence homology to *sfp* gene from Gramicidin operon of *B. brevis* complemented in trans, a defect in the *sfp* gene and was able to initiate surfactin synthesis in a non producer strain *B. subtilis* JH642 with an *sfp⁰* phenotype.[145] Additionally, *Sfp* gene is also responsible for hydrocarbon degradation.[156] *sfp* gene was successfully integrated in chromosome of *B. subtilis* to enhance bioavailability of hydrophobic liquids.[157] Sequencing of *sfp* gene revealed 100% sequence homology to amino acid sequence reported earlier by Nakano, et al.[132] A research team of Morikawa, et al[158] worked on cloning and nucleotide sequencing of regulator gene in *B. pumilis*. Studies indicated that out of three large

ORFs (ORF1, 2, 3), ORF3 was essential for surfactin synthesis. Additionally, production of anti-microbial substances or other secondary metabolites is associated with resistance to the producing organism. Tsuge, et al[144] proposed function of gene *yerP* as a determinant of self resistance to surfactin in *B. subtilis* 168. YerP was homologous to the resistance, nodulation and cell division (RND) family of proteins, which confers resistance to wide range of noxious compounds to the secreting organism. Mutagenesis with mini-Tn10 transposon indicated that the transposon had inserted itself in the *yerP* gene in surfactin susceptible mutant. The molecular machinery for BS synthesis in *B. licheniformis* is similar to that in surfactin synthesis.[159,160] A recombinant strain of *B. licheniformis* KGL11 was constructed by inserting the surfactin synthetase enzyme. This mutant produced 12 times the BS of parent strain.[161,162] With better understanding of the molecular phenomena, many attempts were aimed to enhance BS/BE production. Mulligan, et al[163] were successful in obtaining a threefold higher BS production over wild type employing recombinant *B. subtilis* with modified peptide synthetase. A plasmid pC112 with lpa-14, a gene was used to construct a recombinant strain of *B. subtilis* MI113. High yield of surfactin was achieved by fermentation technology.[164] Another recombinant strain of *Bacillus subtilis* MI113 (pC115), was constructed from *B. subtilis* RB14C. This recombinant strain had a gene responsible for surfactin, iturin production and produced new surfactin variants along with usual surfactin when cultured in solid-state fermentation employing soybean curd residue (okara) as substrate.[165] Along with large number of research papers published, enormous patents on BS production appear to date.[38] Carrera, et al[166,167] filed U.S. patents (5,264,363; 5,227,294) on *B. subtilis* ATCC 55033 mutant strain which produced 4-6 times better BS over wild type. Another US patent (7,011,969) on *B. subtilis* SD901 strain mutated with N-methyl-N'-nitro-N-nitrosoguanidine resulted in 4-25 times more surfactin production.[168] Such studies are opening arrays for improved BS production technologies. Various mutant/recombinant strains of *Bacillus* spp. have been constructed for better quality and optimum quantity of surfactin production (Table 3).

Serratia *Species*

Followed by *Acinetobacter*, *Pseudomonas* and *Bacillus* strains, *Serratia* is one of the well-studied bacterium in terms of molecular genetic studies of BS production. *Serratia*, a Gram-negative organism is known to produce extracellular surface active[172] and surface translocating agents.[173] *S. marcescens* produces a cyclic lipopeptide BS 'Serrawettin' which contains 3-hydroxy-C10 FA side chain. BS production is correlated with populational surface migration.[174] The mobility (swarming/sliding motility) and cell density of a population is monitored; depending on this information, regulatory systems control gene expression. This helps the microbial community in interacting with its surrounding.[175,176] The SpnIR QSS is responsible for regulation of flagellum- independent population surface migration and synthesis of BS (prodigiosin) in *S. marcescens* SS-1.[173] Later on, Wei, et al[177,178] confirmed that *spnIR* quorum-sensing genes were located on a Tn3 family transposon, Tn*TIR*. They also proved that SpnR negatively regulated transposition frequency of Tn*TIR*. This group for the first time reported direct evidence of involvement of a *luxIR*-type QSS in regulation of transposition frequency.

BS production is controlled by auto-induction system which subsequently helps in swarming of cells.[176] *S. marcescens* ATCC 274 produces temperature dependant serrawettin W1[cyclo-(D-3- hydroxydecanoyl –L-seryl)$_2$]. Presence of *swr*W gene encoding serrawettin W1 aminolipid synthetase was identified in *S. marcescens* 274 by transposon mutagenesis. The swrW had all four domains of nonribosomal peptide synthetase (NRP), responsible for condensation, adenylation, thiolation and thioesterisation. The swrW NRP is unimodular and specifies only lysine.[179] The authors also proposed a pathway for serrawettin synthesis based on their findings. Parallel production of serrawettin and pigment production in *S. marcescens* 274 is coded by an ORF namely pswP. Synthesis of serrawettin is believed to be through non ribosomal peptide synthetases (NRPSs) system which is a product of the *pswP* gene. A single mutation in the gene is responsible for parallel disruption of both, pigment as well as BS production in *S. marcescens*.[180] In another study, screening of serrawettin W1 overproducing mini Tn5 insertional mutants

Table 3. *Employment of molecular tools for construction of recombinant/mutant strains of Bacillus spp.*

Organism	Mutation	Objective	Significant Feature	Reference
Bacillus	Transformants	Integration of *sfp* gene in chromosome	Improved avaibility of hydrocarbon.	156,157
B. subtilis ATCC21332	Recombinant	Modification of peptide synthetase	3 fold yield than the parent	
B. subtilis MI 113	Recombinant	Insertion of a plasmid pC112 with lpa-14	High yield	164
B. subtilis	Recombinant	Modification in surfactin synthetase	Surfactin without hemolytic activity of erythrocytes	169
B. pumilus		Nucleotide sequence of regulator gene: 3 large ORFs; ORF3 *psf-1* sequences	Surfactin synthesis Similar with operon of *B. brevis*	158
B. licheniformis (Lichenysin)	Recombinant strain	Enzyme complex with surfactin synthetase	Similar with that of surfactin synthetase (*srfA*)	159,160
B. subtilis	M13	The mutated PsrfA fragments were inserted into pT-Klac for construction of plasmids. Promoter activity, pMMN102 was derived from msf33 and pMMN97-101 and -103 were constructed from msf29. pMMN104 with a 10-bp insertion between two ComA boxes. PsrfA of pMMN103 (5-bp insertion between the ComA boxes).	Found that transcription of srfA operon is dependent on the transcriptional activator ComA.	170
B. subtilis (Surfactin and Iturin)	Recombinant MI113(pC115)	Gene responsible for biosurfactant synthesis cloned in *B. subtilis* RB14C	Production of new surfactin variants on soyabean curd residue (okara)	165
B. subtilis (Lipopeptide antibiotic surfactin)	Tn917	Campbell-like recombination at pBR322 homology present in both SPpc2del2::Tn9]7::pSK10A6 DNA and pMMN derivatives *srfB* located between *aroG*, *ald* in genome.	Competence and surfactin production resorted by a single DNA fragment of 1.5 kbp namely *srfB* gene is *comA*	148

continued on next page

Table 3. Continued

Organism	Mutation	Objective	Significant Feature	Reference
B. subtilis (lipoheptapeptide surfactin)	In vivo and in vitro recombination	Peptide synthetase modified by eliminating large internal region of the enzyme with complete amino acid incorporating module. Permissive fusion sites identified for the engineering of peptide synthetase genes	Surfactin with altered antimicrobial activity. The selection of the recombination site is of crucial importance for a successful engineering.	169
B. subtilis	The srfA operon of surfactin synthetase; competence regulatory protein ComS	Construction of B. subtilis strain expressing epitope-tagged srfB. Plasmid pOH9 with carboxy-terminal end of srfB fused to the DNA encoding the influenza virus hemagglutinin 1 (HA1) epitope was constructed.	Found that Srf expression alters with changes in culture pH. ComP acts both positively and negatively in the regulation of ComA and that both activities are controlled by the ComX pheromone.	153
B. subtilis	Oligonucleotide directed mutagenesis	Ser-to-Ala substitutions made in the amino-acylation site of each domain	Part of the srfA contains the region required for competence development and is composed of the first four amino acid-activating domains responsible for the incorporation of Glu, Leu, D-Leu and Val into the peptide moiety of the lipopeptide surfactin. Fourth, Val-activating, domain is required for competence, suggesting that some activity, other than amino-acylation and perhaps unrelated to peptide synthesis, possessed by the fourth domain is involved in the role of srfA in regulating competence development.	139
B. subtilis 168 and 801	Transposon mini-Tn10	Deletion of internal region of the yerP gene of B. subtilis strain 168 yielding a yerP deficient strain 802	The gene yerP determines surfactin self-resistance.	144

continued on next page

Table 3. *Continued*

Organism	Mutation	Objective	Significant Feature	Reference
B. subtilis		Expression of *sfp* gene in *E. coli*, plasmid-amplified in *B. subtilis*	No effect on surfactin production and repression of a *lacZ* transcriptional fusion of the *srfA* operon, which encodes enzymes that catalyze surfactin synthesis. The *sfp* represents an essential component of peptide synthesis and directly or indirectly affects regulation of surfactin biosynthesis.	132
B. subtilis	Recombinant strain	To create *sinR* and *degU* mutant strains bearing multicopy *comS*, plasmid pMMN284 DNA in combination with DNA from strain LAB2274 (D*sinR*::Phleor) or LAB2275 (*degU*::Neor) DNA To create a *comS9*::9*lacZ* D*sinR* strain, DNA from LAB1874 (*comS9*::9*lacZ* Cmr) and LAB2274 (D*sinR* Phleor) was used to transform JH642 cells with selection for Cmr and screening for Phleor.	It was found that *sinR* is required for optimal *comS* expression but not transcription from the *srf* promoter and that SinR at high concentrations represses *srf* transcription initiation.	138
B. subtilis		The peptidyl carrier protein (PCP) domains of surfactin synthetase by transferring the 4-phosphopantetheinyl moiety of coenzyme A (CoA) to a serine residue conserved in all PCPs.	Several residues of Sfp involved in CoA interactions are not conserved and CoA binding may vary between members of this super family.	171

suggested a down regulating mechanism for BS production. The transposon was inserted between the *hexS* gene. *hexS* is a suppressive gene controlling production, therefore insertion and deactivation resulted in enhanced production of exolipids. Thus, target specific repression of *hexS* gene product in transcription is elucidated.[181] Such abortion of repression can be useful for large scale and economical production of surface active agents. Production of BS and thereby surface migration in *S. marcescens* SS-1 is controlled by N-acylhomoserine lactones (AHLs) of QSS located on a mobile transposon.[173,177] Production of BS is under negative control. *S. marcescens* SS-1 produces four AHLs via spnI. The production is regulated by SpnR in *spnI/spnR* QSS. The SpnR is a homologue of the transcriptional regulator LuxR.[173] Furthermore, deletion of this *spnR* gene to produce an isogenic mutant strain *S. marcescens* SMΔR was found to enhance BS activity.[174] Upstream of *spnI* is a gene *spnT* encoding a 464 amino acid protein.[173] The *spnT* is cotranscribed with *spnI* and also functions as a negative regulator of BS production and sliding motility. Thus mobility and horizontal transfer of these genes was proved by Wei, et al.[178] Similar correlation of genes (*swr*/QS) and enzyme involvement in BS production and swarming motility exists in *S. liquefaciens*.[182,183] This interdependence is obligatory for *S. liquefaciens* MG1 to develop swarming colony. The gene *swrI* encodes a similar putative AHL synthase for synthesis of extracellular signal molecules *N*-butanoyl-L-homoserine lactone (BHL) and *N*-hexanoyl-L-homoserine lactone. Expression of *swrA*, encoding serrawettin synthetase, is a homoserine lactone (HSL) and is dependent on QSS.[176,183] The flagellar master operon (*flhDC*) and AHL are involved in flagellar mobility and cell density regulation.

Mutant strain of *S. liquefaciens* was developed by transposon mutagenesis to construct a non-swarming mutant deficient in serrawettin W2 production. Sequence analysis indicated homology with gene *swrA* that encodes a putative peptide synthetase. Expression of *swrA* is controlled by QSS. Transposon mutagenesis involving the promoter less *luxAB* reporter confirmed action of *swrA* gene via QSS in production of the lipopeptide BS. The gene *swrA* encodes a putative peptide synthetase.[183] Microbes are able to change their cell surface hydrophobicity during different growth phases, morphogenesis and differentiation.[184] Cell surface hydrophobicity is affected by cell bound and extracellular factors viz., serraphobin (capacity to bind with hexadecane) and serratamolide (act as wetting agent). Serratamolide negative mutants revealed that serratamolide increases cell surface hydrophobicity.[185] Various BS producing, mutant/recombinant strains of *Serratia* have been constructed employing molecular approaches (Table 4).

Molecular Genetics of Glycolipid Synthesis in Fungi and Yeast

Candida

Sophorolipids (SLs) are one of the most common glycolipids produced by *Candida* species.[19,186-190] SL is composed of sophorose disaccharide glycosidically linked to a hydroxy FA. Genes involved in biosynthesis of SLs were identified, characterized and cloned by several workers.[188,191,192] Mono-oxygenase enzyme, cytochrome P450 dependant on NADPH (nicotinamide adenine dinucleotide phosphate) is essential for FA conversion. The *CPR* (cytochrome P450 reductase) gene of *Candida bombicola* was isolated using degenerate PCR and genomic walking. The CPR gene is made up of 687 amino acids. Heterologous expression in *Escherichia coli* proved functionality of the gene. The recombinant protein had NADPH-dependent cytochrome *c* reducing activity.[193] The genes of cytochrome P450 are diverse among them and also within the genome of a single organism. The phenomenon responsible for induction and expression of these genes was unknown.[194] Specific glycosyltransferase I leads to the coupling of glycosidic linkage of glucose and FA. Glycosyltransferase II carries out subsequent glycosidic coupling. Both glycosyltransferases have been partially purified.[195-197] Like other microorganisms *C. bombicola* produces glycolipid when grown on alkanes. Cytochrome P450 monooxygenase obtains reducing equivalents from NADPH cytochrome P450 reductase (CPR). The *CPR* gene of *C. bombicola* was isolated, sequenced and expressed in *E. coli*. The recombinant protein shows NADPH-dependent 'cytochrome c' reducing activity.[19,186]

Table 4. Employment of molecular tools for construction of recombinant/mutant strains of Serratia spp.

Organism	Mutation	Objective	Significant Feature	Reference
S. marcescens SS-1 SpnR-defective isogenic mutant, SMΔR	Homologous recombination	Isogenic *spnR* insertion deletion mutant of *Serratia marcescens* SS-1 where a 2 kb Sm-resistant DNA	SMΔR strain exhibited better ability for surface tension reduction and diesel emulsification than SS-1 strain did, it is reasonable to assume that the SMΔR strain produced more biosurfactant. Thus, deletion of *spnR* gene may enhance biosurfactant production from the *S. marcescens* strain.	174
S. marcescens	Mini-Tn5	Purified protein encoded in his (6)-hexS bind to DNA fragments of the upstream region of *pigA* and *swrW* genes and not to that of the *pswP* gene.	Over production of exolipids; Plasmid carrying hexS yielded low prodigiosin and serrawettin W1 with reduced activity of exoenzymes (protease, chitinase and DNAse) except phospholipase C.	181
S. liquefaciens MG1	Tn5	Transposon carrying a promoterless *luxAB* reporter the *luxAB* transposon most likely been integrated into a gene, designated *swrA*, is essential for surfactant production.	The gene *swrA*, encodes a putative peptide synthetase. Expression of *swrA* is controlled by quorum sensing.	183

Mycobacterium, Corynebacteria, Rhodococcus

Trehalose lipid (TL) contain carbohydrates and long-chain aliphatic acids/hydroxy aliphatic acids and are most effective BS produced by *Mycobacteria, Corynebacteria* and *Rhodococcus* species.[27] Finerty[198] studied genes responsible for glycolipid biosynthesis in *Rhodococcus* sp. H13-A. A Genomic library was generated using *E. coli-Rhodococcus* shuttle vector pMVS301. Tn917 transpositional mutagenesis in *Rhodococcus*, was employed for isolation and analysis of sporulation and developmental genes in strains of *Bacillus*.

Pseudozyma, Ustilago maydis

Mannosylerythritol lipid (MEL) are produced by genus *Pseudozyma*. A yeast strain *P. antarctica* produces MEL. Genetic study was conducted on prospective genes involved in MEL production.[199] Under nitrogen limitation, *Ustilago maydis*, a dimorphic basidiomycete produces two different classes of glycolipids, ustilagic acids and ustilipids. Ustilagic acids contain cellobiose linked O-glycosidically to 15, 16 dihydroxyhexadecanoic acid, while ustilipids are derived from β-D-mannopyranosyl-D-erythritol and belong to the class of mannosylerythritol lipids.[200] The first report of molecular characterization of glycolipid production using mutants came very recently in 2005 by Hewald, et al.[200] They identified two genes *emt1* and *cyp1* responsible for production of extracellular glycolipids by the fungus. Gene *cyp1* codes for cytochrome P450 monooxygenase and is involved in synthesing 15, 16 dihydroxyhexadecanoic acid. *U. maydis Emt1* codes for a protein which resembles eukaryotic prokaryotic glycosyltransferases and transfers GDP-mannose to form mannosyl –D-erythritol. DNA micro-array analysis revealed that *emt1* is part of a gene cluster which comprises five open reading frames. Three proteins namely Mac1, Mac2 and Mat1, contain short sequence motifs characteristic for acyl- and acetyltransferases. Mac1 and Mac2 are essential for MEL production and are involved in acylation of MEL. Enzyme Mat1 acts as an acetyl coenzyme which is dependent on acetyltransferase. Mat1 displays relaxed regioselectivity and is able to acetylate MEL at both, the C-4 and C-6 hydroxyl groups.[201] Fifth protein is an export protein of the major facilitator family. This is the first report on presence of a gene cluster for production of extracellular glycolipids in a fungus. With these studies, authors introduce the possibility of transfer of genes between species or recent progenitors, for secondary metabolite production in fungal species.

Exploitation of Biosurfactant Molecular Genetics in Biotechnological Applications

The inherent genetic machinery controls phenotypic expression for any particular organism. Understanding of this molecular machinery and its mechanism will play pivotal role in tailoring efficient microbes for potential, economic products. There has been an ever increasing progress in biotechnology in recent years, which has generated enormous opportunities. Initially biotechnological tools were aimed at hyperproducing mutant/recombinant strains. Mutant of *P. aeruginosa* PTCC 1637 produced 10 times BS to that of wild type. Those of *B. subtilis* MI113 and *B. licheniformis* KGL11 enhanced production by 8 and 12 times respectively. Remarkably *B. subtilis* SD901 mutant produced 4-25 times higher yield.[202] Recombinant and/or mutant strains provide huge impetus for further studies (Tables 1, 3 and 4). Biotechnological applications have been recently extended to initial screening methodology of BS producers. The best example is represented from the work by Hsieh, et al.[143] The *sfp* locus was used for PCR based detection of BS producing *B. amyloliquefaciens* and *B. circulans*. Such methods would authenticate the conventional screening methods enlisted in the brief review of Bodour and Miller-Maier.[203] On similar lines, *P. rugulosa* NBRC 10877 was identified as MEL producer on the basis of rDNA sequence.[204] Direct search for genes involved (Fig. 4) would be faster and less laborious. Newer invention like those of Whiteley, et al[205] could be used to identify modulators and genes of QSS signals in bacteria. Novel indicator strains and vectors have been engineered. Techniques like electroporation are useful in transformation studies and have been used successfully in *Pseudozyma*.[206,207] The cationic liposome bearing MEL (produced by *C. antartica*) has been demonstrated to increase dramatically gene transfection efficiency into mammalian cells. Similar studies have been reported by Inoh, et al[208] in 2004. Thus, molecular tools would help to regulate and modify biosynthetic pathways to improve BS production technologies. Such significant findings can be used to upgrade lab scale studies towards field application. Advent of techniques in identification, isolation and manipulation of structural genes involved in BS biosynthesis has made it easier to improve existing BS production technologies. The first genetically engineered bioluminescent strain *P. fluorescens* HK44, with a plasmid containing pUTK21 (naphthalene degradation), transposon and introduced *lux* gene fused within a promoter for naphthalene catabolic genes was released for bioremediation process. The strain HK44 was capable of generating bioluminescence in response to soil hydrocarbon bioavailability. Authors suggested that *lux*-based bioreporter microorganisms can prove a practical alternative in determination of biodegradation in situ, with the process being well-monitored and controlled.[209]

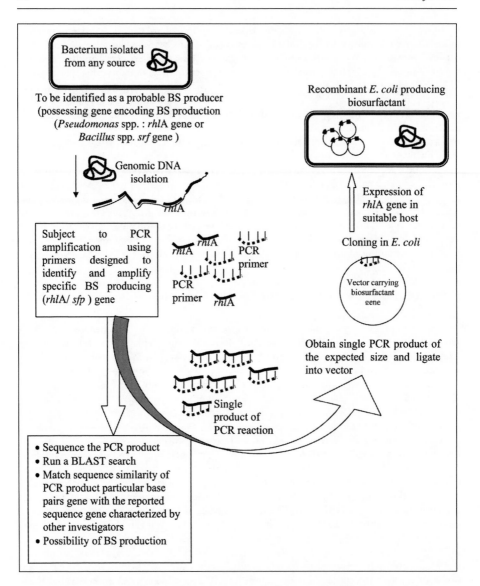

Figure 4. Molecular approach for screening of biosurfactant producers.

It is possible to use naturally occurring molecular tools for investigation purpose. Three cryptic plasmids from both *A. calcoaceticus* BD413, BD4 were isolated, characterized, sequenced and used in the construction of *E. coli* shuttle plasmids. Studies were done to clone and express the alcohol dehydrogenase regulon from *A. lwoffii* RAG-1. Gene expression and transformation in emulsan production and cell surface esterase activity in *A. lwoffii* RAG-1 were also analyzed.[210] The gene (*alnA*) was cloned, sequenced and over expressed in *E. coli*. The recombinant emulsifier protein (AlnA) exhibited 70% emulsifying activity as compared to that of native protein and 2.4 times more than that of the alasan complex. Thus, for the first time Toren, et al[74] in the year 2002, successfully produced a recombinant surface-active protein using a defined gene. The existing molecular knowledge has opened gateways in drug discovery and manipulations. Protein products from microbes can be used for formulation of newer antibiotics and/or life saving drugs. Dams-Kozlowska and Kaplan,[58] introduced a promising and new approach for bioengineering emulsan analogs which has novel application in the field of medicine as biological adjuvants for vaccine and drug delivery.[211,212] Research team of Symmank, et al[169] genetically tailored peptide synthetase, which produced surfactin with reduced haemolytic activity. Rhamnolipid was synthesized in a heterologous host of *P. putida* by cloning *rhlAB* with *rhlRI* from the pathogenic producer strain *P. aeruginosa*.[213] These discoveries are highly commendable and certainly provide promising approach towards conversion of pathogenic to avirulent strains. It appears that, although there is no dearth to the data accumulated which is constantly building up; its actual filed implementation is in a stage of infancy. Thus, maximum exploitation of molecular mechanisms will not only add to our existing understanding of BS production; but will also help bridge the gap between research and actual application.

Conclusion

Irrespective of structural complexity, molecular mechanisms involved in polymer synthesis have been revealed. Among the low molecular BS, the genetic mechanisms in *Pseudomonas* and *Bacillus* have been clearly elucidated. The BS production in both microbes is under the influence of QSS. Different genes are involved and interplay of these genes ensures efficient BS synthesis. Mere choosing of substrates, optimization of physicochemical parameters are not enough. Understanding the genetic mechanisms will help in accelerating research towards achieving economical production. Continued research is adding to the ever expanding knowledge of this field and will certainly prove to be a boon for surfactant industry. Although the utility of genetically modified organisms seems to be farfetched due to environmental constraints; Nevertheless, an understanding of the genetic mechanisms and molecular biology of production of biosurfactants will help us in better understanding of the production phenomena. This will form the basis for further manipulation of conditions resulting in optimal and faster production of these surface active agents. More concerted efforts are needed for an optimal exploitation of generated information. A strong foundation of molecular mechanisms will help in an application oriented outlook at the surfactant industry.

Future Prospects

Over the decades, valuable information on molecular genetics of BS/BE has been generated and this strong foundation would facilitate application oriented output of the surfactant industry. Promising biotechnological advances have expanded the applicability of BS in therapeutics, cosmetics, agriculture, food, beverages and bioremediation. Interaction among experts from diverse fields like microbiology, physiology, biochemistry, molecular biology and genetics is necessary. With the knowledge at hand, BS with desired qualities can be produced. Mutants and recombinants can be generated to achieve desired yield and properties of BS. Potent but harmless strains can be constructed by employing biotechnological advances. However, meticulous and concerted efforts in unfolding the molecular phenomena of BS production in yeast and fungi are essential. PCR based detection methods can be used to authenticate newer BS producers obtained by conventional screening methodologies. Additionally, switch on/off regulatory mechanisms if involved in BS production need to be discovered and investigated.

Acknowledgements

Surekha K. Satpute thanks UGC (F.17-37/98(SA-I)}, Govt. of India, for financial assistance. Smita S. Bhuyan would like to thank Department of Biotechnology, New Delhi, India for financial assistance (DBT project BT/PR 3304/AAQ/03/155/2002 sanctioned to Professor B.A. Chopade).

References

1. Patel P, Desai AJ. Biosurfactant production by Pseudomonas aeruginosa GS3 from molasses. Lett Appl Microbiol 1997; 25:91-94.
2. Makkar RS, Comeotra SS. Utilization of molasses for biosurfactant production by two Bacillus strains at thermophilic conditions. J Am Oil Chem Soc 1997; 74:887-889.
3. Raza ZA, Khan MS, Khalid ZM. Physicochemical and surface-active properties of biosurfactant produced using molasses by a Pseudomonas aeruginosa mutant. J Environ Sci Health Part A 2007; 42:73-80.
4. Rodrigues L, Banat IM, Teixeira J et al. Biosurfactants: potential applications in medicine. J Antimicrobial Chemotherapy 2006; 57:609-618.
5. Soberon-Chavez G, Aguirre-Ramirez M, Ordonez L. Is Pseudomonas aeruginosa only "Sensing Quorum"? Crit Rev Microbiol 2005; 31(3):171-182.
6. Gautam KK, Tyagi VK. Microbial surfactants: A review. J Oleo Sci 2006; 55(4):155-166.
7. Kokare CR, Kadam SS, Mahadik KR et al. Studies on bioemulsifier production from marine Streptomyces sp. S1 Indian J Biotechnol 2007; 6(1):78-84.
8. Satpute SK, Bhawsar BD, Dhakephalkar PK et al. Assessment of different screening methods for selecting biosurfactant producing marine bacteria. Indian J Marine Sciences 2008; 37(3):243-250.
9. Satpute SK, Dhakephalkar PK, Chopade BA. Biosurfactants and bioemulsifiers in hydrocarbon biodegradation and spilled oil bioremediation. Indo-Italian brain storming workshop on technology transfer for industrial applications of novel methods and materials for environmental problem 2005; 1-18.
10. Fiechter A. Biosurfactant moving towards industrial applications. Trends Biotechnol 1992; 10:208-217.
11. Desai AJ, Patel RN. Advances in biosurfactant production: A step forward to commercial applications. J Sci Ind Res 1994; 53:619-629.
12. Desai JD, Banat IM. Microbial production of surfactants and their commercial potential. Microbiol Mol Biol Rev 1997; 61(1):47-64.
13. Peypoux F, Bonmatin JM, Wallach J. Recent trends in the biochemistry of surfactin. Appl Microbiol Biotechnol 1999; 51:553-563.
14. Lang S, Wullbrandt D. Rhamnose lipids-biosynthesis, microbial production and application potential. Appl Microbiol Biotechnol 1999; 51:22-32.
15. Maier RM, Soberon-Chavez G. Pseudomonas aeruginosa rhamnolipids: biosynthesis and potential applications. Appl Microbiol Biotechnol 2000; 54:625-633.
16. Ron E, Rosenberg EZ. Natural role of biosurfactants. J Environ Microbiol 2001; 3(4):229-236.
17. Bodour AA, Maier RM. Biosurfactant: types, screening methods and applications. In: Bitton G, ed. Encyclopedia of Environmental Microbiology. New York: John Wiley & Sons, 2002:750-770.
18. Maier RM. Biosurfactant: evolution and diversity in bacteria. Adv Appl Microbiol 2003; 52:101-121.
19. Inge NA, Bogaert V, Saerens K et al. Microbial production and application of sophorolipids. Appl Microbiol Biotechnol 2007; 76:23-34.
20. Sullivan E. Molecular genetics of biosurfactant production. Curr Opinion Biotechnol 1998; 9:263-269.
21. Margesin R, Schinner F. Bioremediation (natural attenuation and biostimulation) of diesel-oil contaminated soil in an alpine glacier skiing area. Appl Environ Microbiol 2001; 67:3127-3133.
22. Olivera NL, Commendatore MG, Delgado O et al. Microbial characterization and hydrocarbon biodegradation potential of natural bilge waste microflora. J Ind Microbiol Biotechnol 2003; 30:542-548.
23. Gunther NW, Nun'ez A, Fett W et al. Production of rhamnolipids by Pseudomonas chlororaphis, a nonpathogenic bacterium. Appl Environ Microbiol 2005; 71(5):2288-2293.
24. Turkovskaya OV, Dmitrieva TV, Muratova AY. A biosurfactant-Producing Pseudomonas aeruginosa Strain. Appl Biochem Microbiol 2001; 37(1):71-75.
25. Hommel RK, Ratledge C. Biosynthetic mechanisms of low molecular weight surfactants and their precursor molecules. In: Kosaric N, eds. Biosurfactant: Production, Properties, Applications. New York: Marcel Dekker, Inc., 1993:3-63.
26. Syldatk C, Wagner F. Production of biosurfactants. In: Kosaric N, Cairns WL, Gray, NCC, eds. Bio-Surfactants and Biotechnology. New York: Marcel Dekker, Inc., 1987:89-120.
27. Kitamoto D, Isoda H, Nakahara T. Functions and potential applications of glycolipid biosurfactant—from energy-saving materials to gene delivery carriers. J Biosci Bioengg 2002; 94:187-201.
28. Wei YH, Chu IM. Mn^{2+} improves surfactin production by Bacillus subtilis Biotechnol Lett 2002; 24:479-482.
29. Bonilla M, Olivaro C, Corona M et al. Production and characterization of a new bioemulsifier from Pseudomonas putida ML2. J Appl Microbiol 2005; 98:456-463.
30. Maneerat S, Takeshi B, Kazuo H et al. A novel crude oil emulsifier excreted in the culture supernatant of a marine bacterium, Myroides sp. strain SM1. Appl Microbiol Biotechno 2006; 70(2):254-259.

31. Shete AM. Studies on isolation, biochemical and physiological characteristics, antibiotic and bioemulsifier production and plasmid genetics of marine Acinetobacter 2003. A Ph.D. Thesis submitted to the University of Pune, Pune, India.
32. Dubey K, Juwarkar A. Determination of genetic basis for biosurfactant production in distillery and curd whey wastes utilizing Pseudomonas aeruginosa strain B2. Indian J Biotechnol 2004; 3(1):74-81.
33. Bobgelmez-Tinaz G. Quorum sensing in Gram-negative bacteria. Turk J Biol 2003; 7:85-93.
34. Chopade BA. Genetics of antibiotic resistance in Acinetobacter calcoaceticus. 1986. Ph.D. thesis submitted to University of Nottingham, England, Great Britain.
35. Patil JR, Chopade BA. Distribution and in vitro antimicrobial susceptibility of Acinetobacter species on the skin of healthy humans. Natl Med J India 2001; 14:204-208.
36. Patil JR, Chopade BA. Studies on bioemulsifier production by Acinetobacter strains isolated from healthy human skin. J Appl Microbiol 2001; 91(2):290-298.
37. Saha SC, Chopade BA. Effect of food preservatives on Acinetobacter genospecies isolated from meat. J Food Sci Technol 2002; 39(1):26-32.
38. Shete AM, Wadhawa GW, Banat IM et al. Mapping of patents on bioemulsifier and biosurfactant: A review. J Sci Indust Res 2006; 65:91-115.
39. Sar N, Rosenberg E. Emulsifier production by Acinetobacter calcoaceticus strains. Curr Microbiol 1983; 9:309-314.
40. Foght JM, Gutnick DL, Westlake DWS. Effect of emulsan on biodegradation of crude oil by pure and mixed bacterial cultures. Appl Environ Microbiol 1989; 55:36-42.
41. Patil, JR, Chopade BA. Bioemulsifier production by Acinetobacter strains isolated from healthy human skin. United States 2005. Patent No. 20050163739.
42. Belsky I, Gutnick DL, Rosenberg E. Emulsifier of Arthrobacter RAG-1: determination of emulsifier-bound fatty acids. FEBS Lett 1979; 101:175-178.
43. Rosenberg E, Zuckerberg A, Rubinovitz C et al. Emulsifier of Arthrobacter RAG-1: isolation and emulsifying properties. Appl Environ Microbiol 1979; 37:402-408.
44. Zuckerberg A, Diver A, Peeri Z et al. Emulsifier of Arthrobacter RAG-1: chemical and physical properties. Appl Environ Microbiol 1979; 37:414-420.
45. Gorkovenko A, Zhang J, Gross RA et al. Bioengineering of emulsifier structure: emulsan analogs. Can J Microbiol 1997; 43:384-390.
46. Whitfield C, Roberts IS. Structure, assembly and regulation of expression of capsules in Escherichia coli. Mol Microbiol 1999; 31:1307-1319.
47. Whitfield C, Paiment A. Biosynthesis and assembly of group 1capsular polysaccharides in Escherichia coli and related extracellular polysaccharides in other bacteria. Carbohyd Res 2003; 338:2491-2502.
48. Nakar D, Gutnick DL. Analysis of the wee gene cluster responsible for the biosynthesis of the polymeric bioemulsifier from the oil-degrading strain Acinetobacter lwoffii RAG-1. Microbiol 2001; 147:1937-1946.
49. Nakar D, Gutnick DL. Involvement of a protein tyrosine kinase in production of the polymeric bioemulsifier emulsan from the oil-degrading strain Acinetobacter lwoffii RAG-1. J Bacteriol 2003; 185(3):1001-1009.
50. Nesper J, Hill CM, Paiment A et al. Translocation of group 1 capsular polysaccharide in Escherichia coli serotype K30. Structural and functional analysis of the outer membrane lipoprotein Wza. J Biol Chem 2003; 278:49763-49772.
51. Gorkovenko A, Zhang J, Gross RA et al. Biosynthesis of emulsan analogs: direct incorporation of exogenous fatty acids. Proc Am Chem Soc Div Polym Sci Eng 1995; 72:92-93.
52. Gorkovenko A, Zhang J, Gross RA et al. Control of unsaturated fatty acid substitutes in emulsans. Carbohydr Polym 1999; 39:79-84.
53. Zhang J, Gorkovenko A, Gross RA et al. Incorporation of 2-hydroxyl fatty acids by Acinetobacter calcoaceticus RAG-1 to tailor emulsan structure. Int J Bio Macromol 1997; 20:9-21.
54. Johri AK, Blank W, Kaplan DL. Bioengineered emulsans from Acinetobacter calcoaceticus RAG-1 transposon mutants. Appl Microbiol Biotechnol 2002; 59:217-223.
55. Kaplan DL, Fuhrman J, Gross RA. Emulsan adjuvant immunization formulations and use. United States Patent 2004. Application No. 20040265340.
56. Shabtai Y, Gutnick DL. Enhanced emulsan production in mutants of Acinetobacter calcoaceticus RAG-1 selected for resistance to cetyltrimethylammonium bromide. Appl Environ Microbiol 1986; 52:146-151.
57. Alon RN, Gutnick DL. Esterase from the oil degrading Acinetobacter lwoffii RAG-1: sequence analysis and over expression in Escherichia coli. FEMS Microbiol Lett 1993; 12:275-280.
58. Dams-Kozlowska H, Kaplan DL. Protein engineering of wzc to generate new emulsan analogs. Appl Environ Microbiol 2007; 73(12):4020-4028.

59. Elkeles A, Rosenberg E, Ron EZ. Production and secretion of the polysaccharide biodispersan of Acinetobacter calcoaceticus A2 in protein secretion mutants. Appl Environ Microbiol 1994; 60(12):4642-4645.

60. Bach H, Berdichevsky Y, Gutnick D. An exocellular protein from the oil-degrading microbe Acinetobacter venetianus RAG-1 enhances the emulsifying activity of the polymeric bioemulsifier emulsan. Appl Environ Microbiol 2003; 69(5):2608-2615.

61. Tahzibi A, Kamal F, Assadi MM. Improved production of rhamnolipids by a Pseudomonas aeruginosa mutant. Iran Biomed J 2004; 8(1):25-31.

62. de Souza JT, de Boer M, de Waard P et al. Biochemical, Genetic and Zoosporicidal Properties of Cyclic Lipopeptide Surfactants Produced by Pseudomonas fluorescens. Appl Environ Microbiol 2003; 69(12):7161-7172.

63. Zosim Z, Rosenberg E, Gutnick DL. Changes in hydrocarbon emulsification specificity of the polymeric bioemulsifier emulsan: effects of alkanols. Colloid Polym Sci 1986; 264:218-223.

64. Shabtai Y, Gutnick DL. Exocellular esterase and emulsan release from the cell surface of Acinetobacter calcoaceticus. J Bacteriol 1985; 161:1176-1181.

65. Franco AV, Liu D, Reeves PR. The Wzz (cld) protein in Escherichia coli: amino acid sequence variation determines O-antigen chain length specificity. J Bacteriol 1998; 180:670-2675.

66. Daniels C, Morona R. Analysis of Shigella flexneri wzz (Rol) function by mutagenesis and cross-linking: wzz is able to oligomerize. Mol Microbiol 1999; 34:181-194.

67. Leahy JG, Jones-Meehan JM, Pullas EL et al. Transposon mutagenesis in Acinetobacter calcoaceticus RAG-1. J Bacteriol 1993; 175:1838-1840.

68. Reddy PG, Allon R, Mevarech M et al. Cloning and expression in Escherichia coli of an esterase-coding gene from the oil degrading bacterium Acinetobacter calcoaceticus RAG-1. Gene 1989; 76:145-152.

69. Barkay T, Navon-Venezia S, Ron EZ et al. Enhancement of solubilization and biodegradation of polyaromatic hydrocarbons by the bioemulsifier alasan. Appl Environ Microbiol 1999; 65:2697-2702.

70. Navon-Venezia Z, Zosim A, Gottlieb R et al. Alasan, a new bioemulsifier from Acinetobacter radioresistens. Appl Environ Microbiol 1995; 61(9):3240-3244.

71. Bekerman R, Segal G, Ron EZ et al. The AlnB protein of the bioemulsan alasan is a peroxiredoxin. Appl Microbiol Biotechnol 2005; 66:536-541.

72. Toren A, Navon-Venezia S, Ron EZ et al. Emulsifying activity of purified alasan proteins from Acinetobacter radioresistens KA53. Appl Environ Microbiol 2001; 67:1102-1106.

73. Toren A, Orr E, Paitan Y et al. The Active Component of the Bioemulsifier Alasan from Acinetobacter radioresistens KA53 is an OmpA-Like Protein. J Bacteriol 2002; 184(1):165-170.

74. Toren A, Segal G, Ron EZ et al. Structure–function studies of the recombinant protein bioemulsifier AlnA. Environ Microbiol 2002; 4(5):257-261.

75. Ofori-Darko E, Zavros Y, Rieder G et al. An OmpA-like protein from Acinetobacter spp. stimulates gastrin and interleukin-8 promoters. Infect Immun 2000; 68:3657-3666.

76. Rusansky S, Avigad R, Michaeli S et al. Effects of mixed nitrogen sources on biodegradation of phenol by immobilized Acinetobacter sp. strain W-17. Appl Environ Microbiol 1987; 53:1918-1923.

77. Rosenberg E, Rubinovitz C, Gottlieb A et al. Production of biodispersan by Acinetobacter calcoaceticus A2. Appl Environ Microbiol 1988; 54:317-322.

78. Rosenberg E, Rubinovitz C, Legmann R et al. Purification and chemical properties of Acinetobacter calcoaceticus A2 biodispersan. Appl Environ Microbiol 1988; 54:323-326.

79. Rosenberg E, Schwartz Z, Tenenbaum A et al. Microbial polymer that changes the surface properties of limestone; effect of biodispersan in grinding limestone and making paper. J Dispersion Sci Technol 1989; 10:241-250.

80. Kaplan N, Rosenberg E. Exopolysaccharide distribution of and bioemulsifier production by Acinetobacter calcoaceticus BD4 and BD413. Appl Environ Microbiol 1982; 44:1335-1341.

81. Ilan O, Bloch Y, Frankel G et al. Protein tyrosine kinases in bacterial pathogens are associated with virulence and production of exopolysaccharide. The EMBO J 1999; 18:3241-3248.

82. Jarvis FG, Johnson MJ. A glycolipid produced by Pseudomonas aeruginosa. J Am Chem Soc 1949; 71:4124-4126.

83. Bergstrom S, Theorell H, Davide H. On a metabolic product of Pseudomonas pyocyanea, pyolipic acid, active against Mycobacterium tuberculosis. Arkiv Kemi 1947; 23A(13):1-15.

84. Hauser G, Karnovsky ML. Rhamnose and rhamnolipid biosynthesis by Pseudomonas aeruginosa. J Biol Chem 1957; 224:91-105.

85. Burger MM, Glaser L, Burton RM. The enzymatic synthesis of a rhamnose containing glycolipid by extracts of Pseudomonas aeruginosa. J Biol Chem 1963; 238:2595-2602.

86. Lang S, Wagner F. Structure and properties of biosurfactants. In: Kosaric N, Cairns WL, Gray NCC, eds. Biosurfactants and Biotechnology. New York: Marcel Dekker, 1987:21-47.

87. Rendell NB, Taylor GW, Somerville M et al. Characterization of Pseudomonas rhamnolipids. Biochem Biophys Acta 1990; 16:189-193.
88. Ochsner UA, Fiechter A, Reiser J. Isolation, characterization and expression in Escherichia coli of the Pseudomonas aeruginosa rhlA genes encoding rhamnosylatransferas involved in rhamnolipid biosurfactant sysnthesis genes. J Biol Chem 1994; 269:19787-19795.
89. Ochsner UA, Koch AK, Fiechter A et al. Isolation and characterization of a regulatory gene affecting rhamnolipid biosurfactant synthesis in Pseudomonas aeruginosa. J Bacteriol 1994; 176(7):2044-2054.
90. Deziel E, Lepine F, Milot S et al. rhlA is required for the production of a novel biosurfactant promoting swarming motility in Pseudomonas aeruginosa: 3-(3-hydroxy-alkanoyloxy) alkanoic acids (HAAs), the precursors of rhamnolipids. Microbiol 2003; 149:2005-2013.
91. Rahim R, Ochsner UA, Olvera C et al. Cloning and functional characterization of the Pseudomonas aeruginosa rhlC gene that encodes rhamnosyltransferase 2, an enzyme responsible for di-rhamnolipid biosynthesis. Mol Microbiol 2001; 40(3):708-718.
92. Pamp SJ, Tolker-Nielsen T. Multiple roles of biosurfactant in structural biofilm development by Pseudomonas aeruginosa. J Bacteriol 2007; 189:2531-2539.
93. Latifi A, Winson MK, Foglino M et al. Multiple homologues of LuxR and LuxI control expression of virulence determinants and secondary metabolites through quorum sensing in Pseudomonas aeruginosa PAO1. Mol Microbiol 1995; 17:333-343.
94. Stover CK, Pham XQ, Erwin AL et al. Complete genome sequence of Pseudomonas aeruginosa PAO1, an opportunistic pathogen. Nature 2000; 31:959-964.
95. Mulligan CN, Gibbs BF. Correlation of nitrogen metabolism with biosurfactant production by Pseudomonas aeruginosa. Appl Environ Microbiol 1989; 55:3016-3019.
96. Bazire A, Dheilly A, Diab F et al. Osmotic stress and phosphate limitation alter production of cell-to-cell signal molecules and rhamnolipid biosurfactant by Pseudomonas aeruginosa. FEMS Microbiol Lett 2005; 253(1):125-131.
97. Ochsner UA, Reiser J, Fiechter A et al. Production of Pseudomonas aeruginosa rhamnolipid biosurfactant in heterologous hosts. Appl Environ Microbiol 1995; 61:3503-3506.
98. Pesci EC, Pearson JP, Seed PC et al. Regulation of las and rhl quorum sensing in Pseudomonas aeruginosa. J Bacteriol 1997; 179:3127-3132.
99. Lazdunski AM, Ventre I, Sturgis JN. Regulatory circuits and communication in Gram-negative bacteria. Nat Rev Microbiol 2004; 2:581-592.
100. Ochsner UA, Reiser J. Autoinducer-mediated regulation of rhamnolipid biosurfactant synthesis in Pseudomonas aeruginosa. Proc Natl Acad Sci USA 1995; 92:6424-6428.
101. Albus AM, Pesci EC, Runyen-Janecky LJ et al. Vfr control quorum sensing in Pseudomonas aeruginosa. J Bacteriol 1997; 179:3928-3935.
102. Latifi A, Foglino M, Tanaka K et al. A hierachical quorum sensing cascade in Pseudomonas aeruginosa links the transcriptional activators LasR and RhlR (VsmR) to expression of the stationary-phase sigma factor RpoS. Mol Microbiol 1996; 21:1137-1146.
103. Medina G, Jua′rez K, Dı′az R et al. Transcriptional regulation of Pseudomonas aeruginosa rhlR, encoding a quorum-sensing regulatory protein. Microbiol 2003; 149:3073-3081.
104. Holden PA, LaMontagne MG, Bruce AK et al. Assesing the role Pseudomonas aeruginosa: surface active gene expression in hexadecane biodegradation in sand. Appl Environ Microbiol 2002; 68(5):2509-2518.
105. Schlictman D, Kubo M, Shankar S et al. Regulation of nucleoside diphosphate kinase and secretable virulence factors in Pseudomonas aeruginosa: Roles of algR2 and algH. J Bacteriol 1995; 177(9):2469-2474.
106. Lequette Y, Greenberg EP. Timing and localization of rhamnolipid synthesis gene expression in Pseudomonas aeruginosa biofilms. J Bacteriol 2005; 187(1):37-44.
107. Campos-Garci′AJ, Caro AD, Na′Jera R et al. The Pseudomonas aeruginosa rhlG gene encodes an NADPH dependent β-Ketoacyl reductase which is specifically involved in rhamnolipid synthesis. J Bacteriol 1998; 180(17):4442-4451.
108. Branny P, Pearson JP, Pesci EC et al. Inhibition of quorum sensing by a Pseudomonas aeruginosa dksA homologue. J Bacteriol 2001; 183(5):1531-1539.
109. Dubern JF, Lagendijk EL, Lugtenberg BJJ et al. The heat shock genes dnaK, dnaJ and grpE are involved in regulation of putisolvin biosynthesis in Pseudomonas putida PCL1445. J Bacteriol 2005; 187(17):5967-5976.
110. Huber B, Riedel K, Hentzer M et al. The cep quorum-sensing system of Burkholderia cepacia H111 controls biofilm formation and swarming motility. Microbiol 2001; 147:2517-2528.
111. Noordman WH, Janssen DB. Rhamnolipid stimulates uptake of hydrophobic compounds by Pseudomonas aeruginosa. Appl Environ Microbiol 2002; 68:4502-4508.

112. Raza ZA, Khan MS, Khalid ZM et al. Production kinetics and tensioactive characteristics of biosur-
     factant from a Pseudomonas aeruginosa mutant grown on waste frying oils. Biotechnol Lett 2006;
     28(20):1623-1631.
113. Raza ZA, Khan MS, Khalid ZM et al. Production of Biosurfactant using different hydrocarbons by
     Pseudomonas aeruginosa EBN-8 mutant. Z Naturforsch 2006; 61c:87-94.
114. Mulligan CN, Mahmourides G, Gibbs BF. Biosurfactant production by chloramphenicol-tolerant strain
     of Pseudomonas aeruginosa. J Biotechnol 1989; 12:37-44.
115. Mulligan CN, Mahmourides G, Gibbs BF. The influence of phosphate metabolism on biosurfactant
     production by Pseudomonas aeruginosa. J Biotechnol 1989; 12:199-210.
116. Beal R, Betts WB. Role of rhamnolipid biosurfactant in the uptake and mineralization of hexadecane
     in Pseudomonas aeruginosa. J Bacteriol 2000; 89:158-168.
117. Shrive GS, Inguva S, Gunnam S. Rhamnolipid biosurfactant enhancement of hexadecane biodegradation
     by Pseudomonas aeruginosa. Mol Marine Biol Biotechnol 1995; 4:331-337.
118. Koch AK, Kappeli O, Fiechter A et al. Hydrocarbon assimilation and biosurfactant production in
     Pseudomonas aeruginosa mutants. J Bacteriol 1991; 173(13):4212-4219.
119. Al-Tahhan RA, Sandrin TR, Bodour AA et al. Rhamnolipid-induced removal of lipopolysaccharide from
     pseudomonas aeruginosa: effect on cell surface properties and interaction with hydrophobic substrates.
     Appl Environ Microbiol 2000; 66(8):3262-3268.
120. Iqbal S, Khalid ZM, Malik KA. Enhanced biodegradation and emulsification of crude oil and hyper-
     production of biosurfactant by a gamma ray-induced mutant of Pseudomonas aeruginosa. Lett Appl
     Microbiol 1995; 21(3):176-179.
121. Raza ZA, Khan MS, Khalid ZM. Evaluation of distant carbon sources in biosurfactant production by
     a gamma ray-induced Pseudomonas putida mutant. Process Biochem 2007; 42(4):686-692.
122. Koch AK, Reiser J, Kappeli O et al. Genetic construction of lactose-utilizing strains of Pseudomonas
     aeruginosa and their application in biosurfactant production. Biotechnol 1988; 6:1335-1339.
123. Flemming CA, Leung KT, Lee H et al. Survival of lux-lac-marked biosurfactant-producing Pseudomonas
     aeruginosa UG2L in soil monitored by nonselective plating and PCR. Appl Environ Microbiol 1994;
     60(5):1606-1613.
124. Arima K, Kakinuma A, Tamura G. Surfactin, a crystalline lipopeptide surfactant produced by Bacillus
     subtilis: isolation, characterization and its inhibition of fibrin clot formation. Biochem Biophys Res
     Commun 1968; 31:488-494.
125. Cooper DG, Goldenberg BG. Surface-active agents from two Bacillus species. Appl Environ Microbiol
     1987; 53:224-229.
126. Banat IM. The isolation of a thermophilic biosurfactant producing Bacillus Sp. Biotechnol Lett 1993;
     15(6):591-594.
127. Kluge B, Vater J, Salnikow J et al. Studies on the biosynthesis of surfactin, a lipopeptide antibiotic from
     Bacillus subtilis ATCC 21332. FEBS Lett 1988; 231:107-110.
128. Nakano MM, Marahiel MA, Zuber P. Identification of a genetic locus required for biosynthesis of the
     lipopeptide antibiotic surfactin in Bacillus subtilis. J Bacteriol 1988; 170(12):5662-5668.
129. D'Souza C, Nakano M, Corbel N et al. Amino acid site mutations in amino—acid-activating domains
     of surfactin synthetase; Effects on surfactin production and competence development in Bacillus subtilis.
     J Bacteriol 1993; 173(11):3502-3510.
130. Galli G, Rodriguez F, Cosmina P et al. Characterization of the surfactin synthetase multi-enzyme
     complex. Biochem Biophys Acta 1994; 1205:19-28.
131. de Ferra F, Rodriguez F, Tortora O et al. Engineering of Peptide Synthetases key role of the thioesterase-like
     domain for efficient production of recombinant peptides. J Biol Chem 1997; 272(40):25304-25309.
132. Nakano MM, Corbell N, Besson J et al. Isolation and characterization of sfp: a gene that functions in
     the production of the lipopeptide biosurfactant, surfactin, in Bacillus subtilis. Mol Gen Genet 1992;
     232(2):313-321.
133. Solomon JM, Lazazzera BA, Grossman AD. Purification and characterization of an extracellular pep-
     tide factor that affects two different developmental pathways in Bacillus subtilis. Genes Dev 1996;
     10:2014-2024.
134. Solomon JM, Grossman AD. Who's competent and when: regulation of natural genetic competence in
     bacteria. Trends Genet 1996; 12:150-155.
135. Magnuson R, Solomon J, Grossman AD. Biochemical and genetic characterization of a competence
     pheromone from B. subtilis. Cell 1994; 77(2):207-216.
136. Lazazzera BA, Solomon JM, Grossman AD. An exported peptide functions intracellularly to contribute
     to cell density signaling in B. subtilis. Cell 1997; 89:917-925.
137. Luttinger A, Hahn J, Dubnau D. Polynucleotide phosphorylase is necessary for competence development
     in Bacillus subtilis. Mol Microbiol 1996; 19:343-356.

138. Liu L, Nakano MM, Lee OH et al. Plasmid-amplified comS enhances genetic competence and suppresses sinR in Bacillus subtilis. J Bacteriol 1996; 178:5144-5152.
139. D'Souza C, Nakano MM, Zuber P. Identification of comS, a gene of the srfA operon that regulates the establishment of genetic competence in Bacillus subtilis. Proc Natl Acad Sci USA 1994; 91(20):9397-9401.
140. Fabret C, Quentin Y, Guiseppi A et al. Analysis of errors in finished DNA sequences: the surfactin operon of Bacillus subtilis as an example. Microbiol 1995; 141:345-350.
141. Cosmina P, Rodriguez F, De Ferra F et al. Sequence and analysis of the genetic locus responsible for surfactin synthesis in Bacillus subtilis. Mol Microbiol 1993; 8:821-831.
142. Nakano MM, Magnuson R, Myers A et al. srfA is an operon required for surfactin production, competence development and efficient sporulation in Bacillus subtilis. J Bacteriol 1991; 173(5):1770-1778.
143. Hsieh FC, Li MC, Lin TC et al. Rapid detection and characterization of surfactin-producing Bacillus subtilis and closely related species based on PCR. Curr Microbiol 2004; 49:186-191.
144. Tsuge K, Ohata Y, Shoda M. Gene yerP, Involved in surfactin self-resistance in Bacillus subtilis. Antimicrob Agents Chemother 2001; 45(12):3566-3573.
145. Borchert S, Stachelhaus T, Arahiel MA. Induction of surfactin production in Bacillus subtilis by gsp, a gene located upstream of the gramicidin s operon in Bacillus brevis. J Bacteriol 1994; 176(8):2458-2462.
146. Fuma S, Fujishima Y, Corbell N et al. Nucleotide sequence of 5' portion of srfA that contains the region required for competence establishment in Bacillus subtilis. Nucleic Acids Research 1993; 21(1):93-97.
147. Nakano MM, Xia LA, Zuber P. Transcription initiation region of the srfA operon, which is controlled by the comP-comA signal transduction system in Bacillus subtilis. J Bacteriol 1991; 173(17):5487-5493.
148. Nakano MM, Zuber P. Cloning and characterization of srfB, a regulatory gene involved in surfactin production and competence in Bacillus subtilis. J Bacteriol 1989; 171(10):5347-5353.
149. Steller S, Sokoll A, Wilde C et al. Initiation of surfactin biosynthesis and role of Srf-Dthioesterase protein. Biochem 2004; 43:11331-11343.
150. Stein T. Bacillus subtilis antibiotics: structures, syntheses and specific functions. Mol Microbiol 2005; 56(4):845-857.
151. Hamoen LW, Venema G, kuipers OP. Controlling competence in Bacillus subtilis; shared use of regulators. Microbiol 2003; 149:9-17.
152. Hamon MA, Lazazzera BA. The sporulation transcription factor ApoOA is required for biofilm development in Bacillus subtilis. Mol Microbiol 2001; 42:1199-1209.
153. Cosby WM, Vollenbroich D, Lee OH et al. Altered srf expression in Bacillus subtilis resulting from changes in culture pH is dependent on the Spo0K oligopeptide permease and the ComQX system of extracellular control. J Bacteriol 1998; 180(6):1438-1445.
154. Perego M, Higgins CF, Pearce SR et al. The oligopeptide transport system of Bacillus subtilis plays a role in the initiation of sporulation. Mol Microbiol 1991; 5:173-185.
155. Rudner DZ, Ledeaux JR, Ireton K et al. The spo0K locus of Bacillus subtilis is homologous to the oligopeptide permease locus and is required for sporulation and competence. J Bacteriol 1991; 173:1388-1398.
156. Kim HS, Kim SB, Park SH et al. Expression of sfp gene and hydrocarbon degradation by Bacillus subtilis. Biotechnol Lett 2000; 22:1431-1436.
157. Lee YK, Kim SB, Park CS et al. Chromosomal integration of sfp gene in Bacillus subtilis to enhance bioavailability of hydrophobic liquids. Appl Microbiol Biotechnol 2005; 67(6):789-794.
158. Morikawa M, Ito M, Imanaka T. Isolation of a new surfactin producer Bacillus pumilus A-1 and cloning and nucleotide sequence of the regulator gene, psf-1. J Ferm Bioengg 1992; 74(5):255-261.
159. Yakimov MM, Timmis KM, Wray V et al. Characterization of a new lipopeptide surfactant produced by thermotolerant and halotolerant subsurface Bacillus licheniformis BAS50. Appl Environ Microbiol 1995; 61:1706-1713.
160. Yakimov MM, Golyshin PN. ComA-dependant transcriptional activation of lichenysin A synthetase promoter in Bacillus subtilis cells. Biotechnol Prog 1997; 13:757-761.
161. Yakimov MM, Giuliano L, Timmis KN et al. Recombinant acylheptapeptide lichenysin: high level of production by Bacillus subtilis cells. J Mol Microbiol Biotechnol 2000; 2:217-224.
162. Lin SC, Lin KG, Lo CC et al. Enhanced biosurfactant production by a Bacillus licheniformis mutant. Enzyme Microb Technol 1998; 23:267-273.
163. Mulligan CN, Chow TYK, Gibbs BF. Surfactin production by a Bacillus subtilis mutant. Appl Microbiol Biotechnol 1989; 31:486-489.
164. Ohno A, Ano T, Shoda M. Production of a lipopeptide antibiotic, surfactin, by recombinant Bacillus subtilis in solid state fermentation. Biotechnol Bioeng 1995; 47:209-214.
165. Nakayama S, Takahashi S, Hirai M et al. Isolation of new variants of surfactin by a recombinant Bacillus subtilis. Appl Microbiol Biotechnol 1997; 48:80-82.

166. Carrera P, Cosmina P, Grandi G. Eniricerche SPA., Milan, Italy. Mutant of Bacillus subtilis, United States Patent 1993. Application No. 5264363.

167. Carrera P, Cosmina P, Grandi G. Eniricerche SPA., Milan, Italy. Method of producing surfactin with the use of mutant of Bacillus subtilis. United States Patent 1993. Application No. 5227294.

168. Yoneda T, Yoshiaki M, Kazuo F et al. Showa Denko KK (JP), Tokyo, Japan. Production process of surfactin, United States Patent 2006. Application No. 7011969.

169. Symmank H, Franke P, Saenger W et al. Modification of biologically active peptides: production of a novel lipohexapeptide after engineering of Bacillus subtilis surfactin synthetase. Protein Engg 2002; 115(11):913-921.

170. Nakano MM, Zuber P. Mutational analysis of the regulatory region of the srfA operon in Bacillus subtilis. J Bacteriol 1993; 175(10):3188-3191.

171. Reuter K, Mofid MR, Marahiel MA et al. Crystal structure of the surfactin synthetase-activating enzyme Sfp: a prototype of the 4'-phosphopantetheinyl transferase superfamily. The EMBO J 1999; 18(23):6823-6831.

172. Matsuyama T, Sogawa M, Yanot I. Direct colony thin-layer chromatography and rapid characterization of Serratia marcescens mutants defective in production of wetting agents. Appl Environ Microbiol 1987; 53(5):1186-1188.

173. Horng YT, Deng SC, Daykin M et al. The LuxR family protein SpnR functions as a negative regulator of N-acylhomoserine lactone-dependent quorum sensing in Serratia marcescens. Mol Microbiol 2002; 45:1655-1671.

174. Wei Y, Lai HC, Chen SU et al. Biosurfactant production by Serratia marcescens SS-1 and its isogenic strain SMΔR defective in SpnR, a quorum-sensing LuxR family protein. Biotechnol Lett 2004; 26:799-802.

175. Williams P, Camara M, Hardman A et al. Quorum sensing and the population-dependent control of virulence. Philos Trans R Soc London B Biol Sci 2000; 355:667-680.

176. Matsuyama T, Bhasin A, Harshey RM. Mutational analysis of flagellum-independent surface spreading of Serratia marcescens 274 on a low-agar medium. J Bacteriol 1995; 177:987-991.

177. Wei J, Soo PC, Horng YT et al. Regulatory roles of spnT, a novel gene located within transposon TnTIR. Biochem Biophy Res Comm 2006; 348:1038-1046.

178. Wei J, Tsai YH, Horng YT et al. A mobile quorum-sensing system in Serratia marcescens. J Bacteriol 2006; 188(4):1518-1525.

179. Li H, Tanikawa T, Sato Y et al. Serratia marcescens gene required for surfactant serrawettin W1 production encodes putative aminolipid synthetase belonging to nonribosomal peptide synthetase family. Microbiol Immunol 2005; 49(4):303-310.

180. Sunaga S, Li H, Sato Y et al. Identification and characterization of the pswP gene required for the parallel production of prodigiosin and serrawettin W1 in Serratia marcescens. Microbiol Immunol 2004; 48(10):723-728.

181. Tanikawa T, Nakagawa Y, Matsuyama T. Transcriptional downregulator HexS controlling prodigiosin and serrawettin W1 biosynthesis in Serratia marcescens. Microbiol Immunol 2006; 50(8):587-596.

182. Riedel K, Talker-Huiber D, Givskov M et al. Identification and characterization of a GDSL esterase gene located proximal to the swr quorum-sensing system of Serratia liquefaciens MG1. Appl Environ Microbiol 2003; 69(7):3901-3910.

183. Lindum PW, Anthoni U, Christophersen C et al. n-acyl-l-homoserine lactone autoinducers control production of an extracellular lipopeptide biosurfactant required for swarming motility of Serratia liquefaciens MG1. J Bacteriol 1998; 180(23):6384-6388.

184. Rosenberg M, Kjelleberg S. Hydrophobic interactions in bacterial adhesion. Adv Microb Ecol 1986; 9:353-393.

185. Ullrich C, Kluge B, Palacz Z et al. Cell-free biosynthesis of surfactin, a cyclic lipopeptide produced by Bacillus subtilis. Biochem 1991; 30:6503-6508.

186. Inge NA, Bogaert V, Develter D et al. Cloning and characterization of the NADPH cytochrome P450 reductase gene (CPR) from Candida bombicola. FEMS Yeast Res 2007; 7(6):922-928.

187. Solaiman DK, Ashby RD, Nunez A. Production of sophorolipids by Candida bombicola grown on soy molasses as substrate. Biotech Lett 2004; 26:1241-1245.

188. Solaiman D, Ashby RD, Foglia TA. Characterization and manipulation of genes in the biosynthesis of sophorolipids and poly (hydroxyalkanoates). In: Proceedings of the United States-Japan Cooperative program in natural resources, protein resources panel Annual Meeting 2004. 215-219.

189. Solaiman D, Ashby RD, Foglia TA et al. Biosurfactants from microbial fermentation of renewable substrates [abstract]. Industrial application of renewable resources—A Conference on Sustainable Technologies, American Oil Chemists' Society 2004. 14.

190. Hommel RK, Huse K. Regulation of sophorose lipid production by Candida apicola. Biotechnol Lett 1993; 33:853-858.

191. Ashby RD, Solaiman D, Foglia TA. The use of fatty acid-esters to enhance free acid sophorolipid synthesis. Biotechnol Lett 2006; 28:253-260.
192. Zerkowski JA, Solaiman D. Polyhydroxy fatty acids derived from sophorolipids. J Amer Oil Chemists Soc 2007; 84(5):463-471.
193. Van Bogaert INN, Develter D, Soetaert W et al. Cloning and characterization of the NADPH cytochrome P450 reductase gene (CPR) from Candida bombicola. FEMS Yeast Res 2007; 7(6):922-928.
194. Nebert DW, Gonzalez FJ. P450 genes: structure, evolution and regulation. Ann Rev Biochem 1987; 56:945-993.
195. Esders TW, Light RJ. Characterization and in vivo production of three glycolipids from Candida bogoriensis: 13-glucopyranosylglucopyranosyloxydocosanoic acid and its mono- and diacetylated derivatives. J Lipid Res 1972; 13:663-671.
196. Esders TW, Light RJ. Glucosyl- and Acetyltransferases involved in the biosynthesis of glycolipids from Candida bogoriensis. J Biol Chem 1972; 247:1375-1386.
197. Bucholtz ML, Light RJ. Acetylation of 13-sophorosyloxydocosanoic acid by an acetyltransferase purified from Candida bogoriensis. J Biol Chem 1976; 251(2):424-430.
198. Finerty WR. Genetics and biochemistry of biosurfactant synthesis in Arthrobacter species H-13-A Progress Report (Arthrobacter H-13-A): 1988. DOE/ER/10683-6.
199. Konishi M, Morita T, Fukuoka T et al. Production of different types of mannosylerythritol lipids as biosurfactant by the newly isolated yeast strains belonging to the genus Pseudozyma. Appl Microbiol Biotechnol 2007; 75:521-531.
200. Hewald S, Josephs K, Bo¨lker M. Genetic analysis of biosurfactant production in Ustilago maydis. Appl Environ Microbiol 2005; 71(6):3033-3040.
201. Hewald S, Linne U, Scherer M et al. Identification of a gene cluster for biosynthesis of mannosylerythritol lipids in the basidiomycetous fungus Ustilago maydis. Appl Environ Microbiol 2006; 72(8):5469-5477.
202. Mukherjee S, Das P, Sen R. Towards commercial production of microbial surfactants. TRENDS Biotechnol 2006; 24(11):509-515.
203. Bodour AA, Miller-Maier R. x) Biosurfactants: types, screening methods and applications: In: Bitton G, ed. Encyclopedia of Environmental Microbiology. 1st ed. Hoboken: John Wiley and Sons, Inc., 2000:750-770.
204. Morita T, Konishi M, Fukuoka T et al. Discovery of Pseudozyma rugulosa NBRC10877 as a novel producer of the glycolipid biosurfactants, mannosylerythritol lipids based on rDNA sequence. Appl Microbiol Biotechnol 2006; 73(2):305-313.
205. Whiteley M, Lee KM, Greenberg EP. Identification of genes controlled by quorum sensing in Pseudomonas aeruginosa. PNAS 1999; 96(24):13904-13909.
206. Morita T, Habe H, Fukuoka T et al. Gene expression profiling and genetic engineering of a basidiomycetous yeast, Pseudozyma antarctica, which produces multifunctional and environmentally-friendly surfactants (biosurfactant). The XXIIIrd International conference on yeast genetics and molecular biology melbourne 2007. Australia 1-6.
207. Morita T, Konishi K, Fukuoka T et al. Microbial conversion of glycerol in to glycolipid biosurfactant, mannosylerythritol lipids by basidiomycete yeast Pseudozyma antarctica, JCM 1037. J Biosci Bioeng 2007; 104(1):78-81.
208. Inoh Y, Kitamoto D, Hirashima N et al. Biosurfactant MEL-A dramatically increases gene transfection via membrane fusion. J Control Release 2004; 94(2-3):423-431.
209. Ripp S, Nivens DE, Werner C et al. Controlled field release of a bioluminescent genetically engineered microorganism for bioremediation process monitoring and control. Environ Sci Technol 2000; 34:846-853.
210. Minast W, Gutnick DL. Isolation, characterization and sequence analysis of cryptic plasmids from Acinetobacter calcoaceticus and their use in the construction of Escherichia coli shuttle plasmids. Appl Environ Microbiol 1993; 59(9):2807-2816.
211. Panilaitis B, Johri A, Blank W et al. Adjuvant activity of emulsan, a secreted lipopolysaccharide from Acinetobacter calcoaceticus. Clin Diagn Lab Immunol 2002; 9:1240-1247.
212. Castro GR, Kamdar RR, Panilaitis B et al. Triggered release of proteins from emulsan-alginate beads. J Control Release 2005; 109:149-157.
213. Cha M, Lee N, Kim M et al. Heterologous production of Pseudomonas aeruginosa EMS1 biosurfactant in Pseudomonas putida. Bioresour Technol 2008; 99(7):2192-2199.

CHAPTER 3

Interaction of Dirhamnolipid Biosurfactants with Phospholipid Membranes:
A Molecular Level Study

Antonio Ortiz,* Francisco J. Aranda and Jose A. Teruel

Abstract

Rhamnolipids are bacterial biosurfactants produced by *Pseudomonas spp*. These compounds have been shown to present several interesting biological activities and to have potential applications as therapeutics agents. It has been suggested that the interaction with the membrane could be the ultimate responsible for these actions. Therefore it is of great interest to get insight into the molecular mechanism of the interaction of purified rhamnolipids with the various phospholipid components of biological membranes. In this work, the CMC of a purified bacterial dirhamnolipid was determined both by isothermal titration calorimetry and surface tension measurements. The partition coefficients from water to membranes of different compositions, as well as the corresponding thermodynamic parameters, indicated that membrane partitioning was an entropically driven process. Interaction of dirhamnolipid with phospholipids was studied by means of calorimetry, FTIR and X-ray diffraction. It is shown this interaction had various effects that might constitute the molecular basis to explain the former activities: domain formation with lateral phase separation, increased motional disorder of the phospholipid acyl chains and dehydration of the aqueous interface. Our results suggest that dirhamnolipid, having a large polar headgroup and a smaller hydrophobic portion, behaves as an inverted-cone shaped molecule, conferring positive curvature to membranes, which might be behind its disrupting effects on membranes.

Introduction

A number of microorganisms, including bacteria, yeasts and fungi, produce a series of surface active compounds which are known as biosurfactants. These amphiphilic compounds present a wide structural diversity, most of them being of lipidic nature. Because of their interesting chemical and biological properties, there is an increasing interest in considering biosurfactants as potential alternatives to chemically synthesized compounds.[1-4]

Pseudomonas aeruginosa is a Gram-negative bacterium notorious for its environmental versatility, ability to cause disease in particular susceptible individuals and its resistance to antibiotics. The bacterium is capable of utilizing various organic compounds as food sources, thus giving it an exceptional ability to colonize ecological niches where nutrients are limited. *Pseudomonas aeruginosa* produces rhamnolipids when grown under the appropriate conditions.[5] Rhamnolipids are a group of glycolipid biosurfactants composed of a hydrophilic head constituted by one or two rhamnose molecules, called

*Corresponding Author: Antonio Ortiz—Departamento de Bioquímica y Biología Molecular-A, Facultad de Veterinaria, Universidad de Murcia, E-30100 Murcia, Spain. Email: ortizbq@um.es

Biosurfactants, edited by Ramkrishna Sen. ©2010 Landes Bioscience and Springer Science+Business Media.

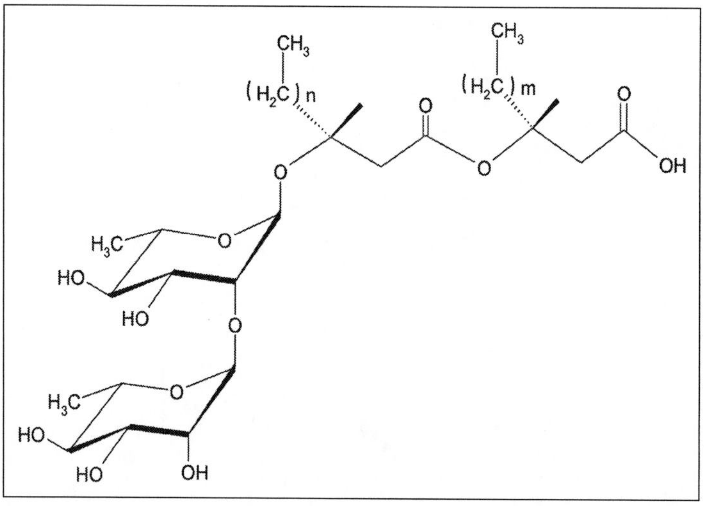

Figure 1. The chemical structure of the diRL compounds produced by *Pseudomonas aeruginosa*. For Rha-Rha-C_{10}-C_{10} m, n = 6 and for Rha-Rha-C_{10}-C_{12} m = 8 and n = 6.

respectively monorhamnolipid and dirhamnolipid (diRL) and a hydrophobic tail formed by one or two fatty acids (Fig. 1). The type of the rhamnolipids produced depends on the bacterial strain, the carbon source used and the culture conditions.[6] Rhamnolipids represent one of the most important classes of biosurfactants because of various advantageous characteristics. Concerning its production, they show high yields as compared to other biosurfactants and several raw materials can be used as carbon sources.[6-8] Rhamnolipids are surface-active compounds, reducing the surface tension of water to values close to 30 mN/m.[9] The CMC of pure rhamnolipids and its mixtures depends greatly on the chemical composition of the various species, ranging from 50 to 200 mg/l.[11]

Rhamnolipids have been shown to present several interesting activities from the biological point of view. They behave as exotoxins, restricting the growth of *Bacillus subtilis*,[12,13] and presenting zoosporicidal activity on various species of zoosporic phytopathogens.[14] It is widely accepted that the majority of the mentioned activities must be related to the action of the rhamnolipids on the lipid constituent of biological membranes, as it has been shown for other biosurfactants which affect the structure of phospholipid membranes.[15,16] The compounds secreted by *Pseudomonas aeruginosa* constitute a heterogeneous mixture of mono- and dirhamnolipids which has been used in most of the published works. However it is interesting to investigate the individual contribution of each homologue to the biological properties of the mixture in order to obtain a rhamnolipid with the desired properties for specific uses. We will show in this chapter that a purified diRL influences the physicochemical characteristics of phospholipid membranes.[17,18] and the molecular interactions with phospholipid membranes will be described.

Critical Micellar Concentration of diRL

Surfactants can assemble into a wide list of morphologically different structures.[19] The complex aggregation behaviour of a purified diRL biosurfactant produced by *Pseudomonas aeruginosa* in aqueous media has been studied in a previous work,[11] showing a concentration dependent micelle-to-vesicle transformation.

The CMC of rhamnolipids has been determined for various mixtures of heterogeneous composition, including mono- and dirhamnolipids.[10,20] We recently carried out the first determination of the CMC of a purified diRL biosurfactant produced by *Pseudomonas aeruginosa*. The CMC of the purified diRL was first determined by surface tension (γ) measurements[21] as shown in Figure 2 (panel A). A dilute solution of the biosurfactant had a value of γ close to that of pure water (75 mN/m). As

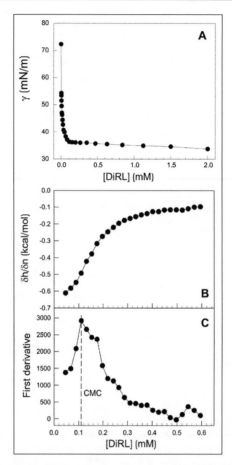

Figure 2. Determination of the critical micelle concentration of diRL by surface tension measurements (A) and isothermal titration calorimetry (B,C). A) A plot of the surface tension (γ) as a function of the diRL concentration for a series of diRL solutions prepared in 150 mM NaCl, 5 mM Hepes, pH 7.4 buffer at 25°C. B,C) A typical ITC demicellization experiment. B) The heats of injection per mole of injected diRL obtained upon injection of a series of 10 μl aliquots of a 3 mM diRL solution prepared in 150 mM NaCl, 5 mM Hepes, pH 7.4 buffer into the same buffer at 25°C (δh/δn) as a function of the diRL concentration in the calorimeter cell. C) First derivative of the plot presented in panel B. The diRL concentration corresponding to the maximum ordinate is the CMC.

the concentration of diRL was increased γ was decreasing to reach a value of ca. 36 mN/m at 0.11 mM diRL and kept essentially constant for higher concentrations. Thus the CMC was 0.11 mM as measured by this procedure, in good agreement with the ITC dilution experiments shown below.

The CMC of the purified diRL was also determined by ITC dilution experiments as shown in Figure 2 (panels B and C). Figure 2B presents the integrated heat flow curves obtained upon injection of a concentrated diRL solution into buffer at 25°C. Each injection of the biosurfactant solution was accompanied by an exothermic heat of reaction due to the rupture of the micelles into monomers and the integration of the corresponding peaks yielded the heat of reaction, δh, which was divided by the number of moles injected, δn, to yield the molar heat of demicellization. This was plotted as a function of the total concentration of diRL, showing a typical sigmoidal shape. The first derivative of this curve had a maximum at 0.11 mM diRL, which corresponded to the value of the CMC[22] (Fig. 2C).

The literature values for the CMC of different rhamnolipid heterogeneous mixtures ranged from 53 to 230 mg/l.[10,20] The value of 0.11 mM (71.5 mg/l) that we obtained for our pure diRL was of the same order of these values. As compared to other relevant biosurfactants, like surfactin (CMC 0.075 mM), the CMC of diRL was relatively high, which already suggested that this biosurfactant will most probably behave as a weak detergent in aqueous solution.

Partitioning of DiRL into Phospholipid Membranes

The thermodynamics of the binding of diRL to phospholipid membranes was determined by ITC experiments in which a lipid dispersion was titrated to a biosurfactant solution at a concentration below the CMC, i.e., in the monomer state.[21] In these experiments, small unilamelar vesicles (SUV) of different compositions were injected into a diRL solution in buffer. The partition of the surfactant into the membrane was endothermic in this case and opposite to the heat of dilution which was exothermic. The integration of the calorimeter peaks yielded the heats of reaction, δh, which were then divided by the amount of lipid injected, δn. A plot of $\delta h/\delta n$ versus the total concentration of lipid allowed the simultaneous determination of the partition constant, K; the membrane partition enthalpy ΔH and the heat of dilution, q_{dil}. In the case of SUV made of pure POPC at pH 7.4, K was 23.4 mM^{-1}, ΔH was +0.9 kcal/mol and q_{dil} was −0.2 kcal/mol (Table 1). In the case of pure diRL the product K · CMC = 2.5 indicated that diRL should behave as a weak detergent and it will most probably prefer membrane penetration over micellization. As a matter of fact we have presented experimental evidence, based on dynamic light scattering and electron microscopy results, that, upon increasing concentration above the CMC, diRL by itself forms bilayer vesicles of heterogeneous size.[11] On the other hand, this behaviour opened the possibility of a number of other applications based on formation of diRL bilayer vesicles.

Effect of Membrane Lipid Composition on Membrane Partitioning

The ITC binding experiments described above were carried out under different conditions and with SUV made of different lipids. The experimental results were fitted as explained before and the data obtained are summarized in Table 1. DiRL is an anionic biosurfactant with a reported pKa value of 5.6.[23] Thus, at pH 7.4, 98.4% of the diRL molecules bear a negative charge, whereas at pH 4.0, 97.5% are neutral. The partition constants, K and the heats of dilution, q_{dil}, of diRL into POPC SUV at pH 7.4 and 4.0 were very similar; however the ΔH changed from +0.9 kcal/mol (endothermic) at pH 7.4 to −1.0 kcal/mol (exothermic) at pH 4.0. Since at both pH values K were very similar, the result was just a slight reduction of the term $T\Delta S$ from 9.2 to 7.3 kcal/mol (Table 2), which might not be high enough to explain the differences in the membrane binding mechanism of negatively charged vs neutral diRL.

Incorporation of cholesterol into POPC resulted in a drastic reduction of the partition constant (Table 1). This result might be a consequence of the increase in the motional order of the phospholipid acyl chains and the general stabilization of the membrane caused by cholesterol[24,25] which resulted in a tighter lipid packing[26] and made binding of the surfactant more difficult.

Table 1. Partition constant, enthalpy change and heat of dilution for the membrane partitioning of diRL into different SUV systems

System	K (mM^{-1})	ΔH (kcal/mol)	q_{dil} (kcal/mol)
POPC pH 7.4	23.4 ± 2.9	0.9 ± 0.05	−0.2 ± 0.01
POPC pH 4.0	25.3 ± 3.0	−1.0 ± 0.05	−0.1 ± 0.01
POPC/Chol (1:1)	8.6 ± 0.8	2.1 ± 0.1	−0.01 ± 0.01
POPC/POPE (1:1)	28.4 ± 4.2	1.2 ± 0.1	−0.02 ± 0.02
POPC/lysoPC (2:1)	9.4 ± 1.1	1.8 ± 0.2	−0.3 ± 0.03

**Table 2.   Thermodynamic parameters for the membrane partitioning of diRL into
different SUV systems**

System	ΔH (kcal mol^{-1})	ΔG^0 (kcal mol^{-1})	$T\Delta S$ (kcal mol^{-1})
POPC pH 7.4	0.9 ± 0.05	−8.3	9.2
POPC pH 4.0	−1.0 ± 0.05	−8.4	7.3
POPC/Chol (1:1)	2.1 ± 0.1	−7.7	9.8
POPC/POPE (1:1)	1.2 ± 0.1	−8.4	9.6
POPC/lysoPC (2:1)	1.8 ± 0.2	−7.8	9.6

Since K was strongly reduced and ΔH was increased from +0.9 to +2.1 kcal/mol, the term $T\Delta S$ remained essentially unchanged (Table 2), indicating that the presence of cholesterol reduced diRL partitioning but did not modify the mechanism of diRL binding to these membranes as compared to pure POPC.

Table 1 also shows that the partition of diRL into POPC membranes which contained 50 mol% of POPE was more favourable, whereas the addition of lysoPC to the membrane resulted in a large reduction of the partition constant. Thus, the presence of POPE facilitated diRL membrane binding whereas lysoPC seemed to have an opposite effect. The thermodynamic parameters for the membrane partitioning of diRL into the different SUV systems are detailed in Table 2. The values of ΔH were very close in all cases and ranged from −1.0 to +2.1 kcal/mol. Interestingly, at pH 4.0 ΔH was exothermic, whereas in all the other cases it was endothermic. However in all cases the process was thermodynamically favourable ($\Delta G < 0$) and, despite the small differences in ΔH, the large entropy term $T\Delta S$ (ca. +10 kcal/mol) constituted the driving force for the partition of monomeric diRL into phospholipid membranes.

Modulation of the Thermotropic Behavior of Phospholipids by diRL

The influence of diRL on the thermotropic gel to liquid crystalline phase transition of saturated phosphatidylcholines bearing acyl chains with 14 (DMPC), 16 (DPPC) and 18 (DSPC) carbon atoms was studied by means of differential scanning calorimetry (DSC). Figure 3 (panel A) shows the thermograms obtained for DMPC as an illustrative example. In the absence of diRL, phosphatidylcholines exhibited two endotherms upon heating: a lower temperature lower enthalpy pretransition and a higher temperature higher enthalpy main transition. In the thermograms of pure phospholipids, the higher temperature tall peaks corresponded to the chain melting transition[27] and the lower temperature small peaks corresponded to the pretransition, which related to the untilting of the phospholipid acyl chains.[28] The thermotropic pretransition of the different phosphatidylcholines was greatly affected by the presence of a very low concentration of diRL, being already abolished at a diRL mol fraction of 0.01. Increasing concentrations of diRL progressively made the transition less cooperative as demonstrated by the increase in width of the main transition and caused a shift to lower temperatures, with the appearance of a second endothermic component in the thermograms. The effect of diRL on the main phase transition was qualitatively similar for the different phosphatidylcholines; however it was larger in the case of the shorter chain homologue DMPC where the broadening of the transition and the separation between both endotherms were more evident (Fig. 3A). These effects could be explained by the establishment of a molecular interaction between the phospholipid acyl chains and the diRL molecule, intercalation of the diRL molecule between the phospholipids and disruption of the phospholipid packing, reducing the cooperativity of the transition and shifting the temperature to lower values. The appearance of a second melting component in the thermograms when the concentration of diRL was increased can be explained by the formation of diRL enriched domains. At increasing concentrations of diRL the shape of the main transition peak became asymmetric. The asymmetric line shape indicated that the phase transition was no longer two-state or that there were multiple two-state transitions.[27] Making the reasonable assumption that there were two coexisting phases and each one underwent a two-state transition, the lower temperature endotherm could be attributed to phospholipids in diRL rich regions or those phospholipids that were near the diRL molecules and were highly perturbed. The higher temperature endotherm could be attributed to lipids in diRL poor regions or those which were far away from the diRL molecules and thus had less perturbed acyl chains. DSC also allowed us to characterize in detail the influence of diRL on the phase behaviour of DEPE. Figure 3 (panel B) shows heating thermograms of aqueous dipersions of DEPE and diRL at different mol fractions. Pure DEPE presented a highly cooperative endothermic gel to liquid-crystalline phase transition at 37.2°C and a lamellar to inverted hexagonal-H_{II} transition at 65°C. Increasing the concentration of the diRL gave rise to a progressive broadening of the gel to liquid-crystalline phase transition whose temperature shifted to lower values. At 0.03 mol fraction a new phase transition started to show up at a temperature around 17°C which became more prominent as the concentration of the biosurfactant was increased. In addition several other minor transitions were observed as shoulders of the main ones indicating, in any case, a complex behaviour. Incorporation of diRL into DEPE also affected the lamellar to hexagonal-H_{II} phase transition, which was progressively shifted to higher temperatures with a simultaneous decrease of ΔH, being not detectable at a diRL concentration as low as a mol fraction of 0.05. The DSC thermograms shown in Figure 3B indicated that diRL incorporated into DEPE bilayers and interacted with the phospholipid, decreasing the cooperativity of the gel to liquid-crystalline phase transition and giving rise to the formation of domains within the membrane with lower transition temperatures, as explained above for DMPC.

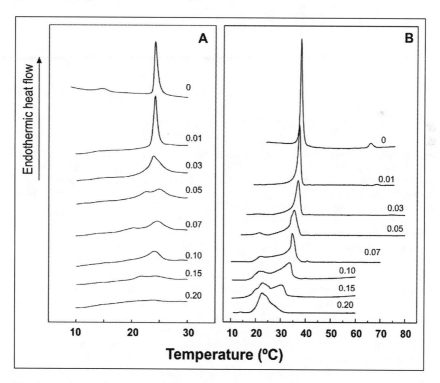

Figure 3. DSC heating thermograms for DMPC (A) and DEPE (B) containing diRL at different concentrations. The mol fraction of DiRL is indicated on the curves. The thermograms are normalized to the same amount of lipid.

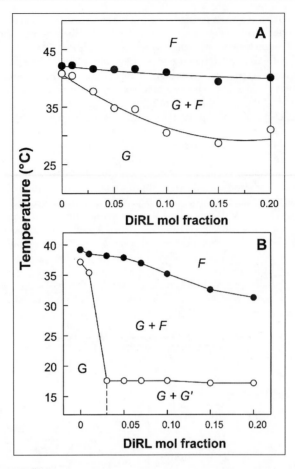

Figure 4. Partial phase diagram for the phospholipid component in mixtures of DMPC (A) and DEPE (B) with DiRL. Open and closed circles were obtained from the onset and completion temperatures of the main gel to liquid-crystalline phase transitions shown in Figure 3 and correspond to the *solidus* and *fluidus* lines respectively. G and G' represent lamellar gel phases and F the lamellar liquid-crystalline (fluid) phase.

Using the thermal data from the DSC scans shown in Figure 3, partial phase diagrams for the phospholipid component were constructed (Fig. 4). The phase diagrams obtained for all phosphatidylcholines under study were similar to that of DMPC (Fig. 4A), showing that the *solidus* lines displayed a near ideal behaviour, i.e., the temperature decreased as more diRL was present in the system. This indicated that phosphatidylcholine and diRL were miscible in the gel phase and that the intercalation of diRL molecules into the phospholipid palisade perturbed its thermotropic properties. However, differences in the behaviour of the *fluidus* line could be observed depending on the acyl chain length of the particular phosphaticylcholine.

The scenario observed for the DEPE/diRL system was somehow different (Fig. 4B). Increasing the concentration of biosurfactant produced a decrease in the *fluidus* line which behaved in a near ideal manner. However the *solidus* line sharply dropped from 37.2 to 17.2°C at a mol fraction of 0.03, remaining horizontal for the rest of the diagram and indicating gel phase immiscibility. The complex behaviour observed in this mixtures, with a eutectic point at a mol fraction =0.03 and a solid-phase immiscibility for diRL concentrations above this value, indicated that in the gel phase there was formation of a diRL/DEPE complex with a diRL mol fraction =0.03, which separated from the bulk of the membrane and coexisted with another gel phase of different stoichiometry (region G + G'). Upon heating, i.e., in the fluid phase, the membrane became homogeneous with a good miscibility of both lipids. Thus, above the *fluidus* line, there was a continuous series of homogeneously distributed diRL/DEPE mixtures.

Effect of diRL on Phospholipid Polymorphism

Phospholipids, when organized into multilamellar structures, should give rise to reflections with relative distances of 1:1/2:1/3.[29] Figure 5 shows the small angle X-ray diffraction pattern profiles corresponding to DMPC and DEPE containing diRL at different temperatures. Pure DMPC presented three reflections with relative distances of 1:1/2:1/3, which was consistent with their expected multilamellar organization.[30] This technique not only defined the macroscopic structure itself, but also provided the interlamellar repeat distance in the lamellar phase. The largest first order reflection component corresponded to the interlamellar repeat distance (d-value), which was comprised of the bilayer thickness and the thickness of the water layer between bilayers.[31] DMPC gave rise to a first order reflection with a d-value of 66.3 Å in the gel state and 62.0 Å in the liquid crystalline state (Fig. 5). Samples containing 0.03 mol fraction of diRL gave rise to two or three reflections which related as 1:1/2:1/3 in the whole range of temperatures under study, confirming that the presence of diRL at this concentration did not alter the lamellar structural organization of phosphatidylcholines. However, the interlamellar repeat distance was found to be between 5 and 13 Å larger (depending on phosphatidylcholine acyl chain and temperature) in the presence of a 0.03 mol fraction of diRL than in the absence of glycolipid, which could be a consequence of the increase of the water layer between the phospholipids bilayers or it could be due to an effective increase of the bilayer thickness. It is interesting to note that the presence of diRL broadened the reflections and lowered their intensities, indicating that it progressively reduced the long-range order in the multilamellar system.

Incorporation of diRL into DEPE systems did not alter the lamellar organization of this phospholipid neither below nor above the gel to-liquid-crystalline phase transition; however there was a slight decrease of the interlamellar repeat distance from 65.7 to 63.5 Å at 15°C and from 53.5 to 51.2 Å at 50°C (Fig. 5). Only one lamellar reflection was observed at temperatures both below and above the gel to liquid-crystalline phase transition. At 70°C pure DEPE samples showed three reflections which related as $1:1/\sqrt{3}:1\sqrt{/4}$, which corresponded to the lattice parameter ratio of an inverted hexagonal-H_{II} phase. However, addition of a diRL mol fraction of 0.10 made DEPE to adopt a lamellar organization

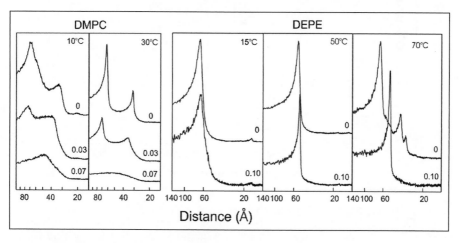

Figure 5. Small angle X-ray diffraction profiles of DMPC and DEPE systems containing different mol fractions of diRL (numbers on the curves), at various temperatures below and above the gel-to-liquid crystalline phase transition.

at this same temperature, with a yet smaller interlamellar repeat distance of 49.8 Å. With respect to the formation of the inverted hexagonal-H_{II} phase it was clear that diRL displaced this transition to higher values, i.e., it precluded H_{II} phase formation or, in other words, stabilized the bilayer organization (Fig. 3). This was confirmed by small angle X-ray diffraction (Fig. 5) which showed that, at 70°C, diRL containing samples still adopted a lamellar organization, as compared to pure DEPE which was H_{II}. This result can be explained by the dynamic shape theory commented above,[32] clearly indicating that diRL behaves as an inverted cone shaped molecule, opposing the cone shape of DEPE and acting as a lamellar stabilizer (Fig. 7). Surfactin, a lipopeptide biosurfactant produced by *Bacillus subtilis*, has been also shown to similarly destabilize the H_{II} phase in DEPE systems.[15]

DiRL Affects Phospholipid Acyl Chain Mobility

The effect of diRL on the phosphatidylcholine acyl chains was examined by monitoring the changes occurring in the CH_2 stretching vibration bands. The CH_2 stretching region of the infrared spectrum of phosphatidylcholines contains two major bands centred near 2850 and 2920 cm^{-1}, which arise from the symmetric and asymmetric methylene stretching vibrations, respectively. With most phospholipid bilayers, these vibrations give rise to relatively sharp absorption peaks at temperatures below the phospholipid gel to liquid-crystalline phase transition and when the phospholipid hydrocarbon chains melt, the absorption bands broaden and shift upward in frequency by 2-3 cm^{-1}. Such behaviour is characteristic of hydrocarbon chain melting phenomena and results from an increase in hydrocarbon conformational disorder and molecular mobility at the chain melting phase transition.[33] These changes in frequency were observed with pure phospholipids and their mixtures with diRL (Fig. 6) along temperatures ranges comparable to those of the thermotropic events detected by DSC

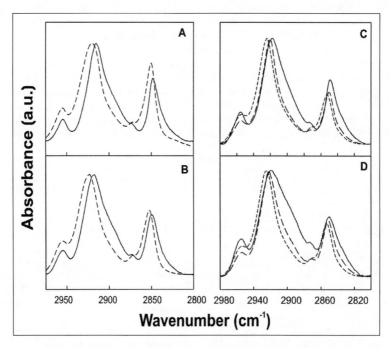

Figure 6. FTIR spectra of the CH_2 stretching absorption bands of mixtures of phospholipids with diRL. The left part of the figure corresponds to pure DMPC (solid line) and DMPC containing 0.07 mol fraction DiRL (dashed line) at 10°C (gel phase) (A) and 30°C (liquid crystalline phase) (B). The right part of the figure shows the spectra of pure DEPE (solid line) and DEPE containing 0.10 mol fraction of diRL (long dashed line) and 0.20 mol fraction of diRL (short dashed line) at 15°C (C) and 50°C (D).

(Fig. 3). This observation provided evidence that all the thermotropic events observed in the DSC experiments involved the melting of the phospholipids hydrocarbon chains. Figure 6 compares the infrared CH_2 stretching bands of the gel and liquid crystalline phases of pure DMPC with that of DMPC containing 0.07 mol fraction of diRL. It was observed that both in the gel (Fig. 6A) and liquid crystalline (Fig. 6B) states, band maxima of the CH_2 stretching vibrations exhibited by the DMPC/diRL system occurred at higher frequencies than those of the pure DMPC. These results suggested that the incorporation of diRL into DMPC bilayers resulted in an overall increase in hydrocarbon chain disorder in both states. This disordering effect was less marked when diRL was incorporated into DPPC and disappeared when it was incorporated into DSPC systems (not shown). Thus, phosphatidylcholines with shorter acyl chains were less able to accommodate the diRL molecule into the phospholipid palisade, being more sensitive to the presence of the glycolipid.

Incorporation of increasing concentrations of the biosurfactant (0.1 and 0.2 mol fraction) into DEPE membranes at 15°C shifted the antisymmetric stretching band from 2917 to 2920 and 2924 cm^{-1} respectively and the symmetric stretching was displaced from 2849 to 2850 and 2853 cm^{-1} (Fig. 6C). These displacements were even higher than those observed in pure DEPE as a consequence of the gel to liquid-crystalline phase transition. At 50°C, i.e., in the fluid phase, the effect was similar, with shifts from 2919 to 2921 and 2923 cm^{-1} respectively in the antisymmetric stretching and from 2850 to 2851 and 2853 cm^{-1} respectively in the symmetric stretching band (Fig. 6D). Thus, incorporation of diRL into DEPE bilayers increased the population of *gauche* conformers both in the gel and the liquid-crystalline phase, causing an additional disordering of the phospholipid acyl chains even in the fluid phase. This alteration also took place at the level of the aqueous interface as observed by the effects on the $C = O$ stretching band (not shown).

Conclusion

Rhamnolipids from *Pseudomonas aeruginosa* have been shown to present antimicrobial activity against a wide variety of microorganisms including Gram-negative and Gram-positive species[34] and to be cytolytic for human monocyte-derived macrophages, particularly the dirhamnolipid species.[35] Its zoorosporicidal activity against phytopatogens has been also described[14] and it was suggested that intercalation of rhamnolipids into the plasma membrane would cause its final destruction. Furthermore, a purified dirhamnolipid from *Burkholderia pseudomallei* has been described to be haemolytic for erythrocytes of various species.[36] The question is: which is the molecular basis for all these interesting biological activities? The marked amphiphilic character of the diRL molecule (Fig. 1) suggest that they must be the consequence of a direct interaction of the rhamnolipids with the target membranes and the consequent alteration of its barrier properties, as it has been shown before for another relevant biosurfactant like surfactin.[37] The results we have presented here show that diRL interaction with phospholipids has various effects that might constitute the molecular basis to explain the former activities: domain formation with lateral phase separation, increased motional disorder of the phospholipid acyl chains and dehydration of the aqueous interface.

Our data also suggest that diRL, having a large polar headgroup and a smaller hydrophobic portion, behaves as an inverted-cone shaped molecule, conferring positive curvature to membranes. This means that the molecular shape of diRL is somehow complementary to that of phosphatidylethanolamine, which facilitates diRL membrane insertion when present in a bilayer and similar to the shape of lysoPC, which impedes diRL membrane insertion (Fig. 7).[32] Many antibacterial compounds act by promoting a negative membrane curvature which can lead to the collapse of the phosphatidylethanolamine-rich bacterial cytoplasmic membrane.[38,39] The mechanism of antimicrobial activity of dirhamnolipid seems to be different, since we have shown that diRL has a bilayer stabilizing effect impeding the formation of the inverted hexagonal H_{II} phase in phosphatidylethanolamine systems.[11] Recent studies on the mechanism of antimicrobial activity have shown that several antimicrobial compounds which, like dirhamnolipid, induce a positive curvature strain of the membrane, disrupt cell membranes through the formation of a transient pore.[40-42] New research has to be carried out to study the effect of diRL on membrane permeability

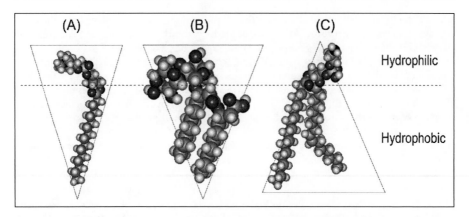

Figure 7. A comparative view of the molecular shapes of lysoPC (A), diRL (B) and PE (C). The structures correspond to 1-palmitoyl-2-hydroxy-*sn*-glycero-3-phosphocholine (lysoPC), Rha-Rha-C$_{10}$-C$_{10}$ (DiRL) and 1-palmitoyl-2-oleoyl-*sn*-glycero-3-phosphoethanolamine (POPE).

and to get insight into its mechanism of antimicrobial activity. These studies will be important in order to elucidate whether diRL acts through a detergent-like mechanism, or permeabilization takes place by means of membrane pore formation.

References

1. Desai JD, Banat IM. Microbial production of surfactants and their commercial potential. Microbiol Mol Biol Rev 1997; 61:47-64.
2. Cameotra SS, Makkar RS. Synthesis of biosurfactants in extreme conditions. Appl Microbiol Biotechnol 1998; 50:520-529.
3. Singh P, Cameotra SS. Potential applications of microbial surfactants in biomedical sciences. Trends Biotechnol 2004; 22:142-146.
4. Rodrigues L, Banat IM, Teixeira J et al. Biosurfactants: potential applications in medicine. J Antimicrob Chemother 2006; 57:609-618.
5. Jarvis FG, Johnson MJ. A glycolipid produced by Pseudomonas aeruginosa. J Am Chem Soc 1949; 71:4124-4126.
6. Soberón-Chávez G, Lépine F, Déziel E. Production of rhamnolipids by Pseudomonas aeruginosa. Appl Microbiol Biotechnol 2005; 14:1-8.
7. Lang S, Wullbrandt D. Rhamnose lipids—biosynthesis, microbial production and applications potential. Appl Microbiol Biotechnol 1999; 51:22-32.
8. Banat IM, Makkar RS, Cameotra SS. Potential applications of microbial surfactants. Appl Microbiol Biotechnol 2000; 53:495-508.
9. Parra JL, Guinea J, Manresa A et al. Chemical characterization and physicochemical behaviour of bio-surfactants. J Am Oil Chem Soc 1989; 66:141-145.
10. Benincasa M, Abalos A, Oliveira I et al. Chemical structure, surface properties and biological activities of the biosurfactant produced by Pseudomonas aeruginosa LBI from soapstock. Antonie van Leeuwenhoek 2004; 85:1-8.
11. Sánchez M, Aranda FJ, Espuny MJ et al. Aggregation behaviour of a dirhamnolipid biosurfactant secreted by Pseudomonas aeruginosa in aqueous media. J Colloid Interface Sci 2007; 307:246-253.
12. Lang S, Katsiwela E, Wagner F. Antimicrobial effects of biosurfactants. Fat Sci Technol 1989; 91:363-366.
13. Lang S, Wagner F. Biological activities of biosurfactants. In: Kosaric N, ed. Biosurfactants. New York: Dekker, 1993:251-268.
14. Stanghellini ME, Miller RM. Biosurfactants—their identity and potential efficacy in the biological control of zoosporic plant pathogens. Plant Dis 1997; 81:4-12.
15. Grau A, Gómez-Fernández JC, Peypoux F et al. A study of the interactions of surfactin with phospho-lipid vesicles. Biochim Biophys Acta 1999; 1418:307-319.
16. Grau A, Ortiz A, De Godos A et al. A biophysical study of the interaction of the lipopeptide antibiotic iturin A with aqueous phospholipid bilayers. Arch Biochem Biophys 2000; 377:315-323.

17. Sánchez M, Teruel JA, Espuny MJ et al. Modulation of the physical properties of dielaidoylphosphatidylethanolamine membranes by a dirhamnolipid biosurfactant produced by Pseudomonas aeruginosa. Chem Phys Lipids 2006; 142:118-127.

18. Ortiz A, Teruel JA, Espuny MJ et al. Effects of dirhamnolipid on the structural properties of phosphatidylcholine membranes. Int J Pharm 2006; 325:99-107.

19. Svenson S. Controlling surfactant self-assembly. Curr Opin Coll Int Sci 2002; 9:201-212.

20. Mata-Sandoval J, Karns J, Torrens A. High-performance liquid chromatography method for the characterization of rhamnolipids mixture produced by Pseudomonas aeruginosa UG2 on corn oil. J Chromatogr 1999; 864:211-220.

21. Aranda FJ, Espuny MJ, Marqués A et al. Thermodynamics of the interaction of a dirhamnolipid biosurfactant secreted by Pseudomonas aeruginosa with phospholipid membranes. Langmuir 2007; 23:2700-2705.

22. Heerklotz H, Seelig J. Detergent-like action of the antibiotic peptide surfactin on lipid membranes. Biophys J 2001; 81:1547-1554.

23. Ishigami Y, Gama Y, Nagahora H et al. The pH sensitive conversión of molecular aggregates of rhamnolipid biosurfactant. Chem Lett 1987; 5:763-766.

24. Stockton GW, Smith ICP. A deuterium nuclear magnetic resonance study of the condensing effect of cholesterol on egg phosphatidylcholine bilayer membranes. I. Perdeuterated fatty acid probes. Chem Phys Lipids 1976; 17:251-263.

25. Henriksen J, Rowat AC, Brief E et al. Universal behavior of membranes with sterols. Biophys J 2006; 90:1639-49.

26. Urbina JA, Pekerar S, Le HB et al. Molecular order and dynamics of phosphatidylcholine bilayer membranes in the presence of cholesterol, ergosterol and lanosterol: a comparative study using 2H-, 13C- and 31P-NMR spectroscopy. Biochim Biophys Acta 1995; 13:163-76.

27. Lee AG. In: Aloia RC, ed. Membrane Fluidity in Biology. New York: Academic Press, 1983:43-88.

28. Lewis RNAH, Mannock DA, McElhaney RN. Membrane lipid molecular structure and polymorphism. Curr Top Membr 1997; 44:25-102.

29. Luzzati V. X-ray diffraction studies of lipid-water systems. In: Chapman D, ed. Biological Membranes. New York: Academic Press, 1968:71-123.

30. Seddon J, Cevc G. Lipid polymorphism: structure and stability of lyotropic mesophases of phospholipids. In: Cev G, ed. Phospholipid Handbook. New York: Dekker, 1993:403-454.

31. Rappolt M, Hickel A, Brigenzu F et al. Mechanism of the lamellar/inverse hexagonal phase transition examined by high resolution X-ray diffraction. Biophys J 2003; 84:3111-3122.

32. Cullis PR, De Kruijff B. Lipid polymorphism and the functional roles of lipids in biological membranes. Biochim Biophys Acta 1979; 559:399-420.

33. Casal H, Mantsch HH. Polymorphic phase behaviour of phospholipid membranes studied by infrared spectroscopy. Biochim Biophys Acta 1984; 779:381-401.

34. Haba E, Pinazo A, Jauregui O et al. Physicochemical characterization and antimicrobial properties of rhamnolipids produced by Pseudomonas aeruginosa 47T2 NCBIM 40044. Biotech Bioeng 2003; 81:316-322.

35. McClure CD, Schiller NL. Effects of Pseudomonas aeruginosa rhamnolipids on human monocyte-derived macrophages. J Leukoc Biol 1992; 51:97-102.

36. Häubler S, Nimtz M, Domke T et al. Purification and characterization of a cytotoxic exolipid of Burkholderia pseudomallei. Inf Imm 1998; 66:1588-1593.

37. Carrillo C, Teruel JA, Aranda FJ et al. Molecular mechanism of membrane permeabilization by the peptide antibiotic surfactin. Biochim Biophys Acta 2003; 1611:91-97.

38. El Jastimi R, Lafleur M. Nisin promotes the formation of nonlamellar invertid phases in unsaturated phosphatidylethanolamines. Biochim Biophys Acta 1999; 1418:97-105.

39. Willumeit R, Kumpugdee M, Funari SS et al. Structural rearrangement of model membranes by the peptide antibiotic NK-2. Biochim Biophys Acta 2005; 1699:125-134.

40. Henzler-Wildman KA, Lee DK, Ramamoorthy A. Mechanism of lipid bilayer disruption by the human antimicrobial peptide, LL-37. Biochemistry 2003; 42:6545-6558.

41. Hallock KJ, Lee DK, Ramamoorthy A. MSI-78, an analogue of the magainin antimicrobial peptides, disrupts lipid bilayer structure via positive curvature strain. Biophys J 2003; 84:3052-3060.

42. Thennarasu S, Lee DK, Tan A et al. Antimicrobial activity and membrane selective interactions of a synthetic lipopeptide MSI-843. Biochim Biohys Acta 2005; 1711:49-58.

CHAPTER 4

Microbial Surfactants and Their Potential Applications:
An Overview

Ashis K. Mukherjee* and Kishore Das

Abstract

Biosurfactant or microbial surfactants produced by microbes are structurally diverse and heterogeneous groups of surface-active amphipathic molecules. They are capable of reducing surface and interfacial tension and have a wide range of industrial and environmental applications. The present chapter reviews the biochemical properties of different classes of microbial surfactants and their potential application in different industrial sectors.

Introduction

Surfactants are amphipathic molecules that partition preferentially at the interface between fluid phases such as oil/water or air/water interfaces. These properties of surfactants capable them of reducing surface and interfacial tension and make surfactant an excellent detergency, emulsifier, foaming and dispersing agents.

With increasing environmental awareness and emphasis on a sustainable society in harmony with the global environment, during the recent years, natural surfactants produced by living cells are getting much more attention as compared to the synthetic chemical surfactants. Among the natural surfactants, those produced by microbial origin, known as microbial surfactants or biosurfactants are the most promising. They are defined as "structurally diverse/heterogeneous groups of surface-active molecules synthesized by microorganisms".[1,2] Considering the important properties and a wide range of applications of biosurfactants, during recent years much more attention has been given to understand the biochemical properties and physiological role of different classes of biosurfactant on the producing microorganism as well as commercial application of biosurfactants.[3]

Classification of Biosurfactants

Based on their chemical composition and types of microbes producing them, biosurfactant are divided into five broad groups viz., glycolipids, lipopeptides and lipoproteins, phospholipids, hydroxylated and crossed-linked and fatty acids, polymeric surfactants and particulate surfactants.[4,5]

Glycolipids

Glycolipids are carbohydrates like mono-, di-, tri- and tetrasaccharides that include glucose, mannose, galactose, glucuronic acid, rhamnose and galactose sulphate combined with long chain aliphatic acids or hydroxy aliphatic acids. The best examples of glycolipids include trehalose lipids,

*Corresponding Author: Ashis K. Mukherjee—Department of Molecular Biology and Biotechnology, Tezpur University, Tezpur-784 028, Assam, India. Email: akm@tezu.ernet.in

Biosurfactants, edited by Ramkrishna Sen. ©2010 Landes Bioscience and Springer Science+Business Media.

rhamnolipids, sophorolipids, diglycosyl diglycerides and mannosylerythritol lipids. Other types of glycolipids have been reported in the literature such as glycoglycerolipid,[6] sugar-based bioemulsifiers,[7,8] mannosylerythritol lipid A and many different hexose lipids.[9]

Trehalose Lipids

Several structural types of microbial trehalose lipid biosurfactants have been reported. Disaccharide trehalose linked at C-6 and C-6′ to mycolic acids is associated with most species of *Mycobacterium*, *Nocardia* and *Corynebacterium*.[4,10] Mycolic acids are long-chain, α-branched -β- hydroxy fatty acids. Trehalolipids from different organisms differ in the size and structure of mycolic acid, the number of carbon atoms and the degree of unsaturation.[4,11] In 2002, Philp and his colleagues[12] reported the production of trehalose lipids from alkanotrophic *Rhodococcus ruber* on gaseous alkanes propane and butane.

Rhamnolipids

Certain species of *Pseudomonas* are characterized to produce large amounts biosurfactant containing one or two molecules of rhamnose linked to one or two molecules of β-hydroxydecanoic acid.[13-16] In 1965, Edward and Hayashi[17] have reported formation of glycolipid, type R-1 containing two rhamnose and two β hydroxydecanoic units by *Pseudomonas aeruginosa*. A second kind of rhamnolipid (R-2) containing one rhamnose unit was reported by Itoh et al.[18] Gas-chromatographic analysis of hydroxyl fatty acids rhamnolipid produced by *P. aeruginosa* DAUPE 614 showed that positions of the fatty acids in the lipid moiety were variable.[16]

Sophorolipids

Sophorolipids consist of a dimeric carbohydrate sophorose attached with a long chain hydroxy fatty acid and are mainly produced by yeasts such as *Torulopsis bombicola*, *T. apicola*[19] and *Wickerhamiella domericqiae*.[20] Sophorolipids have the capacity to lower the surface tension of water from 72.8 mN/m to 40 to 30 mN/m, with a critical micelle concentration of 40 to 100 mg/l.[21] It has been shown that *T. petrophilum* produces sophorolipids on water insoluble substrates such as alkanes and vegetable oil.[22] Moreover, it has been reported that critical micelle concentration (CMC) and the solubilization ratio of the sophorolipids biosurfactant were found to be in a good range compared with synthetic surfactants.[23]

Mannosylerythritol Lipids

This glycolipid biosurfactant consists of a sugar called mannosylerythritol and are synthesized by yeast like *Candida antarctica*[24,25] and *Candida* sp. SY 16.[26] The fatty acid component of biosurfactant was determined to be hexanoic, dodecanoic, tetradecanoic or tetradecenoic acids.[26] Mannosylerythritol lipids synthesized by *Candida* sp. SY 16[26] lowered the surface tension of water to 29 dyne/cm at critical micelle concentration of 10 mg/l and the minimum interfacial tension was 0.1 dyne/cm against kerosene.[26] Fukuoka et al[27] have characterized the surface active properties of a new glycolipid biosurfactant, mono acylated mannosylerythritol lipid produced by *Psdozyma antarctica* and *P. rugulosa*.

Lipopeptides

Surfactin

Surfactin, a cyclic lipopeptide is one of the most effective biosurfactants known so far, which was first reported in *B. subtilis* ATCC-21332.[28] Because of its exceptional surfactant activity it is named as surfactin.[29] Surfactin can lower the surface tension from 72 to 27.9 mN/m[30] and have a critical micelle concentration of 0.017 g/l.[31] The surfactin groups of compounds are shown to be a cyclic lipoheptapeptides which contain a β-hydroxy fatty acid in its side chain.[32] Recent studies indicate that surfactin shows potent antiviral, antimycoplasma, antitumoral, anticoagulant activities as well as inhibitors of enzymes.[30,33] Although, such properties of surfactins qualify them for potential applications in medicine or biotechnology, they have not been exploited extensively till date.

Iturin

Iturin A, the first compound discovered of the iturin group and its best known member, was isolated from a *Bacillus subtilis* strain taken from the soil in Ituri (Zaire) and its structure was elucidated.[34] The subsequent isolation from other strains of *Bacillus subtilis* of five other lipopeptides such as iturin A_L, mycosubtilin, bacillomycin L, D, F and L_C (or bacillopeptin), all having a common pattern of chemical constitution, led to the adoption of the generic name of "iturins" for this group of lipopeptides.[35] The iturin group of compounds are cyclic lipoheptapeptides which contain a β- amino fatty acid in its side chain. Lipopeptids belonging to the iturin family are potent antifungal agents which can also be used as biopesticides for plant protection.[32,36,37]

Fengycin

Fengycin is a lipodecapeptide containing β- hydroxy fatty acid in its side chain and comprises of C_{15} to C_{17} variants which have a characteristic Ala-Val dimorphy at position 6 in the peptide ring.[32,38] Wang et al[39] have demonstrated the identification of fengycin homologues produced by *B. subtilis* by using electrospray ionization mass spectrometry (ESI-MS) technique.

Lichenysin

Lichenysin, produced by *Bacillus licheniformis* exhibits similar structure and physiochemical properties to that of surfactin.[40] *B. licheniformis* also produce several other surface active agents which act synergistically and exhibit excellent temperature, pH and salt stability.[40] Lichenysin A produced by *Bacillus licheniformis* strain BAS50, is characterized to contain a long chain beta-hydroxy fatty acid molecule.[41] Lichenysin is reported to be stable over a wide range of pH, temperature and NaCl concentration and promotes dispersion of colloidal 3- silicon carbide and aluminum nitride slurries much more efficiently than chemical agents.[42] It has also been reported that lichenysin is a more efficient cation chelator compared with surfactin.[43]

Fatty Acid Biosurfactant

Certain hydrocarbon degrading microbes produce extracellular free fatty acids when grown on alkanes and exhibit good surfactant activity. The fatty acid biosurfactants are saturated fatty acids in the range of C_{12} to C_{14} and complex fatty acids containing hydroxyl groups and alkyl branches.[44,45] It was shown that *Arthobacter* strain AK-19[46] and *P. aeruginosa* 44T1[47] accumulated up to 40-80% (w/w) of such lipids when cultivated on hexadecane and olive oil respectively.

Polymeric Biosurfactants

Polymeric biosurfactants are high molecular weight biopolymers, which exhibit properties like high viscosity, tensile strength and resistance to shear. The following are the examples of different classes of polymeric biosurfactants.

Emulsan

Acinetobacter calcoaceticus RAG-1 produces a potent extracellular polymeric bioemulsifier called emulsan[48] which is characterized as a polyanionic amphipathic heteropolysaccharide. The heteropolysaccharide backbone consists of repeating units of trisaccharide of N- acetyl-D-galactosamine, N-acetylgalactosamine uronic acid and an unidentified N- acetylamino sugar.[49] Removal of the protein fraction yields a product, apoemulsan, which exhibits much lower emulsifying activity on hydrophobic substrates such as n-hexadecane. One of the key proteins associated with the emulsan complex is a cell surface esterase.[50]

Biodispersan

A. calcoaceticus A-2 produces an extracellular, nondialyzable surface-active dispersing substance called biodispersan.[51] The surface active component of biodispersan is an anionic heteropolysaccharide, with an average molecular weight of 51,400 and contains four reducing sugars namely glucosamine, 6- methylaminohexose, galactosamine uronic acids and an unidentified amino sugar.[51] Elkeles and his colleagues[52] have suggested that mutants of strain *A. calcoaceticus* A-2 that were defective in protein secretion are potentially useful for the production of biodispersan.

Alasan

Alasan is an anionic alanine- containing heteropolysaccharide protein biosurfactant produced by *A. radioresistens* KA-53.[53] Alasan produced by *A. radioresistens* KA-53 was reported to solubilise and degrade polyaromatic hydrocarbons.[54] The surface active component of alasan is a 35.77 kD protein called as AlnA. This surface-active protein AlnA have a high amino acid sequence homology to *Escherichia coli* outer membrane protein A (OmpA), but however OmpA does not possess any emulsifying activity.[55]

Three of alasan proteins were purified from *A. radioresistens* KA-53 are having molecular masses of 16, 31 and 45 kD and it was demonstrated that the 45-kD protein had the highest specific emulsifying activity, 11% higher than the intact alasan complex.[56] The 16- and 31-kD proteins gave relatively low emulsifying activities, but they were significantly higher than that of apo-alasan.[56]

Liposan

C. lipolytica produce an extracellular water soluble emulsifier called Liposan which is composed of 83% (w/v) carbohydrate and 17% (w/v) protein.[57] The carbohydrate portion is a heteropolysaccharide consisting of glucose, galactose, galactosamine and galacturonic acid.[57]

Emulsifying Biopolymer from Fungus

The production of large amounts of mannoprotein by *Saccharomyces cerevisiae* exhibiting excellent emulsifier activity toward several oils, alkanes and organic solvents had been reported.[58] The purified emulsifier contains 44% mannose and 17% protein. A manose- fatty acid complex from alkane grown *C. tropicalis* was isolated.[59] This complex stabilizes hexadecane-in-water emulsion.

Emulsifying Protein

An emulsifying peptidoglycolipid containing 52 amino acids, 11 fatty acids and a sugar unit produced by *P. aeruginosa* P-20 has been reported by Koronelli et al.[60] Also, a bioemulsifier, composed of 50% carbohydrate, 19.6% protein and 10% lipid produced by *P. fluorescens* was reported.[61]

Particulate Biosurfactant

Some examples of particulate biosurfactant are extracellular membranes vesicles of microbial cells, which help in emulsification of hydrocarbon. Accumulation of extracellular membrane vesicles having 20-50 mm diameter and a bouyant density of 1.158 g/cm^2 has been reported in *Acinetobacter* sp. HO1-N cells.[62] The purified vesicles are composed of protein, phospholipid and lipopolysaccharide.

Potential Applications of Biosurfactant

Biosurfactants are becoming important biotechnology products for industrial and medical applications due to their specific modes of action, low toxicity, relative ease of preparation and widespread applicability.[63-65] Biosurfactants also exhibit natural physiological roles in increasing bioavailability of hydrophobic molecules and can complex with heavy metals, promoting improved degradation of chemical contaminants.[66] They can be used as emulsifiers, de-emulsifiers, wetting and foaming agents, functional food ingredients and as detergents in petroleum, petrochemicals, environmental management, agrochemicals, foods and beverages, cosmetics and pharmaceuticals, commercial laundry detergents and in the mining and metallurgical industries.[67-71]

Role of Microbial Surfactants in Bioremediation of Oil Pollutants

Oil-contamination of soil is a common problem and its physical treatment methods or remediation techniques can be difficult or economically not feasible. One of the most economically feasible methods includes in situ bioremediation by the use of microorganisms which is the partial simplification or complete destruction of the molecular structure of environmental pollutants.[64,70-72] Permeability of the microbial cell membrane might be adversely affected by the use of synthetic surfactant, which would interfere with the capacity of a microorganisms to biodegrade.[73] Microbial surfactants are generally much less toxic than chemical surfactants, but are as effective and more readily biodegradable. Using microorganisms that produce their own biosurfactants capable of degrading pollutants can further lower treatment costs.

Numerous attempts have been made to successfully remediate the oil contaminated soil by using microbial inoculation and by biosurfactant treatment. The rhamnolipid biosurfactant produced by *P. aeruginosa* stimulates the uptake of hydrophobic compounds finally leading to its degradation.[74] Similarly, Das and Mukherjee[71] have demonstrated the crude petroleum-oil biodegradation efficiency of biosurfactant producing *B. subtilis* DM-04 and *P. aeruginosa* M and NM strains isolated from the petroleum oil contaminated soil from North-East India. Study has shown that all the three bacteria are efficient biosurfactant producers in petroleum oil-contaminated soil which offers the advantage of a continuous supply of natural, nontoxic and biodegradable biosurfactants by bacteria at low cost for solubilizing the hydrophobic oil hydrocarbons prior to biodegradation. In an another study, it was shown that the biosurfactant secreted by the *B. subtilis* and *P. aeruginosa* strains enhanced the apparent solubility of pyrene (a toxic polyaromatic hydrocarbon) by factors 5 to 7, and also influenced the bacterial cell surface hydrophobicity resulting in higher uptake and utilization of pyrene by bacteria.[70]

Application of Biosurfactant in Petroleum Industry

Biosurfactant in Oil Clean Up of Storage Tanks

Due to excellent emulsifying properties of biosurfactants, they are used as detergents in cleaning up hydrocarbon/crude oil storage tank. Banat et al[75] reported the ability of biosurfactants produced by a bacterial strain (Pet 1006) for cleaning up oil storage tanks and to recover hydrocarbons from emulsified sludge. In a test for cleaning up of oil storage tank, about 91% crude oil could be recovered from the total sludge. Such clean up process is highly desirable as it is economically rewarding and environmentally friendly.[76]

Microbial Surfactants in Microbial Enhanced Oil Recovery (MEOR)

Approximately 30% of the oil present in a reservoir can be recovered using current enhanced oil recovery (EOR) technology.[77] The low permeability or the high viscosity of the oil, as well as, high interfacial tensions between the water and oil may also result in high capillary forces retaining the oil in the reservoir rock leading to poor recovery of oil.[64,78] Due to failure of primary and secondary recovery techniques to recover the oil from reservoirs, interests have evolved in tertiary recovery techniques (MEOR) by utilizing microorganisms and/or their biosurfactant.[79]

There are several strategies involving the use of biosurfactant in MEOR. The first strategy involves injection of biosurfactant-producing microorganisms into a reservoir through the well, with subsequent in-situ propagation of microbes through the reservoir rock.[80] The second strategy involves the injection of selected nutrients into a reservoir, to favor and encourage the growth of indigenous biosurfactant-producing microorganisms. The third mechanism involves the production of biosurfactants in bioreactors ex situ and subsequent injection into the reservoir.

Laboratory studies on MEOR usually utilize core samples and columns containing the desired substrate. Fermentative culture broth containing biosurfactant from *Rhodococcus* ST-5[81] and the thermophilic *Bacillus* AB-2[82] could release 80% and 95% oil from sand-pack columns respectively. Studies from our lab have shown that biosurfactant from the *B. subtilis* strains can release appreciable amount of crude kerosene oil from sand pack column reinforcing it's potential application in MEOR.[83]

Field studies involving MEOR increases the production of oil by 250% using *Clostridium acetobutylicum*.[84] MEOR investigations in carbonate reservoirs showed an increase of 60-120% in oil production in Hungary.[85] Recently it has been demonstrated that biosurfactant produced by *Bacillus* strains inside a limestone petroleum reservoir may be promising candidates for MEOR.[86]

Use of Biosurfactants in Food Industries

Biosurfactants have several applications in food industries such as to control the agglomeration of fat globules, stabilize aerated systems, improve texture and shelf-life of starch-containing products, modify rheological properties of wheat dough and improve consistency and texture of fat-based products.[63,65,87] In the food industry, biosurfactants are used as emulsifiers in the processing of raw materials whereas in bakery and meat products they influence the rheological characteristics of flour or the emulsification of partially broken fat tissue.[88] An improvement of dough stability, texture, volume and conservation of bakery products was obtained by the addition of rhamnolipid surfactants.[89] Recently, a bioemulsifier isolated from a marine strain of *Enterobacter cloaceae* was used as a potential viscosity enhancement agent of interest in food industry especially due to the good viscosity observed at acidic pH allowing its use in food products containing edible acids like citric acid or ascorbic acid.[90]

Use of Biosurfactants in Agricultural Sectors

Surface active compounds like polymeric fatty acids, or short-chained alkyl sulfonates are used in agricultural sector for hydrophilization of heavy soil. Good wettability and equal distribution are the preconditions for loosening the soil. Hydrate formation between emulsifiers and water helps in soil improvement.[87]

Biodegradation of the chlorinated pesticide α- and β-endosulfan by using the biosurfactant from *B. subtilis* MTCC2423 was reported by Banat et al.[91] The use of biosurfactant leads to around 40% biodegradation of the said pesticides.[91] This furnishes another example of the role of microbial surfactant in environment protection.

The rhamnolipid biosurfactant, mostly produced by the genus *Pseudomonas* is known to possess potent antimicrobial activity.[92] For example, Zonix™ biogungicide, which is a trade product of mixture of two rhamnolipid biosurfactants (known as technical grade active ingredient-TGAI) has been claimed as biofungicide to prevent and control pathogenic fungi on horticultural and agricultural crops. Further, no adverse effects on humans or the environment are anticipated from aggregate exposure to rhamnolipid biosurfactants. Fengycins are also reported to possess antifungal activity and, therefore may be employed in biocontrol of plant diseases.[93,94]

Application of Biosurfactant as a Substitute of Synthetic Chemical Surfactant in Commercial Laundry Detergents

Almost all surfactants, an important component used in modern day commercial laundry detergents, are chemically synthesized and exert toxicity to fresh water living organisms. Furthermore, these components often produce undesirable effects. Therefore, growing public disquiet about the environmental hazards and risks associated with chemical surfactants has stimulated the search for ecofriendly, natural substitutes of chemical surfactants in laundry detergents.

A recent study from our laboratory has shown that cyclic lipopeptide (CLP) biosurfactants produced by *B. subtilis* strains were stable over a pH range of 7.0-12.0 and heating them at 80°C for 60 min did not result in any loss of their surface-active property.[69] Crude CLP biosurfactants showed good emulsion formation capability with vegetable oils and demonstrated excellent compatibility and stability with commercial laundry detergents favoring their inclusion in laundry detergents formulations.[69]

Biosurfactant as Biopesticide

Conventional arthropod control strategy involves application of broad-spectrum chemicals and pesticides, which often produce undesirable effects. Further, emergence of pesticide resistant insect populations as well as rising prices of new chemical pesticides have stimulated the search for new eco-friendly vector control tools. Eventually, biocontrol of insect pests and vectors is becoming one of the most promising alternatives to chemical pesticides. Studies have shown that the lipopeptide biosurfactant produced by *B. subtilis* exhibit insecticide activity against fruit fly *Drosophila melanogaster*.[95]

Since mosquitoes continue to pose a serious public health problem throughout the world, therefore, the mosquito larvicidal potency of cyclic lipopeptides (CLPs) secreted by two *B. subtilis* strains were determined in our laboratory.[68] LC_{50} of the crude CLPs secreted by *B. subtilis* DM-03 and DM-04 strains against 3rd instar larvae of *Culex quinquefasciatus* was 120.0 ± 5.0 mg/l and 300.0 ± 8.0 mg/l respectively post 24 h of treatment. Physico-chemical factors such as pH of water, incubation temperature, heating and exposure to sunlight did not influence the larvicidal potency of these CLPs.[68] Further, *B. subtilis* CLPs were insensitive to UV or sunlight exposure demonstrating the greater UV radiation stability of *B. subtilis* lipopeptides as compared to bactoculicide (Bti) and *B. sphaericus* insecticidal toxins. Moreover, the crude CLPs secreted by *B. subtilis* strain can withstand many environmental stresses like extreme pH, sunlight/UV radiation etc. and they did not impart toxicity to the tested aquatic vertebrate *Labeo rohita* up to a concentration that induced mortality to the mosquito larvae.[68] These properties can be exploited for the formulation of a safer, novel biopesticide for effective control of mosquito larvae.

Use of Biosurfactants in Pharmaceutical Sectors and Molecular Biology Research

Rhamnolipids produced by *P. aeruginosa*,[67] lipopeptides produced by *B. subtilis*[30,96] and *B. licheniformis*[97] and mannosylerythritol lipids from *C. antarctica*[25] have been reported to have antimicrobial activities. Rhamnolipid biosurfactant produced by *P. aeruginosa* was recently reported to have potential algicidal activity against some harmful algae.[98] Surfactin was reported to have properties like hemolysis and inhibiting fibrin clot formation that indicates its potential use in the pharmaceutical sector.[33] Iturin produced by *B. subtilis* was reported to have antifungal properties.[33,99] Pumilacidin, a surfactin analog was reported to have inhibitory effect against herpes simplex virus 1 (HSV-1), H^+, K^+- Atpase and gastic ulcer in vivo. Itokawa et al[100] reported the potential application of surfactin against human immunodeficiency virus 1(HIV-1) showing this class of biosurfactant is a deserving candidate for the development of rational anti-HIV drug. Takizawa et al[101] reported significant stimulation of the proliferation of bone marrow cells from BALB/c female mice by lipopeptide biosurfactant produced by *S. amethystogenes*. The reports on antibiotic effects and inhibition of HIV virus growth in white blood corpuscles have opened up new arena in the potential application of these microbial surface active compounds in pharmaceutical sector.[33,100]

Gene transfection is a fundamental technology for molecular and cell biology and also clinical gene therapy. Recently it was found that a biosurfactant, monnosylerythritol lipid (MEL)-A, dramatically increased the efficiency in transfection of plasmid DNA mediated by cationic liposomes.[102]

Conclusion

During the recent years there is an increasing environmental awareness and therefore, it might be reasonable to assume that microbial surfactants have a promising role to play in the years to come. Considering the importance of biosurfactants, there is an urgent need to gain a greater understanding of the physiology, genetics and biochemistry of biosurfactant-producing strains and to improve the process technology to reduce production costs for commercial level production of biosurfactant. Therefore, an extensive cooperation among different science disciplines is needed in order to fully characterize the biochemical properties of biosurfactant and exploration of their potential applications in different industrial sectors.

References

1. Cooper DG. Biosurfactants. Microbiol Sci 1986; 3:145-149.
2. Banat IM. Biosurfactants production and possible uses in microbial enhanced oil recovery and oil pollution remediation: A review. Bioresource Technol 1995; 51:1-12.
3. Mukherjee S, Das P, Sen R. Towards commercial production of microbial surfactants. Trends in Biotechnology 2006; 24:509-515.
4. Lang S, Wagner F. Structure and properties of biosurfactants. In: Kosaric N, Cairns WL, Gray NCC, eds. Biosurfactants and Biotechnology. New York: Marcel Dekker, Inc, 1987:21-47.

5. Maier RM. Biosurfactant: Evolution and diversity in bacteria. Adv Appl Microbiol 2003; 52:101-121.
6. Nakata K. Two glycolipids increase in the bioremediation of halogenated aromatic compounds. J Biosci Bioeng 2000; 89:577-581.
7. Kim HS, Lim EJ, Lee SO et al. Purification and characterization of biosurfactants from nocardia sp. L-417. Biotechnol Appl Biochem 2000; 31:249-253.
8. Van Hoogmoed CG, van der Kuijl-Booij M, van der Mei HC et al. Inhibition of streptococcus mutans NS adhesion to glass with and without a salivary conditioning film by biosurfactant-releasing streptococcus mitis strains. Appl Environ Microbiol 2000; 66:659-663.
9. Golyshin PM, Fredrickson HL, Giuliano L et al. Effect of novel biosurfactants on biodegradation of polychlorinated biphenyls by pure and mixed bacterial cultures. Microbiologica 1999; 22:257-267.
10. Desai JD, Banat IM. Microbial production of surfactants and their commercial potential. Microbiol Mol Bio Rev 1997; 61:47-64.
11. Cooper DG, Liss SN, Longay R et al. Surface activities of mycobacterium and pseudomonas. J Ferment Technol 1989; 59:97-101.
12. Philp JC, Kuyukina MS, Ivshina IB et al. Alkanotripic rhodococcus ruber as a biosurfactant producer. Appl Microbiol Biotechnol 2002; 59:318-324.
13. Benincasa M, Abalos A, Oliveria I et al. Chemical structure, surface properties and biological activities of the biosurfactant produced by pseudomonas aeruginosa LBI from soapstock. Antonie van Leeuwenhoek 2004; 85:1-8.
14. Nitschke M, Costa SG, Contiero J. Rhamnolipid surfactants: an update on the general aspects of these remarkable biomolecules. Biotechnol Prog 2005; 21:1593-1600.
15. Pornsunthorntawee O, Wongpanit P, Chavadej S et al. Structural and physicochemical characterization of crude biosurfactant produced by pseudomonas aeruginosa SP4 isolated from petroleum-contaminated soil. Bioresour Technol 2008; 99:1589-1595.
16. Monteiro SA, Sassaki GL, de Souza LM et al. Molecular and structural characterization of the biosurfactant produced by pseudomonas aeruginosa DAUPE 614. Chem Phys Lipids 2007; 147:1-13.
17. Edward JR, Hayashi JA. Structure of a rhamnolipid from pseudomonas aeruginosa. Arch Biochem Biophys 1965; 111:415-421.
18. Itoh S, Honda H, Tomita F et al. Rhamnolipids produced by pseudomonas aeruginosa grown on n-paraffin. J Antibiot 1971; 24:855-859.
19. Tullock P, Hill A, Spencer JFT. A new type of marocyclic lactone from torulopsis apicola. J Chem Soc Chem Commun 1967; 584-586.
20. Chen J, Song X, Zhang H et al. Production, structure elucidation and anticancer properties of sophorolipid from wickerhamiella domercqiae. Enzyme Microb Technol 2006; 39:501-506.
21. Van Bogaert IN, Saerens K, De Muynck C et al. Microbial production and application of sophorolipids. Appl Microbiol Biotechnol 2007; 76:23-34.
22. Rau U, Hammen S, Heckmann R et al. Sophorolipids: a source for novel compounds. Ind Crops Prod 2001; 13:85-92.
23. Schippers C, Gessner K, Müller T et al. Microbial degradation of phenanthrene by addition of a sophorolipid mixture. J Biotechnol 2000; 83:189-198.
24. Crich D, de la Mora MA, Cruz R. Synthesis of the mannosyl erythritol lipid MEL A; confirmation of the configuration of the meso-erythritol moiety. Tetrahedron 2002; 58:35-44.
25. Kitamoto D, Yanagishita H, Shinbo T et al. Surface active properties and antimicrobial activities of mannosylerythritol lipids as biosurfactants produced by candida antarctica. J Biotechnol 1993; 29:91-96.
26. Kim HS, Yoon BD, Choung DH et al. Characterization of a biosurfactant, mannosylerythritol lipid produced from candida sp. SY16. Appl Microbiol Biotechnol 1999; 52:713-721.
27. Fukuoka T, Morita T, Konishi M et al. Characterization of new glycolipid biosurfactants, tri-acylated mannosylerythritol lipids, produced by pseudozyma yeasts. Biotechnol Lett 2007; 29:1111-1118.
28. Arima K, Kakinuma A, Tamura G. Surfactin, a crystalline peptide lipid surfactant produced by bacillus subtilis: isolation, characterization and its inhibition of fibrin clot formation. Biochem Biophys Res Commun 1968; 31:488-494.
29. Peypoux F, Bonmatin JM, Wallach J. Recent trends in the biochemistry of surfactin. Appl Microbiol Biotechnol 1999; 51:553-563.
30. Mukherjee AK, Das K. Correlation between diverse cyclic lipopeptides production and regulation of growth and substrate utilization by bacillus subtilis strains in a particular habitat. FEMS Microbiol Eco 2005; 54:479-489.
31. Sen R, Swaminathan T. Characterization of concentration and purification parameters and operating conditions for the small-scale recovery of surfactin. Process Biochem 2005; 40:2953-2958.
32. Vater J, Kablitz B, Wilde C et al. Matrix- assisted laser desorption ionization- time of flight mass spectrometry of lipopeptide biosurfactants in whole cells and culture filtrates of bacillus subtilis C-1 isolated from petroleum sludge. Appl Environ Microbiol 2002; 68:6210-6219.

33. Rodrigues LR, Banat IM, Teixeria JA et al. Biosurfactants: Potential applications in medicine. J Antimicrob Chemother 2006; 57:609-618.
34. Peypoux F, Besson F, Michel G et al. Structure de l'iturine C de bacillus subtilis. Tetrahedron 1978; 38:1147-1152.
35. Kajimura Y, Sugiyama M, Kaneda M. Bacillopeptins, new cyclic lipopeptide antibiotics from bacillus subtilis FR-2. J Antibiot (Tokyo) 1995; 48:1095-1103.
36. Romero D, de Vicente A, Olmos JL et al. Effect of lipopeptides of antagonistic strains of bacillus subtilis on the morphology and ultrastructure of the cucurbit fungal pathogen podosphaera fusca. J Appl Microbiol 2007; 103:969-976.
37. Mizumoto S, Hirai M, Shoda M. Enhanced iturin a production by bacillus subtilis and its effect on suppression of the plant pathogen rhizoctonia solani. Appl Microbiol Biotechnol 2007; 75:1267-1274.
38. Schneider J, Taraz K, Budzikiewicz H et al. The structure of two fengycins from bacillus subtilis S499. Z Naturforsch 1999; 54:859-865.
39. Wang J, Liu J, Wang X et al. Application of electrospray ionization mass spectrometry in rapid typing of fengycin homologues produced by bacillus subtilis. Lett Appl Microbiol 2004; 39:98-102.
40. McInerney MJ, Javaheri M, Nagle DP. Properties of the biosurfactant produced by bacillus licheniformis strain JF-2. J Ind Microbiol 1990; 5:95-102.
41. Yakimov MM, Fredrickson HL, Timmis KN. Effect of heterogeneity of hydrophobic moieties on surface activity of lichenysin A, a lipopeptide biosurfactant from bacillus licheniformis BAS50. Biotechnol Appl Biochem 1996; 23:13-18.
42. Horowitz S, Currie JK. Novel dispersants of silicon carbide and aluminium nitrate. J Dispersion Sci Technol 1990; 11:637-659.
43. Grangemard I, Wallach J, Maget-Dana R et al. Lichenysin: a more efficient cation chelator than surfactin. Appl Biochem Biotechnol 2001; 90:199-210.
44. MacDonald CR, Cooper DG, Zajic JE. Surface-active lipids from nocardia erythropolis grown on hydrocarbons. Appl Environ Microbiol 1981; 41:117-123.
45. Kretschmer A, Bock H, Wagner F. Chemical and physical characterization of interfacial-active lipids from rhodococcus erthropolis grown on n-alkane. Appl Environ Microbiol 1982; 44:864-870.
46. Wayman M, Jenkins AD, Kormady AG. Biotechnology for oil and fat industry. J Am Oil Chem Soc 1984; 61:129-131.
47. Robert M, Mercade ME, Bosch MP et al. Effect of the carbon source on biosurfactant production by pseudomonas aeruginosa 44T. Biotechnol Lett 1989; 11:871-874.
48. Rosenberg E, Zuckerberg A, Rubinovitz C et al. Emulsifier arthrobacter RAG-1: isolation and emulsifying properties. Appl Environ Microbiol 1979; 37:402-408.
49. Zukerberg A, Diver A, Peeri Z et al. Emulsifier of arthrobacter RAG-1: chemical and physical properties. Appl Environ Microbiol 1979; 37:414-420.
50. Bach H, Berdichevsky Y, Gutnick D. An exocellular protein from the oil-degrading microbe acinetobacter venetianus RAG-1 enhances the emulsifying activity of the polymeric bioemulsifier emulsan. Appl Environ Microbiol 2003; 69:2608-2615.
51. Rosenberg E, Rubinovitz C, Legmann R et al. Purification and chemical properties of acinetobacter calcoaceticus A2 biodispersan. Appl Environ Microbiol 1988; 54:323-326.
52. Elkeles A, Rosenberg E, Ron EZ. Production and secretion of the polysaccharide biodispersan of acinetobacter calcoaceticus A2 in protein secretion mutants. Appl Environ Microbiol 1994; 60:4642-4645.
53. Navonvenezia S, Zosim Z, Gottieb A et al. Alasan, a new bioemulsifier from acinetobacter radioresistens. Appl Environ Microbiol 1995; 61:3240-3244.
54. Barkay T, Navon-Venezia S, Ron EZ et al. Enhancement of solubilization and biodegradation of polyaromatic hydrocarbons by the bioemulsifier alasan. Appl Environ Microbiol 1999; 65:2697-2702.
55. Toren A, Segal G, Ron EZ et al. Structure-function studies of the recombinant protein bioemulsifier AlnA. Environ Microbiol 2002; 4:257-261.
56. Toren A, Navon-Venezia S, Ron EZ et al. Emulsifying activities of purified alasan proteins from acinetobacter radioresistens KA53. Appl Environ Microbiol 2001; 67:1102-1106.
57. Cirigliano MC, Carman GM. Isolation of a bioemulsifier from candida lipolytica. Appl Environ Microbiol 1984; 48:747-750.
58. Cameron DR, Cooper DG, Neufeld RJ. The mannoprotein of saccharomyces cerevisiae is an effective bioemulsifier. Appl Environ Microbiol 1988; 54:1420-1425.
59. Kappeli O, Walther P, Muller M et al. Structure of cell surface of the yeast candida tropicalis and its relation to hydrocarbon transport. Arch Microbiol 1984; 138:279-282.
60. Koronelli TV, Komarova TI, Denisov YV. Chemical composition and role of peptidoglycolipid of pseudomonas aeruginosa. Mikrobiologiya 1983; 52:767-770.
61. Desai AJ, Patel KM, Desai JD. Emulsifier production by pseudomonas fluorescence during the growth on hydrocarbon. Curr Sci 1988; 57:500-501.

62. Kappeli O, Finnerty WR. Partition of alkane by an extracellular vesicle derived from hexadecane-grown acinetobacter. J Bacteriol 1979; 140:707-712.
63. Nitschke M, Costa SGVAO. Biosurfactants in food industry. Trends Food Sci Technol 2007; 18:252-259.
64. Singh A, Van Hamme JD, Ward OP. Surfactants in microbiology and biotechnology: part2. Application aspects. Biotechnol Adv 2007; 25:99-121.
65. Makkar R, Cameotra SS. An update on the use of unconventional substrates for biosurfactant production and their application. Appl Microbiol Biotechnol 2002; 58:428-434.
66. Van Hamme JD, Singh A, Ward OP. Physiological aspect. Part1 in a series of papers devoted to surfactants in microbiology and biotechnology. Biotechnol Adv 2006; 24:604-620.
67. Das K, Mukherjee AK. Characterization of biochemical properties and biological activities of biosurfactants produced by pseudomonas aeruginosa mucoid and nonmucoid strains. Appl Microbiol Biotechnol 2005; 69:192-199.
68. Das K, Mukherjee AK. Assessment of mosquito larvicidal potency of cyclic lipopeptides produced by bacillus subtilis strains. Acta Tropica 2006; 97:168-173.
69. Mukherjee AK. Potential application of cyclic lipopeptide biosurfactants produced by bacillus subtilis strains in laundry detergent formulations. Lett Appl Microbiol 2007; 45:330-335.
70. Das K, Mukherjee AK. Differential utilization of pyrene as the sole source of carbon by bacillus subtilis and pseudomonas aeruginosa strains: role of biosurfactants in enhancing bioavailability. J Appl Microbiol 2007; 102:195-203.
71. Das K, Mukherjee AK. Crude petroleum-oil biodegradation efficiency of bacillus subtilis and pseudomonas aeruginosa strains isolated from petroleum oil contaminated soil from north-east india. Bioresource Technol 2007; 98:1339-1345.
72. Mulligan CN. Environmental applications of biosurfactants. Environ Pollution 2005; 133:183-198.
73. Hunt PG, Robinson KG, Ghosh MM. The role of biosurfactants in biotic degradation of hydrophobic organic compounds. In: Hinchee RE, Alleman BC, Hoeppel RE et al, eds. Hydrocarbon Bioremediation. Boca Raton: Lewis Publishers, 1994:318-322.
74. Noordman WH, Janssen DB. Rhamnolipid stimulates uptake of hydrophobic compounds by pseudomonas aeruginosa. Appl Environ Microbiol 2002; 68:4502-4508.
75. Banat IM, Samarah N, Murad M et al. Biosurfactant production and use in oil tank clean-up. World J Microbiol Biotechnol 1991; 7:80-88.
76. Lillienberg L, Hogstedt B, Nilson L. Health-effects of tank cleaners. Amer Ind Hygiene Assoc J 1992; 53:95-102.
77. Singer ME, Vogt Finnerty WR. Microbial metabolism of straight and branched alkanes. In: Atlas R, ed. Petroleum Microbiology. New York: Collier Mac Millan, 1984:1-59.
78. Van Dyke MI, Lee H, Trevors JT. Applications of microbial surfactants. Biotech Adv 1991; 9:241-252.
79. Morkes J. Oil-spills-whose technology will clean up. R and D Mazagine 1993; 35:54-56.
80. Bubela B. A comparison of strategies for enhanced oil recovery using in situ and ex situ produced biosurfactants. Surfactant Science Series 1987; 25:143-161.
81. Abu-Ruwaida AS, Banat IM, Haditirto S et al. Isolation of biosurfactant-producing bacteria-product characterization and evaluation. Acta Biotechnologica 1991; 11:315-324.
82. Banat IM. The isolation of a thermophilic biosurfactant producing bacillus sp. Biotech Lett 1993; 15:591-594.
83. Das K, Mukherjee AK. Comparison of lipopeptide biosurfactants production by bacillus subtilis strains in submerged and solid state fermentation systems using a cheap carbon source: some industrial application of biosurfactants. Process Biochem 2007; 42:1191-1199.
84. Tanner RS, Udegbunam EO, McInerney MJ et al. Microbially enhanced oil recovery from carbonate reservoirs. Geomicrobiol J 1991; 9:169-195.
85. Hitzman DO. Petroleum microbiology and the history of its role in enhanced oil recovery. In: Donaldson EC, Clark JB, eds. Proc 1982. International Conf: Microbial enhancement of oil recovery. Springfield: NTIS, 1983:163-218.
86. Youssef N, Simpson DR, Duncan KE et al. In situ biosurfactant production by bacillus strains injected into a limestone petroleum reservoir. Environ Microbiol 2007; 73:1239-1247.
87. Kachholz T, Schlingmann M. Possible food and agricultural application of microbial surfactants: an assessment. In: Kosaric N, Cairns WL, Grey NCC, eds. Biosurfactant and Biotechnology, Vol 25. New York: Marcel Dekker Inc, 1987:183-208.
88. Vater PJ. Lipopeptides in food application. In: Kosaric N, ed. Biosurfactant—Production, Properties and Applications. New York: Marcel Dekker Inc, 1986:419-446.
89. Van Haesendonck IPH, Vanzeveren ECA. Rhamnolipids in bakery products. W.O. 2004/040984, International application patent (PCT), 2004.

90. Iyer A, Mody K, Jha B. Emulsifying properties of a marine bacterial exopolysaccharide. Enzyme Microbial Technol 2006; 38:220-222.
91. Ashwati N, Kumar A, Makkar RS et al. Biodegradation of soil-applied endosulfan in the presence of a biosurfactant. J. Environ Sci Health B 1999; 34:793-803.
92. Kulkarni M, Chaudhari R, Chaudhari A. Novel tensio-active microbial compounds for biocontrol applications. In: Ciancio A, Mukerji KG, eds. General Concepts in Integrated Pest and Disease Management. Springer Netherlands 2007:295-304.
93. Ongena M, Jacques P, Touré Y et al. Involvement of fengycin-type lipopeptides in the multifaceted biocontrol potential of bacillus subtilis. Appl Microbiol Biotechnol 2005; 69:29-38.
94. Ramarathnam R, Bo S, Chen Y et al. Molecular and biochemical detection of fengycin- and bacillomycin D-producing bacillus spp., antagonistic to fungal pathogens of canola and wheat. Can J Microbiol 2007; 53:901-911.
95. Assie LK, Deleu M, Arnaud L et al. Insecticide activity of surfactins and iturins from a biopesticide bacillus subtilis cohn (S499 strain). Meded Rijksuniv Gent Fak Landbouwkd Toegep Biol Wet 2002; 67:647-655.
96. Vollenbroich D, Ö zel M, Vater J et al. Mechanism of inactivation of enveloped viruses by the biosurfactant surfactin from bacillus subtilis. Biologicals 1997; 25:289-297.
97. Yakimov MM, Timmis KN, Wray V et al. Characterization of a new lipopeptide surfactant produced by thermotolerant and halotolerant subsurface bacillus licheniformis BAS 50. Appl Environ Microbiol 1995; 61:1706-1713.
98. Wang X, Gong L, Liang S et al. Algicidal activity of rhamnolipid biosurfactants produced by pseudomonas aeruginosa. Harmful Algae 2005; 4:433-443.
99. Thimon L, Peypoux F, Wallach J et al. Effect of the lipopeptide antibiotic iturin A, on morphology and membrane ultrastructure of yeast cells. FEMS Microbiol Lett 1995; 128:101-106.
100. Itokawa H, Miyashita T, Morita H et al. Structural and conformational studies of [Ile7] and [Leu7] surfactins from bacillus subtilis. Chem Pharm Bul 1994; 42:604-607.
101. Takizawa M, Hida T, Horiguchi T et al. Tan-1511 A, B and C, microbial lipopeptides with G-CSF and GM-CSF inducing activity. J Antibiot 1995; 48:579-588.
102. Inoh Y, Kitamoto D, Hirashima N et al. Biosurfactant MEL-A dramatically increases gene transfection via membrane fusion. J Control Release 2004; 94:423-431.

Chapter 5

Microbial Biosurfactants and Biodegradation

Owen P. Ward*

Abstract

Microbial biosurfactants are amphipathic molecules having typical molecular weights of 500-1500 Da, made up of peptides, saccharides or lipids or their combinations. In biodegradation processes they mediate solubilisation, mobilization and/or accession of hydrophobic substrates to microbes. They may be located on the cell surface or be secreted into the extracellular medium and they facilitate uptake of hydrophobic molecules through direct cellular contact with hydrophobic solids or droplets or through micellarisation. They are also involved in cell physiological processes such as biofilm formation and detachment, and in diverse biofilm associated processes such as wastewater treatment and microbial pathogenesis. The protection of contaminants in biosurfactants micelles may also inhibit uptake of contaminants by microbes. In bioremediation processes biosurfactants may facilitate release of contaminants from soil, but soils also tend to bind surfactants strongly which makes their role in contaminant desorption more complex. A greater understanding of the underlying roles played by biosurfactants in microbial physiology and in biodegradative processes is developing through advances in cell and molecular biology.

Introduction

Microorganisms synthesize an extensive array of biosurfactants, amphipathic molecules that typically concentrate at the interfaces between hydrophobic and hydrophilic phases or surfaces, be they solids, liquids or gasses. As with chemical surfactants, they function to reduce surface or interfacial tensions to form emulsions, and they have the ability to form molecular aggregates including micelles. These biosurfactants vary in their chemical structures and charges and also vary with microbial source. Molecular weights of microbial biosurfactants generally range from 500-1500Da.[1] Among biosurfactants, the lower molecular weight glycolipids and glycopeptides are typically more effective in reducing surface and interfacial tensions while high molecular weight amphipathic polysaccharides and proteins as well as lipopolysaccharides and lipoproteins are oil-in-water stabilizers.[2,3] The minimum biosurfactant concentration required to form micelles, the critical micelle concentration (cmc) typically ranges from 1-200 mg/L.

The cell membrane or cell wall of microbes represents the cell's primary interface with the environment and the diversity of microbial species and their unique capacities to physiologically respond to and interact at different environmental interfaces is often mediated by cell-associated or secreted extracellular biosurfactants. In that regard the most fundamental requirement for cell survival and proliferation of microbial species relates to nutrient supply from the cell's external environment. Hence biosurfactants play diverse roles in facilitating that supply by mediating

*Owen P. Ward—Department of Biology, University of Waterloo, Waterloo, Ontario N2L 3G1, Canada. Email: opward@uwaterloo.ca

Biosurfactants, edited by Ramkrishna Sen. ©2010 Landes Bioscience and Springer Science+Business Media.

solubilisation, mobilization, accession and/or biodegradation of synthetic organic molecules. They may also facilitate cell uptake of extracellular natural organic or indeed inorganic nutrients, or nutrients associated with other living cells through various types of cell-cell interaction including pathogenesis. These interfacial processes may result in formation of microbial cellular aggregates, including microbial biofilms and microbial pellets. These interfacial phenomena may occur naturally and passively in the environment or may be promoted or engineered in bioprocesses, most notably in bioremediation and biological waste treatment processes. Biosurfactants may also impact on the physiology of microbes by exhibiting toxic or inhibitory effects, either directly or indirectly, through pseudosolubilisation of chemicals which may be toxic to specific microbial species.

Biosurfactant-mediated microbial biodegradation processes are particularly common in biodegradation of synthetic organic contaminants given that all cellular processes require high water activity (A_w) while the vast majority of synthetic organic chemicals and the dominant source of these chemicals (petroleum) are hydrophobic.

In the discussion below we will explore the mechanisms by which microbes use biosurfactants to facilitate their access to and biotransformation/biodegradation of hydrophobic contaminants in aqueous media and in soil environments and address in particular the concepts of direct cell contact with hydrophobic molecules and the process of micellarization. We will also consider microbial physiological alterations related to biosurfactant production and/or activity. In order to more fully understand some of these concepts we will also draw on some examples of impacts of chemical surfactants on basic or applied aspects of these topics. Because microbial biofilms are such important multicellular structures which participate in biodegradation processes we will consider the roles biosurfactants play in biofilm formation and detachment.

Accession of Hydrophobic Contaminants in Aqueous Media

The water insoluble nature of petroleum hydrocarbons and most petrochemicals presents a barrier to their microbial degradation, given that microbes generally exist in aqueous phases. In order therefore for microbes to metabolise hydrocarbons their access to these hydrophobic molecules must be facilitated. Two general mechanisms facilitating this access are recognized: direct interaction between the microbes and the particulate or liquid droplet hydrophobic substance and interaction with pseudosolubilized oil or molecules in the form of a surfactant-generated oil-in-water or water-in-oil emulsion. In the latter process, extracellular biosurfactants produced/ secreted by the microorganism, promote emulsion formation which may support cellular uptake of the hydrophobic substrate and many microbial strains which utilize hydrophobic substrates have the capacity to produce these biosurfactants.

In the case of oil degradation by *Pseudomonas* species, these organisms typically synthesize biosurfactants which solubilize hydrocarbons such as hexadecane through micellarization thereby facilitating access.[4] The other mechanism used by microorganisms, by directly associating with solid or liquid hydrophobic surfaces may also be considered in the context of biosurfactants except in this case the pseudosolubilisation mechanism may occur at the cell surface, the hydrophobic nature of which promotes interaction with the contaminant particle or droplet surface. For example, an oil-metabolising *Rhodococcus* species was found to directly associate with crude oil droplets.[5]

However, mechanisms of uptake are complicated and may be strain and/or biosurfactant specific. The mechanisms of uptake of hexadecane by *Acinetobacter calcoaceticus* RAG1, *Rhodoccus erythropolis* ATCC 19558 and *R. erythropolis* BCG112 appeared to be different to that of *Pseudomonas aeruginosa* UG2.[6] Rhamnolipid biosurfactant stimulated degradation of hexadecane by *P. aeruginosa* UG2, the rhamnolipid-producing organism, but did not promote biodegradation by other biosurfactant-producing strains, *A. calcoaceticus* RAG1, *R. erythropolis* ATCC 19558 or *R. erythropolis* BCG112. In addition the biosurfactants produced by these other strains did not stimulate their biodegradation of hexadecane.

In general studies of modes of hydrocarbon uptake by bacteria in the environment, Bouchez-Naretali et al[7] found that 61% of the isolates were from the group of species,

Corynebacteria/Mycobacteria/Nocardia. Forty seven percent of the strains used direct interfacial mechanisms of hydrocarbon uptake while 53% produced biosurfactants in hexane-continning media. Of the latter 53%, 11% were considered to employ biosurfactant-mediated micelle transfer as the uptake mechanism while the remaining 42% involved biosurfactant-induced interfacial uptake.

However, it would be too simplistic to conclude the mechanism of contaminant uptake for a particular strain was either just direct-insoluble contaminant uptake or pseudosolubilisation. Elegant studies on hydrocarbon uptake mechanism by *P. aeruginosa* were conducted by Beal and Betts.[8] A rhamnolipid producing strain (PG202) increased apparent solubility of hexadecane in the culture medium (from 1.84 to 22.76 ppm). While rates of substrate uptake and mineralization by this strain were indeed higher than those observed in a rhamnolipid deficient strain (UO299), the difference was lower than expected. Cell surface hydrophobicity increased in both strains when grown on hexadecane as compared to growth on hydrophilic substrates suggesting that, in addition to rhamnolipid promoting uptake of hexadecane in the PG202 strain, both strains used direct contact with hydrophobic droplets as a mechanism of substrate accession. Thus both uptake mechanisms are used by strain PG202.

Prabhu and Phale[9] observed that although production of biosurfactant by *Pseudomonas* strain PP2 was constitutive and growth associated, greater production occurred with phenanthrene as growth substrate as compared to glucose or benzoate. These authors also observed that cells grown on hydrocarbons exhibited greater hydrophobicity and also concluded that hydrocarbon uptake by this strain was due to both the increase in cell surface hydrophobicity and biosurfactant effects.

While the latter pure culture studies indicate that hydrocarbon uptake at least by some rhamnolipid-producing *Pseudomonas* strains appears to be mediated by a combination of biosurfactant secretion as well as development of a more hydrophobic cell surface the dominant accession mechanisms used by *Pseudomonas* and *Rhodococcus* species appear to be different. When an oil-degrading *Pseudomonas* sp. and an oil-degrading *Rhodoccus* species were separately cultured in aqueous media supplemented with crude oil, the *Pseudomonas* was observed to exist predominantly in the aqueous phase and did not associate with oil droplets whereas the *Rhodococcus* species was observed to concentrate at the oil-water interface.[5] Greatest degradation was observed when a coculture of the strains was used. It was presumed that in the coculture the *Pseudomonas* predominantly utilizes hydrocarbon which was pseudosolubilised into the aqueous phase by biosurfactant while the *Rhodococcus* predominantly utilized hydrocarbon by directly contact with the oil droplet at the oil-water interface. In somewhat analogous studies Kumar et al[10] observed enhanced biodegradation of oil by combining a hydrocarbon degrading *Pseudomonas putida* with a biosurfactant producing bacterium in both aqueous and soil media as compare with use of the isolates separately. The in situ biosurfactant production promoted both oil emulsification and altered the process of bacterial adhesion to the hydrocarbons.

In a different scenario, where microbes have hydrophobic surfaces which enable them to interact directly by surface contact with hydrophobic contaminants addition of biosurfactants or chemical surfactants can counteract this interaction with potential to reduce rates of uptake and transformation of the contaminants by the microbes. *Rhodoccus* sp. strain F9-D79 grew in media containing crude oil by attachment to oil droplets at the oil-water interface and produced a capsule containing mycolic acid.[5] Igepal-CO630 inhibited these cells from adhering to the oil-water interface, causing them to disperse into the aqueous phase. It was suggested that the surfactant removed the cells from the oil phase through disruption of the cell-oil hydrophobic interactions as a result of emulsification and/or that the surfactant may have interacted with mycolic residues in the outer regions of the cell envelope to change the cell surface properties from being predominantly hydrophobic to predominantly hydrophilic.

A cell free high molecular weight biosurfactant produced by *Pseudomonas marginalis* contained a combination of protein and lipopolysaccharide.[11-14] The phenanthrene solubilizing ability of this biosurfactant was observed by the clearing effect observed by application of the surfactant to an agar surface coated with an opaque film of the PAH. Incorporation of this biosurfactant into liquid media containing a cloudy PAH suspension prevented flocculation and settling out of the PAH particles. Transformation of PAHs by *P. marginalis* resting cells was enhanced by addition of the biosurfactant.

Biosurfactants may mediate a quite different process in the de-emulsification of crude oil emulsions.[15] Oilfield emulsions, both oil-in-water and water-in-oil, are found at various stages of oil production and recovery and it is necessary to break these emulsions to produce pipeline quality oil (typically <1% water).[16] The amphipathic nature of microbial biosurfactants and/or the hydrophobic properties of microbial cell surfaces may be exploited to displace emulsifiers present at the oil-water interface of petroleum emulsions to break the emulsion. Microbial polymers including polysaccharides, glycolipids including rhamnolipids and glycoproteins have been shown to exhibit de-emulsification properties.[17] While this process might not be perceived as biodegradative, the microbial cultures applied to the emulsions utilize hydrocarbon components to support growth and biosurfactant production.[18] Indeed such biodegradations of hydrocarbon components at the water/oil interface may also contribute to the de-emulsification process.

Impact of Micellization on Access

Biosurfactants, like their chemical counterparts, are amphipathic molecules which means they contain both hydrophilic and hydrophobic substituents or ends. Above a certain biosurfactant concentration (cmc) the molecules begin to aggregate into micelles. When micelles form in aqueous media in the presence of a hydrophobic contaminant the hydrophobic ends of the biosurfactant molecules associate with and solubilize the hydrophobic contaminant in the centre of the micelle while the hydrophilic ends of the biosurfactant molecules remain on the outside of the micelle in contact with the aqueous phase. Thus biosurfactants or chemical surfactants may inhibit degradation of contaminants by creation of these micelles or shells around the contaminants in effect isolating them from the biodegrading microbes.

Makkar and Rockne[19] have compared performance of chemical surfactants and biosurfactants in biodegradation of polycyclic aromatic hydrocarbons (PAHs). In some cases chemical surfactants have been shown to inhibit PAH degradation and this has been attributed either to surfactant toxicity, surfactant degradation or protective effects on PAHs within surfactant micelles. The failure of many biosurfactants to produce true micelles has been reported to promote bioavailability of biosurfactant-associated PAHs to biodegrading bacteria by direct transfer. It was concluded that emulsan from *A. calcoaceticus* RAG-1 caused inhibition of biodegradation of saturated hydrocarbon compounds by creating a hydrophilic shell around the oil droplets.[50] Shin et al[21,22] and others have observed that pseudosolubilisation of phenanthrene by biosurfactants, such as rhamnolipids, does not necessarily make it all available to biodegrading organisms, such as *P. putida* CRE7. They demonstrated that a significant amount of the phenanthrene was present in high molecular weight phenanthrene-biosurfactant aggregates.

Trehalose lipid biosurfactants at concentrations above its cmc enhanced apparent solubility of phenanthrene and increased both its rates and extent of degradation in aqueous media and in a soil system containing loamy sand with some organic matter.[23] In contrast rate but not extent of mineralization was increased in a soil-water slurry. Perhaps the slurry afforded greater opportunity for phenanthrene to diffuse into pores in soil particles inaccessible to degrading organisms and perhaps even to biosurfactant.

In the case of polychlorinated biphenyls (PCBs) microbial biotransformation, at chemical surfactant concentrations above the cmc, the presence of an anionic surfactant promoted while non-ionic surfactants inhibited transformation as compared to no surfactant controls.[24] The inhibitory effect of the non-ionic surfactant on PCB biodegradation could be eliminated by dilution of the surfactant-PCB solution to a concentration close to the cmc, suggesting that full micelle formation protected the PCB contaminant from microbial transformation.

On the otherhand, Moran et al[25] observed that the biosurfactant surfactin, produced by *Bacillus subtilis*, at concentrations below its cmc neither affected growth on, nor biodegradation of HC wastes by an indigenous microbial community. At concentrations above the CMC biodegradation of aliphatic hydrocarbons were increased from 20.9-35.5%, with the impact being more pronounced with long chain alkanes. More importantly, the biosurfactant promoted biodegradation of 41% of aromatic hydrocarbons, which were not degraded at all in the absence of biosurfactant. When chemical surfactants of various chemical classes were investigated for their effect on biodegradation of crude oil by a mixed culture of the nonylphenol ethoxylate surfactant substantially increased oil biodegradation.[26] Surfactants from other chemical classes had no affect or were inhibitory to degradation.

Accession of Hydrophobic Contaminants in Soil

Soil is an important medium for pollutants and contaminant persistence is influenced strongly by formation of bound pollutant residues.[27] Indeed the majority of the vast range of bioremediation processes which have been implemented involve microbial-mediated soil clean up. As microbial growth and metabolic degradation processes only operate in the presence of water, soil bioremediation processes have to have adequate amounts of water present in the soil to support these processes.

Contaminants first appear to bind to soil surfaces through reversible sorbtion. This can be observed in the laboratory by spiking of soil with contaminants and observing generally good removal efficiencies in surfactant washing or biodegradation experiments. However, over time soil sorbtion increases and bioavailability decreases partially perhaps as a result of the contaminants penetrating deeper into soil crevices and micropores which restrict accessd by microbes or even biosurfactants. The contaminant may also become chemically altered, for example, through chemical or biological oxidation processes, rendering it more resistant to desorbtion and/or biodegradation. Harms and Bosma[28] have characterized the covalent attachment of chlorinated phenols and othere substances to humic matter following reactions mediated by peroxidases, certain metals or reactive oxygen atoms. Crawford et al[29] have considered the roles of oxidizing and reducing molecular species in soil on abiological transformation of xenobiotic compounds. The phenomenon of decreased bioavailability of contaminants in soil over time is often described as weathering. Hence, soil spiking as a laboratory bioremediation feasibility test is a poor predictor of bioremediation field performance where there is a significant duration between contamination and remediation. Hydrophobic contaminants tend to sorb strongly to organic matter.[30]

Chemical and bio surfactants have sometimes been successfully used to promote desorbtion of hydrophobic pollutants from soil. While biosurfactants, produced by hydrophobic contaminant-biodegrading microbes, are presumed to mediate soil bioremediation processes, these systems are much more complex than the systems discussed above for aqueous media without soil. In addition to the tendencies for contaminants to sorb to soil, the surfactants themselves tend to sorb strongly to soil. This limits the application of rhamnolipids, for example, in bioremediation of soil. Consequently much higher chemical or biosurfactant concentrations are required to promote pseudosolubilisation of hydrophobic contaminants present in soil as compared to requirements for solubilisation in aqueous media alone. Indeed examples involving chemical surfactants show that the surfactant concentration required for soil biotreatment may have to be increased by an order of magnitude as compared to the amount of surfactant required for biotreatment in an aqueous system.[24,31]

Monorhamnose lipid sorbtion is concentration-dependent and its relative tendency to sorb to different clays, metal oxides and organic matter have been characterized such that performance may be predicted. The monorhamnose surfactant sorbs more strongly to soil when present alone rather than in a mixture also containing the dirhamnose moiety.[32]

Robinson et al[33] reported 45-fold enhancement of mineralisation of non-aqueous and soil-bound PCB congener 4,4'CB by *Alcaligenes eutrophus* as a result of addition of rhamnolipid R1 at concentrations above its cmc. In contrast, rhamnolipid amendment had little effect on the anaerobic reductive dechlorination of spiked PCBs in soil, possible due to the lack of weathering of the contaminants.[34]

The complex interactions occurring in soil between such a diversity of hydrophobic molecules and such a diversity of soil particulate types makes definition and characterization of the roles of biosurfactants in bioremediation difficult to interpret. Furthermore, as discussed above the complex interactions occurring between selected biosurfactants and the diversity of soil types makes definition and characterization of effects biosurfactant concentration for pseudosolubilisation obscure. Controlled laboratory experiments suggest that careful characterization of the physical and chemical properties of the contaminants and the polluted medium offers potential to implement biosurfactant-mediated bioremediation processes for target contaminants in soil.

The biosurfactant produced by *Candida antarctica* from n-undecane substrate a) promoted emulsification and biodegradation of n-alkanes; b) altered the hydrophobicity and zeta potential of the cell surface thereby promoting hydrophobic contaminant attachment to the cells and c) also altered the zeta potential of porous media causing improved attachment of the cells to this support.[35]

Addition of chemical surfactants to aqueous slurries containing particulate matter can cause disruption of hydrophobic-hydrophobic interactions, for example between the contaminant and the contaminated solid medium. This is illustrated by studying the effect of surfactants on sorption of oil onto the surfaces of hydrophobic polystyrene beads. In the absence of surfactants, polystyrene strongly absorbs petroleum oil or other hydrophobic contaminants, including PCBs. Sorbtion of these contaminants is reduced by non-ionic surfactants such as Igepal CO-630.[36]

A number of researchers have attributed long term bioremediation ineffectiveness of rhamnolipid application to the biodegradation of the biosurfactant. For example, when rhamnolipids were applied to aquifer soil containing weathered diesel fuel, the biosurfactant was preferentially degraded over the contaminant.[37] One strategy which was found to be effective in overcoming this biosurfactant degradation is to pulse apply the surfactant over time.[38] It was concluded that prolonged biodegradation of oil fractions mediated by biosurfactant isolated from *P. aeruginosa* USB-CS1 was limited by loss of surface activity of the biosurfactant after 30 days, likely due to its biodegradation.[39]

Severe metal contamination in soil can inhibit the microbial activity required to bioremediate organic contaminants. Rhamnolipids can complex with metals such as cadmium or lead and counteract completely or partially metal inhibition of degradation of naphthalene or phenanthrene.[38] *Pseudomonas* sp. S8A, which was isolated from mine-tailings contaminated soil exhibited resistance to cadmium (to 200 mg/L) and lead (to 300 mg/L), produced biosurfactant.[40] Two morphologically distinct colony subtypes, characterized as small/round and large/flat were observed and it was demonstrated. Cadmium caused immediate appearance of the large morphotype and this morphotype produced larger quantities of biosurfactant than the small morphotype. The concentrations of rhamnolipid required to promote organic contaminant biodegradation are generally much lower than the levels required for metal complexation[32] and this may limit the economic feasibility of this approach.

Physiological and Morphological Changes Due to Surfactant Activity

Not surprisingly, amphoteric substances, such as surfactants, can impact on cell morphology. Significant morphological changes result when *Pseudomonas nautica* 617 is transferred from a water soluble substrate (acetate) to a hydrophobic substrate(eicosane).[41] Extracellular vesicles and filaments were observed to develop on the cell surface and biosurfactant production was observed. Beal and Betts[8] observed that cell surface hydrophobicity increased in both the rhamnolipid-producing *P. aeruginosa* strain (PG202) and in a rhamnolipid deficient strain (UO299), when these cultures were grown on hexadecane as compared to growth on hydrophilic substrates suggesting both strains could access hydrophobic substrates by direct contact. *Pseudomonas* strain PP2 cells grown on phenanthrene rather than on glucose or benzoate, exhibited greater hydrophobicity.[9] The phenanthrene-grown cells also exhibited greater production of biosurfactant. Perhaps, at least in part, it is the release of these amphoteric biosurfactant molecules from the cell surface that renders the cell surface more hydrophobic. On the other hand Zhang and Miller[42] showed that addition of rhamnolipids increased cell hydrophobicity of slow octadecane-degrading cells of *P. aeruginosa*. They also observed that the rate of increase of cell hydrophobicity was dependent on rhamnolipid concentration and correlated directly with rate of octadecane biodegradation. In the case of fast octadecane degraders, rhamnolipid had no affect on cell hydrophobicity.

An acidic form (dR-A) and methyl ester form (dR-Me) of the dirhamnose lipid exhibited contrasting surfactant properties with dR-Me and dR-A decreasing interfacial tension between hexadecane and water to <0.1 and 5 dynes/cm, respectively.[43] The methyl ester form enhanced degradation of a liquid (hexadecane) and solid (octadecane) alkane by seven different microbial strains. In the case of a further strain, characterized by its very high cell envelope hydrophobicity, the dR-A enhanced degradation of the liquid alkane but inhibited degradation of the solid. dR-A exhibited a lesser enhancement of degradation of hexadecane by the strains. In the case of octadecane, dR-A only enhanced degradation of octadecane by cells having low hydrophobicity.

While certain chemically synthesized surfactants have often been cited as being toxic to microorganisms, this claim has rarely been made against biosurfactants. When two strains isolated from a diesel-contaminated site in Korea were cultured in phenanthrene-containing media in the presence and absence of rhamnolipid, the strains exhibited good cell growth and phenanthrene degradation in the no-biosurfactant controls, whereas growth and phenanthrene degradation appeared to be inhibited in rhamnolipid-supplemented cultures.[22] Rhamnolipid was subsequently shown to cause substantial toxic effects to one of the strains (3Y), but was not toxic to the other (4-3). The results suggested different mechanisms were involved for each strain, namely that the rhamnolipid itself was toxic to 3Y whereas the toxicity of the pseudosolubilized phenanthrene or the increased toxicity of the biosurfactant in the presence of phenanthrene inhibited growth and phenanthrene biodegradation by 4-3.

Biofilm Formation and Detachment

Biofilms are complex aggregations of microbes characterized by the excretion of polymeric matrix substances with adhesion and protective properties. Biofilms typically develop on surfaces and exhibit characteristics of microbial, genetic and structural diversity although some biofilms may contain a single species. The microbial composition may include bacteria, archaea, fungi, algae and protozoa.

In simple biodegradative processes biofilms are essential components of the food chain in aquatic environments. In industrial processes biofilms are essential elements in wastewater and sewage treatment and biofilms also mediate environmental processes such as degradation of petroleum oil or other chemical contaminants in water, soils and sludges.[43] Biofilms are the essential biodegradative component in air biofilters.[44-46] Biofilms also participate in a wide range of plant and animal pathogenic processes, which are also arguably biodegradative processes mediated mainly by microbial carbohydrases in the case of plants[47] or by microbial proteases or other enzymes in the case of mammalian tissues or cells.[48] For example, biofilms are reported to participate in the infective processes in urinary tract, middle ear, dental plaque and gingivitis infections.[49]

Initial attachments of microbes at the start of biofilm formation is due to weak van der Waals forces. Later the biofilm is strengthened by microbial polymeric substances including pili.[50,51] Biofilms exhibit co-operative metabolic capabilities among the member organisms and they also are characterized by having increased resistence to detergents and antibiotics.[53] It has been suggested that the greater antibiotic resistance of some biofilm surface bacteria, described as 'persisters', is due to their low level of metabolic activity.[53]

The influence of biosurfactants in biofilm attachment/detachment processes may also provide insights into the roles of biosurfactants in biodegradation processes. *P. aeruginosa*, an opportunistic human pathogen, has been used as a model strain for study of biofilm development. When it is cultured as a biofilm in flow chambers, mushroom-shaped multicellular structures, including cap- and stalk-forming subpopulations, have been observed to develop[54] and it has been proposed that intramicrocolony channels and interstitial voids facilitate nutrient supply and metabolite removal.[55] Among the biosurfactants produced by *P. aeruginosa*, 3-(3-hydroxyalkanoyloxy) alcanoic acid (HAA), monorhamnolipid and dirhamnolipid are the most common. HAA synthesis is mediated by the RhlA enzyme and is converted to monorhamnolipid by the RhlB enzyme, which in turn is converted to the dirhamnolipid by the RhlB enzyme.[56-58] Biosurfactant production, mediated by the RhlA enzyme, play a role in maintenance of the channels within the biofilm and occurs in microcolonies early in biofilm development and in the mushroom stalks of more established biofilm structures.[59] A bacterial migration process mediated by pili has implicated in formation of the mushroom cap and it has been recently shown that biosurfactant production facilitates this migration.[60]

Detachment of bacteria from biofilms is characterized as a dynamic process which is regulated by certain genes in response to specific environmental signals. Certain variants of _P. aeruginosa_ exhibited properties of accelerated biofilm detachment under specific conditions and the detachment mechanism is mediated by rhamnolipid biosurfactant.[61] This detachment process is also characterized as restoring antibiotic sensitivity to these strains which raises the question as to how biosurfactant production influences antibiotic resistance. The biofilm detachment process alters biofilm structure by cavity formation.

P. putida PCL1445 produces two cyclic lipopeptide biosurfactants, putisolvins I and II which also have roles in biofilm formation and degradation.[62] Synthesis of these particular biosurfactants is positively regulated by a two component signaling system. There are surely potential opportunities to apply biosurfactant amendments or control their production to alter the characteristics of biofilms as they relate to implementing boiodegradation processes. Correspondingly, a mutated strain of PCL1445, _P. putida_ PCL1436 which appeared to have a modified ORF corresponding to lipopeptide synthetases, lacked the putisolvin I and II biosurfactants. This nonbiosurfactantant-producing mutant aggregated earlier and produced stronger biofilms than the wild-type putisolvin-producing strain PCL1445.[63] These biosurfactants inhibited biofilm formation.

Conclusion

Clearly, biosurfactants play signigicant roles in a diverse range of biodegradation processes. They are essential mediators in processes for bioremediation or biotransformation of hydrophobic contaminants in aqueous media, in oil-water emulsions and in soil, where they facilitate the accession of the contaminants by the degrading microbes. They also participate in crude oil de-emulsification processes. Many biodegradation processes are facilited by microbes immobilized in biofilms, including many wastewater treatment processes and microbes present in biofilms are also implicated in a variety of mammalian and plant infective processes. It has been clearly demonstrated that biosurfactant activity plays a role in biofilm formation and also in biofilm detachment. While some progress has been made in our understanding of the roles of biosurfactants in the biochemistry and physiology of these processes, the precise mechanisms are still not well-understood. It is expected that further research, supported by advances in cellular and molecular biology, will substantially add to our knowledge of these complex processes in the coming years. This greater understanding will greatly assist our ability to optimise, better exploit and control these biosurfactant-mediated biodegradation processes.

References

1. VanHamme JD, Singh A, Ward OP. Surfactants in microbiology and biotechnology: Part 1. Physiological Aspects Biotechnol Adv 2006; 24:604-620.
2. Gutnick DL and Shabtai Y. Exopolysaccharide bioemulsifiers. In: Kosaric N, Cairns WL, Gray NCC, eds. Biosurfactants and Biotechnology. New York: Dekker, 1987:211-246.
3. Lin SC. Biosurfactants: recent advances. J Chem Technol Biotechnol 1996; 66:109-120.
4. Sekelsy AM, Shreve GS. Kinetic model of biosurfactant-enhanced hexadecane biodegradation by pseudomonad aeruginosa. Biotechnol Bioeng 1999; 63:401-409.
5. VanHamme JD, Ward OP. Physical and metabolic interactions of pseudomonas sp. strain-B45 and rhodococcus sp. F9-D79 during growth on crude oil and the effect of chemical surfactants thereon. Appl Environ Microbiol 2001; 67:4874-4879.
6. Noordman WH, Janssen DB. Rhamnolipid stimulates uptake of hydrophobic compounds by pseudomonas aeruginosa. Appl Environ Microbiol 2002; 68:4502-4508.

7. Bouchez-Naietali M, Rakatozafy H, Marchal R et al. Diversity of bacterial strains degrading hexadecane in relation to the mode of substrate uptake. J Appl Microbiol 1999; 86:421-428.

8. Beal R, Betts W. Role of rhamnolipid biosurfactants in the uptake and mineralization of hexadecane in pseudomonas aeruginosa. J Appl Microbiol 2000; 89:158-168.

9. Prabhu Y, Phale PS. Biodegradation of phenanthrene by pseudomonas sp. strain PP2: Novel metabolic pathway, role of biosurfactant and cell surface hydrophobicity in hydrocarbon assimilation. Appl Microbiol Biotechnol 2003; 61:342-351.

10. Kumar M, Leon V, De Sisto Materano A et al. Enhancement of oil degradation by coculture of hydrocarbon degrading and biosurfactant producing bacteria. Pol J Microbiol 2006; 55:139-146.

11. Burd G, Ward OP. Bacterial degradation of polycyclic aromatic hydrocarbons on agar plates: the role of biosurfactants. Biotech Techs 1996; 10:371-374.

12. Burd G, Ward OP. Involvement of a surface active high-molecular weight factor in degradation of polycyclic aromatic hydrocarbons. Can J Microbiol 1996; 42:791-797.

13. Burd G, Ward OP. Physicochemical properties of PM-factor, a surface-active agent produced by pseudomonas marginalis. Can J Microbiol 1996; 42:243-251.

14. Burd G, Ward OP. Energy-dependent production of particulate biosurfactant by p. marginalis. Can J Microbiol 1997; 43:391-394.

15. Singh A, VanHamme JD, Ward OP. Surfactants in microbiology and biotechnology: Part 2. Application aspects. Biotechnol Adv 2007; 25:99-121.

16. Manning FC, Thompson, RE. Oilfield Processing. Crude Oil Tulsa: Penwell 1995; 2:1-434.

17. Das M. Characterization of de-emulsification capabilities of a micrococcus sp. Bioresource Technol 2001; 79:15-22.

18. Ward OP, Singh A. Biological process for breaking oil-water emulsions. United States Patent 2001; (6)171:500 B1.

19. Makkar RS, Rockne KJ. Comparison of synthetic surfactants and biosurfactants in enhancing biodegradation of polycyclic aromatic hydrocarbons. Environ Toxicol Chem 2003; 22:2280-2292.

20. Foght JM, Gutnick DL, Westlake DWS. Effect of emulsan on biodegradation of crude oil by pure and mixed bacterial cultures. Appl Environ Microbiol 1989; 55:36-42.

21. Shin KH, Kim KW, Seagren EA. Combined effects of pH and biosurfactant addition on solubilization and biodegradation of phenanthrene. Appl Microbiol Biotechnol 2004; 65:336-343.

22. Shin KH, Ahn Y, Kim KW. Toxic effect of biosurfactant addition on the biodegradation of phenanthrene. Environ Toxicol Chem 2005; 24:2768-2774.

23. Chang JS, Radosevich M, Jin Y et al. Enhancement of phenanthrene solubilization and biodegradation by trehalose lipid biosurfactants. Environ Toxicol Chem 2004; 23:2816-2822.

24. Billingsley KA, Backus SM, Ward OP. Effects of surfactants on aqueous solubilization of PCB congeners and on their biodegradation by Pseudomonas strain LB400. Appl Microbiol Biotechnol 1999; 52:255-260.

25. Moran AC, Olivera N, Commendatore M et al. Enhancement of hydrocarbon waste biodegradation by addition of a biosurfactant from Bacillus subtilis O9. Biodegradation 2000; 11:65-71.

26. VanHamme JD, Ward OP. Influence of chemical surfactants on the biodegradation of crude oil by a mixed bacterial culture. Can J Microbiol 1999; 45:130-137.

27. Mackay D. Multimedia environmental models: the fugacity approach. Boca Raton: Lewis CRC 2001.

28. Harms H, Bosma TNP. Mass transfer limitation of microbial growth and pollutant degradation. J Indust Microbiol Biotechnol 1997; 18:97-105.

29. Crawford RL, Hess TF, Paszczynski A. Combined biological and abiological degradation of xenobiotic compounds. In: Singh A, Ward OP, eds. Soil Biology, Biodegradation and Bioremediation. Berlin: Springer-Verlag 2004; 2:251-278.

30. Haderlein SB, Schwartzenbach RP. Adsorbtion of substituted nitrobenzenes and nitrophenols to mineral surfaces. Environ Sci Technol 1993; 37:316-326.

31. Billingsley KA, Backus SM, Wilson S et al. Remediation of PCBs in soil by surfactant washing and biodegradation in the wash by Pseudomonas sp. LB400. Biotechnol Letts 2002; 24:1827-1832.

32. Ochoa-Loza FJ, Noordman WH, Jannsen DB et al. Effect of clays, metal oxides and organic matter on rhamnolipid biosurfactant sorption by soil. Chemosphere 2007; 66:1634-1642.

33. Robinson KG, Ghosh MM, Shi Z. Mineralization enhancement of non-aqueous phase and soil-bound PCB using biosurfactant. Water Sci Technol 1995; 34:303-309.

34. Royal CL, Preston DR, Sekelsky AM et al. Reductive dechlorination of polychlorinated biphenyls in landfill leachate. Internat Biodeter Biodeg 2003; 51:61-66.

35. Hua Z, Chen J, Lun S et al. Influence of biosurfactants produced by candida antarctica on surface properties of microorganism and biodegradation of n-alkanes. Water Res 2003; 37:4143-4150.

36. Ward OP, Singh A, Billingsley KA. Treatment of soil contaminated with hazardous residues. United States Patent 2001; (6)251:058 B1.

37. Bregnard TP-A, Hoehener P, Zeyer J. Bioavailability and biodegradation of weathered diesel fuel in aquifer material under denitrifying conditions. Environ Toxicol Chem 1998; 17:1222-1229.
38. Maslin P, Maier RM. Rhamnolipid-enhanced mineralization of phenanthrene in organic-metal cocontaminated soils. Bioremediation J 2000; 4:295-308.
39. Rocha C, Infante C. Enhanced oily sludge biodegradation by a tensio-active agent isolated from pseudomonas aeruginosa USB-CS1. Appl Microbiol Biotechnol 1997; 47:615-619.
40. Kassab DM, Roane TM. Differential responses of a mine tailings pseudomonas isolate to cadmium and lead exposures. Biodegradation 2006; 17:379-387.
41. Husain DR, Goutx M, Bezac C et al. Morphological adaptation of pseudomonas nautica strain 617 to growth on eicosane and modes of eicosane uptake. Letts Appl Microbiol 1997; 24:55-58.
42. Zhang Y, Miller RM. Effect of rhamnolipid (biosurfactant) structure on solubilization and biodegradation of n-alkanes. Appl Environ Microbiol 1995; 61:2247-2251.
43. Martins dos Santos VAP, Yakimov, MM, Timmins KN et al. Genomic insights into oil biodegradation in marine systems. In Diaz E, ed. Microbial Biodegradation: Genomics and Molecular Biology Caister Academic Press 2008; Chapter 9.
44. Godvind R, Narayan S. Selection of bioreactor media for odor control. In: Shareefdeen Z, Singh A, eds. Biotechnology for Odor and Air Pollution Control. Berlin: Springer 2005:65-100.
45. Data I Allen DG. Biofilter Technology. In: Shareefdeen Z, Singh A, eds. Biotechnology for Odor and Air Pollution Control. Berlin: Springer, 2005:126-145.
46. Singh A, Ward OP. In: Shareefdeen Z, Singh A, eds. Biotechnology for Odor and Air Pollution Control Berlin: Springer 2005:101-121.
47. Ward OP, Moo-Young M. Critical reviews in biotechnology.
48. Ward OP, Rao MB, Kulkarni A. Proteases. In: Schaechter M ed. Encyclopedia of Microbiology, 3rd Ed. Oxford: Elsevier, 2009.
49. Rogers AH. Molecular oral microbiology. Norwich, UK. Caiser Academic Press 2008; 1-292.
50. Allison D. Community structure and co-operation in biofilms. Cambridge: Cambridge University Press 2000;
51. Allison DG. The biofilm matrix. Biofouling 2003; 19:139-150.
52. Stewart P, Costerton J. Antibiotic resistance of bacteria in biofilms. Lancet 2001; 358:135-138.
53. Lewis K. Riddle of biofilm resistance. Antimicrob Agents Chemother 2001; 45:999-1007.
54. Klausen M, Heydorn A, Ragas P et al. Biofilm formation by Pseudomonas aeruginosa wild type, flagella and type IV pili mutants. Molec Microbiol 2003; 48:1511-1524.
55. Stoodley P, DeBeer D, Lewandowski Z. Liquid flow in biofilm systems. Appl Environ Microbiol 1994; 60:2711-2716.
56. Deziel E, Lepine F, Dennie D et al. Liquid chromatography/mass spectrometry analysis of mixtures of rhamnolipids produced by Pseudomonas aeruginosa strain 57RP grown on mannitol or naphthalene. Biochim Biophys Acta 1999; 1440:244-252.
57. Ochsner UA, Fiechter A, Reiser J. Isolation, characterization and expression in escherichia coli of the Pseudomonas aeruginosa rhlAB genes encoding a rhamnosyltransferase involved in rhamnolipid biosurfactant synthesis. J Biol Chem 1994; 269:19787-19795.
58. Rahim R, Ochsner UA, Olvera C et al. Cloning and functional characterization of the pseudomonas aeruginosa rhlC gene that encodes rhamnosyltransferase 2, an enzyme responsible for di-rhamnolipid biosynthesis. Molec Microbiol 2001; 40:708-718.
59. Lequette Y, Greenberg EP. Timing and localization of rhamnolipid synthesis gene expression in Pseudomonas aeruginosa biofilms. J Bacteriol 2005; 187:37-44.
60. Pamp SJ, Tolker-Nielsen T. Multiple roles of biosurfactants in structural biofilm development by Pseudomonas aeruginosa . J Bacteriol 2007; 189:2531-2539.
61. Boles BR, Thoendel M, Singh PK. Rhamnolipids mediate detachment of pseudomonas aeruginosa from biofilms. Molec Microbiol 2005; 57:1210-1223.
62. Dubern J-F, Lagendijk EL, Lugtenberg BJJ et al. The Heat Shock Genes dnaK, dnaJ and grpE Are Involved in Regulation of Putisolvin Biosynthesis in Pseudomonas putida PCL1445. J Bacteriol 2005; 187:5967-5976.
63. Kuiper I, Lagendijk EL, Pickford R et al. Characterization of two pseudomonas putida lipopeptide biosurfactants, putisolvin I and II, which inhibit biofilm formation and break down existing biofilms. Molec Microbiol 2004; 51:97-113.

CHAPTER 6

Biomedical and Therapeutic Applications of Biosurfactants

Lígia R. Rodrigues* and José A. Teixeira

Abstract

During the last years, several applications of biosurfactants with medical purposes have been reported. Biosurfactants are considered relevant molecules for applications in combating many diseases and as therapeutic agents due to their antibacterial, antifungal and antiviral activities. Furthermore, their role as anti-adhesive agents against several pathogens illustrate their utility as suitable anti-adhesive coating agents for medical insertional materials leading to a reduction of a large number of hospital infections without the use of synthetic drugs and chemicals. Biomedical and therapeutic perspectives of biosurfactants applications are presented and discussed in this chapter.

Introduction

Biosurfactants are microbial compounds that exhibit pronounced surface and emulsifying activities. These compounds comprise a wide range of chemical structures, such as glycolipids, lipopeptides, polysaccharide-protein complexes, phospholipids, fatty acids and neutral lipids.[1-7] Therefore, it is reasonable to expect diverse properties and physiological functions for different groups of biosurfactants. Comparing with chemical surfactants, these compounds have several advantages such as lower toxicity, higher biodegradability and effectiveness at extreme temperatures or pH values.[6-10] Although these compounds present interesting features as compared with their chemical counterparts, many of the envisaged applications depend considerably on whether they can be produced economically. Hence, much effort in process optimization and at the engineering and biological levels has been carried out. Biosurfactants production from inexpensive waste substrates and low cost raw materials, thereby decreasing their production cost,[11-18] has been reported. Furthermore, these molecules can be tailor-made to suit different applications by changing the growth substrate or growth conditions.[19-20] Most biosurfactants are considered secondary metabolites, though, some may play essential roles for the survival of the producing-microorganisms either through facilitating nutrient transport, microbe-host interactions or as biocide agents.[6] Biosurfactant roles include increasing the surface area and bioavailability of hydrophobic water-insoluble substrates, heavy metal binding, bacterial pathogenesis, quorum sensing and biofilm formation.[21] An interface is any boundary between two different phases and microbial life may be more common at interfaces as evidenced by microbial biofilms, surface films and aggregates. Given that, all microbial life is impacted by interfacial phenomena and biosurfactants are a common mechanism by which microorganisms deal with interfacial challenges.[6] Biosurfactants are amphipatic molecules with both hydrophilic and hydrophobic moieties that partition preferentially at the interface between fluid phases that have different degrees of polarity and hydrogen bonding, such as oil and water, or air and water interfaces. In addition to this behaviour,

*Corresponding Author: Lígia R. Rodrigues—IBB, Centre of Biological Engineering, Universidade do Minho, Campus de Gualtar, 4710-057 Braga, Portugal.
Email: lrmr@deb.uminho.pt

Biosurfactants, edited by Ramkrishna Sen. ©2010 Landes Bioscience and Springer Science+Business Media.

their diversity, environmentally friendly nature, suitability for large-scale production and selectivity, has driven most of the research in biosurfactants field for environmental applications.[7,22-25] Legal aspects such as stricter regulations concerning environmental pollution by industrial activities and health regulations will also strongly influence the chances of biodegradable biosurfactants replacing their chemical counterparts.[7,10,19,22-25]

Regardless of the potential and biological origin of biosurfactants few studies were carried out on applications related to biomedical applications.[11,26-30] Nevertheless, some biosurfactants have proven to be suitable alternatives to synthetic medicines and antimicrobial agents and may therefore be used as safe and effective therapeutic agents (Table 1).

The biosurfactants potential applications in the medical field, as well as their main mechanisms of interaction are discussed in this chapter.

Biomedical and Therapeutic Applications of Biosurfactants

As discussed above a broad range of chemical structures have been attributed to biosurfactants.[1-2,4-5] Some of these biosurfactants were described for their potential as biological active compounds and applicability in the medical field. Therefore, they are a suitable alternative to synthetic medicines and antimicrobial agents and may be used as safe and effective therapeutic agents.[21,25] Recently, there has been an increasing interest in the effect of biosurfactants on human and animal cells and cell lines.[28,42,83] Lipopeptides produced by *Bacillus subtilis*[36] and *Bacillus licheniformis*,[19,49-51] mannosylerythritol lipids produced by *Candida antartica*[53] and rhamnolipids produced by *Pseudomonas aeruginosa*,[33-34] have been shown to have antimicrobial activities.

Biological Activity

Glycolipids

Glycolipids are the most common group of biosurfactants of which the most effective regarding surface active properties are the trehalose lipids obtained from *Mycobacterium* and related bacteria, the rhamnolipids obtained from *Pseudomonas* sp. and the sophorolipids obtained from yeasts. Otto and coworkers[12] described the production of sophorose lipids using deproteinized whey concentrate as substrate by a two-stage process. Several antimicrobial, immunological and neurological properties have been attributed to mannosylerythritol lipid (MEL), a yeast glycolipid biosurfactant, produced from vegetable oils by *Candida* strains.[62,84] Kitamoto et al[53] showed that MEL exhibits antimicrobial activity particularly against Gram-positive bacteria. Isoda et al[54] investigated the biological activities of seven extracellular microbial glycolipids including MEL-A, MEL-B, polyol lipid, rhamnolipid, sophorose lipid and succinoyl trehalose lipid STL-1 and STL-3. Except for rhamnolipid, all the other tested glycolipids induced cell differentiation instead of cell proliferation in the human promyelocytic leukaemia cell line HL60. These glycolipids induced the human myelogenous leukaemia cell line K562 and the human basophilic leukaemia cell line Ku812 to differentiate into monocytes, granulocytes and megakaryocytes. STL and MEL differentiation-inducing activity was attributed to a specific interaction with the plasma membrane instead of a simple detergent-like effect.

In addition, the effects of several kinds of microbial extracellular glycolipids on neutrite initiation in PC12 cells were investigated.[55] The PC12 cell line derived from a rat pheochromocytoma, provides a relatively simple and homogeneous system for studying various aspects of neuronal differentiation, because PC12 cells can survive and proliferate without requiring the presence of neutrotrophic factors. A significant neutrite outgrowth was observed as a consequence of the addition of MEL-A, MEL-B and sophorose lipid (SL) to PC12 cells. MEL-A increased acetylcholinesterase activity to an extent similar to nerve growth factor (NGF). MEL-A induced neutrite outgrowth after treatment of PC12 cells with an anti-NGF receptor antibody that obstructed the NGF action. It was shown that MEL-A and NGF induce differentitation of PC12 cells through different mechanisms. Moreover, MEL was found to induce the outgrowth of neutrites, enhance the activity of acetylcholinesterase and increase the levels of galactosylceramide from PC12 pheochromocytoma cells.[56]

Table 1. Examples of biosurfactant applications in the medical field (adapted from Rodrigues et aP⁸)

Microorganism	Biosurfactant Type	Activity/Application	Reference
Pseudomonas aeruginosa	Rhamnolipid	• Antimicrobial activity against *Mycobacterium tuberculosis*	31-35
		• Anti-adhesive activity against several bacterial and yeast strains isolated from voice prostheses	
		• Induced dose-dependent hemolysis and coagulation of platelet-poor plasma but is not detrimental to chicken lung, liver, heart and kidney tissues	
Bacillus subtilis	Surfactin	• Antimicrobial and antifungal activities	36-43
		• Inhibition of fibrin clot formation	
		• Hemolysis and formation of ion channels in lipid membranes	
		• Antitumor activity against Ehrlich's ascite carcinoma cells	
		• Antiviral activity against human immunodeficiency virus 1 (HIV-1)	
		• Induction of apoptosis in human leukemia K562	
Bacillus subtilis	Pumilacidin (surfactin analog)	• Antiviral activity against herpes simplex virus 1 (HSV-1)	44
		• Inhibitory activity against H⁺, K⁺-ATPase and protection against gastric ulcers in vivo	
Bacillus subtilis	Iturin	• Antimicrobial activity and antifungal activity against profound mycosis	5,45-48
		• Effect on the morphology and membrane structure of yeast cells	
		• Increase in the electrical conductance of biomolecular lipid membranes	

continued on next page

Table 1. *Continued*

Microorganism	Biosurfactant Type	Activity/Application	Reference
Bacillus licheniformis	Lichenysin	• Nontoxic and nonpyrogenic immunological adjuvant	
		• Antibacterial activity	49-52
		• Chelating properties that might explain the membrane disrupting effect of lipopeptides	
Candida antartica	Mannosylerythritol lipids	• Antimicrobial, immunological and neurological properties	
		• Induction of cell differentiation in the human promyelocytic leukemia cell line HL60	53-66
		• Induction of neuronal differentiation in PC12 cells	
		• Enhancement of gene transfection efficiency	
Rodococcus erythropolis	Treahalose lipid	• Antiviral activity against HSV and influenza virus	67-68
Streptococcus thermo-philus	Glycolipid	• Anti-adhesive activity against several bacterial and yeast strains isolated from voice prostheses	69-73
Streptococcus mitis	Not identified	• Anti-adhesive activity against *Streptococcus mutans*	74-75
Lactobacillus	Surlactin	• Anti-adhesive activity against several pathogens including enteric bacteria	76-81
Lactococcus lactis	Not identified	• Anti-adhesive activity against several bacterial and yeast strains isolated from voice prostheses	70, 82

Glycolipids have also been implicated with growth arrest, apoptosis and the differentiation of mouse malignant melanoma cells.[57-58] Exposure of B16 cells to MEL resulted in the condensation of the chromatin, DNA fragmentation and sub-G1 arrest (the sequence of events of apoptosis). Furthermore, MEL was reported to markedly inhibit the growth of mouse melanoma B16 cells in a dose-dependent manner. Moreover, MEL exposure stimulated the expression of differentiation markers of melanoma cells, such as tyrosinase activity and the enhanced production of melanin, which is an indication that MEL triggered both apoptotic and cell differentiation programs. In addition, exposure of PC12 cells to MEL enhanced the activity of acetylcholinesterase and interrupted the cell cycle at the G1 phase, with resulting outgrowth of neutrites and partial cellular differentiation.[59] MEL has been implicated in the induction of neuronal differentiation in PC12 cells and therefore provides the basis for the use of glycolipids as therapeutical agents for cancer treatment. Nevertheless, further studies of the molecular basis of the signalling cascade that follows exposure of PC12 cells to MEL may ultimately lead to a better understanding of the processes that result in the outgrowth of neutrites and the commitment to differentiation of PC12 cells.

In other studies, four analogs of STL-3 at their critical micelle concentration were evaluated for their ability to inhibit growth and induce differentiation of HL60 human promyelocytic leukaemia cells.[85] It was found that the effect of STL-3 and its analogs on HL60 cells was dependent on the hydrophobic moiety of STL-3. Furthermore, a high binding-affinity of MEL towards human immunoglobulin G (HIgG) was shown by Im et al.[86] They suggested the possibility of using MEL-A as an alternative ligand for immunoglobulins. In subsequent studies they evaluated the potential of MEL (-A, -B and -C) attached to PHEMA beads (poly(2-hydroxyethyl methacrylate)), for binding, affinity to HIgG.[87] Of these three composite compounds, those bearing MEL-A exhibited the highest binding capacity to HIgG. More significantly, the bound HIgG was efficiently recovered (approximately 90%) under significantly mild elution conditions, with phosphate buffer at pH 7, indicating a great potential of the glycolipids as an affinity ligand material. Other researchers also demonstrated that MEL-A assembled monolayers would be useful as noble affinity ligand system for various immunoglobulins.[64-65] Inoh et al[88-89] reported that MEL-A significantly increased the efficiency of gene transfection mediated by cationic liposomes with a cationic cholesterol derivative. Among the cationic liposomes tested, the liposome bearing cholesteryl-3β-carboxyamindoethylene-*N*-hydroxyethylamine and MEL-A showed the best efficiency for delivery of plasmids encoding luciferase (ρGL3) into the target cells (NIH3T3, COS-7 and HeLa). The properties, production and applications of MEL were widely studied by Kitamoto and coworkers[90] and by Ueno et al,[60-61] particularly the exceptional interfacial properties and differentiation-inducing activities of MEL. They also focused on the excellent biological and self-assembling actions of MEL and examined the effect of MEL-A on the gene transfection using cationic liposomes. These results were also demonstrated by other researchers that studied the transfection efficiency in human cervix carcinoma HeLa cells[66] and the potential of these liposomes as vectors for herpes simplex virus thymidine kinase gene therapy.[63]

The succinoyl-trehalose lipid produced by *Rhodococcus erythropolis* has also been reported to inhibit HSV and influenza virus.[67-68] The deficiency of pulmonary surfactant which is responsible for respiration failure in premature infants[91] may be corrected through the isolation of genes for protein molecules of this surfactant and cloning in bacteria for possible fermentative production and use in medical application.[33] Sano et al[92] demonstrated the different actions of pulmonary surfactant protein A upon distinct serotypes of LPS which is the major constituent of the outer membrane of Gram-negative bacteria.

Lipopeptides

Several features and biological activities have been reported for lipopeptides, mainly for iturin A and surfactin. They have been described as antibiotics, antiviral and antitumor agents, immunomodulators or specific toxins and enzyme inhibitors. Ahimou et al[5] reported that lipopeptide profile and bacterial hydrophobicity vary greatly with the producing strains, iturin A being the only lipopeptide type produced by all *B. subtilis* strains. Surfactin was found to be more efficient than iturin A in modifying the *B. subtilis* surface hydrophobic character. Morikawa et al[1] identified and characterized a biosurfactant, arthrofactin, produced by *Arthrobacter* species, which was found to be seven times more effective than surfactin. Jenny and coworkers[49] determined the structural analysis and characterized surface activities of biosurfactants produced by *B. licheniformis*, while several researchers described their continuous production.[50,93] Yakimov and coworkers[51] demonstrated the antibacterial activity of lichenysin A, a biosurfactant produced by *B. licheniformis* that favourably compares to others surfactants. More recently Grangemard et al[52] reported the chelating properties of lichenysin, which might explain the membrane disrupting effect of lipopeptides.

In another study, Carrillo and its collaborators[94] proposed a molecular mechanism of membrane permeabilization by surfactin, which may explain surfactin induced pore formation underlying the antibiotic and haemolytic action of these lipopeptides. This study also suggested that the membrane barrier properties are likely to be damaged in the areas where surfactin oligomers interact with the phospholipids, at concentrations much below the onset for solubilisation. Such properties can cause structural fluctuations that may well be the primary mode of the antibiotic action of this lipopeptide. Surfactin type peptides that can rapidly act on membrane integrity rather than other vital cellular processes may perhaps constitute the next generation of antibiotics. Lipopeptide surfactin has been found to interact with artificial and biomembrane systems, for example bacterial protoplasts or enveloped viruses.[36] Several biological activities have been attributed to surfactin including the induction of ion channels formation in lipid bilayer membranes,[40] the inhibition of fibrin clot formation and haemolysis,[39] the inhibition of cyclic adenosine monophosphate (cAMP), the inhibition of platelet and spleen cytosolic phospholipase A2 (PLA2)[95] and antimicrobial, antiviral and antitumor activity against Ehrlich's ascite carcinoma cells.[38,95] According to the differences in their amino acid sequences, different types of surfactins (A, B and C) have been identified. Surfactin C was found to enhance the activation of prourokinase (plasminogen activator) and the conformational change in plasminogen, leading to increased fibrinolysis in vitro and in vivo.[96] The plasminogen-plasmin system is involved in blood clot dissolution, as well as in a variety of physiological and pathological processes requiring localized proteolysis. In a rat pulmonary embolism model, surfactin C increases plasma clot lyses when injected in combination with prourokinase.[83] The results gathered in this study point to the possible use of surfactin in thrombolytic therapy related to pulmonary, myocardial and cerebral disorders.

Vollenbroich and coworkers[36] showed that a surfactin treatment improved proliferation rates and lead to changes in the morphology of mammalian cells that had been contaminated with mycoplasma. Furthermore, the low cytotoxicity of surfactin to mammalian cells allowed specific inactivation of mycoplasmas without significant damaging effects on cell metabolism.[42,43] Additionally, surfactin and surfactin analogs have been reported as antiviral agents, namely it was demonstrated a significant inhibitory effect of pumilacidin on herpes simplex virus 1 (HSV-1)[44] and an inhibitory activity against H+, K+-ATPase and protection against gastric ulcers in vivo. The potential of surfactin against human immunodeficiency virus 1 (HIV-1) was reported by Itokawa et al.[41] The antiviral action of surfactin was suggested to be due to physicochemical interactions between the membrane-active surfactant and the virus lipid membrane, which causes permeability changes and at higher concentrations leads finally to the disintegration of the mycoplasma membrane system by a detergent effect.[37] Furthermore, surfactin was found to be active against Semliki Forest virus, herpes simplex virus, suid herpes virus, vesicular stomatitis virus, simian immunodeficiency virus, feline calicivirus and murine encephalomyocarditis virus.[37]

Moreover, Kim and coworkers[95] demonstrated that surfactin is a selective inhibitor for cytosolic PLA2 and a putative anti-inflammatory agent through the inhibitory effect produced by direct interaction with cytosolic PLA2 and that inhibition of cytosolic PLA2 activity may suppress inflammatory responses.

Another lipopeptide, iturin A, produced by *B. subtilis* was reported to have effective antifungal properties[5,46] which affects the morphology and membrane structure of yeast cells. This lipopeptide was shown to pass through the cell wall and disrupt the plasma membrane with the formation of small vesicles and the aggregation of intramembranous particles. Iturin also passes through the plasma membrane and interacts with the nuclear membrane and probably with membranes of other cytoplasmic organelles. This lipopeptide has been proposed as an effective antifungal agent for profound mycosis.[47] Other members of the iturin group, including bacillomycin D and bacillomycin Lc were also found to have antimicrobial activity against *Aspergillus flavus*, but the different lipid chain length apparently affected the activity of the lipopeptide against other fungi.[97] Thus, the members of the iturin-like biosurfactant group are considered alternative antifungal agents.

Possible applications of biosurfactants as emulsifying aids for drug transport to the infection site, for supplementing pulmonary surfactant and as adjuvants for vaccines were suggested by Kosaric.[98] Mittenbuhler et al[48] showed that bacterial lipopeptides constitute powerful nontoxic and nonpyrogenic immunological adjuvants when mixed with conventional antigens. A marked enhancement of the humoral immune response was obtained with the low molecular mass antigens iturin AL, herbicolin A and microcystin (MLR) coupled to poly-L-lysine (MLR-PLL) in rabbits and in chickens. Conjugates of lipopeptide—Th-cell epitopes also constituted effective adjuvants for the in vitro immunization of either human mononuclear cells or mouse B cells with MLR-PLL and result in a significantly increased yield of antibody-secreting hybridomas.

Other Biosurfactants

Nielsen and coworkers[99] reported viscosinamide, a cyclic depsipeptide, as a new antifungal surface active agent produced by *Pseudomonas fluorescens* and with different properties as compared to the biosurfactant viscosin, known to be produced from the same species and to have antibiotic activity.[100] Massetolides A-H, also cyclic depsipeptides, were isolated from *Pseudomonas* species, derived from a marine habitat and found to exhibit in vitro antimicrobial activity against *Mycobacterium tuberculosis* and *Mycobacterium avium-intracellulare*.[31]

Precursors and degeneration products of sphingolipids biosurfactants were found to inhibit the interaction of *Streptococcus mitis* with buccal epithelial cells and of *Staphylococcus aureus* with nasal mucosal cells.[101] Gram-positive *Bacillus pumilis* cells were found to produce pumilacidin A, B, C, D, E, F and G which exhibited antiviral activity against herpes simplex virus 1 (HSV-1), inhibitory activity against H^+, K^+-ATPase and were found to be protective against gastric ulcers[44] probably through inhibiting microbial activity contributing to these ulcers.

Although there is an increasing potential for the application of biosurfactants in the biomedical field, some of these molecules may constitute a risk for humans. For instance, *P. aeruginosa* is a bacterium responsible for severe nosocomial infections, life-threatening infections in immunocompromised persons and chronic infections in cystic fibrosis patients; thus rhamnolipids have to be well-investigated prior to such uses. *P. aeruginosa* strain's virulence depends on a large number of cell-associated and extracellular factors.[102-104] Cell-to-cell signalling systems control the expression and allow a coordinated, cell-density-dependent production of many extracellular virulence factors. The possible role of cell-to-cell signalling in the pathogenesis of *P. aeruginosa* infections and a rationale for targeting cell-to-cell signalling systems in the development of new therapeutic approaches was discussed by Van Delden and Iglewski.[102] Synthesis of rhamnolipids is regulated by a very complex genetic regulatory system that also controls different *P. aeruginosa* virulence-associated traits.[34] The possible application of rhamnolipids in the pharmaceutical industry is still being studied by some researchers.[35,105] The cosmetic and health care industries use large amounts of surfactants for a wide variety of products including insect repellents, antacids, acne pads, contact lens solutions, hair colour and care products, deodorants, nail care products, lipstick, eye shadow, mascara, toothpaste, denture cleaners, lubricated condoms, baby products, foot care products, antiseptics, shaving and depilatory products.[8] Biosurfactants are known to have advantages over synthetic surfactants such as low irritancy or anti-irritating effects and compatibility with skin. Rhamnolipids in particular are being used as cosmetic additives and have been patented to make some liposomes and emulsions,[103-104] both of which are important in the cosmetic industry.

Anti-Adhesive Activity

Biosurfactants have been found to inhibit the adhesion of pathogenic organisms to solid surfaces or to infection sites, thus prior adhesion of biosurfactants to solid surfaces of implant materials might constitute a new and effective means of combating colonization by pathogenic microorganisms.[21] Precoating vinyl urethral catheters by running the surfactin solution through them before inoculation with media resulted in a decrease of the amount of biofilm formed by *Salmonella typhimurium, Salmonella enterica, Escherichia coli* and *Proteus mirabilis*.[106] Given the importance of opportunistic infections with *Salmonella* species, including urinary tract infections of AIDS patients, these results have great potential for practical applications.

A role for biosurfactants as defence weapons in post adhesion competition with other strains or species has to date been suggested only for biosurfactants released by *S. mitis* strains against *Streptococcus mutans* adhesion[74-75] and for biosurfactants released by lactobacilli against adhesion of uropathogens.[77-78] The biosurfactant surlactin,[79] produced by several *Lactobacillus* isolates, was suggested as a suitable anti-adhesive coating for catheter materials. The role of *Lactobacillus* species in the female urogenital tract as a barrier to infection is of considerable interest.[107] These organisms are believed to contribute to the control of vaginal microbiota by competing with other microorganisms for adherence to epithelial cells and by producing biosurfactants. There are reports of inhibition of biofilm formation by uropathogens and yeast on silicone rubber with biosurfactants produced by *Lactobacillus acidophilus*.[108-109] Heinemann and coworkers showed that *Lactobacillus fermentum* RC-14 releases surface-active components that can inhibit adhesion of uropathogenic bacteria, including *Enterococcus faecalis*.[110] Velraeds et al[80] also reported on the inhibition of adhesion of pathogenic enteric bacteria by a biosurfactant produced by a *Lactobacillus* strain and later showed that the biosurfactant caused an important, dose-related inhibition of the initial deposition rate of *E. coli* and other bacteria adherent on both hydrophobic and hydrophilic substrata.[76]

Dairy *S. thermophilus* strains were found to be biosurfactant-producers and Busscher et al[72-73] showed that this biosurfactant inhibited adhesion onto silicone rubber and growth of several bacterial and yeast strains isolated from explanted voice prostheses. Efforts in the development of strategies to prevent the microbial colonization of silicone rubber voice prostheses have been reported by Rodrigues et al.[71,82] The ability of biosurfactants obtained from the probiotic strains, *L. lactis* 53 and *S. thermophilus* A, to inhibit adhesion of four bacterial and two yeast strains isolated from explanted voice prostheses to precoated silicone rubber was evaluated. The results obtained showed that the biosurfactants were effective in decreasing the initial deposition rates, as well as the number of bacterial cells adhering after 4 h, for all microorganisms tested. Over 90% reductions in the initial deposition rates were achieved for most of the bacterial strains tested. Recently, the authors also demonstrated that a rhamnolipid biosurfactant containing solution may be useful for use as a biodetergent solution for prostheses cleaning, prolonging their lifetime and directly benefiting laryngectomized patients. Gotek et al[81] assessed the adhesive properties of several biosurfactant-producers *Lactobacillus* spp. strains to a monolayer of intestinal epithelium in vitro, represented by the Caco2 cell line. All tested *Lactobacillus* strains showed adhesion to Caco2 cells. A 50% reduction in the population of *Klebsiella pneumoniae* 2 cells adhering to the surface previously impregnated with a solution of biosurfactants synthesised by *Lactobacillus casei rhamnosus* CCM 1825, after the 3-hour contact with the tested surface was also observed.

The role for surfactants in the defence against infection and inflammation in the human body is a well-known phenomenon. The pulmonary surfactant is a lipoprotein complex synthesized and secreted by the epithelial lung cells into the extracellular space, where it lowers the surface tension at the air-liquid interface of the lung and represents a key factor against infections and inflammatory lung diseases.[91]

Antimicrobial Activity

The antimicrobial activity of several biosurfactants has been reported in the literature for many different applications.[111] For instance, the antimicrobial activity of two biosurfactants obtained from probiotic bacteria, *L. lactis* 53 and *S. thermophilus* A, against a variety of bacterial and yeast strains isolated from explanted voice prostheses was evaluated.[70] In another study, Reid et al[112-113] emphasized a possible probiotic role for the biosurfactant-producing lactobacilli in the restoration and maintenance of healthy urogenital and intestinal tracts, conferring protection against pathogens and suggested a reliable alternative treatment and preventive regimen to antibiotics in the future. The first clinical evidence that probiotic lactobacilli can be delivered to the vagina following oral intake was provided[113] and although only a limited set of strains have any proven clinical effect or scientific basis, there are sufficient data to suggest that this approach could provide a valuable alternative to antibiotic prophylaxis and treatment of infection. By the use of a rat model of surgical implant infection, Gan et al[114] determined that the probiotic strain, *L. fermentum* RC-14 and its secreted biosurfactant reduced infections associated with surgical implants, which are mainly caused by *S. aureus* through inhibition of growth and reduction of adherence to surgical implants. A recent in vitro study of *Lactobacillus plantarum* 299v and *L. rhamnosus* GG showed that these probiotic strains could inhibit the adhesion of *E. coli* to intestinal epithelial cells by stimulating epithelial expression of mucins.[115] These strains however were also found to be biosurfactant producers.[14] These observations generally indicated that biosurfactants might also contain signalling factors that interact with host and/or bacterial cells leading to the inhibition of infections. Moreover they support the assertion of possible role in preventing microbial adhesion[76,116] and their potential in developing anti-adhesion biological coatings for implant materials.[32]

Conclusion

Interest in the use of biosurfactants in the medical field has been increasing in the last years as a result of many studies published on their unique features. Biosurfactants are not only useful as antibacterial, antifungal and antiviral agents, but also have potential for use as major immuno-modulatory molecules, adhesive agents and even in vaccines and gene therapy. They have been used for gene tranfection, as ligands for binding immunoglobulins, as adjuvants for antigens and also as inhibitors for fibrin clot formation and activators of fibrin clot lyses. Promising alternatives to produce potent biosurfactants with altered antimicrobial profiles and decreased toxicity against mammalian cells may be exploited by genetic alteration of biosurfactants. Furthermore, biosurfactants have the potential to be used as anti-adhesive biological coatings for biomaterials, thus reducing hospital infections and use of synthetic drugs and chemicals. They may also be incorporated into probiotic preparations to combat urogenital tract infections and pulmonary immunotherapy.

Regardless of the enormous potential of biosurfactants in this field, their use still remains limited, possibly due to their high production and extraction cost and lack of information on their toxicity towards human systems. Further research on human cells and natural microbiota are required to validate the use of biosurfactants in several biomedical and health related areas. Nevertheless, there appears to be great potential for their use in the medical science arena waiting to be fully exploited.

References

1. Morikawa M, Daido H, Takao T et al. A new lipopeptide biosurfactant produced by Arthrobacter sp. strain MIS38. J Bacteriol 1993; 175:6459-6466.
2. Lin S. Biosurfactants: recent advances. J Chem Tech Biotechnol 1996; 66:109-120.
3. Desai JD, Banat IM. Microbial production of surfactants and their commercial potential. Microbiol Mol Biol Rev 1997; 61:47-64.
4. Angelova B, Schmauder H-P. Lipophilic compounds in biotechnology—interactions with cells and technological problems. J Biotechnol 1999; 67:13-32.
5. Ahimou F, Jacques P, Deleu M. Surfactin and iturin a effects on bacillus subtilis surface hydrophobicity. Enz Microb Technol 2001; 27:749-754.
6. Van Hamme JD, Singh A, Ward OP. Physiological aspects. Part 1 in a series of papers devoted to surfactants in microbiology and biotechnology. Biotech Adv 2006; 24:604-620.
7. Singh A, Van Hamme JD, Ward OP. Surfactants in microbiology and biotechnology: Part 2. Application aspects. Biotech Adv 2007; 25:99-121.
8. Kosaric N. Biosurfactants in industry. J Am Oil Chem Soc 1992; 64:1731-1737.

9. Cameotra S, Makkar R. Synthesis of biosurfactants in extreme conditions. Appl Microbiol Biotechnol 1998; 50:520-529.
10. Mukherjee S, Das P, Sen R. Towards commercial production of microbial surfactants. Trends Biotechnol 2006; 24:509-515.
11. Makkar R, Cameotra S. An update on the use of unconventional substrates for biosurfactant production and their new applications. Appl Microbiol Biotechnol 2002; 58:428-434.
12. Otto RT, Daniel H-J, Pekin G et al. Production of sophorolipids from whey II.—Product composition, surface active properties, cytotoxicity and stability against hydrolases by enzimatic treatment. Appl Microbiol Biotechnol 1999; 52:495-501.
13. Rodrigues LR, Teixeira JA, Oliveira R. Low cost fermentative medium for biosurfactant production by probiotic bacteria. Biochem Eng J 2006; 32:135-142.
14. Rodrigues LR, Moldes A, Teixeira JA et al. Kinetic study of fermentative biosurfactant production by lactobacillus strains. Biochem Eng J 2006; 28:109-116.
15. Das K, Mukherjee AK. Comparison of lipopeptide biosurfactants production by Bacillus subtilis strains in submerged and solid state fermentation systems using a cheap carbon source: some industrial applications of biosurfactants. Process Biochem 2007; 42:1191-1199.
16. Joshi S, Bharucha C, Jha S et al. Biosurfactant production using molasses and whey under thermophilic conditions. Biores Technol 2008; 99:195-199.
17. Rivera OMP, Moldes AB, Torrado AM et al. Lactic acid and biosurfactants production from hydrolyzed distilled grap marc. Process Biochem 2007; 42:1010-1020.
18. Moldes AB, Torrado AM, Barral MT et al. Evaluation of biosurfactant production from various agricultural residues by lactobacillus pentosus. J Agr Food Chem 2007; 55:4481-4486.
19. Fiechter A. Biosurfactants: moving towards industrial application. Trends Biotechnol 1992; 10:208-218.
20. Rodrigues LR, Teixeira JA, Oliveira R et al. Response surface optimization of the medium components for the production of biosurfactants by probiotic bacteria. Process Biochem 2006; 41:1-10.
21. Singh P, Cameotra S. Potential applications of microbial surfactants in biomedical sciences. Trends Biotechnol 2004; 22:142-146.
22. Banat IM. Biosurfactants production and use in microbial enhanced oil recovery and pollution remediation: A review. Biores Technol 1995; 51:1-12.
23. Banat IM. Biosurfactants characterization and use in pollution removal: State of the art. A review. Acta Biotechnol 1995; 15:25167.
24. Mulligan CN. Environmental application for biosurfactants. Environ Pollut 2005; 133:183-198.
25. Banat IM, Makkar R, Cameotra S. Potential commercial applications of microbial surfactants. Appl Microbiol Biotechnol 2000; 53:495-508.
26. Benincasa M, Abalos A, Oliveira I et al. Chemical structure, surface properties and biological activities of the biosurfactant produced by pseudomonas aeruginosa LB1 from soapstock. Antonie Van Leeuwenhoek 2004; 85:1-8.
27. Flasz A, Rocha CA, Mosquera B et al. A comparative study of the toxicity of a synthetic surfactant and one produced by Pseudomonas aeruginosa ATCC 55925. Med Sci Res 1998; 6:181-185.
28. Rodrigues LR, Banat IM, Teixeira JÁ et al. Biosurfactants: Potential applications in medicine. J Antimicrob Chemother 2006; 57:609-618.
29. Rodrigues LR, Banat IM, Teixeira JA et al. Strategies for the prevention of microbial biofilm formation on silicone rubber voice prostheses. J Biomed Mater Res B Appl Biomater 2007; 81B:358-370.
30. Maier RM. Biosurfactant: evolution and diversity in bacteria. Adv Appl Microbiol 2003; 52:101–121.
31. Gerard J, Lloyd R, Barsby T et al. Massetolides A-H, antimycobacterial cyclic depsipeptides produced by two pseudomonads isolated from marine habitats. J Nat Prod 1997; 60:223-229.
32. Rodrigues LR, Banat IM, Van der Mei HC et al. Interference in adhesion of bacteria and yeasts isolated from explanted voice prostheses to silicone rubber by rhamnolipid biosurfactants. J Appl Microbiol 2005; 100:470-480.
33. Lang S, Wullbrandt D. Rhamnose lipids—biosynthesis, microbial production and application potential. Appl Microbiol Biotechnol 1999; 51:22-32.
34. Maier R, Soberon Chavez G. Pseudomonas aeruginosa rhamnolipids: biosynthesis and potential applications. Appl Microbiol Biotechnol 2000; 54:625-633.
35. Das K, Mukherjee AK. Characterization of biochemical properties and biological activities of biosurfactants produced by pseudomonas aeruginosa mucoid and nonmucoid strains isolated from hydrocarbon-contaminated soil samples. Appl Microbiol Biotechnol 2005; 69:192-199.
36. Vollenbroich D, Pauli G, Ozel M et al. Antimycoplasma properties and applications in cell culture of surfactin, a lipopeptide antibiotic from bacillus subtilis. Appl Env Microbiol 1997; 63:44-49.

37. Vollenbroich D, Ozel M, Vater J et al. Mechanism of inactivation of enveloped viruses by the biosurfactant surfactin from bacillus subtilis. Biologicals 1997; 25:289-297.

38. Kameda Y, Ouchira S, Matsui Kkanatomo S et al. Antitumor activity of bacillus natto V. Isolation and characterization of surfactin in the culture medium of bacillus natto KMD 2311. Chem Pharmacol Bull 1974; 22:938-944.

39. Bernheimer A, Avigad L. Nature and properties of a cytolytic agent produced by Bacillus subtilis. J Gen Microbiol 1970; 61:361-69.

40. Sheppard JD, Jumarie C, Cooper DG et al. Ionic channels induced by surfactin in plannar lipid bilayer membranes. Biochim Biophys Acta 1991; 1064:13-23.

41. Itokawa H, Miyashita T, Morita H et al. Structural and conformational studies of [Ile7] and [Leu7] surfactins from bacillus subtilis. Chem Pharmacol Bull 1994; 42:604-607.

42. Wang CL, Ng TB, Yuan F et al. Induction of apoptosis in human leukemia K562 cells by cyclic lipopeptide from bacillus subtilis natto T-2. Peptides 2007; 28:1344-1350.

43. Dehghan Noudeh G, Housaindokht M, Bazzaz BSF. Isolation, characterization and investigation of surface and haemolytic activities of a lipopeptide biosurfactant produced by Bacillus subtitlis ATCC 6633. J Microbiol 2005; 43:272-276.

44. Naruse N, Tenmyo O, Kobaru S et al. Pumilacidin, a complex of new antiviral antibiotics: production, isolation, chemical properties, structure and biological activity. J Antibiot 1990; 43:267-280.

45. Besson F, Peypoux F, Michel G et al. Characterization of iturin A in antibiotics from various strains of Bacillus subtilis. J Antibiot 1976; 29:1043-1049.

46. Thimon L, Peypoux F, Wallach J et al. Effect of lipopeptide antibiotic, iturin A, on morphology and membrane ultrastructure of yeast cells. FEMS Microbiol Lett 1995; 128:101-106.

47. Tanaka Y, Takashi T, Kazuhik U et al. Method of producing iturin A and antifungal agent for profound mycosis. Biotechnol Adv 1997; 15:234-235.

48. Mittenbuhler K, Loleit M, Baier W et al. Drug specific antibodies: T-cell epitope-lipopeptide conjugates are potent adjuvants for small antigens in vivo and in vitro. Int J Immunopharmacol 1997; 19:277-287.

49. Jenny K, Kappeli O, Fietcher A. Biosurfactants from bacillus licheniformis: structural analysis and characterization. Appl Microbiol Biotechnol 1991; 36:5-13.

50. Lin S, Carswell K, Sharma M. Continuous production of the lipopeptide biosurfactant of bacillus licheniformis JF-2. Appl Microbiol Biotechnol 1994; 41:281-285.

51. Yakimov M, Timmis K, Wray V et al. Characterization of a new lipopeptide surfactant produced by thermotolerant and halotolerant subsurface Bacillus licheniformis BAS50. Appl Env Microbiol 1995; 61:1706-1713.

52. Grangemard I, Wallach J, Maget Dana R et al. Lichenysin: A more efficient cation chelator than surfactin. Appl Biochem Biotechnol 2001; 90:199-210.

53. Kitamoto D, Yanagishita H, Shinbo T et al. Surface active properties and antimicrobial activities of mannosylerythritol lipids as biosurfactants produced by Candida antarctica. J Biotechnol 1993; 29:91-96.

54. Isoda H, Kitamoto D, Shinmoto H et al. Microbial extracellular glycolipid induction of differentiation and inhibition of protein kinase C activity of human promyelocytic leukaemia cell line HL60. Biosci Biotechnol Biochem 1997; 61:609-614.

55. Isoda H, Shinmoto H, Matsumura M et al. The neurite-initiating effect of microbial extracellular glycolipids in PC12 cells. Cytotechnol 1999; 31:163-170.

56. Shibahara M, Zhao X, Wakamatsu Y et al. Mannosylerythritol lipid increases levels of galactoceramide in and neutrite outgrowth from PC12 pheochromocytoma cells. Cytotechnol 2000; 33:247-251.

57. Zhao X, Geltinger C, Kishikawa S et al. Tretament of mouse melanoma cells with phorbol 12-myristate 13-acetate counteracts mannosylerythritol lipid-induced growth arrest and apoptosis. Cytotechnol 2000; 33:123-130.

58. Zhao X, Wakamatsu Y, Shibahara M et al. Mannosylerythritol lipid is a potent inducer of apoptosis and differentiation of mouse melanoma cells in culture. Cancer Res 1999; 59:482-486.

59. Wakamatsu Y, Zhao X, Jin C et al. Mannosylerythritol lipid induces characteristics of neuronal differentiation in PC12 cells through an ERK-related signal cascade. Eur J Biochem 2001; 268:374-383.

60. Ueno Y, Hirashima N, Inoh Y et al. Characterization of biosurfactant-containing liposomes and their efficiency for gene transfection. Biol Pharmaceut Bull 2007; 30:169-172.

61. Ueno Y, Inoh Y, Furuno T et al. NBD-conjugated biosurfactant (MEL-A) shows a new pathway for transfection. J Contr Release 2007; 123:247-253.

62. Shah V, Badia D, Ratsep P. Sophorolipids having enhanced antibacterial activity. Antimicrob Agents Chemother 2007; 51:397-400.

63. Maitani Y, Yano S, Hattori Y et al. Liposome vector containing biosurfactant-complexed DNA as herpes simplex virus thymidine kinase gene delivery system. J Liposome Res 2006; 16:359-372.

64. Konishi M, Imura T, Fukuoka T et al. A yeast glycolipid biosurfactant, mannosylerytritol lipid, shows high binding affinity towards lectins on a self-assembled monolayer system. Biotechnol Lett 2007; 29:473-480.
65. Ito S, Imura T, Fukuoka T et al. Kinetic studies on the interactions between glycolipid biosurfactant assembled monolayers and various classes of immunoglobulins using surface plasmon resonance. Colloids Surf B Biointerfaces 2007; 58:165-171.
66. Igarashi S, Hattori Y, Maitani Y. Biosurfactant MEL-A enhances cellular association and gene transfection by cationic liposome. J Contr Release 2006; 112:362-368.
67. Uchida Y, Misava S, Nakahara T et al. Factor affecting the production of succinotrehalose lipids by rodococcus erythropolis SD-74 grown on n-alkanes. Agr Biol Chem 1989; 53:765-769.
68. Uchida Y, Tsuchiya R, Chino M et al. Extracellular accumulation of mono and di succinyl trehalose lipids by a strain of rodococcus erythropolis grown on n-alkanes. Agr Biol Chem 1989; 53:757-763.
69. Busscher HJ, Neu T, Van der Mei HC. Biosurfactant production by thermophilic dairy streptococci. Appl Microbiol Biotechnol 1994; 41:4-7.
70. Rodrigues LR, Van der Mei HC, Teixeira J et al. The influence of biosurfactants from probiotic bacteria on the formation of voice prosthetic biofilms. Appl Env Microbiol 2004; 70:4408-4410.
71. Rodrigues LR, Van der Mei HC, Banat IM et al. Inhibition of microbial adhesion to silicone rubber treated with biosurfactant from streptococcus thermophilus A. FEMS Immunol Med Microbiol 2004; 6:107-125.
72. Busscher HJ, Van Hoogmoed CG, Geertsema Doornbusch GI et al. Streptococcus thermophilus and its biosurfactants inhibit adhesion by candida spp on silicone rubber. Appl Env Microbiol 1997; 63:3810-3817.
73. Busscher HJ, Van de Belt-Gritter B, Westerhof M et al. Microbial interference in the colonization of silicone rubber implant surfaces in the oropharynx: Streptococcus thermophilus against a mixed fungal/ bacterial biofilm. In: Rosenberg E, ed. Microbial Ecology and Infectious Disease. Washington DC: American Society for Microbiology, 1999:66-74.
74. Pratt Terpstra IH, Weerkamp AH, Busscher HJ. Microbial factors in a thermodynamic approach of oral streptococcal adhesion to solid substrata. J Col Int Sci 1989; 129:568-574.
75. Van Hoogmoed CG, Van der Kuijl Booij M, Van der Mei HC et al. Inhibition of streptococcus mutans NS adhesion to glass with and without a salivary conditioning film by biosurfactant-releasing streptococcus mitis strain. Appl Env Microbiol 2000; 66:659-663.
76. Velraeds M, Van der Mei HC, Reid G et al. Inibition of initial adhesion of uropathogenic enterococcus faecalis to solid substrata by an adsorbed biosurfactant layer from Lactobacillus acidophilus. Urology 1997; 49:790-794.
77. Reid G, Zalai C, Gardiner G. Urogenital Lactobacilli probiotics, reliability and regulatory issues. J Dairy Sci 1984; 84:164-169.
78. Reid G, Heinemann C, Velraeds M et al. Biosurfactants produced by lactobacillus. Methods Enzymol 1999; 310:426-433.
79. Velraeds M, Van der Mei HC, Reid G et al. Physicochemical and biochemical characterization of biosurfactants released by Lactobacillus strains. Colloids Surf B Biointerfaces 1996; 8:51-61.
80. Velraeds M, Van der Mei HC, Reid G et al. Inhibition of initial adhesion of uropathogenic enterococcus faecalis by biosurfactants from lactobacillus isolates. Appl Env Microbiol 1996; 62:1958-1963.
81. Gotek P, Bednarski W, Lewandowska M. Characterization of adhesive properties of lactobacillus strains synthesising biosurfactants. Polish J Nat Sci 2007; 22:333-342.
82. Rodrigues LR, Van der Mei HC, Teixeira J et al. Biosurfactant from lactococcus lactis 53 inhibit microbial adhesion on silicone rubber. Appl Microbiol Biotechnol 2004; 66:306-311.
83. Kikuchi T, Hasumi K. Enhancement of reciprocal activation of prourokinase plasminogen by the bacterial lipopeptide surfactins and iturins. J Antibiot 2003; 56:34-37.
84. Van Bogaert INA, Saerens K, De Muynck C et al. Microbial production and application of sophorolipids. Appl Microbiol Biotechnol 2007; 76:23-34.
85. Sudo T, Zhao X, Wakamatsu Y et al. Induction of the differentiation of human HL-60 promyelocytic leukemia cell line by succinoyl trehalose lipids. Cytotechnol 2000; 33:259-264.
86. Im J, Nakane T, Yanagishita H et al. Mannosylerythritol lipid, a yeast extracellular glycolip, shows high binding affinity towards human immunoglobulin G. BMC Biotechnol 2001;1:1-5.
87. Im JH, Yanagishita H, Ikegami T et al. Mannosylerythritol lipids, yeast glycolipid biosurfactants, are potential affinity ligand materials for human immunoglobulin G. J Biomed Mat Res 2003; 65:379-385.
88. Inoh Y, Kitamoto D, Hirashima N et al. Biosurfactants of MEL-A increase gene transfection mediated by cationic liposomes. Biochem Biophys Res Comm 2001; 289:57-61.
89. Inoh Y, Kitamoto D, Hirashima N et al. Biosurfactant MEL-A dramatically increases gene transfection via membrane fusion. J Contr Release 2004; 94:423-431.

90. Kitamoto D, Isoda H, Nakahara T. Functions and potential applications of glycolipid biosurfactants—from energy-saving materials to gene delivery carriers. J Biosci Bioeng 2002; 94:187-201.
91. Wright JR. Pulmonary surfactant: a front line of lung host defense. J Clin Inv 2003; 111:1453-1455.
92. Sano H, Sohma H, Muta T et al. Pulmonary surfactant protein A modulates the cellular response to smooth and rough lipopolysaccharides by interaction with CD14. J Immunol 1999; 163:387-395.
93. Sen R, Swaminathan T. Characterization of concentration and purification parameters and operating conditions for the small-scale recovery of surfactin. Proc Biochem 2005; 40:2953-2958.
94. Carrillo C, Teruel J, Aranda F et al. Molecular mechanism of membrane permeabilization by the peptide antibiotic surfactin. Biochim Biophys Acta 2003; 1611:91-97.
95. Kim K, Jung SY, Lee DK et al. Suppression of inflammatory responses by surfactin, a selective inhibitor of platelet cytosolic phospholipase A2. Biochem Pharmacol 1998; 55:975-985.
96. Kikuchi T, Hasumi K. Enhancement of plasminogen activation by surfactin C: augmentation of fibrinolysis in vitro and in vivo. Biochim Biophys Acta 2002; 1596:234-245.
97. Moyne AL, Shelby R, Cleveland TE et al. Bacillomycin D: an iturin with antifungal activity against aspergillus flavus. J Appl Microbiol 2001; 90:622-629.
98. Kosaric N. Biosurfactants. In: Rehm HJ, Reed G, Puhler A et al, eds. Biotechnology. P. Weinheim VCH 1996:659-717.
99. Nielsen T, Christophersen C, Anthoni U et al. Viscosinamide, a new cyclic depsipeptide with surfactant and antifungal properties produced by pseudomonas fluorescens DR54. J Appl Microbiol1999; 86:80-90.
100. Neu T, Hartner T, Poralla K. Surface active properties of viscosin: a peptidolipid antibiotic. Appl Microbiol Biotechnol 1990; 32:518-20.
101. Bidel DJ, Aly R, Shinefield HR. Inhibition of microbial adherence by sphinganine. Can J Microbiol 1992; 38:983-985.
102. Van Delden C, Iglewski B. Cell-to-cell signaling and pseudomonas aeruginosa infections. Emerg Infect Dis 1998; 4:551-560.
103. Ishigami Y, Suzuki S. Development of biochemicals—functionalization of biosurfactants and natural dyes. Prog Organ Coat 1997; 31:51-61.
104. Ramisse F, Delden C, Gidenne S et al. Decreased virulence of a strain of pseudomonas aeruginosa O12 overexpressing a chromosomal type 1 b-lactamase could be due to reduced expression of cell-to-cell signalling dependent virulence factors. FEMS Immunol Med Microbiol 2000; 28:241-245.
105. Sotirova A, Spasova D, Vasileva Tonkova E et al. Effects of rhamnolipid-biosurfactant on cell surface of pseudomonas aeruginosa. Microbiol Res 2007; In press.
106. Mireles JR, Toguchi A, Harshey RM. Salmonella enterica serovar typhimurium swarming mutants with altered biofilm formation abilities: surfactin inhibits biofilm formation. J Bacteriol 2001; 183:5848-5854.
107. Boris S, Barbés C. Role played by lactobacilli in controlling the population of vaginal pathogens. Microbes Infect 2000; 2:543-546.
108. Velraeds M, Van de Belt Gritter B, Van der Mei HC et al. Interference in initial adhesion of uropathogenic bacteria and yeasts to silicone rubber by a Lactobacillus acidophilus biosurfactant. J Med Microbiol 1998; 47:1081-1085.
109. Reid G. In vitro testing of Lactobacillus acidophilus NCFM as a possible probiotic for the urogenital tract. Int Dairy J 2000; 10:415-419.
110. Heinemann C, Van Hylckama V, Janssen D et al. Purification and characterization of a surface-binding protein from Lactobacillus fermentum RC-14 that inhibits adhesion of Enterococcus faecalis 1131. FEMS Microbiol Lett 2000; 190:177-180.
111. Cameotra S, Makkar R. Recent applications of biosurfactants as biological and immunological molecules. Curr Opin Microbiol 2004; 7:262-266.
112. Reid G, Bruce A, Smeianov V. The role of Lactobacilli in preventing urogenital and intestinal infections. Inter Dairy J 1998; 8:555-562.
113. Reid G, Bruce A, Fraser N et al. Oral probiotics can resolve urogenital infections. FEMS Immunol Med Microbiol 2001; 30:49-52.
114. Gan B, Kim J, Reid G et al. Lactobacillus fermentum RC-14 inhibits staphylococcus aureus infection of surgical implants in rats. J Infect Dis 2002; 185:1369-1372.
115. Mack DR, Michail S, Wei S et al. Probiotics inhibit enteropathogenic E. coli adherence in vitro by inducing intestinal mucin gene expression. Am J Physiol 1999; 276:941-950.
116. Millsap K, Reid G, Van der Mei HC et al. Adhesion of Lactobacillus *species* in urine and phosphate buffer to silicone rubber and glass under flow. Biomaterials 1996; 18:87-91.

CHAPTER 7

Microbial Surfactants of Marine Origin:
Potentials and Prospects

Palashpriya Das, Soumen Mukherjee, C. Sivapathasekaran
and Ramkrishna Sen*

Abstract

Marine environment occupies the vast majority of the earth's surface and is a rich source of highly potent and active compounds. In recent years, microbial surfactants and emulsifiers have been reported from marine microflora. Surfactant and emulsifier molecules having diverse chemical nature such as exopolysaccharides, carbohydrate-lipid-protein complexes or glycolipopeptide, glycolipids, lipopeptides, phospholipids and ornithine lipids have been reported from various marine bacteria. These surface-active agents have been found to possess good emulsification and stabilization potentials for various lipophilic compounds such as aliphatic, aromatic and polyaromatic hydrocarbons and their uptake and degradation by the microorganisms. Few biosurfactant types such as glycolipids and lipopeptides have also been found to possess valuable biological activities. Surface-active agents from marine environments thus have tremendous potential to be used in industrial processes, for environmental remediation and as drugs.

Introduction

Biosurfactants are surface-active agents of microbial origin. They have both hydrophobic and hydrophilic domains in the same molecule, due to which, they partition at the interfaces between liquid phases. The major classes of biosurfactants include glycolipids, lipopeptides and lipoprotein, phospholipids and fatty acids, polymeric biosurfactants and particulate biosurfactants.[1] They outperform their chemical counterparts in various aspects such as their lesser toxicity, stability at extremes of temperature, pH and salinity, higher biodegradability hence ecological acceptability and ability to be synthesized from cheap renewable resources.[2] Broadly, these molecules can be classified into two groups viz. low molecular weight and high molecular weight biosurfactants. The low molecular weight biosurfactants (Mw: 1-2 KDa) are generally glycolipids or lipopeptides and are more effective in lowering the interfacial and surface tension. The high molecular weight group of biosurfactants (Mw > 1 MDa), which are mostly amphipathic polysaccharides, proteins, lipopolysaccharides and lipoproteins are effective stabilizers of oil-in-water emulsions.[3] Several groups of researchers have suggested that biosurfactants are important for microbial growth and survival in the environment.[4,5] However, the reason behind the production of biosurfactants by these microorganisms is not always so obvious. Some proposed physiological roles of biosurfactants include increasing the surface area and bioavailability of hydrophobic water-insoluble substrates, heavy metal binding, bacterial pathogenesis, quorum sensing and biofilm formation.[5] For example, viscosinamide production by *Pseudomonas fluorescens* strain is coupled to primary metabolism and

*Corresponding Author: Ramkrishna Sen—Bioprocess and Bioproduct Laboratory, Department of Biotechnology, Indian Institute of Technology Kharagpur, West Bengal 721302, India. Email: rksen@yahoo.com or rksen@hijli.iitkgp.ernet.in

Biosurfactants, edited by Ramkrishna Sen. ©2010 Landes Bioscience and Springer Science+Business Media.

cell proliferation in the producing bacteria.[6] Rhamnolipid is necessary for normal biofilm formation by *Pseudomonas aeruginosa*.[7] Hence, it might be reasonable to assume that different groups of biosurfactants have different natural roles in the growth of the producing microorganisms. Therefore, two closely related organisms belonging to the same genus and species, but present in two different habitats, may produce different biosurfactant isoforms to sustain their growth in that particular environment; one group of biosurfactants would have an advantage in a specific ecological niche, whereas another group of emulsifier would be more appropriate for a different niche.[5] Because of their unique physicochemical properties these compounds find potential industrial and environmental applications. They also have potential therapeutic applications as antibacterial, antiviral and antifungal agents.[8] The biosurfactant producing microorganisms reported till date are mostly obtained from terrestrial sources. The marine environment which occupies nearly about three-fourth of the earth's surface is a robust reservoir of diverse microflora including biosurfactant producers. Few reports on biosurfactants from marine microbes have been described later in the text. Most of the biosurfactants of marine origin have been evaluated for their environmental remediation application potentials but their therapeutic potentials have not been exploited extensively. Hence the scientific community is on an incessant quest for marine compounds with therapeutic applications by keeping in mind the great diversity of structures obtained from this source.

In the recent years, several types of biosurfactants such as exopolysaccharides, glycolipopeptides, carbohydrate-lipid-protein complexes, glycolipids as well as lipopeptide, have been isolated from various genera of microorganisms of marine origin (Table 1). A detailed description of these microbial surfactants, their composition, structure and their potential application in environmental and therapeutic fields follows.

Marine Biosurfactants and Bioemulsifiers

Exopolysaccharide Biosurfactants

The exopolysaccharide biosurfactants form an important group of marine biosurfactants. Microbial genera such as *Alcaligenes, Pseudomonas, Halomonas* and *Antarctobacter* have been reported as the main producers of this type of biosurfactants. For example, tetradecan degrading *Alcaligenes* sp. PHY 9L.86 was isolated from hydrocarbon polluted sea-surface water. This marine bacterium produced surface active exopolysaccharides (extracellular carbohydrates) and lipids which caused foam formation and emulsification of the culture medium.[9] The extracellular lipid concentration was found to attain a maximum value of 7.91 mg L^{-1} in the early stationary phase, whereas maximum concentration of exopolysaccharides reached 12.63 mg L^{-1} at the stationary phase. The extracellular lipids produced by this strain was composed mainly of phospholipids, free fatty acids, triglycerides, monoglycerides and wax esters amongst which the percentage of free fatty acids (73%) was the highest. Electron microscopy revealed the presence of fibrillar structures made up of exopolysaccharides around the microorganism which were connected to the lipid vesicles having a possible role in emulsification and hydrocarbon degradation. The capacity for assimilation and degradation of the hydrocarbons depended on the availability of these surface active compounds. Another EPS producing strain, *Pseudomonas putida* ML2, isolated from hydrocarbon-polluted sediment, produced emulsifiers during growth on a hydrophobic substrate, naphthalene, in the exponential and the stationary phase of growth.[10] The crude EPS emulsifier had a molecular mass between 10-80 kDa and contained no proteins. The monosaccharide composition was rhamnose, glucose and glucosamine in a molar ratio of 3:2:1. Similarly, another EPS bioemulsifier producer *Planococcus maitriensis* Anita I was isolated from seawater collected from coastal area of Gujrat, India.[11] The EPS obtained from this strain contained 12.06% carbohydrate, 24.44% protein, 11% uronic acid and 3.03% sulfate. Similarly, marine strain *Antarctobacter* sp. produced emulsifiers AE22 starting from the late exponential phase of its growth.[12] The carbohydrate content of AE22 was 15.4 ± 0.2% dry mass. Sugar analysis showed that this polymer contained hexoses (rhamnose, fucose, galactose, glucose and mannose)

Table 1. Marine biosurfactants/bioemulsifiers, their producer microorganisms and chemical nature

Type of Biosurfactant/Bioemulsifier	Producer Organism	Chemical Composition	Ref.
Extracellular polysaccharide-Lipid	Alcaligenes sp. PHY 9L-86	EPS and lipid (phospholipids, free fatty acids, triglycerides, monoglycerides and wax esters)	9
Extracellular polysaccharide	Pseudomonas putida ML2	Monosaccharides (rhamnose: glucose: glucosamine :: 3:2:1)	10
Extracellular polysaccharide	Planococcus maitriensis Anita I	Carbohydrate (12.06%), protein (24.44%), uronic acid (11%) and sulfate (3.03%)	11
Extracellular polysaccharide	Antarctobacter sp.	Carbohydrates—rhamnose, fucose, galactose, glucose and mannose, galactosamine, glucosamine and muramic acid, galacturonic acid and glucuronic acid Amino acids—aspartic acid, glycine and alanine	12
Extracellular polysaccharide	Halomonas sp. TG39, Halomonas sp. TG 67	Carbohydrates—Rhamnose, glucuronic acid, galactose, glucosamine and mannose Amino acids—aspartic acid, glutamic acid, glycine and alanine	13
Glycolipopeptide	Corynebacterium kutscheri	Carbohydrate (40%), lipid (27%), protein (29%)	14
Glycolipopeptide	Yarrowia lipolytica	Fatty acids—palmitic acid (35.8%), stearic acid (21.4%), lauric acid (8.8%) and oleic acid (6.9%) Carbohydrates—arabinose : galactose : glucose : mannose :: 1:6:17:31	15
Glycolipopeptide	Yarrowia lipolytica	lipid-carbohydrate-protein complex having 75% lipid (palmitic acid being the major lipid), 20% carbohydrate (mannose and galactose) and 5% protein (amino acids like aspartic acid, alanine and threonine).	16
Glycolipopeptide	Halomonas sp. ANT-3b	Carbohydrates—Mannose : galactose : glucose :: 1.71: 1.00: 2.96. Lipid—Caprylic acid : Myristic acid : Palmitic acid : palmitoleic acid : oleic acid ::18.85:1.0: 9.68: 5.69:1.26	17
Glycolipid	Pseudomonas aeruginosa A41	Not available	18

continued on next page

Table 1. *Continued*

Type of Biosurfactant/Bioemulsifier	Producer Organism	Chemical Composition	Ref.
Glycolipid	Bacterial strain MM1	Sugar—glucose Lipid part -3-OH-decanoic acids	19
Glycolipid	*Nocardioides* sp.	Sugar—rhamnose	20
Glycolipid	*Pantoea* sp.	Not available	21
Glycolipid	*Rhodococcus erythropolis*	12 types of free fatty acids (C_{10}–C_{22}) are present with docosenoic acid ($C_{22}H_{42}O_2$) as the most abundant component. Sugar—glucose and trehalose	22
Glycolipid	*Aeromonas* sp.	38% carbohydrate and an unidentified lipid	23
Glycolipid and phospholipids	*Alcanivorax borkumensis*	The main component of the glycolipid part is 18-(1-β-glucopyranosyl)-6,10,14-triheptyl-4,8,12,16-tetroxy-3-aza-7,11,15-trioxa-pentaeicosanoic acid. Phospholipid part had phosphatidylglycerol, palmitic, hexadecenoic and octadecenoic acid.	24
Lipopeptide	*Pseudomonas* sp. isolates MK90e85 and MK91CC8	Cyclic depsipeptides (massetolides and viscosin)	25
Lipopeptide	*Bacillus pumilus* KMM 150	Cyclic depsipeptides (Amino acids -leucine: valine: aspartic acid: glutamic acid:: 4: 1: 1: 1). The fatty acid component—3β-hydroxypentadecanoic acid (C_{15}-β-hydroxy acid and C_{13}-C_{14}- β-hydroxy acid)	26
Lipopeptide	*Bacillus pumilus* KMM 1364	Lipid part consisted of C_{15}, C_{16} and C_{17} fatty acids. Peptide part -Asx: Glx: Leu: Val or Ile (1:1:4:1)	27
Lipopeptide	*Bacillus circulans*	Not available	28, 8
Lipopeptide	*Brevibacillus laterosporus* PNG-276	Amino acid sequence in the pentapeptide chain: Tyr-Ser-Leu-Trp-Arg.	29
Aminolipid	*Myroides* sp. strain SM1	L-ornithine lipids	30, 31

amino sugars (galactosamine, glucosamine and muramic acid) and uronic acids (galacturonic acid and glucuronic acid). Fucose ($16.2 \pm 0.2\%$), glucosamine ($31.9 \pm 0.4\%$) and glucuronic acid ($20.3 \pm 0.7\%$) were the most abundant sugars present in this bioemulsifier. The amino acid content of this biopolymer was $5.0 \pm 0.2\%$ dry mass and three amino acids—aspartic acid, glycine and alanine contributed to 37.3% of the total amino acid content. The active fraction of the extracellular emulsifier AE22 had a molecular mass of more than 2000 kDa. Similar high molecular mass emulsifiers have also been reported from bacterial strains like TG39 and TG67 later characterized as *Halomonas* sp.[13] These cultures showed profuse growth and emulsifier production during the exponential growth phase and the emulsions formed were stable even up to 6 months. The carbohydrate content of the biopolymers from TG39 was $17.3 \pm 1.0\%$ which consisted mainly of rhamnose ($31.7 \pm 2.1\%$), glucuronic acid ($27.9 \pm 1.9\%$) and galactose ($15.3 \pm 0.5\%$) while the carbohydrate content in TG67 bioemulsifiers was $22.7 \pm 0.8\%$ and had glucuronic acid ($58.8 \pm 0.4\%$), glucosamine ($10.9 \pm 0.1\%$) and mannose ($11.5 \pm 0.5\%$) as the major components. The amino acid analysis revealed that the total amino acid content in bioemulsifiers from TG39 and TG67 were $26.6 \pm 1.0\%$ and $40.5 \pm 1.6\%$ respectively and contained four major amino acids viz. aspartic acid, glutamic acid, glycine and alanine. However, no fatty acids were detected in its structural composition. The emulsifiers from both the strains upon chromatography resolved into multiple fractions. TG39 emulsifiers separated into three main components having molecular mass more than 2000 kDa, 150 kDa and 16.5 kDa respectively, whereas TG67 emulsifiers fractionated into two major components with molecular mass of 1300 kDa and 56 kDa respectively.

Glycolipopeptides and Carbohydrate-Lipid-Protein Complexes

Another important class of biosurfactants and emulsifiers from marine bacteria are the carbohydrate-lipid-protein complexes or glycolipopeptides being produced from bacteria like *Corynebacterium* sp. and *Halomonas* sp. as well as yeasts like *Yarrowia* sp. A strain of *Corynebacterium kutscheri* isolated from Tuticorin harbor, India utilized substrates like waste motor lubricant oil and peanut oil cake and produced glycolipopeptide type of biosurfactant having a chemical composition of carbohydrates (40%), lipid (27%) and protein (29%).[14] The maximum biosurfactant concentrations achieved in the early stationary phase of the growth were 3.85 g L^{-1} and 6.4 g L^{-1} using waste motor lubricant oil and peanut oil cake respectively. The biosurfactant thus produced emulsified various hydrocarbons, vegetable oils and polyaromatic hydrocarbons. Yansan is another bioemulsifier being produced by a strain of *Yarrowia lipolytica*, isolated from Guanabara Bay in Brazil, during cultivation in glucose based YPD medium.[15] Although the emulsifier was isolated in the late stationary phase, significant emulsifying capacity was also observed in cell free supernatant from the exponential phase. The protein content in this bioemulsifier was found to be 15% while the lipid content was below 1%. The fatty acids present in the lipid were palmitic acid (35.8%), stearic acid (21.4%), lauric acid (8.8%) and oleic acid (6.9%). The monosaccharide composition of this bioemulsifier was arabinose, galactose, glucose and mannose in a ratio of 1:6:17:31. The molecular weight of this bioemulsifier was approximately 20 kDa. The CMC value of Yansan was found to be 0.5 g L^{-1} and the minimum surface tension attained at CMC was 50mN m^{-1}. Yet another emulsifier producer strain, *Yarrowia lipolytica* NCIM 3589 being isolated from an oil contaminated sample produced emulsifiers in the stationary phase of its growth.[16] The isolated emulsifier was found to be a lipid-carbohydrate-protein complex having 75% lipid, 20% carbohydrate and 5% protein. 80% of the lipid part comprised of palmitic acid, mannose and galactose constituted the carbohydrate part while the major amino acids present were aspartic acid, alanine and threonine. The emulsifier was found to stabilize oil-in-water emulsions with several aromatic hydrocarbons.

Glycolipids

Glycolipid biosurfactants are the types in which the molecules consist of a hydrophilic glyco part consisting of few sugar molecules and a hydrophobic lipid portion. Various microbial genera like *Halomonas*, *Pantoea*, *Nocardioides*, *Rhodococcus* to name a few are the ones which produce glycolipids type of biosurfactants. The *n*-hexadecane degrading biosurfactant producer *Halomonas* sp. ANT-3b being isolated from Ross sea, Antarctica, showed best growth and emulsifier production at low temperature of 15˚C using *n*-hexadecane as the sole source of carbon.[17] The molecular weight of the major component of the glycolipid emulsifier was determined to be 18 kDa. The monosaccharide present in the emulsifier was mannose, galactose and glucose in a molar ratio of 1.71: 1.00: 2.96. The lipid part of this glycolipid biosurfactant consisted in terms of molar ratio—caprylic acid: myristic acid: palmitic acid: palmitoleic acid: oleic acid (3:1.5:1). Similarly, *Pseudomonas aeruginosa* A41 isolated from the gulf of Thailand produced rhamnolipids, another glycolipid biosurfactant.[18] The biosurfactant yield steadily increased even after attaining the stationary phase thereby lowering the surface tension of the culture media from 55-70 mN/m to 27.8-30 mN/m for a variety of carbon substrates such as coconut oil, palm oil, olive oil, lauric acid, myristic acid, palmitic acid, strearic acid, oleic acid and linoleic acid. Highest yield of rhamnolipids (6.58 g L^{-1}) was obtained using olive oil as the carbon substrate. Although the rhamnolipid yield using palm oil as the carbon source was lower (2.91 g L^{-1}), it was found to be best in surface tension reduction. In general it was found that substrates with shorter fatty acid chains ($C_{12}>C_{14}>C_{16}$) and those having unsaturation ($C_{18:2}$) resulted in biosurfactant production with higher rhamnose content and greater oil displacement activity. Yet another bacterial strain MM1 isolated from the Isle of Borkum produced an anionic glucose lipid in batch fermentation experiments.[19] After fermentation for 91 h, the maximum biosurfactant concentration of 1.7 g L^{-1}, was achieved. HPLC revealed the sugar part of this glycolipid as glucose whereas lipid part of this molecule consisted of 3-OH-decanoic acids. The glucose lipid produced by this strain had a CMC value of 25 mg L^{-1} and was able to reduce the surface tension of water from 72 mN m^{-1} to a minimum value of 30 mN m^{-1}. Another glycolipid biosurfactant producing strain *Nocardioides* sp. was isolated from the Antarctic soil.[20] The secretion of rhamnose in the n-paraffin media coupled with a decrease in the surface tension of the medium to 35 mN m^{-1} after 16 days of growth indicated the production of rhamnolipids. The cell free supernatant contained 0.18 ± 0.06 g L^{-1} proteins, 0.45 ± 0.15 g L^{-1} lipids and 1.1 ± 0.19 g L^{-1} carbohydrates. The biosurfactant product obtained caused hemolysis and inhibited *Bacillus subtilis* cells. It was also able to emulsify n-parrafin and several other aromatic hydrocarbons. Similarly, facultative anaerobe *Pantoea* sp. strain A-13 isolated from Frazier Islands, Antarctica produced glycolipid biosurfactants when grown on n-paraffins or kerosene as the sole source of carbon.[21] Enhanced production of these glycolipids (0.8-1.2 g L^{-1}) was detected at the stationary phase of the growth evident by increase in emulsification activity and rhamnose concentration. These glycolipids produced after 12 days of fermentation reduced the surface tension of the culture medium to 37 mN m^{-1}. A CMC value of 40 mg L^{-1} was determined for these biosurfactants. At early stationary phase of the growth, the cell surface hydrophobicity was found to higher ($43.9 \pm 1.9\%$ to $57.5 \pm 3.2\%$) for hydrocarbon grown cells, than that of glucose grown cells ($27.2 \pm 1.8\%$). Another glycolipid biosurfactant producer was *Rhodococcus erythropolis* 3C-9 being isolated from a soil sample obtained from Island of Xiamen, located on the west bank of the Taiwan Strait.[22] The strain was selected amongst the hexadecane degraders due to its high capacity of oil degradation and emulsification. The culture did not produce biosurfactants when cultivated on water-miscible substrates like glucose, sucrose or glycerol and required alkanes to induce biosurfactant production. The biosurfactant produced by this strain using n-hexane as the sole carbon source lowered the surface tension to a minimum value of 33.4 mN m^{-1}. However, it was found that the resting cells of this strain were unable to produce any biosurfactant. Fatty acid analysis of the crude biosurfactant showed that there were 12 types of free fatty acids (C_{10}-C_{22}) present, most of which were straight chain. These fatty acids were mostly unsaturated with docosenoic acid ($C_{22}H_{42}O_2$) as the most abundant (37.03%) component. Thin layer chromatography (TLC) separated the glycolipids of the biosurfactant into two components, lipid 1 ($Rf_1 = 0.51$) and lipid 2 ($Rf_2 = 0.15$). Staining with specific reagents on the TLC plates confirmed that both the fractions were glycolipids. The hydrophilic sugar moiety of glycolipid 1 (GL1) was found to be glucose while that for glycolipid 2 (GL2) was trehalose. The hydrophobic part of the GL1 consisted of seven straight chain fatty acids ranging from C_{12}-C_{18}. Amongst these the C_{12} unsaturated fatty acid

$(C_{12}H_{22}O_2)$ was found to be the most abundant component (32.93%). The hydrophobic moiety of GL2 also consisted of seven straight chain fatty acids ranging from C_{10}-C_{18}. However the most abundant (35.81%) component was a C_{16} saturated fatty acid $(C_{16}H_{32}O_2)$. Another glycolipid type of biosurfactant was obtained from a marine *Aeromonas* sp. collected from tropical estuarine water.[23] The compound contained 38% carbohydrate, an unidentified lipid but no protein and thus was classified as a glycolipid. The strain showed good growth and biosurfactant production when crude oil, diesel or hexadecane were used as carbon substrates. However, glucose was found to be the best substrate for biosurfactant production. Although the biosurfactant was detected as early as day 4 of fermentation using crude oil as carbon substrate, maximum cell density and biosurfactant production was obtained on the day 8. Yet another glycolipid producer, *Alcanivorax borkumensis* DSM 11573, isolated from oil contaminated marine environments produced glucose lipid during the logarithmic phase of growth.[24] This strain produced medium polarity components which were glycolipids and highly polar components which were determined to be phospholipids. The glycolipid fraction contained 10 medium polar glycolipid fractions with m/z 916, 888, 860. The main glycolipid of the *A. borkumensis* was found to 18-(1-β-glucopyranosyl)-6,10,14-triheptyl-4,8,12,16-tetroxy-3-aza-7,11,15-trioxa-pentaeicosanoic acid. The highly polar phospholipids had three major fractions having m/z 720, 746 and 748. The hydrophilic parts of these molecules had phosphatidylglycerol while the fatty acid part consisted of palmitic acid, hexadecenoic acid and octadecenoic acid.

Lipopeptides

Another major class of biosurfactants are lipopeptides. These molecules have a hydrophilic peptide head group and a hydrophobic lipid tail. Several species of marine microorganisms such as *Bacillus*, *Pseudomonas* and *Myroides* have been reported to produce this type of surfactants. For example, two marine isolates MK90e85 and MK91CC8, identified as *Pseudomonas* sp. produced antimycobacterial cyclic depsipeptides and viscosin.[25] The marine isolate MK90e85 which was obtained from a red alga produced massetolides A, B, C and D while the other isolate MK91CC8 obtained from a marine tubeworm produced massetolides E, F, G, H and viscosin. Massetolide A, which was an optically active molecule, had a mass of 1141 Da and a molecular formula of $C_{55}H_{97}N_9O_{16}$. Massetolide A and viscosin showed antimicrobial action against *Mycobacterium tuberculosis* and *Mycobacterium avium-intracellulare*. Several *Bacillus* sp. from marine environment also have been reported to produce surface-active compounds. A mixture of cyclic depsipeptides originally named as *bacircines* was obtained from the cultures of *Bacillus pumilus* KMM 150 isolated from an Australian marine sponge *Ircinia* sp.[26] The culture growing at a temperature of 24-26°C on a mineral salts medium produced a mixture of cyclic depsipeptides with molecular masses of 1007, 1021, 1035 Daltons. The *bacircines* 4 and 5 could be described by the empirical formula $C_{53}H_{93}N_7O_{13}$ and had the molecular mass of 1035 Daltons. These had the amino acid composition of Leu: Val: Asp: Glu in the ratio of 4: 1: 1: 1. The fatty acid component of these compounds was identified as 3β-hydroxypentadecanoic acid (C_{15}-β-hydroxy acid). Contrastingly, *bacircines* 1, 2 and 3 had molecular masses of 1007, 1021 and 1021 respectively. The amino acid composition was similar to that of *bacircines* 4 and 5; however the lipophilic part of these molecules were different. Instead this group of compounds had C_{13}-C_{14}- β-hydroxy acid as the lipophilic side chain. Similarly, the marine bacterium *Bacillus pumilus* KMM 1364 isolated from the surface of the ascidian *Halocynthia aurantium* produced a mixture of analogues of lipopeptide surfactin.[27] Eight different compounds were separated by RP-HPLC which gave positive ninhydrin test. Amino acid analysis revealed that seven amino acids were present: Asx: Glx: Leu: Val or Ile in molar ratios 1:1:4:1. These major components of lipopeptide molecules had molecular masses of 1035, 1049, 1063, 1077. The variations in the molecular masses of these components were caused due to differences in the methylene groups of the lipid or peptide part of the compound. The structural difference of these compounds from surfactin, a well-known lipopeptide biosurfactant, was due to the substitution of valine by leucine at position 4 in the peptide chain of the molecule. The lipid part of the molecule consisted of C_{15}, C_{16} and C_{17} fatty acids. These surfactins were quite different from similar molecules reported earlier[26] and thus production of various isoforms not only depends on the culture conditions but also on the bacterial strain. These variations in molecular structures may confer certain bioactive properties to these molecules. Recently we reported a marine *Bacillus circulans* that was isolated from sea water sample from Andaman and Nicobar Islands. The crude lipopeptide biosurfactants obtained from this culture was resolved into six major fractions using RP-HPLC. Only one of these fractions was found to possess profound antimicrobial action against various Gram-positive and Gram-negative bacterial strains. Mild antimicrobial action was also shown against multi-drug resistant *Staphylococcus aureus* (MRSA) and other MDR strains.[8] The biosurfactants from this strain also increased the bioavailability of hydrophobic polyaromatic hydrocarbons (PAH) such as anthracene and facilitated their biodegradation.[28] Similar lipopeptide compounds have also been reported from other strains. For example, a marine bacterial isolate PNG-276 was obtained from the tissues of an unidentified tubeworm collected from the coast of Loloata Island, Papua, New Guinea and was later identified as *Brevibacillus laterosporus*.[29] The culture produced a lipopeptide, Tauramamide, having a molecular mass of 878.51 Da ($C_{45}H_{68}N_9O_9$). Arginine, tryptophan, leucine, tyrosine and serine residues were identified in its molecular structure among which tyrosine and leucine had D-configuration while Arginine, tryptophan and serine had L configuration. The sequence of amino acids in the pentapeptide chain was Tyr-Ser-Leu-Trp-Arg. Tauramamide and its methyl ester showed antimicrobial action. Other marine bacteria such as *Myroides* sp. strain SM1 produced L-ornithine lipids which were able to emulsify weathered crude oil.[30] The crude biosurfactant secreted in the culture medium was extracted through solvent extraction and purified by normal and reverse phase silica gel column chromatography. The mass determination by FAB-MS showed that the purified fraction had a mixture of compounds of variable carbon chain lengths. Both the cell suspension and the culture supernatant were able to emulsify weathered crude oil and *n*-hexadecane which indicated that the emulsifiers produced are secreted into culture supernatant as well as they remained attached to the cell walls. The results indicated that the microorganism was able to colonize on the surface of the emulsified droplets of the weathered crude oil.[31]

Environmental and Industrial Potentials

The marine biosurfactants have proved their potential in environmental bioremediation. Studies suggested that these biosurfactants can be used for cleaning the environments polluted with crude oil or polyaromatic hydrocarbons. Besides their applications in environmental cleaning, these molecules have also been found to be useful for industrial emulsification and stabilization processes (Table 2).

The high molecular weight emulsifiers such as the exopolysaccharide type of biosurfactants isolated from various marine bacteria showed their efficacy in environmental cleaning and potential for industrial application. For example, the exopolysaccharide producer marine bacterium *Alcaligenes* sp. PHY 9L.86 used 0.1% tetradecan as the sole carbon and energy source. This culture was able to degrade 98% of the hydrocarbon substrate within 48 h of its growth. The high degradation efficiency showed by this marine bacterium may be exploited in the remediation of the crude oil contaminated sites.[9] Similarly, bioemulsifier producer *Pseudomonas putida* ML2 was also able to grow on polyaromatic hydrocarbon like naphthalene and produce biosurfactants and hence can play a role in solubilization of aliphatic, aromatic and polyaromatic hydrocarbons.[10] EPS produced by salt tolerant strain *Planococcus maitriensis* Anita I showed a positive oil spreading test even at a low concentration of 0.1% and this oil dispersing potential was retained even at acidic and alkaline pH ranges. The oil dispersal capacity of this EPS was found comparable to Tween 80 and was even better than Triton X. The EPS product also possessed good emulsification properties and could emulsify various hydrocarbons and vegetable oils. Strikingly, its emulsion with Silicone, Paraffin and jatropa oil showed 100% stability up to 45 days and hence strain or its biosurfactant/bioemulsifier can find potential applications in industrial applications as well as in enhanced oil recovery.[11] Emulsifier AE22 produced by *Antarctobacter* sp. was found to form stable emulsions with various food oils at neutral and acidic pH values. The results indicated that the

Table 2. Environmental remediation potentials and industrial application potential of various marine biosurfactants/bioemulsifiers

Type of Biosurfactant/ Bioemulsifier	Producer Organism	Environmental Remediation/Industrial Potentials	Ref.
Extracellular polysaccharide-Lipid	*Alcaligenes* sp. PHY 9L-86	Degradation of tetradecan	9
Extracellular polysaccharide	*Pseudomonas putida* ML2	Degradation of aliphatic and polyaromatic hydrocarbons	10
Extracellular polysaccharide	*Planococcus maitriensis* Anita I	Good emulsification property and oil dispersion potential	11
Extracellular polysaccharide	*Antarctobacter* sp.	Emulsification of food oils and as metal adsorbent	12
Extracellular polysaccharide	*Halomonas* sp. TG39, *Halomonas* sp. TG 67	Emulsification of food oils and in emulsion stabilization	13
Glycolipopeptide	*Corynebacterium kutscheri*	Emulsification and degradation of hydrocarbons	14
Glycolipopeptide	*Yarrowia lipolytica*	Emulsification of aromatic hydrocarbons and perfluourocarbons	15
Glycolipopeptide	*Yarrowia lipolytica*	Thermostable emulsifier stabilizing oil-in-water emulsions with several aromatic hydrocarbons	16
Glycolipopeptide	*Halomonas* sp. ANT-3b	Remediation of the oil spills in cold environments	17
Glycolipid	*Pseudomonas aeruginosa* A41	Enhanced oil recovery	18
Glycolipid	Bacterial strain MM1	Removal of marine oil pollution	19
Glycolipid	*Nocardioides* sp.	Emulsification of n-paraffin and other aromatic hydrocarbons	20
Glycolipid	*Rhodococcus erythropolis*	Oil solubilization and degradation, enhance oil degradation by other oil degrading bacteria without causing any harm to them.	22
Glycolipid	*Pantoea* sp.	Emulsification of a large number of hydrocarbons	21
Glycolipid	*Aeromonas* sp.	Thermostable emulsifier emulsifying various hydrocarbon substrates	23
Glycolipid and phospholipids	*Alcanivorax borkumensis*	Cleaning of oil spills	24
Lipopeptide	*Bacillus circulans*	Polyaromatic hydrocarbon solubilization and utilization	28
Aminolipid	*Myroides* sp. strain SM1	Emulsification of weathered crude oil Thermostable bioemulsifier causing emulsification of weathered crude oil and n-hexadecane	30, 31

AE22 biopolymer can be a better stabilizing agent than an emulsifying agent, a characteristic of natural hydrocolloid polymers. These stabilizing and emulsification properties may find extensive applications in healthcare and food oil formulations. The AE22 may also be applied as a biosorbent for treatment of contaminated environments.[12] Similarly emulsifiers from *Halomonas* sp. TG39 and TG67 showed good emulsification activity with different edible oils as well as with hexadecane and these emulsions remained stable for several months. Both the emulsifiers were also able to show stable emulsification under both neutral and acidic conditions. However, the emulsification capacity at acidic pH was found to be lower (< 45%) than neutral pH. Heat treatment was also found to increase the emulsification activity of these bioemulsifiers. The emulsifying and stabilizing properties of these extracellular bioemulsifiers suggest their potential use for commercial purposes. These novel emulsifiers may substitute the presently used emulsifiers that have limited emulsification and stabilization potentials.[13] Emulsifiers produced by *Corynebacterium kutscheri* emulsified various hydrocarbons. This culture was able to degrade crude oil most efficiently with added fertilizers. The potential of this strain of *Corynebacterium* and its biosurfactant product to emulsify and degrade hydrocarbons may prove to be potent in environmental remediation purposes.[14] Similarly emulsifiers from *Yarrowia lipolytica* called Yansan showed high emulsification activity with hydrocarbons such as hexadecane, aromatic hydrocarbons such as toluene, xylene and styrene and perfluourocarbons (PFC). The emulsification activity was retained in a wide pH range (3-9) and was fairly pH independent. This emulsifier has potential application in bioremediation and formulation of perfluourocarbons based emulsions.[15] In a similar way emulsifiers from *Yarrowia lipolytica* NCIM 3589 were found to stabilize oil-in-water emulsions with several aromatic hydrocarbons such as benzene, xylene, toluene and 1-methyl naphthalene. However, interestingly, the emulsion was not stable with *n*-alkanes, though the bacterium used these as the sole carbon source. The emulsifier was stable and retained its activity in a wide range of pH values 2-10. It was also found to retain its activity at 80°C for 7 h and at 100°C for 3 h.[16]

Low molecular weight biosurfactants such as glycolipids from marine microorganisms also have great potential for industrial emulsification and environmental remediation applications. For example, Glycolipid producer *Halomonas* sp. ANT-3b, was able to degrade *n*-hexadecane and use it as the sole source of carbon to produce biosurfactants. Hence this strain can be successfully used in remediation of the oil spills especially in cold environments.[17] Similarly, strain *Pseudomonas aeruginosa* A41 produced rhamnolipid biosurfactants, that showed good stability and activity in wide ranges of temperature (40-121°C), pH (2-12) and NaCl concentrations (0-5%). Hence this marine glycolipid producer can be used for environmental cleaning in various extreme conditions and for enhanced oil recovery purposes.[18] The glycolipids produced by MM1 were also found to be effective emulsifiers and also non toxic in nature. Hence these glycolipids can be effectively used for the removal of marine oil pollution without harming the marine ecology.[19] In a similar manner glycolipids produced by actinomyces *Nocardioides* sp. was able to emulsify n-paraffin and several other aromatic hydrocarbons and thus could be used for the remediation of the polluted sites.[20] The cell surface hydrophobicity is an important factor that determines the microbial adhesion on surfaces including hydrophobic substrates. It is also an important step in bioremediation as this step is required for the introduction of the molecular oxygen. The cell surface of facultative anaerobe *Pantoea* sp. strain A-13 becomes more hydrophobic when grown in hydrocarbons than that when grown in water miscible substrates like glucose. The glycolipid was able to emulsify a large number of hydrocarbons and showed high emulsification activity against Benzene. The emulsification activity was shown in a wide pH range, the highest being at alkaline pH value. Although the biosurfactant showed good emulsification at mesophilic conditions (30-37°C) the emulsification power was fairly good at thermophilic conditions (45°C).[21] Another glycolipid producer strain *Rhodococcus erythropolis* was able to utilize a wide range of *n*-alkanes (C_5-C_{36}), the growth of this strain was better using C_{14}-C_{36} *n*-alkanes, compared using shorter alkane chains i.e., C_5, C_6, C_7 and C_9 n-alkanes. The study suggested that the *Rhodococcus erythropolis* 3C-9 biosurfactants enhanced oil degradation by other oil degrading bacteria without causing any harm to them. The potential of this strain and its biosurfactants in oil solubilization and degradation makes them a promising candidate for use in oil spill cleanup operations.[22] In a similar manner, glycolipids produced by *Aeromonas* sp. were able to emulsify various hydrocarbon substrates. The activity of this glycolipid biosurfactant was enhanced at slightly alkaline pH (8.0) and NaCl concentration (5%). Activity was found to be highest at 40°C and decreased on further increasing temperature. However, about 77% of activity was still retained after a temperature treatment at 100°C for 120 min. In general the emulsification activity was better with aliphatic hydrocarbons than aromatic hydrocarbons.[23] Similarly, the crude oil devouring glycolipid producer *Alcanivorax borkumensis* DSM 11573 has the substrate specificity for the straight chain alkanes and can serve in cleaning the oil spills.[24] Lipopeptide biosurfactants have also been reported for their emulsification potential. For example *Bacillus circulans* isolated from marine samples produced lipopeptide biosurfactants that could emulsify various hydrocarbons such as diesel, petrol, kerosene, benzene and hexadecane. Although the microorganism was not able to uptake anthracene as a sole source of carbon, it was able to do so in presence of another carbon source such as glycerol. The biosurfactants produced by the bacterium utilizing glycerol increased the bioavailability of the hydrophobic anthracene and facilitated its uptake by the cells, thus affecting its bioremediation. Thus, this strain and its biosurfactant can find potential application in the remediation of the hydrocarbon and PAH contaminated environments.[28] Other low molecular weight biosurfactants such as L-ornithine lipids produced by *Myroides* sp. strain SM1 were able to emulsify weathered crude oil. The cell surface hydrophobicity studies indicated that the cells had maximum affinity for weathered crude oil (85.48%) than toluene (48.40%) and xylene (28.07%) than any other hydrocarbons. In general the affinity of cells was more towards aromatic hydrocarbons (highly nonpolar) than aliphatic hydrocarbons. The culture was unable to utilize any hydrocarbon as the sole source of carbon although it was able to emulsify them. This emulsifier was found to be stable in the temperature range of 30-121°C and pH values ranging from 5-12.[30,31]

Biological Action of the Marine Biosurfactants

The microbial surfactants have been reported to posses several properties of therapeutic and biomedical importance. The biosurfactants obtained from marine microbes, however, have not been assessed extensively for their biological activities. However, a few reports on the biological activities of marine surfactants demonstrate their potential to act as therapeutic agents (Table 3). For example the glycolipid obtained from bacterial strain MM1 was found to be nontoxic against a panel of marine microorganisms such as marine bacteria, microalgae and flagellates. Hence these glycolipids can be effectively used for various biomedical applications.[19] Another glycolipid obtained from *Nocardioides* sp. caused hemolysis and inhibited *Bacillus subtilis* cells. The biosurfactant was able to modify the cell surface hydrophobicity of the other bacterial strains which indicated their role in attachment and detachment of bacteria on certain surfaces.[20] Similarly *Pseudomonas* sp MK90e85 and MK91CC8 produced antimycobacterial cyclic depsipeptides and viscosin. Massetolide A and viscosin showed antimicrobial action against *Mycobacterium tuberculosis* and *Mycobacterium avium-intracellulare*. Massetolide A showed a MIC value of 5-10 μg ml^{-1} against *M. tuberculosis* and 2.5-5 μg ml^{-1} against *M. avium-intracellulare*. Similarly, Viscosin had a MIC value of 10-20 μg ml^{-1} against *M. tuberculosis* and 10-20 μg ml^{-1} against *M. avium-intracellulare*. Massetolide A was also found to be nontoxic to mice at a dose of 10 mg kg^{-1} body weight. Thus these potent bioactive molecules from marine environments can prove to be effective in treating infections caused by *Mycobacterium* sp.[25] Thus these microbial surfactants can be developed as antimicrobial agents for clinical applications. *Bacircines*, yet another mixture of cyclic depsipeptides obtained from the cultures of Bacillus pumilus KMM 150 caused anomalies in the developmental process of ova of the *Echinus* and stopped blastomere fission. The bacircines had cytotoxic effect at more than 2.5-10 μg mL^{-1}. As these possess cytotoxic effect they can be potential agents in anticancer therapy. The ovicidal and cytotoxic effect of this compound against cells in the early stages of development can be of potential use as contraceptive agent or an agent for safe termination of

Table 3. Biological activities displayed by various marine biosurfactants/ bioemulsifiers

Type of Biosurfactant/ Bioemulsifier	Producer Organism	Biological Activity	Ref.
Glycolipid	Bacterial strain MM1	The toxicity tests indicated that these biosurfactants have no toxic effects against the marine microorganisms such as marine bacteria, microalgae and flagellates.	19
Glycolipid	*Nocardioides* sp.	Caused hemolysis and inhibited *Bacillus subtilis* cells.	20
		Modification of cell surface hydrophobicity of the other bacterial strains thus affecting adhesion of bacteria on certain surfaces.	
Lipopeptide	*Pseudomonas* sp. isolates MK90e85 and MK91CC8	Antimicrobial action against *Mycobacterium tuberculosis* and *Mycobacterium avium-intracellulare*.	25
Lipopeptide	*Bacillus pumilus* KMM 150	Caused anomalies in the developmental process of ova of the *Echinus*.	26
		The ovicidal and cytotoxic effect against cells in the early stages of development can be of potential use as contraceptive agent or an agent for safe termination of unwanted pregnancy.	
Lipopeptide	*Bacillus circulans*	Antimicrobial activity against common laboratory strains and multidrug resistant strains.	8
Lipopeptide	*Brevibacillus laterosporus* PNG-276	Antimicrobial action against multi-drug resistant *Staphylococcus aureus* (MRSA) and Gram-positive human pathogen *Enterococcus* sp.	29

unwanted pregnancy.[26] Other lipopeptides obtained from marine microbes also demonstrated a strong antimicrobial action. For example, the biologically active fraction of the marine *Bacillus circulans* biosurfactant was obtained through RP-HPLC. The bioactive fraction was found to be antimicrobial action against various Gram-positive and Gram-negative bacterium such as *Micrococcus flavus, Bacillus pumilis, Mycobacterium smegmatis, Escherichia coli, Serratia marcescens, Proteus vulgaris, Citrobacter freundii, Proteus mirabilis, Alcaligenes faecalis, Acetobacter calcoaceticus, Bordetella bronchiseptica, Klebsiella aerogenes* and *Enterobacter cloacae*. The lipopeptide biosurfactant showed MIC values as low as 10 µg ml^{-1} against microorganisms such as *Proteus vulgaris* and *Alcaligenes faecalis*. Mild antimicrobial action was also shown against multi-drug resistant *Staphylococcus aureus* (MRSA) and other MDR strains. The biosurfactant was also found to be nonhemolytic in nature thus indicating its use as a drug in antimicrobial chemotherapy.[8] Other lipopeptide biosurfactants such as tauramamide from *Brevibacillus laterosporus* PNG-276 also showed profound antimicrobial action. Tauramamide and its methyl ester showed antimicrobial action against Multi-drug resistant *Staphylococcus aureus* (MRSA) and Gram-positive human pathogen *Enterococcus* sp. A low MIC of 0.1 µg ml^{-1} for *Enterococcus* sp. was obtained which suggests that these can prove to be potent new group of antimicrobials against several multi-drug resistant strains.[29]

Conclusion

The marine environment that encompasses a major area of the world's surface is a vast unexploited repertoire of compounds of unique structures and activities. Various biosurfactants and bioemulsifiers from marine microorganisms show their efficacy in emulsification and solubilization of various aliphatic, aromatic and perfluourocarbons (PFC) and thus have tremendous potentials in remediation of contaminated environments and for industrial emulsification. The significant antimicrobial action and other important biological activities displayed by the marine biosurfactants make these potential candidates to be developed as a drug or for other important biomedical applications. The gradually uprising threat of multidrug resistance has led to the incessant search for compounds with new activities and the marine microbial surfactants can be an answer to this. More research inputs are required in this direction so that this virtually inexhaustible resource can be tapped for human welfare.

Acknowledgements

PD acknowledges IIT Kharagpur and SM acknowledges CSIR, New Delhi for their research fellowships. RS and SC acknowledge DBT, Govt. of India for the project grant (BT/PR-6827/AAQ/03/263/2005) in Marine Biotechnology.

References

1. Desai JD, Banat IM. Microbial Surfactants and their commercial potential. Microbiol Mol Biol Rev 1997; 61:47-58.
2. Mukherjee S, Das P, Sen R. Towards commercial production of microbial surfactants. Trends Biotechnol 2006; 24:509-515.
3. Rosenberg E, Ron EZ. High- and Low-molecular-mass Microbial Surfactants. Appl Microbiol Biotechnol 1999; 52:154-162.
4. Maier RM. Biosurfactant: evolution and diversity in bacteria. Adv Appl Microbiol 2003; 52:101-121.
5. Ron EZ, Rosenberg E. Natural roles of biosurfactants. Environ Microbiol 1999; 3:229-236.
6. Nielsen TH, Christophersen C, Anthoni U et al. Viscosinamide, a new cyclic depsipeptide with surfactant and antifungal properties produce by Pseudomonas fluorescens DR 54. J Appl Microbiol 1999; 86:80-90.
7. Davey ME, Caiazza NC, Tootle GAO. Rhamnolipid surfactant production affects bioflims architecture in Pseudomonas aeruginosa PA-01. J Bacteriol 2003; 185:1027-36.
8. Das P, Mukherjee S, Sen R. Antimicrobial potentials of a lipopeptide biosurfactant derived from a marine Bacillus circulans. J Appl Microbiol 2008a; 104:1675-84.
9. Goutx M, Mutaftshiev S, Bertrand JC. Lipid and exopolysaccharide production during hydrocarbon growth of a marine bacterium from the sea surface. Mar Ecol Prog Ser 1987; 40:259-65.
10. Bonilla M, Olivaro C, Corona M et al. Production and characterization of a new bioemulsifier from Pseudomonas putida ML2. J Appl Microbiol 2005; 98:456-63.
11. Kumar AS, Mody K, Jha B. Evaluation of biosurfactant/bioemulsifier production by a marine bacterium. Bull Environ Contam Toxicol 2007; 79:617-21.
12. Gutiérrez T, Mulloy B, Bavington C et al. Partial purification and chemical characterization of a glyco-protein (putative hydrocolloid) emulsifier produced by a marine bacterium. Appl Microbiol Biotechnol 2007; 76:1017-1026.
13. Gutiérrez T, Mulloy B, Black K et al. Glycoprotein emulsifiers from two marine Halomonas species: chemical and physical characterization. J Appl Microbiol 2007; 103:1716-27.
14. Thavasi R, Jayalakshmi S, Balasubramanian T et al. Biosurfactant production by Corynebacterium kutscheri from waste motor lubricant oil and peanut oil cake. Lett Appl Microbiol 2007; 45:686-91.
15. Amaral PFF, Da-Silva JM, Lehocky M et al. Production and characterization of a bioemulsifier from Yarrowia lipolytica. Proc Biochem 2006; 41:1894-98.
16. Zinjarde S, Chinnathambi S, Lachke AH et al. Isolation of an emulsifier from Yarrowia lipolytica NCIM 3589 using a modified mini isoelectric focusing unit. Lett Appl Microbiol 1997; 24:117-21.
17. Pepi M, Cesàro A, Luit G et al. An antarctic psychrotropic bacterium Halomonas sp. ANT-3b, growing on n-hexadecane, produces a new emulsifying glycolipid. FEMS Microbiol Ecol 2005; 53:157-66.
18. Thaniyavarn J, Chongchin A, Wanitsuksombut N et al. Biosurfactant production by Pseudomonas aeruginosa A41 using palm oil as carbon source. J Gen Appl Microbiol 2006; 52:215-22.
19. Passeri A, Schmidt M, Haffner T et al. Marine biosurfactants. IV. Production, characterization and bio-synthesis of an anionic glucose lipid from the marine bacterial strain MM1. Appl Microbiol Biotechnol 1992; 37:281-86.

20. Vasileva-Tonkawa E, Gesheva V. Glycolipids produced by Antarctic Nocardioides sp. during growth on n-paraffin. Process Biochem 2005; 40:2837-91.

21. Vasileva-Tonkova E, Gesheva V. Biosurfactant production by Antarctic facultative anaerobe Pantoea sp. during growth on hydrocarbons. Curr Microbiol 2007; 54:136-41.

22. Peng F, Liu Z, Wang L et al. An oil-degrading bacterium: Rhodococcus erythropolis strain 3C-9 and its biosurfactants. J Appl Microbiol 2007; 102:1603-11.

23. Ilori MO, Amobi CJ, Odocha AC. Factors affecting biosurfactant production by oil degrading Aeromonas spp. isolated from a tropical environment. Chemosphere 2005; 61:985-992.

24. Abraham WR, Meyer H, Yakimov M. Novel glycine containing glucolipids from the alkane using bacterium Alcanivorax borkumensis. Biochim Biophys Acta 1998; 1393:57-62.

25. Gerard J, Lloyd R, Barsby T et al. Massetolides A-H, Antimycobacterial cyclic depsipeptides produced by two Pseudomonads isolated from marine habitats. J Nat Prod 1997; 60:223-29.

26. Kalinovskaya NI, Kuznetsova TA, Rashkes YV et al. Surfactin-like structures of five cyclic depsipeptides from the marine isolate of Bacillus pumilus. Russ Chem Bull 1995; 44:951-55.

27. Kalinovskaya NI, Kuznetsova TA, Ivanova EP et al. Characterization of surfactin-like cyclic depsipeptides synthesized by Bacillus pumilus from ascidian Halocynthia aurantium. Mar Biotechnol 2002; 4:179-88.

28. Das P, Mukherjee S, Sen R. Improved bioavailability and biodegradation of a model polyaromatic hydrocarbon by a biosurfactant producing bacterium of marine origin. Chemosphere 2008b; 72:1229-34.

29. Desjardine K, Pereira A, Wright H et al. Tauramamide, a lipopeptide antibiotic produced in the culture by Brevibacillus laterosporus isolated from a marine habitat: structure elucidation and synthesis. J Nat Prod 2007; 70:1850-1853.

30. Maneerat S, Bamba T, Harada K et al. A novel crude oil emulsifier excreted in the culture supernatant of a marine bacterium, Myroides sp. strain SM1. Appl Microbiol Biotechnol 2006; 70:254-59.

31. Maneerat S, Dikit P. Characterization of cell-associated bioemulsifier from Myroides sp. SM1, a marine bacterium. Songklanakarin J Sci Technol 2007; 29:769-79.

CHAPTER 8

Biomimetic Amphiphiles:
Properties and Potential Use

S.K. Mehta,* Shweta Sharma, Neena Mehta and Swaranjit Singh Cameotra

Abstract

Surfactants are the amphiphilic molecules that tend to alter the interfacial and surface tension. The fundamental property related to the structure of surfactant molecules is their self-aggregation resulting in the formation of association colloids. Apart from the packing of these molecules into closed structures, the structural network also results in formation of extended bilayers, which are thermodynamically stable and lead to existence of biological membranes and vesicles. From biological point of view the development of new knowledge and techniques in the area of vesicles, bilayers and multiplayer membranes and their polymerizable analogue provide new opportunities for research in the respective area. 'Green Surfactants' or the biologically compatible surfactants are in demand to replace some of the existing surfactants and thereby reduce the environmental impact, in general caused by classic surfactants. In this context, the term 'natural surfactants or biosurfactants' is often used to indicate the natural origin of the surfactant molecules. Most important aspect of biosurfactants is their environmental acceptability, because they are readily biodegradable and have low toxicity than synthetic surfactants. Some of the major applications of biosurfactants in pollution and environmental control are microbial enhanced oil recovery, hydrocarbon degradation, hexa-chloro cyclohexane (HCH) degradation and heavy-metal removal from contaminated soil. In this chapter, we tried to make a hierarchy from vital surfactant molecules toward understanding their behavioral aspects and application potential thereby ending into the higher class of broad spectrum 'biosurfactants'. Pertaining to the budding promise offered by these molecules, the selection of the type and size of each structural moiety enables a delicate balance between surface activity and biological function and this represents the most effective approach of harnessing the power of molecular self-assembly.

Introduction

Surfactants are among the most versatile products of the chemical industry appearing in essential biological systems and industrial processes.[1] Our food, cosmetics, medicines, house-hold items, the drilling mud used in prospecting for petroleum and the floatation agents used in benefication of ores, contain a wide range of surfactants. Surfactant is an abbreviation for surface active agent, which literally means: a species, which is active at the interface. In other words, a surfactant is characterized by its tendency to adsorb at the surfaces and interfaces. The term interface denotes a boundary between any two immiscible phases while, the term surface indicates that one of the phases is a gas, generally air.[2,3] The driving force for surfactant adsorption is the lowering of free energy of the phase boundary.

The interfacial free energy per unit area is what we measure when we determine the interfacial tension between two phases. It is the minimum amount of work required to create unit area of

*Corresponding Author: S.K. Mehta—Chemistry Department, Panjab University, Chandigarh 160014, India. Email: skmehta@pu.ac.in

Biosurfactants, edited by Ramkrishna Sen. ©2010 Landes Bioscience
and Springer Science+Business Media.

the interface or to expand it by unit area. When we measure the surface tension of a liquid, we are measuring the interfacial free energy per unit area of the boundary between the liquid and the air above it. When the interface is expanded, the minimum work required to create the additional amount of that interface is the product of the interfacial tension r_I times the increase in the area of the interface: $W_{min} = \eta \times \Delta A$. When the boundary is covered by the surfactant molecules, the surface tension (or the amount of work required to expand that interface) is reduced. The denser the surfactant packing at the interface, larger is the reduction in surface tension.[4-6]

Surfactants may adsorb at all the interfaces listed below:

Solid—Vapor   *Surface*
Solid—Liquid
Solid—Solid
Liquid—Vapor   *Surface*
Liquid—Liquid

However, the discussion will be restricted to the interface involving a liquid phase. The liquid considered here is usually, but not always water. Examples of different interfaces and products in which these interface are important are given in Table 1. In many formulated products several types of interfaces are present at the same time. Water-based paints and paper coating colors are examples of familiar ones, but from the point of view of a colloidal chemist, the complicated systems contain both solid-liquid (dispersed pigment particles) and liquid-liquid (latex or other binder droplets) interfaces.

In addition, foam formation is a common (though unwanted sometimes) phenomenon at the application stage. All types of interface are well-stabilized by the surfactants.[7] The total interfacial area of such systems is so immense that oil-water and solid-water interfaces of one liter of paint may cover several football fields. This can be related to an old, saying by Benjamin Franklin in 1974, reported to the British Royal Society:

"At length at Clapman where there is, on the common, a large pond, which I observed to be one day very rough with the wind, I fetched out a cruet of oil and dropped a little of it on the water. I saw it spread itself with surprising swiftness upon the surface. The oil, though not more than a teaspoonful, produced an instant cam over a space several yards square, which spread amazingly and extended itself gradually until it reached the leeside, making all that quarter of the pond, perhaps half an acre, as smooth as a looking glass."

$$V \sim 2 \text{ ml}, A \sim 2000 \text{ m}^2 \Longrightarrow \text{ thickness of layer} \sim 1 \text{ nm}$$

It was not until over a hundred years later when Lord Rayleigh suspected that the maximum extension of an oil film on water represented a layer within the thickness of a single molecule.

Coming back to surfactant, these molecules have a strong tendency to accumulate at the interfaces and it can be considered as the fundamental property of these species. In principle stronger is the tendency of accumulation better is the surfactant. The degree of surfactant accumulation at a boundary depends upon the surfactant structure and also upon the nature of the two phases that meet at the interface. Therefore the choice of surfactant depends upon the application potential e.g., some surfactants molecules are soluble only at the oil-water interface.

Table 1. Examples of interfaces involving a liquid phase

Interface	Type of System	Product
Solid-liquid	Suspension	Solvent-borne point
Liquid-liquid	Emulsion	Milk, cream
Liquid-vapour	Foam	Shaving cream

Scope

The purpose of this chapter is to provide an insight into the basics of surfactant molecules, their behavior in solution and most importantly the application of these molecules, in special reference to the biological systems.

Surfactants find applications in almost every chemical industry including detergents, paints, dyestuff, cosmetics, agrochemicals, fibers and pharmaceuticals. Therefore, the fundamental understanding of the physical chemistry of surface-active agents, their usual properties and their phase behavior is essential for most chemical industries. In addition, understanding of the basic phenomenon involved in application of surfactants in the preparation of emulsions, suspensions and micro-emulsions etc. is of vital importance in arriving at right system composition. In pharmaceutical science the usage of surfactants is associated with the control release of trapped drugs along with their in-vivo and in-vitro preparation.

Commercially produced surfactants are not pure chemically and within each chemical type there can be tremendous variation. This is understandable since surfactants are prepared from various feedstocks. It is thus advisable to obtain as much information as possible from the manufacturer about the properties of surfactants e.g., its suitability of the job, variation in the batch, toxicity and impurity, if any.

In the chapter emphasis has been given on the basics of surfactants, their classification, the phenomenon of self-assembly, behavior in solution and microbial surfactants in reference to their properties and commercial potential.

Surfactant Basis

'Surfactants are the amphiphiles': the word being derived from the Greek word "amphi" meaning both and the term is related to the point that all surfactant species consist of at least two parts: a nonpolar hydrophobic portion, usually a straight or branched hydrocarbon chain containing ~8-18 carbon atoms, attached to a polar or ionic portion (hydrophilic). The hydrophilic part is referred to as the head group and hydrophobic part as the tail (Fig. 1). The hydrophobic part of the surfactants may be branched or linear and interacts weakly with water molecules in an aqueous environment. The degree of chain branching, the position of the polar group and the length of the chain are important parameters in deciding the physico-chemical properties of the surfactants.

The polar part of surfactant may be ionic or non-ionic in natural. For non-ionic surfactants the size of the head group can be varied at will but in the case of ionic surfactant this parameter is a fixed one. The polar head group interacts strongly with water molecules (via dipole or ion-dipole interactions) which renders the surfactant soluble in water. The cooperative action of dispersion and hydrogen bonding between the water molecules tends to squeeze the hydrocarbon chain out of water and hence these chain are referred to as hydrophobic. It is the balance between the hydrophobic and hydrophilic parts of the molecule that gives these systems, their special property of accumulation at various interfaces and behavior of self-assembly (i.e., micellization).[8]

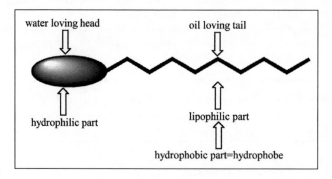

Figure 1. Structure of surfactant molecule.

N⁺.....COOH ⟷ N⁺.....COO⁻ ⟷ NH.....COO⁻

pH<3   isoelectric   pH>6

Scheme 1. pH dependent ionization of surfactant molecules anionics.

Specific Classes of Surfactants

In general surfactants are classified on the basis of the charge of the polar head group and the common practice is to divide the surfactants into anionic, cationic, non-ionic and zwitterions.[9-11] Most ionic surfactants are monovalent but there are also examples of divalent anionic amphiphiles. The most common counterion in anionic surfactants is sodium; however other cations e.g., Li⁺, K⁺, Ca⁺² and protonated amines are used as counterion for specialty purposes. The counterion of cationic surfactants is usually a halide or sulfate. The hydrophobic group is normally a hydrocarbon (alkyl or arylalkyl) but many vary for polydimethylsiloxame or a fluorocarbon. The common non-ionic surfactants are based on ethylene oxide and are referred as ethoxylated surfactants. The amphoteric or the zwitterionic surfactants contain both the cationic and anionic groups. The characteristic feature of these surfactants is their dependence on the pH of the solution in which they are dissolved. In acidic solutions, the molecules acquire a positive charge and behave like cationic surfactants, whereas in alkaline solutions they become negatively charged and behave like an anionic one. A specific pH can be defined at which both ionic groups show equal ionization, specified as the isoelectric point of the molecule (Scheme 1).

Of the four classes of the surfactants, anionics are the most widely used. Important types of anionic surfactants are carboxylates, sulfonates, sulfates and the phosphates. Figure 2 shows the structure of commonly used anionic surfactants.

Important aspects of anionic surfactants are:

1. Major reason for the popularity of the anionic surfactants is their low cost of manufacture.
2. They possess enhanced foaming and spreading properties.
3. Since sulfonate group is a strong acid, the sulfonate surfactants are soluble and effective in acidic as well as in alkaline media and thus they are useful for textile scouring formulations.
4. Sulfates are more hydrophilic than the suflonates.
5. Sodium salts are the most common although salts with diethanolamine, thiethano-lamine and ammonia are used in cosmetics and shampoos.
6. Phosphate surfactants are excellent emulsifiers under strongly alkaline conditions.

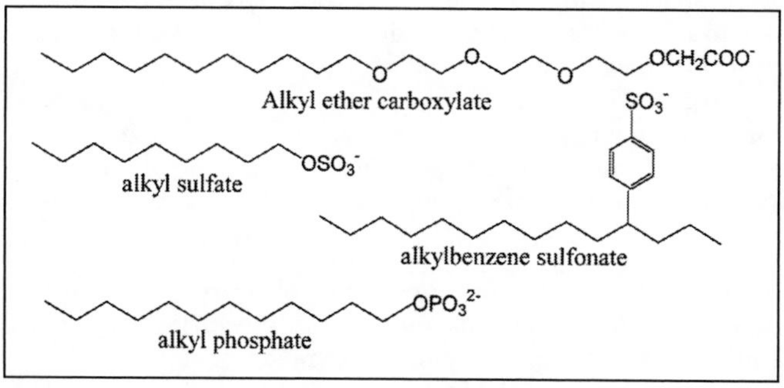

Figure 2. Structures of anionic surfactants.

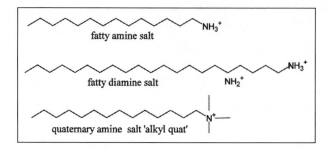

Figure 3. Structure of some cationic surfactants.

Cationics

Most of the uses of cationic surfactants result from their ability to adhere and modify the solid surfaces. Figure 3 represents the structures of some typical cationic surfactants. The common types of cationic surfactants are long chair amines and quaternary amine salts (alkyl 'quat'). Amines function only at the protonated state and thus cannot be used at high pH. The quaternary ammonium compounds are not pH sensitive.

Important facts about cationic surfactants are:

1. They are important as corrosion inhibitors, fuel and lubricating oil additives, germicides and hair conditioners.
2. Other applications include their use as fabric softener, fixatives for anionic dye and drying rate retarder for cationic dye.
3. Cationic surfactants are compatible with non-ionic and zwitterionic surfactants. However their usage is small compared to anionic and non-ionic ones.
4. They adsorb strongly to most surfaces and their main uses are related to in situ surface modification.

Non-Ionics

Non-ionic surfactants have either a polyether or a polyhydroxyl unit as the polar group. In majority of cases, the polar group is a polyether consisting of oxyethylene units, made by the polymerization of ethylene oxide.

The non-ionic surfactants can be specified in terms of the following aspects:

1. These have diverse uses in textiles.
2. The hydrocarbon group is the hydrophobic part of the surfactant while the chains of ethylene oxide group is hydrophilic part. The length of ethylene oxide chain determines the hydrophilicity of the surfactants.
3. Non-ionic surfactants are compatible with all other types of surfactants.
4. Their low foaming tendency can be an advantage to the horticulture industry where they do a good job of breaking water surface tension.
5. They are more effective than the sulfonate surfactants in removing soil from hydrophobic fibres but are inferior to anionic surfactants for soil removal from cotton.
6. The properties of a non-ionic surfactant can be tailored somewhat for a particular use by controlling a relative amount of hydrophilic and hydrophobic characters.

Zwitterionics

Zwitterionic surfactants contain two charged groups of different sign. Whereas the positive charge is almost invariably ammonium, the source of negative charge may vary, although carboxylate is the most common. Common types of zwitterionic surfactants are N-alkyl derivatives of simple amino acids such as glycine (NH_2CH_2COOH), betaines ((CH_2)$_2NCH_2COOH$) and amino-propionic acid ($NH_2CH_2CH_2COOH$). Structures of some of the zwitterionic surfactants are shown in Figure 4.

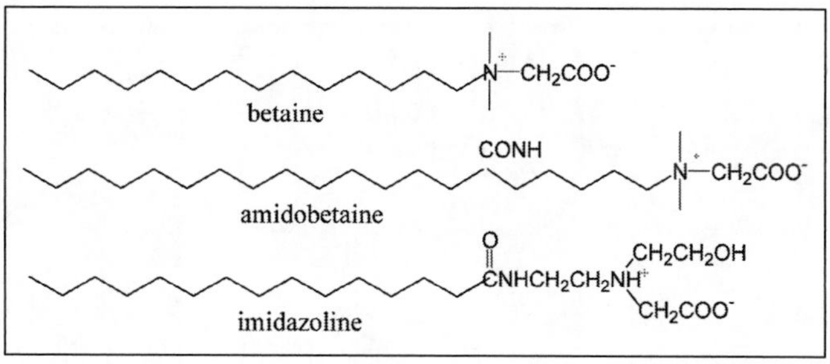

Figure 4. Structure of some zwitterionic surfactants.

Some interesting facts about these surfactants include:
1. These species provide a feel of softness to textile materials.
2. Zwitterionic surfactants are compatible with all other classes of surfactants and are soluble and effective in the presence of high concentrations of electrolytes, acids and alkalies.
3. They exhibit cationic behavior near or below their isoelectric points and anionic behavior at high pH.
4. Their uses in horticulture crop production is very rare.
5. The products from the zwitterionic surfactants are very specifically used to match the properties of specific pesticide formulations and generally are not used in the green house as the stand-alone products.

Surface Active Compounds are Ample in Nature

Nature's own surfactants are the polar lipids and these are abundant in all living organisms. In the biological systems the surface-active agents are used in the similar manner as they are used in the technical systems: to overcome the solubility problems as emulsifiers, as dispersants and to modify the surfaces etc. The examples of polar lipids are given in Figure 5.

A good example of biological surfactants is: bile salts, which are extremely efficient solubilizers of hydrophobic components in the blood. On the other hand the phospolipids packed as ordered bilayer constitute the cell memberane.

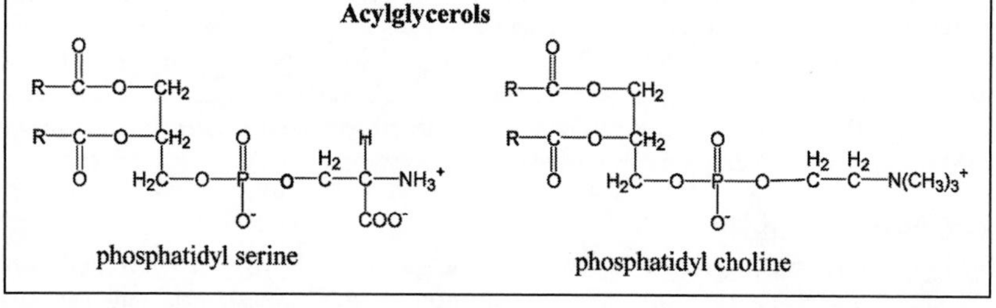

Figure 5. Polar lipids acting as surfactants.

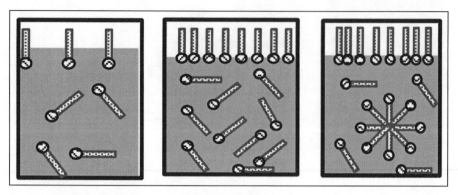

Figure 6. Self-assembly of surfactant monomers.

Self-Assembly Processes

As discussed earlier the characteristic feature of surfactants is their tendency to adsorb at the interface in an oriented fashion.[12-14] This adsorption has been studied to determine:

i. The concentration of surfactant at the interface, since this is a measure of how much of the interface has been covered (and thus changed) by the surfactant: the performance of the surfactant in many interfacial processes (e.g., foaming, detergency, emulsification etc.) depends on its concentration at the interface.

ii. The orientation of the surfactant at the interface, since this determines how the interface will be affected by the adsorption, that is, whether it will become more hydrophilic or more hydrophobic.

iii. The energy changes i.e., free energy (ΔG), enthalpy (ΔH) and entropy (ΔS) in the system, resulting from the adsorption, since these quantities provide information on the type and mechanism of any interactions involving the surfactant at the interface and the efficiency of its operation as a surface-active material.

The nature of surfactant molecules, having both the lyophilic and the lyophobic groups, is responsible for their tendency to accumulate at the interface and thus reduce the free energy of the system in which they interact. Another fundamental property related to the structure of surfactant molecules is their tendency to form self-associated structures, called the '*micelles*'. Micelle formation or the phenomenon of micellization can be viewed as structurally resembling the solid crystals or the crystalline hydrates. Thermodynamically, the formation of micelles favors an increase in solubility of the surfactant molecules. Micelles are generated at very low surfactant concentration in dispersion media (which generally is water).

The concentration at which micelles start to form is called the critical micellization concentration (*cmc*). The *cmc* is an important characteristic of individual surfactant.[15] Figure 6 depicts the self-assembly of surfactant monomers when their concentration exceeds the critical value.

The measurement of bulk properties of solution e.g., surface tension, electric conductivity, light scattering etc. as a function of surfactant concentration at some point reflects the change occurring in the nature of solute species (Fig. 7). This break point corresponds to the *cmc* of a typical surfactant. A *cmc* of 2 mM for any surfactant means that unimer concentration will never exceed this value, regardless of the amount of surfactant added to the solution i.e., after the concentration of 2 mM the surfactant mainly exist in the self-assembled form.

Association Colloids

The various surfactant aggregates in general are categorized as the 'association colloids' where particle size ranges between 10-100 nm. The association colloids formed by the self-aggregation of the surfactant monomers differs from the other colloids in that they are in dynamic equilibrium with the monomers in the solution.

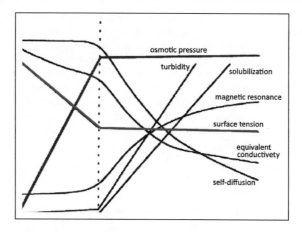

Figure 7. Break point in measured property indicate appearance of *cmc*.

Micelles

McBain[16] proposed the presence of molecular aggregates in soap/surfactant solutions on the basis of the unusual change in the measured bulk property of the system. Micellar colloids represent the dynamic association-dissociation equilibrium. However, ever since the conception of micellization, the structure of micellar aggregates has been a matter of discussion. McBain[16] suggested the formation of two distinct types of micelles: spherical structures composed of ionized salt molecules and lamellar structure comprised of non-ionic aggregates. Subsequently Hartley's[17] model consisted of essentially spherical micelles with diameter equal to approximately twice the length of the hydrocarbon chain. X-ray studies by Harkin's et al[18] suggested the sandwich or the lamellar model. Later Debye and Anacker[19] proposed that micelles are rod shaped rather than spherical or disc like. The cross section of such a rod would be circular, with the polar heads of the detergent lying on the periphery and the hydrocarbon tails filling the interior. The end of the rod would almost certainly have to be rounded and polar. Hartley's (1956) spherical micelle model has been established by Reich[20] from the viewpoint of entropy and the spherical form of micelles is now generally accepted as the actual structure. Figure 8 shows various shapes ascribed to the surfactant aggregates.

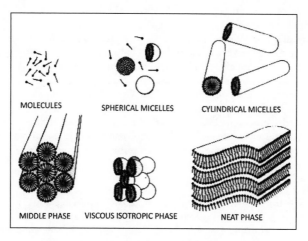

Figure 8. Shapes and the structure of different micelles.

The formation of micelles by ionic-surfactant is ascribed to the balance between the hydrocarbon chain attraction and the ionic repulsion. In general, the net charge of micelles is less than the degree of micellar aggregates indicating the large fraction of counter-ions remains associated with the micelles (These counter-ions form the *stern layer* at the micellar surface). In the case of non-ionic surfactant, the hydrocarbon chain attraction is opposed by the requirement of the hydrophilic group for hydration and space. Therefore, the micellar structure is determined by the equilibrium between repulsive forces among the hydrophilic groups and the short-range attractive forces among hydrophobic groups. In other words, the chemical structure of a given surfactant determines the shape and size of the micelles.

Classical Theories of Micelle Formation

In classical literature two approaches/models for the micellization have been accepted: the mass action model and pseudophase model.[21] In mass action model it is assumed that an equilibrium exists between the surfactant monomers and the micelles e.g., in the case of non-ionic (or unionized) surfactants, the monomer/micelle equilibrium can be written as:

$$NS \text{ (monomers)} \rightleftharpoons M \text{ (micelles)}$$

With a corresponding equilibrium constant, K_m, given by

$$K_m = [M]/[S]^n$$

where n is the number of monomers in the micelles, termed as the aggregation number. In such systems the activity of the surfactants may increase with the total concentration above *cmc*, although the size of that increase may be negligibly small.

In the phase separation or the pseudophase model the micelle is assumed to be a separate but soluble phase, which appears when the surfactant concentration reaches the *cmc*. The *cmc* therefore may be viewed as a solubility limit or the saturation concentration for the monomeric species. According to such a concept the concentration of individual surfactant molecules should not increase beyond that attained at the point of micelle formation. The assumption for the pseudophase model that the activity of the monomeric species remains constant above the *cmc* is related to the observation that the surface tension of a surfactant solution normally remains constant above that concentration.[2]

Micelles and Ahead

The associations of surfactants into simpler structures like spheres, rods and discs allow a direct analysis of the fundamental aspects of their behavior.

However, the amphiphiles which can not pack themselves into closed structures result in the assembly of extended bilayers. Such molecules have relatively small head groups or bulky hydrocarbon network. Although extended bilayers are thermodynamically favorable, there are the conditions under which it is more desirable to form the closer bilayers systems, leading to existence of biological membranes and the vesicles. Considering the impact of surfactants and the membranes on the biological systems, it has been a goal in many allied fields to develop a well-characterized synthetic model of biological membranes and enzymes. From biological point of view the development of new knowledge and techniques in the area of vesicles, bilayers and multiplayer membranes and their polymerizable analogue provide new opportunities for research in the respective area.

Emulsification

Emulsification—the formation of emulsions from two immiscible liquid phases is probably the most versatile property of surface-active agents for practical applications.[22] Paints, polishes, pesticides, mettle cutting oils, margarine, ice-cream, cosmetics, metal cleaners and textile processing oils are all examples of emulsions in one form or the other.

An emulsion is a significantly stable suspension of particles of one liquid (say water) of certain particle size within the second, immiscible liquid (say oil). For this suspension, surfactant due to their polarity acts as a good stabilizing agent. The solution eventually remains transparent and aggregation of surfactants encircling the oil becomes sufficiently large that the oil in the center has the properties similar to that of bulk oil. This oil could be considered to be emulsified by the surfactant and not the solubilized. So, as long as the mixture forms spontaneously, is not turbid and does not separate, it would merit the name microemulsion. Basically the size of dispersed particles count for the three types of formulations: (i) macroemulsions, the opaque emulsions with particle size >400 nm that are easily visible under the microscope, (ii) microemulsions, transparent dispersion with particle size <100 nm and (iii) miniemulsions, a recently suggested type that is blue with particle size between 100-400 nm.

Recently explored are the multiemulsions where the dispersed particles themselves are the emulsions of the all types. Microemulsions has remained the area of significant research because of their wide spread application potential which vary from miniature house hold products to large scale enhanced oil recovery. In the case of microemulsions the dual character of surfactants provides a way to the stable mixing of two entirely different phases (say: water and oil). These two phases in turn provide the microenvironment to the solubilization of external entity, which occupy the space in microemulsion media according to their physico-chemical aspects. The avenue of such formulations has largely been explored in biological applications e.g., in pharmaceuticals where microemulsions act as drug carrier molecules in vivo, in agricultural and house hold products, as dry cleaning fluids, in beverages and as dying agents.

Biosurfactants and Their Potential Uses

The particulate properties of surfactants confer excellent detergency, emulsifying, foaming and dispersing traits, which makes them one of the versatile chemical products.[23] More than 4500 tons of environmentally harmful surfactants (classified as emulsifiers, floatation aids and surfactants) were used in Sweden during 1999. A good surfactant should begin with the user and end up friendly to the environment.[24] 'Green Surfactants' or the biologically compatible surfactants are in demand to replace some of the existing surfactants and thereby reduce the environmental impact. In this context, the term 'natural surfactants or biosurfactants' is often used to indicate the natural origin of the surfactant molecules. Biosurfactants are the amphiphilic compounds produced on living surfaces, mostly on the microbial cell surfaces and contain the hydrophobic and hydrophilic moieties that have the ability to accumulate between the liquid interface, thus reducing the surface and interfacial tension.[25] Originally, biosurfactants attracted attention in the late 1960s and their applications have been greatly extended in the past five decades as an improved alternative to the chemical surfactants (carboxylates, sulphates and esters), preferably in food, pharmaceuticals and the oil industry.[26,27] The reason for their popularity as high-value microbial products is primarily because of their specific action, low toxicity, higher biodegradability, effectiveness at extreme temperatures, wide spread applicability and their structure which provide different properties than that of the classical surfactants.

Activity of Biosurfactants

The activities of biosurfactants can be determined by measuring the change in physico-chemical property, stabilization or destabilization of emulsion and the hydrophilic-lipophilic balance (HLB). When surfactant is added to air/water or oil/water system at increasing concentration, a change in measured property is observed up to a critical level, above which supramolecular structures corresponding to surfactant assemblies are formed. This critical value is called the *cmc* and is the parameter to measure the efficiency of any surfactant.

Biosurfactants may stabilize (emulsifiers) or destabilize (de-emulsifiers) the emulsion. The emulsification activity is determined by the ability of surfactant to generate turbidity due to sus-pended hydrocarbons such as a hexadecane-2-methylnephthalene in an aqueous assay system.[28] The de-emulsification activity is derived by determining the effect of surfactant on a standard emulsion by using a synthetic surfactant.[29]

The HLB value indicates whether a surfactant will promote water-in-oil or the oil-in-water emulsion. Emulsifiers with HLB value less that 6 favor stabilization of water-in-oil emulsification whereas the HLB value in the range 10-18 gives the opposite effect and favor the oil-in-water emulsification.

Classification of Biosurfactants

Unlike chemically synthesized surfactants, which are classified on the basis of polar head-groups, biosurfactants are classified by their chemical composition and microbial origin. Rosenberg and Ron[30] have suggested that biosurfactants can be divided into low-molecular-mass molecules, which efficiently lower the surface and interfacial tension and the high-molecular-mass polymers, which are more effective as emulsion-stabilizing agents. In general, the structure of biosurfactants includes the hydrophilic moiety consisting of amino acids or peptide anions or cations; mono-, di-, polysac-charides; and a hydrophobic moiety consisting of unsaturated or saturated fatty-acids.[31] The major types of biosurfactants and the microbial species of origin are listed in Table 2.

Glycolipids

Most of the biosurfactants are the glycolipids, which are the carbohydrates in combination with long chain aliphatic acids or hydroxyaliphatic acids. The linkage is by means of either ether or an ester group.

Rhamnolipids: In this class one or two molecules of rhamnose are linked to one or two molecules of β-hydroxydecanoic acid and are the best studied glycolipids. While the –OH group of one of the acids is involved in glycosidic linkage with the reducing end of the rhamnose disaccharide, the –OH group of the second acid is involved in ester formation. Production of rhamnose containing glycolipids was first described in *Pseudomonas aeruginosa* by Jarvis and Johnson.[32] L-Rhamnosyl-L-rhamnosyl-β-hydroxydecanoyl-β-hydroxydecanoate (Fig. 9) and L-Rhamnosyl-β-hydroxydecanoyl-β-hydroxydecanoate, referred to as rhamnolipids 1 and 2, respectively, are the principal glycolipids produced by *P. aeruginosa*.

Trehalolipids: Various types of microbial trehalolipid biosurfactants have been reported.[33] Disaccharide trehalose linked at C-6 and C-6′ to mycolic acids is associated with most species of *Mycobaterium*, *Nocardia* and *Corynebacterium*. Mycolic acids are long-chain, α-branched-β-hydroxy fatty acids. Trehalolipids from different organisms differ in the size and structure of mycolic acid, the number of carbon atoms and the degree of unsaturation. Trehalose dimycolate produced by *R. erythropolis* (Fig. 9) has been extensively studied. Trehalose lipids from *R. erythropolis* lowered the surface and interfacial tension in the culture broth to 25-40 and 1-5 mN m^{-1}, respectively.

Sophorolipids: Sophorolipids, which are produced mainly by yeasts such as *T. bombicola*, *T. apicola* and *T. Petrophilum* consist of a dimeric carbohydrate sorphorose linked to a long-chain hydroxyl fatty acid (Fig. 9). These biosurfactants are a mixture of at least six to nine different

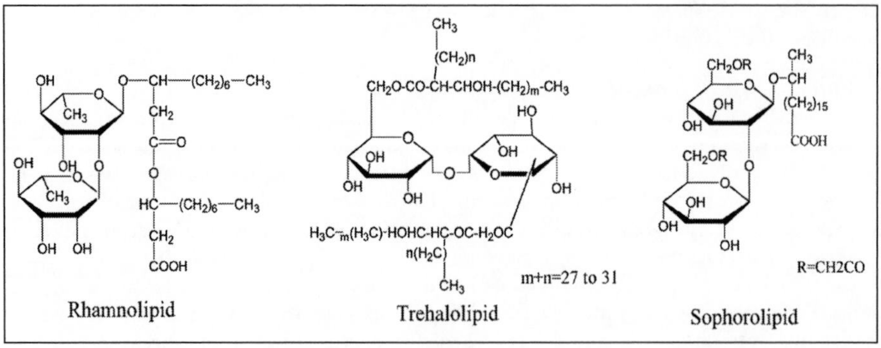

Figure 9. Structures of some common glycolipids.

Table 2. Microbial sources and major types of microbial surfactants

Biosurfactant	Organism	Surface Tension (mN m^{-1})
Glycolipids		
Rhamnolipids	*P. aeruginosa*	29
	Pseudomonas sp.	25-30
Trehalolipids	*R. erythropolis*	32-36
	N. erythropolis	30
	Mycobacterium sp.	38
Sophorolipids	*T. bombicola*	33
	T. apicola	30
	T. petrophilum	
Cellobiolipids	*U. zeae*	
	U. maydis	
Lipopeptides and lipoproteins		
Peptide-lipid	*B. licheniformis*	27
Serrawettin	*S. marcescens*	28-33
Viscosin	*P. fluorescens*	26.5
Surfactin	*B. subtilis*	27-32
Subtilisin	*B. subtilis*	
Gramicidins	*B. brevis*	
Polymyxins	*B. polymyxa*	
Fatty acids, neutral lipids, phospholipids		
Fatty acids	*C. lepus*	30
Neutral lipids	*N. erythropolis*	32
Phospholipids	*T. thiooxidans*	
Polymeric surfactants		
Emulsan	*A. calcoaceticus*	
Biodispersan	*A. calcoaceticus*	
Mannan-lipid-protein	*C. tropicalis*	
Liposan	*C. lipolytica*	
Carbohydrate-protein-lipid	*P. fluorescens*	27
	D. polymorphis	
Protein PA	*P. aeruginosa*	
Particulate biosurfactants		
Vesicles and fimbriae	*A. calcoaceticus*	
Whole cells	Variety of bacteria	

hydrophobic sophorosides. Although sophorolipids can lower the surface and interfacial tension, they are not effective emulsifying agents.

Lipopeptides and Lipoprotiens

A large number of cyclic lipopeptides including decapeptide antibiotics and lipopeptide antibiotics, produced by *Bacillus brevis* and *Bacillus polymyxa*, respectively, possess remarkable surface-active properties. An aminolipid biosurfactant called serratamolide has been isolated from *Serratia marcescens* NS.38. Studies on serratamolide-negative mutants showed that the biosurfactants increased cell hydrophilicity by blocking the hydrophobic sites on the cell surface.

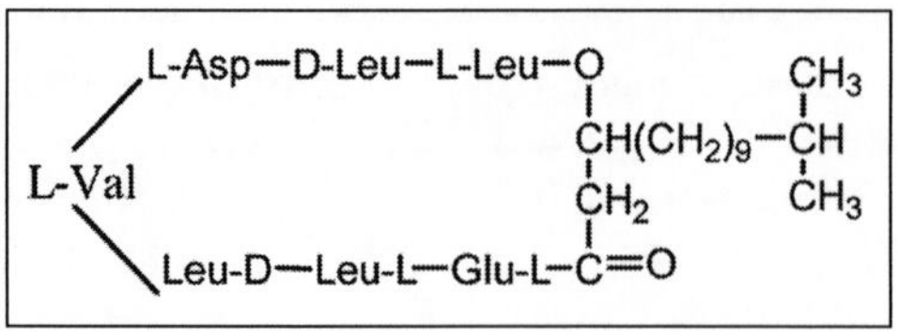

Figure 10. Structure of surfactin obtained from *Baxcillus subtilis*.

The cyclic lipopeptide surfactin (Fig. 10) produced by *B. subtilis* ATCC21332, is one of the most powerful biosurfactant. It lowers the surface tension from 72 to 27.9 mN m^{-1} at concentration as low as 0.005%.

Recently, Yakimov et al[34] have showed the production of a new lipopeptide surfactant, lichenysin A, by *B. licheniformis* BAS-50 containing the long-chain β-hydroxy fatty acids.

Fatty Acids, Neutral Lipids, Phospholipids

Several bacteria and yeasts produce large quantities of fatty acids and phospholipid surfactants during growth on n-alkanes. The HLB is directly related to the length of the hydrocarbon chain in their structure. In *Acinetobactor sp.* strain HO1-N phosphatidylethanolamine (Fig. 11) rich vesicles are produced, which form optically clear microemulsion of alkanes in water.

Phosphatidylethanolamine produced by *R. erythropolis* grown on n-alkane caused a lowering of interfacial tension between water and hexadecane to less than 1 mN m^{-1} and a *cmc* of 30 mg l^{-1}.

Polymeric Surfactants

The best-studied polymeric biosurfactants are emulsan, liposan, mannoprotein and other polysaccharide-protein complexes. *Acinetobacter calcoaceticus* RAG-1 produces a potent polyanionic amphipathic heteropolysaccharide bioemulsifier called emulsan (Fig. 12). Emulsan is a very effective emulsifying agent for hydrocarbon in water even at a concentration as low as 0.001 to 0.01%. It is one of the most powerful emulsion stabilizers known today and resists inversion even at a water-to-oil ratio of 1:4. Biodispersan is an extracellular, nondialyzable dispersing agent produced by *A. calcoaceticus* A2. It is an anionic heteropolysaccharide, with an average molecular weight of 51,400 and contains four reducing sugars.

Liposan is an extracellular water soluble emulsifier synthesized by *Candida lipolytica* and is composed of 83% carbohydrate and 17% protein. The carbohydrate portion is a heteropolysaccharide consisting of glucose, galactose, galactosamine and galacturonic acid.

Particulate Biosurfactants

Extracellular membrane vesicles partition hydrocarbons, to form a microemulsion which plays an important role in alkane uptake by microbial cells. Vesicles of *Acinetobacter sp.* strain HO1-N with a diameter of 20 to 50 nm and a buoyant density of 1.158 g cm^{-3} are composed of protein,

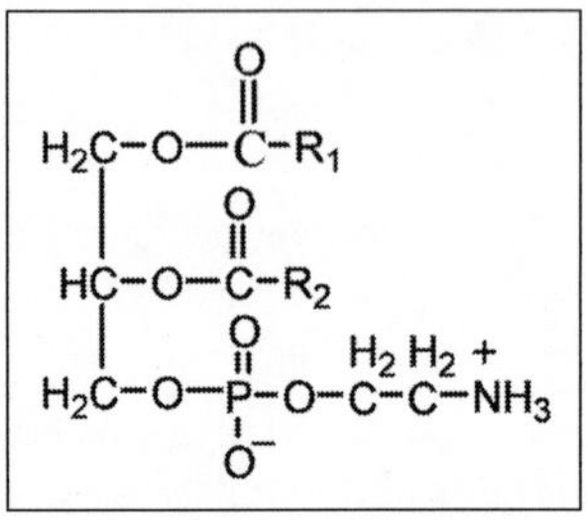

Figure 11. Structure of phosphatidylethanolamine, a microbial surfactant produced by *Acinetobacter sp.*

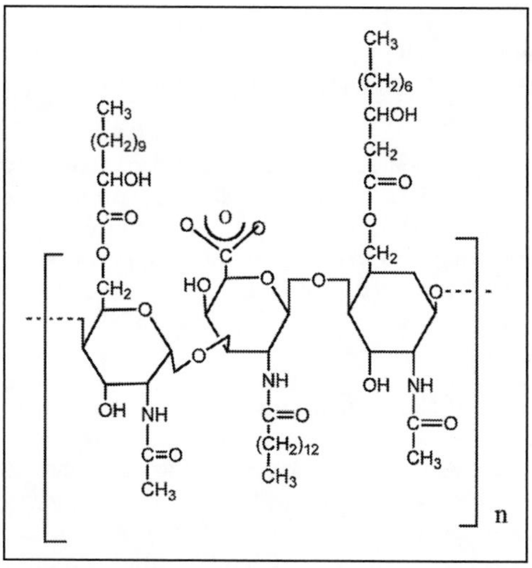

Figure 12. Structure of emulsan, produced by *Acinetobacter calcoaceticus*.

phospholipids and lipopolysaccharide.[35] Surfactant activity in most hydrocarbon-degrading and pathogenic bacteria is attributed to the cell surface components.

Properties of Biosurfactants

Biosurfactants are of increasing interest for commercial use because of the continually growing spectrum of available substances. The main distinctive features of biosurfactants and a brief description of their properties are as given below:

Surface and Interfacial Activity

A good surfactant can lower the surface tension of water from 72 to 35 mN m^{-1} and the interfacial tension of water/hexadecane from 40 to 1 mN m^{-1}. Surfactin from *B. subtilis* can reduce the surface tension of water to 25 mN m^{-1} and interfacial tension of water/hexadecane to <1 mN m^{-1}.[36] Rhamnolipids from *P. aeruginosa* decreases the surface tension of water to 26 mN m^{-1} and the interfacial tension of water/hexadecane to <1 mN m^{-1}.[37]

Temperature, pH and Ionic Strength Tolerance

Many biosurfactants and their surface activities are not affected by environmental conditions such as temperature and pH. McInerney et al[38] reported that lichenysin from *B. licheniformis* JF-2 was not affected by temperature up to 50°C, pH 4.5-9.0 and by NaCl and Ca^{+2} concentrations up to 50 and 25 g l^{-1}, respectively.

Biodegradability

Unlike synthetic surfactants, microbial-produced compounds are easily degraded and particularly suited for environmental applications such as bioremediation and dispersion of oil spills.

Emulsion Forming and Emulsion Breaking

Stable emulsion can be produced with a life span of months and year. Higher molecular-mass biosurfactants are in general better emulsifier that the low-molecular-mass biosurfactants. Sophorolipids from *T. bombicola* have been shown to reduce surface tension, but are not good emulsifiers. By contrast, liposan does not reduce the surface tension, but has been used successfully to emulsify edible oils. Polymeric surfactants offer additional advantages because they coat droplets of oil, thereby forming the stable emulsions. This property is especially useful for making oil/water emulsion for cosmetics and food.

Chemical Diversity

The chemical diversity of naturally produced biosurfactants offer a wide selection of surface-active agents with properties closely related to specific applications.

Low Toxicity

Microbial surfactants are generally considered as the low or nontoxic products and therefore are appropriate for pharmaceutical, cosmetic and food industries. A report suggested that a synthetic anionic surfactant (corexit) displayed an LC50 (concentration lethal to 50% of test species) against Photobacterium phosphoreum ten times lower than rhamnolipids, demonstrating the higher toxicity of chemical-based surfactants. It was also reported that biosurfactants showed higher EC50 (effective concentration to decrease 50% of test population) value than synthetic surfactants.[39]

Potential Applications of Biosurfactants

Most important aspect of biosurfactants is their environmental acceptability, because they are readily biodegradable and have low toxicity than synthetic surfactants. These unique properties of biosurfactants allow their use and possible replacement of chemically synthesized surfactants in a great number of industrial applications. Some of the major applications of biosurfactants in pollution and environmental control are microbial enhanced oil recovery, hydrocarbon degradation, hexa-chloro cyclohexane (HCH) degradation and heavy-metal removal from contaminated soil[40]:

Microbial Enhanced Oil Recovery (MEOR)

An area of considerable potential for biosurfactant application is microbial enhanced oil recovery. In MEOR, microorganisms in reservoir are stimulated to produce polymers and surfactants, which aid MEOR by lowering interfacial tension at the oil—rock interface. To produce microbial surfactants in situ, microorganisms in the reservoir are usually provided with low-cost substrates, such as molasses and inorganic nutrients. However, to be useful for MEOR in situ, bacteria must be able to grow under extreme conditions encountered in oil reservoirs such as high temperature, pressure, salinity and low oxygen level. Several aerobic and anaerobic thermophiles tolerant of pressure and moderate salinity have been isolated which are able to mobilize crude oil in the laboratory.[41]

Hydrocarbon Degradation

Hydrocarbon-utilizing microorganisms excrete a variety of biosurfactants. An important group of such surfactants is mycolic acids which are the α-alkyl, β-hydroxy very long-chain fatty acids contributing to some characteristic properties of a cell such as acid fastness, hydrophobicity, adherability and pathogenicity. This product has many applications in agrochemistry, mineral flotation and bitumen production and processing. Further, the product may be used as an emulsifying and dispersing agent while formulating herbicides, pesticides and growth regulator preparations. The constituent fatty acids of biolipid extract also have antiphytoviral and antifungal activities and therefore, can be applied in controlling plant diseases.[42]

Hydrocarbon Degradation in the Soil Environment

Degradation is dependent on presence in soil of hydrocarbon-degrading species of microorganisms, hydrocarbon composition, oxygen availability, water, temperature, pH and inorganic nutrients. Addition of synthetic surfactants or microbial surfactants results in increased mobility and solubility of hydrocarbon, which is essential for effective microbial degradation.

Lindley and Heydeman[43] have reported that the fungus *Cladosporium resiuae*, grown on alkane mixtures, produces extracellular fatty acids and phospholipids, mainly dodecanoic acid and phosphatidylcholine. Supplement of the growth medium with phosphatidylcholine enhances the alkane degradation rate by 30%. Foght et al[44] has reported that the emulsifier, Emulsan, stimulated aromatic mineralization by pure bacterial cultures, but inhibited the degradation process when mixed cultures were used.

Hydrocarbon Degradation in Aquatic Environment

When oil is spilled in aquatic environment, the lighter hydrocarbon components volatilize while the polar hydrocarbon components dissolve in water. However, because of low solubility (<1 ppm) of oil, most of the oil components will remain on the water surface. The primary means of hydrocarbon removal are photooxidation, evaporation and microbial degradation. Since hydrocarbon-degrading organisms are present in seawater, biodegradation may be one of the most efficient methods of removing pollutants.[45]

Emulsan, a high MW lipopolysaccharide produced by *A. calcaoceticus* RAG-1, has been proposed for a number of applications in the petroleum industry such as to clean oil and sludge from barges and tanks, reduce viscosity of heavy oils, enhance oil recovery and stabilize water-in-oil emulsions in fuels.

Biosurfactant and HCH Degradation

Hexa-chlorocyclohexane (HCH) is still the highest ranking pesticide used in India and many other countries. Of the eight known isomers of HCH, the alpha-form constitutes more than 70% of the technical product, which is not only known insecticidal but also a suspected carcinogen. The poor solubility is one of the limiting factors in the microbial degradation of alpha-HCH. Presence of six chlorines in the molecule is another factor that renders HCH lipophilic and persistent in the biosphere.

It has been reported that addition of biosurfactant from *Pseudomonas* Ptm$^+$ strain facilitied 250-fold increase in dispersion of HCH in water. Addition of either this organism or biosurfactant dislodged surface-borne HCH residues from many types of fruits, seeds and vegetables as well.[46] Laboratory-scale studies have revealed that microbial surfactants are very efficient in cleaning the containers where HCH residues were sticking to the wall.

Some more applications of biosurfactants include:

i. Binding of heavy metals. A rhamnolipid biosurfactant has been shown to be capable of removing Cd, Pb and Zn from soil. The mechanism by which rhamnolipid reduces metal toxicity may involve a combination of rhamnolipid complexation of Cd and rhamnolipid interaction with the cell surface to alter Cd uptake.

ii. Food industry. Lecithin and its derivatives, fatty acid esters containing glycerol, sorbitan or ethylene glycol and ethoxylated derivatives of monoglycerides including a recently synthesized oligopeptide are currently in use as emulsifier in the food industry.

iii. Cosmetic industry. A large number of compounds for cosmetic applications are prepared by enzymatic conversion of hydrophobic molecules by various lipases and whole cells.[47] The cosmetic industry demands surfactants with a minimum shelf life of 3 years. Therefore, saturated acyl groups are preferred over the unsaturated compounds. Monoglycerides, one of the widely used surfactants in the cosmetic industry, has been reported to be produced from glycerol-tallow (1.5:2) with a 90% yield by using *P. fluorescens* lipase treatment.

iv. Medicinal uses. A deficiency of pulmonary surfactant, a phospholipid-protein complex, is responsible for the failure of respiration in prematurely born infants. The isolation of genes for protein molecules of this surfactant and cloning in bacteria has made possible its fermentative production for medical application. 1% emulsion of rhamnolipids is successfully used for the treatment of Nicotiana glutinosa infected with tobacco mosaic virus and for the control of potato virus-x disease.

Association Properties of Biosurfactants

The association properties or self-assembly of biologically based amphiphilic molecules into potentially useful structures has been the area of interest. Owing to their dualistic structure these molecules self-assemble to form wide variety of morphologies including micelles, vesicles, tubes and coacervates. The micellar aggregation of biosurfactants is originated at the critical micellar concentration (*cmc*) and interestingly, they have about 10- to 40-fold lower *cmc* compared to chemical surfactants. This fact narrows the gap between the cost and efficiency of biosurfactants. However, bulkier structure of biosurfactants makes them more prone to the result in the formation of bilayered aggregates prior to the formation of routine microaggregates. It has been found that the single component of glycolipid biosurfactants, mannosyl-erythritol lipid-A (MEL-A) forms the sponge phase (L_3) together with the usual vesicle formation.[48] Later, it has been observed that the addition of phospholipids to glycolipid sponge phase (L_3) induces the formation of thermo-dynamically stable vesicle ($L_{\alpha1}$).[49] The formation of micellar aggregates followed by higher order aggregates for dirhamnolipids (diRL) extracellular biosurfactant has been observed by Sanchez et al[50]. As determined by surface tension measurements, at pH 7.4, the *cmc* of dirhamnolipid is 0.110 mM whereas at pH 4.0 the value falls to 0.010 mM, indicating that the negatively charged diRL has a much higher *cmc* than its neutral species. In comparison to other relevant biosurfactants like surfactin (*cmc* = 0.0075 mM), the *cmc* of diRL is one order higher in magnitude, suggesting that dirhamnolipids behave as weak detergents. At higher concentration the diRL results in the formation of mainly multilamellar vesicles of heterogeneous size.

The chemical character of respective hydrophobic portion and the hydrophilic part allows a wide range of variation in the physical and biological properties. Selection of the type and size of each moiety enables a delicate balance between surface activity and biological function and this represents the most effective approach of harnessing the power of molecular self-assembly.

Toxological and Ecological Aspects of Surfactants

The environmental impact of surfactant volume merging directly to the surrounding has become an important area of concern. The rate of biodegradation of surfactant in combination with the degree of toxicity produced, majorly determines the ecological impact.[51]

Dermatological Aspects

A number of dermatological problems of day life can be related to exposure of skin to surfactant solutions. Many of the formulations contain significant amount of surfactants e.g., cutting fluids, rolling oil emulsion, house-hold cleaning formulations and personal care products. The physiological aspects of surfactant on the skin has been investigated by various dermatological laboratories, starting with the surface of skin and progressing via the horney layer and its barrier function to the deeper layer of the vessel cells. Surfactant classes that are generally known to be mild to the skin include the polyol surfactants (alkyl polyglucosides), zwitterionic surfactant (betaines, amidobetaines and iso-thionates) and many polymeric surfactants. Alcohol ethoxylates are relatively mild but not as mild as the polyol-based non-ionics (the alkyl polyglucoside). In addition, alcohol ethoxylates may undergo oxidation to give by-products (hyperoxide and aldehydes) that are skin irritants.

Anionic surfactants are generally greater skin irritant than non-ionics. For examples, sodium dodecyl sulphate, which is commonly used in toothpaste, has relatively high skin toxicity. In contrast, ether sulphates are milder and are recommended for use in hand dishwashing formula-tions. However, some amphoteric surfactants such as betaines can also reduce the skin irritation of anionics.

Aquatic Toxicity

Aquatic toxicity may be measured on fish, daphnia or algae. Toxicity is given as LC_{50} (for fish) or EC_{50} (for daphnia or algae), where LC and EC stand for lethal and effective concentration, respectively. Values below 1 mg l^{-1} after 96 h testing on fish and algae and 48 h on daphnia are considered toxic.

Bioaccumulation

Bioaccumulation can be measured directly on fish in experimental way but is more often calculated from a model experiment. Partitioning of the surfactant/compound between two phases, organic and water is measured and logarithm of the values, log P, is used. The value of log P usually tells us about the hydrophobicity of the surfactant. A surfactant is considered to be bioaccumulated if:

$$\mathrm{Log\,P_{organic/water}} > 3$$

Most of the surfactant have log P values below 3. Bioaccumulation therefore is not considered to be a critical issue.

Biodegradability

This is the biological process carried by bacteria in nature. Through a series of enzymatic reactions, a surfactant molecule is finally converted into CO_2, H_2O and oxides of other elements. However, stable and persistent compound does not undergo natural biodegradation. For surfactants the rate of biodegradation varies from 1-2 h for fatty acids, 1-2 days for linear alkylbenzene sulfonates and months for branched alkylbenzene sulfonates. The rate of biodegradation depends upon the factors such as concentration, pH and temperature. The temperature effect is the most important factor. The rate at which chemicals are broken down in sewage plants may vary by as much as a factor of five between summer and winter in Northern Europe.

Conclusion

The chapter provides an insight into the basics of surfactant molecules, their behavior in solution and most importantly the application of these molecules. The dualistic structure of surfactant molecules results in the stubble balance between the hydrophobic and hydrophilic interactions. This results in their special property of accumulation at various interfaces and behavior of self-assembly (i.e., micellization).

The properties of surfactant molecules make them the most versatile of process chemicals appearing in wide range of product starting from house-hold usage, to medicinal chemistry and then to industries. The last decade has seen the extension of surfactant applications to high-technology areas such as electronic printing, magnetic recording, microelectronic, biotechnology and diversified medicinal research. In surge of green chemistry, the biologically compatible surfactants are in demand to replace some of the existing chemical surfactants. The reason for the popularity of biosurfactants as high-value microbial products is primarily because of their specific action, low toxicity, higher biodegradability, effectiveness at extreme temperatures, wide spread applicability and their structure which provide different properties than that of the classical surfactants.

Biological surfactants are highly sought after biomolecules as fine specialty chemicals, biological control agents and new generation molecules for pharmaceutical, cosmetic and health care industries.

References

1. Atwood D, Florence AT. Surfactant Systems; Their Chemistry, Pharmacy and Biology. New York: Chapman and Hall, 1983.
2. Rosen MJ. Surfactants and Interfacial Phenomenon. 2nd ed. New York: Wiley, 1978.
3. Tanford C. The Hydrophobic Effect. 2nd ed. New York: Wiley, 1980.
4. Holmberg K, Jonsson B et al. Surfactants and polymers in solution. 2nd ed. Chichester, John Wiley & Sons, 2003.
5. Holmes MC. Intermediate phases of surfactant-water mixtures. Current Opinion in Colloid Interface Sci 1998; 3:485-492.
6. Khan A. Phase science of surfactants. Current Opinion in Colloid Interface Sci 1996; 1:614-623.
7. Rosen MJ, Solash J. Factors affecting initial foam height in the Ross-Miles foam test. J Am Oil Chemists Soc 1969; 46(8):399-402.
8. Wyn-Jones E, Gormally J. Aggregation process in Solutions. Amsterdam: Elsevier, 1983.
9. Schick MJ. ed. Non-ionic surfactants, New York, M. Dekker, 1967.
10. Jungermann E. ed. Cationic surfactants, New York, M. Dekker, 1970.
11. Linfield WM. ed. Anionic surfactants, New York, M. Dekker, 1973.
12. Somasundaran P, Kunjappu JT. In situ investigation of adsorbed surfactants and polymers on solids in solution. Colloids Surfaces 1989; 37:245-268.
13. Griffith JC, Alexander AE. Equilibrium adsorption isotherms for wool/detergent systems: I. The adsorption of sodium dodecyl sulfate by wool. J Colloid Interface Sci 1967; 25:311-316.
14. Giles GH. Surfactant Adsorption at Solid/Liquid Interface, in Anionic Surfactants; Physical Chemistry of Action, Surfactant Science Series, Vol. II, New York: M. Dekker, 1981.
15. Mukerjee P, Mysels KJ. Critical micelle concentration of aqueous surfactant systems, NSRDS-NBS 36, National Bureau of Standards, Washington, D.C. 1971.
16. McBain JW. Colloids and their viscosity. Trans Faraday Soc 1913; 9:99.

17. Hartley GS. Aqueous solutions of paraffin chain salt. Peris: Harmann, 1936.
18. Harkins WD. A cylindrical model for the small soap micelle. J Chem Phys 1948; 16:156-57.
19. Debye P, Anacker EW. Micelle shape from dissymmetry measurements. J Phys Colloid Chem 1951; 55:644-655.
20. Reich I. Factors responsible for the stability of detergent micelles. J Phys Chem 1956; 60:257-262.
21. Moroi Y. Micelles: Theoretical and Applied Aspects. New York: Plenum Press, 1992.
22. Smith AL. Theory and Practice of Emulsion Technology. New York: Academic, 1976.
23. Greek BF. Sales of detergents growing despite recession. Chem Eng News 1991; 69:25-52.
24. Volkering F, Breure AM et al. Microbiological aspects of surfactant use for biological soil remediation Biodegradation 1998; 8:401-417.
25. Karanath NGK, Deo PG et al. Microbial production of biosurfactants and their importance. Curr Sci 1999; 77:116.
26. Desai JD, Banat IM. Microbial production of surfactants and their commercial potential. Microbiol Mol Biol Rev 1997; 61:47-64.
27. Banat IM, Makkar RS et al. Potential commercial applications of microbial surfactants. Appl Microbiol Biotechnol 2000; 53(5):495.
28. Desai AJ, Patel KM et al. Emulsifier production by Pseudomonas fluorescents during the growth on hydrocarbons. Curr Sci 1988; 57:500-501.
29. Rosenberg E. Microbial surfactants. Crit Rev Biotechnol 1986; 3:109-132.
30. Rosenberg E, Ron EZ. High- and low-molecular-mass microbial surfactants. Appl Microbiol Biotechnol 1999; 52(2):154.
31. Gautam KK, Tyagi VK. Microbial surfactants: a review. J Oleo Sci 2006; 55:155-166.
32. Jarvis FG, Johnson MJA. A glycolipid produced by Pseudomonas aeruginosa. J Am Oil Chem Soc 1949; 71:4124-4126.
33. Li ZY, Lang S et al. Formation and identification of interfacial-active glycolipids from resting microbial cells. Appl Environ Microbiol 1984; 48:610-617.
34. Yakimov MM, Timmis KN et al. Characterization of a new lipopeptide surfactant produced by thermotolerant and halotolerant subsurface Bacillus licheniformis BAS50. Appl Environ Microbiol 1995; 61:1706-1713.
35. Kappeli O, Finnerty WR. Partition of alkane by an extracellular vesicle derived from hexadecane-grown Acinetobacter. J Bacteriol 1979; 140:707-712.
36. Cooper DG, MacDonald CR et al. Enhanced production of surfactin from Bacillus subtilis by continuous product removal and metal cation additions. Appl Environ Microbiol 1981; 42:408-412.
37. Hisatsuka K, Nakahara T et al. Formation of rhamnolipid by Pseudomonas aeruginosa and its function in hydrocarbon fermentation. Agric Biol Chem 1971; 35:686-692.
38. Mclnerney MJ, Javaheri M et al. Properties of biosurfactants produced by Bacillus liqueniformis strain JF-2 I. J Microbiol Biotechnol 1990; 5:95-102.
39. Poremba K, Gunkel W et al. Toxicity testing of synthetic and biogenic surfactants on marine microorganisms. Environ Toxicol Water Qual 1991; 6:157-163.
40. Singh A, Van Hamme JD et al. Surfactants in microbiology and biotechnology: Part 2. Application aspects. Biotechnol Adv 2007; 25:99-121.
41. Post FJ, Al-Harjan FA. Surface activity of halobacteria and potentail use in microbial enhanced oil recovery System. Appl Microbiol 1988; 11:97-101.
42. Voigt B, Mueller H et al. Antiphytovirale Aktivität von lipophilen Fraktionen aus der Hefe Lodderomyces elongisporus IMET H 128. Acta Biotechnol 1985; 5:313-317.
43. Lindley ND, Heydemann MT. The uptake of n-alkanes from alkane mixtures during growth of the hydrocarbon-utilizing fungus Cladosporium resinae. Appl Microbiol Biotechnol 1986; 23(5):384-388.
44. Foght JM, Gutnick DL et al. Effect of Emulsan on Biodegradation of Crude Oil by Pure and Mixed Bacterial Cultures. Appl Environ Microbiol 1989; 55:36-42.
45. Atlas RM. Microbial degradation of petroleum hydrocarbons: an environmental. Microbiol Rev 1981; 45(1):180-209.
46. Doris MS, Ramesha N et al. Proceedings of the National Seminar on Advances in Seed Science and Technology, University of Mysore, Mysore, India, 1990, p. 368.
47. Therisod M, Klibanov AM. Facile enzymatic preparation of monoacylated sugars in pyridine. J Am Oil Chem Soc 1986; 108:5638-5640.
48. Imura T, Yanagishita H et al. Coacervate formation from natural glycolipid: one acetyl group on the headgroup triggers coacervate-to-vesicle transition. J Am Chem Soc 2004; 126:10804-10805.
49. Imura T, Yanagishita H et al. Thermodynamically stable vesicle formation from glycolipid biosurfactant sponge phase. Colloids Surfaces B 2005; 43:115-121.
50. Sanchez M, Aranda FJ et al. Aggregation behaviour of a dirhamnolipid biosurfactant secreted by Pseudomonas aeruginosa in aqueous media. J Colloid Interface Sci 2007; 307:246-253.
51. Rosen MJ, Li F et al. The relationship between the interfacial properties of surfactants and their toxicity to aquatic organisms. Environ Sci Technol 2001; 35:954-959.

CHAPTER 9

Applications of Biological Surface Active Compounds in Remediation Technologies

Andrea Franzetti,* Elena Tamburini and Ibrahim M. Banat

Abstract

Many microorganisms synthesize a wide range of surface active compounds (SACs), classified according to their molecular weights, properties and localizations. The low molecular weight SACs or biosurfactants lower the surface tension at the air/water interfaces and the interfacial tension at oil/water interfaces, whereas the high molecular weight SACs, also known as bioemulsifiers, are more effective in stabilizing oil-in-water emulsions. The ability to biosynthesize SACs is, often, coupled with the ability of these microorganisms to grow on immiscible carbon sources, such as hydrocarbons. Different mechanisms are involved in the SACs interactions between microbial cells and immiscible hydrocarbons including: (i) emulsification, (ii) micellarization, (iii) adhesion-deadhesion of microorganisms to and from hydrocarbons and (iv) desorption of contaminants. These naturally occurring phenomena can be exploited by adding bioemulsifiers and biosurfactants into environments where bioremediation/biodegradation rates of organic pollutants is to be enhanced. However, analysis of the current literature show some cases where the complex interactions among SACs, microbial cells, organic substrates and environmental media led to an inhibition of the biodegradation. The understanding of the different physiological roles of SACs in microbial communities is fundamental in order to develop more effective remediation technologies exploiting both synthetic surfactants and microbial SACs. The physio-chemical properties of some microbial SACs have been exploited in hydrocarbon-contaminated soils washing and in mobilisation of soil-bound metal in metal-contaminated soils. Our ability to analyse the microbial diversity in the natural environments will expand our knowledge on microbial SACs with respect to their exploitation for commercial applications and their roles in the physiology of the producing microorganisms.

Microbial Surface Active Compounds

Structures and Properties

Many prokaryotic and eukaryotic microorganisms synthesize a wide range of structurally different amphiphilic molecules containing both hydrophilic and hydrophobic (typically a hydrocarbon) moieties. The structural features of amphiphiles confer them the ability to concentrate and alter the conditions at interfaces. Interface is a term describing a surface which forms a boundary between two different phases, such as gas/liquid, two immiscible liquids, solid/liquid. Due to their

*Corresponding Author: Andrea Franzetti—Department of Environmental Sciences, University of Milano-Bicocca, Piazza della Scienza 1, 20126 Milano, Italy.
Email: andrea.franzetti@unimib.it

Biosurfactants, edited by Ramkrishna Sen. ©2010 Landes Bioscience and Springer Science+Business Media.

superficial properties, amphiphilic microbial metabolites have been usually referred to as Surface Active Compounds (SACs). Neu[1] divided SACs into three different classes: (i) biosurfactants are defined as low molecular weight SACs (e.g., glycolipids, lipopeptides); (ii) amphiphilic polymers are defined as high molecular weight SACs with a hydrophobic region at one end of the molecule (e.g., lipopolysaccharides, lipoteicoic acids); (iii) polyphilic polymers are defined as high molecular weight SACs with hydrophobic groups distributed across the entire polymeric molecule (e.g., hydrophobic polysaccharides, emulsan). The low molecular weight SACs or biosurfactants lower the surface tension at the air/water interfaces and the interfacial tension at oil/water interfaces, whereas the high molecular weight SACs, also called bioemulsifiers, are more effective in stabilizing oil-in-water emulsions.[2]

Comparing the properties of different biosurfactants, surface and interfacial tensions are parameters used as a measure of biosurfactant effectiveness. When a biosurfactant is added to air/water or oil/water systems at increasing concentrations, a reduction of the surface tension is observed up to a critical level, above which the amphiphilic molecules associate readily to form supramolecular structures, such as micelles, bilayers and vesicles.[3] The concentration at which surfactants begin to form micelles is known as the critical micelle concentration (CMC) which is used to evaluate biosurfactant efficiency.

In a heterogeneous system, an emulsion is the mixture of two immiscible liquids which is formed when one liquid phase is dispersed as microscopic droplets in an other continuous phase.[3] The activity of different bioemulsifiers is compared by assaying their ability to stabilize a water/oil emulsion or generate turbidity due to suspended hydrocarbons in an aqueous system.[4,5]

The best studied low molecular weight SACs so far are glycolipids and lipopeptides.[2] Glycolipids are disaccharides acylated with long chain fatty acids or hydroxyl fatty acids. Among them, the best-characterized structural subclasses are rhamnolipids produced by several *Pseudomonas* species, sophorolipids synthesized by different species of the yeast *Candida* (formerly *Torulopsis*) and trehalolipids found in *Rhodococcus* and other actinomycetes.[6,7] Most of the biosurfactants produced by rhodococci are trehalose mycolates consisting of a trehalose residue linked by an ester bond to mycolic acids, long α-alkyl β-hydroxy fatty acids.[8] Lipopeptides are low molecular weight SACs showing potent surface activities. A variety of structurally different variants is produced by several *Bacillus* species. *Bacillus subtilis* produces a cyclic lipopeptide called surfactin or subtilisin which has been reported as the most active biosurfactant discovered todate.[9]

High molecular weight SACs are produced by a wide diversity of Bacteria (Gram-positive and Gram-negative) and Archaea. Most of the emulsifiers are composted by mixtures of hydrophobic and hydrophilic polymers. The most extensively studied bioemulsifiers are the ones produced by different *Acinetobacter* species.[2] An example of well-characterized high molecular weight SAC is Emulsan, an effective emulsifier produced by the *Acinetobacter lwoffii* strain RAG-1 (formerly *Acinetobacter calcoaceticus*). Emulsan is a complex mixture of an anionic heteropolysaccharide and proteins. It presents a polyphilic structure being composed of fatty acids attached, over the entire molecule, to the polysaccharidic backbone. Its emulsification activity is due to the tight affinity of emulsan for oil/water interfaces. Emulsan has been found to exibit high specificity: it is not able to emulsify pure aliphatic, aromatic, or cyclic hydrocarbons but it efficiently emulsifies mixtures containing the appropriate proportions of aliphatic and aromatic (or cyclic) alkanes.[2]

Novel Microbial Surface Active Compounds

Most research on microbial SAC has been confined, mostly, to few well-characterized molecules produced by a small number of microbial genera (*Pseudomonas, Candida, Bacillus, Acinetobacter*). Consequently, our understanding of the diversity, physiological roles and potential applications of microbial SACs is limited to a relatively narrow spectrum of microbial metabolites and biological systems. Only few studies were concerned with the phylogenetic diversity of SAC-producing microorganisms and the majority of the producing microorganisms has been isolated from a narrow range of environments, mainly undisturbed and hydrocarbon contaminated soils or heavy metal contaminated soils.[10-13]

In the last few years, a growing number of new SAC-producing microorganisms have been described although their products often remain uncharacterized in respect to their chemical structures. Bodour et al[14] reported a new glycolipid class, the flavolipids, produced by a *Flavobacterium* strain isolated from soil. Flavolipids exhibit a unique polar moiety which features citric acid and two cadaverine molecules and display strong surfactant and emulsifying activities. The cold-adapted *Halomonas* sp. strain ANT-3b, isolated from Antarctic seawater, has been also recently reported to produce a new high molecular weight glycolipidic bioemulsifier.[15] Bonilla et al[16] also reported the production of an exopolysaccharide with emulsifying activity by a *Pseudomonas* strain which has a significantly different chemical composition to previous reports.

The Roles of SACs in Hydrocarbon Metabolism

Microbial ability to biosynthesize SACs is, often, coupled with their ability to grow on immiscible carbon sources although many produce amphiphilic metabolites from miscible carbon sources.[17] SACs can be intracellular, cell surface bound or extracellular compounds.[1] The kinetics of SAC production differ among various biological systems[3] and are produced by a variety of microorganisms in heterogeneous growth conditions leading to varying roles in the physiology of the producing microorganisms.[9] The physiological roles proposed for microbial SACs have been recently reviewed by Van Hamme et al.[18] SACs appear to play a role in different behaviours which microbial cells carry out when they contact interfaces. Among the roles proposed for microbial SACs are motility (gliding, swarming, de-adhesion from surfaces), cell-cell interactions (biofilm formation, maintenance and maturation, quorum sensing, amensalism, pathogenicity), cellular differentiation, substrate accession as well as avoidance of toxics elements and compounds.

In this chapter, we examine the proposed roles for SACs with respect to the interactions between microbes and hydrocarbons. Particularly, we discuss the different strategies evolved by microorganisms to overcome the low solubility of hydrocarbons, access to hydrocarbons before transportation into cells and adhesion-deadhesion of microbial cells from and to hydrocarbon surfaces.[19,20] Understanding of the different physiological roles of SACs in microbial communities is fundamental in order to develop more effective remediation technologies exploiting both synthetic surfactants and microbial SACs and techniques useful in evaluating the impact of treatments on microbial communities and outcomes of remediation processes.

Microbial Access to Hydrocarbons

Hydrocarbon metabolism is always restricted to water/hydrocarbon interfaces since the oxygenases involved in their catabolic pathways are never extracellular but always membrane-bound enzymes.[19] Thus, microbial growth on hydrocarbons can be limited by the interfacial surfaces leading to a linear growth rather than exponential one. Extracellular biosurfactants and bioemulsifiers increase oil/water interfaces enhancing substrate mass transfer and allowing more microorganisms to contact the hydrocarbon substrates. Emulsifiers increase the hydrocarbon/water interfaces stabilizing oil droplets in the water/oil emulsion. On the other hand, when a surfactant is present in an oil/water system at concentrations above its CMC, the oil solubility, dramatically, increases due to the aggregation of surfactant micelles. The hydrophobic moieties of the surfactant molecules cluster together exposing the hydrophilic ends to the aqueous phase on the exterior. Consequently, the core of micelles becomes a compatible environment for hydrophobic organic molecules. The process is known as pseudosolubilization.[21]

The ability of different microorganisms to access hydrocarbons depends on their cell surface hydrophobicity. High cell-hydrophobicity allows them to directly contact oil drops and solid hydrocarbons while low cell hydrophobicity permits their adhesion to micelles or emulsified oils.[19,20] Three different mechanisms of cell access to hydrocarbons have been postulated: (i) access to water-solubilize hydrocarbons, (ii) direct contact of cells with large oil drops, (iii) contact with pseudosolubilized or emulsified oil. The first mechanism is limited to low molecular weight hydrocarbons since the hydrocarbon solubility, dramatically, decreases with increased molecular weights. In rhodococci, cells are hydrophobic due to the presence of a hydrophobic mycolic acid layer in their cell walls and the major hydrocarbon accession mode is likely to be direct contact of hydrophobic cells with large oil drops (Fig. 1A).[8,21] *Rhodococcus* genus belongs to mycolic acid-containing actinomycetes including also *Gordonia, Nocardia, Corynebacterium, Tsukamurella* and *Mycobacterium* genera. In *Rhodoccoccus* spp., mycolic acids are found attached to the cell wall arabinogalactans and partially free in the form of trehalose mycolates. Arabinogalactan-bound mycolic acids, as well as free trehalose mycolates, are thought to be localized in the outer layer of the cell wall, where they form the basis of an outer lipid permeability barrier.[22] Thus, the cell-associated amphiphilic trehalose mycolates seems to play a structural role in the rhodococci cell wall. On the other hand, the access to hydrocarbons in *Pseudomonas* strains relays on the release in the culture broths of the extracellular surfactants, rhanmolipids, which enhance the hydrocarbon apparent solubility. The hydrophilic surface allows *Pseudomonas* cells to interact with the hydrophilic outer layer of the hydrocarbon-containing micelles (Fig. 1B).[23]

SACs are thought to play a role in regulating the cell surface hydrophobicity thereby controlling adhesion-deadhesion of microbial cells to and from hydrocarbon surfaces.[1,9,24] Microorganisms either increase or decrease their cell hydrophobicity by respectively exposing outwardly or inwardly the hydrophobic moieties of the cell-bound SACs. For example, the cell-surface hydrophobicity of *A. lwoffii* RAG-1 is reduced by the presence of emulsan, a cell-bound bioemulsifier.[2,25] During the exponential phase of growth on oil mixtures, RAG-1 cells are attached to the oil droplets and emulsan is cell-bound in the form of a minicapsule. After bacteria have consumed long chain *n*-alkanes in the oil droplets, RAG-1 cells become starved being unable to metabolize any of the other oil components which leads to the release of emulsan minicapsule from the cell surfaces desorbing starved cells from hydrocarbons and forming a polymeric film on the *n*-alkane-depleted oil droplets. This hydrophilic film layer is laid over the exhausted droplets to which RAG-1 cells cannot attach anymore therefore compelling them to attach to fresh oil droplets.[2]

Altering Access Mode

Franzetti et al[24] recently suggested that some microbial SACs play a role in changing the substrate access mode during the different growth stages on hydrocarbons. They observed that *Gordonia* sp. strain BS29 grown on hydrocarbons synthesizes both cell-bound glycolipid biosurfactants and extracellular bioemulsifiers. During early exponential phase of growth on *n*-hexadecane, BS29 surface is hydrophobic and cells access large oil drops through direct contact (Fig. 1A). During the late exponential phase, the cell surface becomes hydrophilic. This change in surface hydrophobicity may be due to cell-bound SACs which expose their hydrophilic moieties toward the water phase masking the highly hydrophobic character of the mycolic acid layer. Consequentially, the hydrophilic surface allows cells to attach to the hydrophilic outer layer of the emulsified oil droplets (Fig. 1C). Ron and Rosenberg[9] have suggested that there are conceptual difficulties in understanding the evolutionary advantages of producing extracellular bioemulsifiers, since it is impossible to obtain an oil emulsion available only for the producing strain in an open system. However, the population-specific interaction between BS29 and microemulsion (mediated by the regulation of cell hydrophobicity and emulsifier biosynthesis) could allow BS29 to take advantage of the emulsion over the other microbial populations.

Remediation Technologies

SACs have recently been evaluated in bench and field-scale experimentations as substitutes for chemically synthesized surfactants to improve rate of contaminant removal in soil and water remediation processes. Microbial SACs find potential applications within physicochemical technologies for remediation of both organic and metal contaminations, such as in situ soil flushing and ex situ soil washing for remediation of unsaturated zone, pump and treat for aquifer remediation,[26-28] and also in bioremediation technologies to improve the biodegradation rate of organic compounds.[28] A wide range of other different potential commercial exploitations have been described not only for oil industry, such as microbial enhanced oil recovery, oil transportation and tank cleaning, but also in medicine, cosmetics and food industries.[2,29,30]

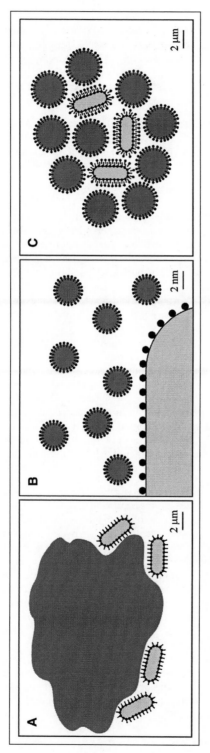

Figure 1. Different hydrocarbon accession modes in microorganisms: direct contact of cells with large oil drops (A), contact with pseudosolubilized oil (B) and emulsified oil (C). Dots and lines represent hydrophilic and hydrophobic moieties of microbial SACs, respectively (not on scale).

Bioremediation

Physicochemical properties of SACs are involved in the interaction between microbial cells and immiscible hydrocarbons by the following mechanisms[9,31]: (i) emulsification, (ii) micellarization, (iii) adhesion-deadhesion of microorganisms to and from hydrocarbons and (iv) desorption of contaminants. These naturally occurring phenomena can be exploited to enhance bioremediation treatments by adding biological SACs (Table 1) and chemical surfactants (Table 2).

Emulsification

Despite their potentials, microbial emulsifiers have been rarely evaluated as enhancers of hydrocarbon biodegradation in bioremediation. Barkay et al[32] showed that Alasan, produced by *Acinetobacter radioresistens* more than doubled the rate of [^{14}C] fluoranthene mineralization and significantly increased the rate of [^{14}C] phenanthrene mineralization by *Sphingomonas paucimobilis* EPA505.

Micellarization

When a surfactant is present at concentrations above its CMC, a significant fraction of the hydrophobic contaminants partitioned in the surfactant micelle cores. This, generally, results in an increase in the bioavailability of the hydrophobic contaminants to the degrading-microorganisms thus enhancing their biodegradation rate.[31] Several researchers demonstrated that rhamnolipid addition to contaminated soils above CMC both accelerated the biodegradation of hexadecane, octadecane, *n*-paraffins, creosotes and other hydrocarbon mixtures and enhanced the bioremediation of petroleum sludges.[33-36] Furthermore, the addition of glycolipids improved the biodegradation of chlorinated hydrocarbons.[37] Pesticide biodegradation was also reported to be promoted by surfactin.[38]

On the other hand, other studies showed the organic contaminants trapped into micelle cores become less bioavailable to the microorganisms resulting in an inhibition of their degradation. Witconol SN70, a non-ionic alcohol ethoxylate surface active compound, inhibited the mineralization of hexadecane and phenanthrene.[39] Doses of four surfactants (Tween 20, sodium dodecyl sulfonate, tetradecyl trimethyl ammonium bromide, Citrikleen) at ≥ CMCs, inhibited mineralization of phenanthrene in a soil-water system.[40] In aqueous media, the biodegradation of four PCB congeners by *Pseudomonas* LB-400 was inhibited by Igepal CO-630, a non-ionic surfactant, at concentrations above its CMC.[41] Also other cases of inhibition of biodegradation due the addition of surfactants have been observed and believed to be due to the surfactants providing a more easily degradable carbon source alternative to the contaminants.[42,43]

Regulation of Adhesion-Deadhesion of Microorganisms to Hydrocarbons

A proposed role for microbial SACs is the regulation of the adhesion-deadhesion of microorganisms to and from hydrocarbons. The exploitation of this natural roles consists in the addition of surfactants to increase the hydrophobicity of degrading microorganisms which allows cells to access to hydrophobic substrates more easily.[44,45] Al-Tahhan et al[46] demonstrated that sub-CMC levels of rhamnolipids caused the release of LPS by *Pseudomonas* spp., a phenomenon that rendered the cell surface more hydrophobic allowing a more efficient uptake of hexadecane. Normann et al[35] demonstrated that rhamnolipid by *P. aeruginosa* UG2 stimulated the degradation of hexadecane by the same organism facilitating the hydrocarbon uptake. This rhamnolipid did not stimulate to the same extent the biodegradation of hexadecane by four other strains (*A. lwoffii* RAG1, *Rhodococcus erythropolis* DSM 43066, *R. erythropolis* ATCC 19558 and strain BCG112), nor was degradation of hexadecane stimulated by addition of their own biosurfactants. More recently, Zhong et al[47] studied the adsorption of dirhamnolipid biosurfactants on cells of *P. aeruginosa*, *B. subtilis* and *Candida lipolytica*. Their results showed that the adsorption was specific to the microorganisms and depended on the physiological status of their cells. Furthermore, biosurfactant adsorption caused the cell surface hydrophobicity to change depending on both the rhamnolipid concentrations and the cell physiological conditions.

Table 1. *Effect of microbial SACs on biodegradation of organic compounds*

Producing Microorganisms	SACs (E/S)[1]	Experimental Systems	Degrading Microorganisms	Pollutants	Effect on Degradation[2]	Mechanisms of Degradation Enhancement/Inhibition	Ref
Acinetobacter radioresitant KA53	Alasan (E)	Liquid cultures	*Sphingomonas paucimobilis* EPA 505	Phenanthrene	E	Increasing phenanthrene solubility	32
Acinetobacter calcoaceticus RAG1	Emulsan (E)	Liquid cultures	*Acinetobacter calcoaceticus* RAG1, *Rhodococcus erythropolis* DSM 43066, *R. erythropolis* ATCC 19958, *Pseudomonas aeruginosa* UG2	Hexadecane	I	Altering accession to hydrocarbon	35
Pseudomonas aeruginosa	Rhamnolipid (S)	Liquid cultures	*Pseudomonas aeruginosa*	Hexadecane	E	Involvement in hexadecane uptake	33
Pseudomonas aeruginosa UG2	Rhamnolipid (S)	Liquid cultures	*Pseudomonas aeruginosa* UG2, PG201 and ATCC 15528	Hexadecane	E	Facilitating the hydrocarbon uptake	35
Pseudomonas aeruginosa UG2	Rhamnolipid (S)	Liquid cultures	*Rhodococcus erythropolis* DSM 43066, *R. erythropolis* ATCC 19958,	Hexadecane	I	Altering accession to hydrocarbon	35
Pseudomonas aeruginosa	Rhamnolipid (S)	Soil microcosms	Soil autochthonous community/ degrading consortium	Petroleum sludge	E	Increasing bioavailability	36
Pseudomonas aeruginosa	Rhamnolipid (S)	Liquid cultures	*Streptomyces* PS1/5	Trifluralin,	E	Increasing bioavailability	37
Pseudomonas aeruginosa	Rhamnolipid (S)	Liquid cultures	*Streptomyces* PS1/5	Atrazine	I	Providing alternative substrate	37
Pseudomonas aeruginosa	Rhamnolipid (S)	Liquid cultures	Degrading consortia from a contaminated cattle dip	Coumaphos	E	Increasing bioavailability	37

continued on next page

Table 1. Continued

Producing Microorganisms	SACs (E/S)[1]	Experimental Systems	Degrading Microorganisms	Pollutants	Effect on Degradation[2]	Mechanisms of Degradation Enhancement/Inhibition	Ref
Pseudomonas aeruginosa	Rhamnolipid (S)	Soil slurry	*Streptomyces PS1/5*	Trifluralin, Atrazine	NA	-	37
Pseudomonas aeruginosa	Rhamnolipid (S)	Soil slurry	Degrading consortia from a contaminated cattle dip	Coumaphos	E	Increasing bioavailability	37
Pseudomonas aeruginosa ATCC 9027	Rhamnolipid (S)	Liquid cultures	Pseudomonas aeruginosa ATCC 9027/ATCC 27853	Hexadecane	E	Increasing cell hydrophobicity	46
Pseudomonas aeruginosa sp.	Rhamnolipid (S)	Liquid cultures	*Pseudomonas aeruginosa*	Hexadecane	E	Increasing cell hydrophobicity/ pseudosolubilisation	44
Pseudomonas aeruginosa sp.	Rhamnolipid (S)	Soil column	Soil autochthonous community	Phenanthrene	E	Desorption of phenatrene from soil	50
Pseudomonas aeruginosa UG2	Rhamnolipid (S)	Silica column	*Pseudomonas aeruginosa UG2*	Hexadecane	E	Desorption of hexadecane from micropores	54
Bacillus subtilis MTCC1427	Surfactin	Liquid cultures/soil: water slurry	Consortium of two bacterial cultures	Endosulfan	E	Increasing bioavailability	38

[1]SACs; E: emulsifier; S: surfactant; [2]Effect on degradation: E: Enhancement; I: Inhibition; NA: not affected.

Table 2. Effect of chemical synthesized surfactants on biodegradation of organic compounds

Surfactant	Experimental System	Degrading MOs	Pollutants	Effect on Degradation[1]	Mechanisms of Degradation Enhancement/Inhibition	Ref
Triton X-100	Liquid culture	*Streptomyces* PS1/5	Trifluralin and Atrazine	I	Lowering bioavailability	37
Triton X-100	Soil slurry	*Streptomyces* PS1/5	Trifluralin and Atrazine	NA	-	37
Triton X-100	Soil slurry	degrading consortia from a contaminated cattle dip	Coumaphos	I	Lowering bioavailability	37
Triton X-100	Liquid cultures	*Mycobacterium* sp;; *Pseudomonas* sp	Anthracene	I	Decreasing cell hydrophobicity— inhibition cell-substrate access	48
Triton X-100	Soil	Soil autochthonous community	Phenanthrene	E	Desorption of phenatrene from soil	53
Triton X-100; PLE10	Liquid cultures	*Pseudomonas* sp. 8909N	Naphthalene	E	Increasing of dissolution rate	51
Brij 56	Liquid cultures	Gram-positive bacterium	Diesel fuel	NA	-	43
Tween 80	Liquid cultures	Gram-positive bacterium	Diesel fuel	E	Pseudosolubilisation	43
Tween 80; Brij 56	Soil slurry	Soil autochthonous community	Diesel fuel	I	Codegradation and soil sorption (Tween 80); toxicity and lowering bioavailability (Brij 56)	43
Witconol SN70	Soil	Soil autochthonous community	Hexadecane, phenanthrene	I	Toxicity/codegradation	39
Tween 20, sodium dodecyl sulfonate, tetradecyl trimethyl ammonium bromide, citrikleen	Liquid cultures/soil water slurry	Degrading consortium	Phenanthrene	I	Toxicity of surfactant and solubilized phenanthrene	40

[1]Effect on degradation; E: Enhancement; I: Inhibition; NA: not affected.

Cases of inhibition of microbial degradation due to surfactant-induced change in surface hydrophobicity have also been reported. Chen et al[48] observed that low concentration (0.09 CMA) of Triton X-100 inhibited the growth on solid anthracene of a *Mycobacterium* sp. strain and a *Pseudomonas* sp. strain. The causes of inhibition were believed to be the sorption of the surfactant onto both microbial cell surfaces and anthracene particles.

Desorption of Contaminants

Organic compounds can often strongly bind to particles on porous materials, such as soils therefore, becoming trapped into micropores. This, usually, does not allow rapid remediation and can lead to extended remediation periods. Several studies have shown that the mass transfer from ab/adsorbed phase to liquid is the controlling mechanism of biodegradation rate.[49] In these cases, biosurfactants can enhance the bioavailability of contaminants even at concentrations below the CMC.[28] Phenomena associated with this mechanism include a reduction of surface and interfacial tensions, capillary force and wettability and an increase of contact angle. At concentrations below CMC, surfactants reduce the surface and interfacial tensions between air/water, oil/water and soil/water systems. In a soil/oil system, surfactants increase the contact angle and reduce the capillary force holding together oil and soil particles due to the reduction of the interfacial force. Surfactants have been used to stimulate the dissolution of non-aqueous phase liquids initially present in soils,[50] the dissolution of solid contaminants[51] and the desorption and transport of soil-sorbed contaminants.[52,53]

Noordman et al[54] investigated the effect of the rhamnolipid biosurfactant on hexadecane degradation in the case of substrate entrapped in small soil pore sizes (6 nm). Even in low mixing conditions, rhamnolipids stimulated the release of entrapped substrates and enhanced uptake by cells.

Soil Washing

Hydrocarbon Contaminated Soils

The prospects of using biosurfactants in hydrocarbon-contaminated soil washing depend on the capacity of these compounds to enhance the desorption and dissolution of the polluting organic compounds and increase the rate of transport of contaminants in soils. The mechanisms involved in the hydrocarbon removal from soils are related to the mechanisms involved in increasing bioavailability for bioremediation purposes. The properties of stabilizing oil/water emulsions and increasing hydrocarbon solubility may enhance both the biodegradation rate and the hydrocarbon removal rate from soils.[55] These mobilization and solubilization effects occur at both concentration below and above the CMC. The application of microbial SACs to remove contaminants from soils is a technology characterized by some minor degree of uncertainty than the SAC-enhanced bioremediation, since only the chemicophysical properties of the biosurfactants and not their effects on cell surface properties and microbial metabolisms drive the removal efficiency.

The use of chemical surfactants has been reported to be efficient in removing hydrocarbons from soils. Lee at al.[56] reported that non ionic surfactants removed more than 80% of total hydrocarbons from soils. Billingsley et al[41] demonstrated interesting differences in the effects of non-ionic and anionic surfactants on the removal and bioavailability of PCBs. Non-ionic surfactants washed more PCBs from soils while the substrate into anionic surfactants micelle cores were more available for biodegradation by a PCB-degrading *Pseudomonas* sp. Microbial SACs often exhibited better capacity of removing hydrocarbons than their synthetic counterparts. The more commonly studied biosurfactants, such as rhamnolipids and surfactin, have been successfully evaluated in washing of soils contaminated by crude oils, PAHs and chlorinated hydrocarbons.[28] In several cases, the removal efficiency was very high (up to 80%) and depended on both the contact time and biosurfactant concentration.[50,57] Rhamnolipids have been reported to release three times as much oil as water alone from the beaches in Alaska after the Exxon Valdez tanker spill.[58] Van Dyke et al[59] have reported that rhamnolipids, at a concentration of 5 g/l, could remove approximately 10% more hydrocarbons from a sandy loam soil than sodium dodecyl sulfate. Biosurfactants appeared to be more effective in increasing the apparent solubility of PAHs by up to five times as compared to chemical surfactants.[60,61] Biosurfactants have also found applications in aquifer remediation due to their ability to reduced interfacial tension between dense the non-aqueous phase liquids and groundwaters.[62,63]

Metal Contaminated Soils

The interactions between surfactants and metals are not fully understood. It is known that surfactants can remove metals from surfaces by different mechanisms. Non ionic metals can form complexes with biosurfactants, enhancing their removal from porous media.[64] Anionic surfactants interact with cationic metals leading to their desorption from surfaces.[27] Nevertheless, also cationic surfactants can play a role by competitive binding to negative charged binding sites. The first studies on biosurfactant-metal complex were carried out by Tan et al[65] They demonstrated the rapid formation of monorhamnolipid-metal complex. Rhamnolipids have been evaluated for their affinity to metal cations.[66] $K^+ < Mg^{2+} < Mn^{2+} < Ni^{2+} < Co^{2+} < Ca^{2+} < Hg^{2+} < Fe^{3+} < Zn^{2+} < Cd^{2+} < Pb^{2+} < Cu^{2+} < Al^{3+}$ are the cations in order (from lowest to highest) of affinity with rhamnolipids. Mulligan and coworkers extensively studied the potential of rhamnolipids, sophorolipids and surfactin in washing of metal-contaminated soils and sediments.[26] Mulligan and Young[67] studied the effect of biosurfactants by *Pseudomonas* sp., *Bacillus* sp. and *Candida* sp. on zinc and copper removal from soils and demonstrated that anionic surfactants are able to selectively remove metals oxide, carbonate and organic fraction from soils. Rhamnolipids successfully removed heavy metals from an oil cocontaminated soil[68] and heavy metal contaminated sediments.[26] Batch soil washing experiments were carried out to evaluate the feasibility of using surfactin for the removal of heavy metals from contaminated soils and sediments. By a series of five soil washings, removals of 70% and 22% of copper and zinc, respectively were reported.[26] Surfactin was able to remove the metals by both sorption at the soil particle interphase and metal complexation.

Future applications of bioemulsifiers in remediation of heavy metals and radionuclides can be now envisaged. Several microbial polysaccharides have been shown to bind heavy metals. Emulsan by *A. lwoffii* RAG-1 forms stable oil-in-water emulsions. In this system, metal ions bind primarily at the oil/water interphase enabling their recovery and concentration from relatively dilute solutions. Cations bound to the emulsion can be completely removed to the water phase when pH was lowered.[69]

Conclusion and Prospects

The heterogeneity of SAC structural types and properties results in a broad spectrum of potential applications in environmental remediation as well as in the oil industry, agriculture, medicine, cosmetic and food industries.[29] Our increasing ability to analyze the microbial diversity in natural environments is expected to expand our knowledge on microbial SACs with respect to their exploitation for commercial applications and their roles in the physiology of the producing microorganisms. During the past few years, high throughput methods have been generated for the systematic screening of SAC-producing microorganisms.[70,71] Unfortunately, only a small percentage of microorganisms can be cultivated from environmental samples using traditional cultivation techniques.[72] In order to overcome the problems associated with cultivation of microorganisms, new cultivation methods have been developed in order to increase the number of culturable bacterial species and investigate the previously inaccessible resources that these microorganisms potentially have.[73]

References

1. Neu T. Significance of bacterial surface-active compounds in interaction of bacteria with interfaces. Microbiol Rev 1996; 60:151-166.
2. Rosenberg E, Ron EZ. High- and low-molecular-mass microbial surfactants. Appl Microbial Biotechnol 1999; 52:154-162.
3. Desai JD, Banat IM. Microbial production of surfactants and their commercial potential. Microbiol Mol Biol Rev 1997; 61:47-64.
4. Cooper DG, Goldenberg BG. Surface-active agents from two Bacillus species. App Environ Microbiol 1987; 53:224-229.

5. Rosenberg E, Zuckerberg A, Rubinovitz C et al. Emulsifier of Arthrobacter RAG-1: isolation and emulsifying properties. Appl Environ Microbiol 1979; 37:402-408.
6. Ito S, Inoue S. Sophorolipids from Torulopsis bombicola: possible relation to alkane uptake. Appl Environ Microbiol 1982; 43:1278-1283.
7. Kretschmer A, Bock H, Wagner F. Chemical and physical characterization of interfacial-active lipids from Rhodococcus erythropolis grown on n-alkanes. Appl Environ Microbiol 1982; 44:864-870.
8. Lang S, Philp JC. Surface-active lipids in rhodococci. Anton Leeuw Int J G 1998; 74:59-70.
9. Ron EZ, Rosenberg E. Natural roles of biosurfactants. Environ Microbiol 2001; 3:229-236.
10. Bodour AA, Drees KP, Maier RM. Distribution of biosurfactant-producing bacteria in undisturbed and contaminated arid southwestern soils. Appl Environ Microbiol 2003; 6:3280-3287.
11. Bento FM, Camargo FA, Okeke BC et al. Diversity of biosurfactant producing microorganisms isolated from soils contaminated with diesel oil. Microbiol Res 2005; 160:249-255.
12. Batista SB, Mounteer AH, Amorim FR et al. Isolation and characterization of biosurfactant/bioemulsifier-producing bacteria from petroleum contaminated sites. Bioresour Technol 2006; 97:868-875.
13. Ruggeri C, Franzetti A, Bestetti G et al. Isolation and screening of surface active compound-producing bacteria on renewable substrates. Proceedings of second international conference on environmental, industrial and applied microbiology. Seville, Spain. In press.
14. Bodour AA, Guerrero-Barajas C, Jiorle BV et al. Structure and characterization of flavolipids, a novel class of biosurfactants produced by Flavobacterium sp. Strain MTN11. Appl Environ Microbiol 2004; 70:114-120.
15. Pepi M, Cesàro A, Liut G et al. An antarctic psychrotrophic bacterium Halomonas sp. ANT-3b, growing on n-hexadecane, produces a new emulsyfying glycolipid. FEMS Microbiol Ecol 2005; 53:157-166.
16. Bonilla M, Olivaro C, Corona M et al. Production and characterization of a new bioemulsifier from Pseudomonas putida ML2. J Appl Microbiol 2005; 98:456-463.
17. Makkar RS, Cameotra SS. An update on the use of unconventional substrates for biosurfactant production and their new application. Appl Microbiol Biotechnol 2002; 58:428-434.
18. Van Hamme JD, Singh A, Ward OP. Physiological aspects. Part 1 in a series of papers devoted to surfactants in microbiology and biotechnology. Biotechnol Adv 2006; 24:604-620.
19. Van Hamme JD, Singh A, Ward OP. Recent advances in petroleum microbiology. Microbiol Mol Biol R 2003; 6:503-549.
20. Bouchez-Naitali M, Rakatozafy H, Marchal R et al. Diversity of bacterial strains degrading hexadecane in relation to the mode of substrate uptake. J Appl Microbiol 1999; 8:421-428.
21. Urum K, Pekdemir T. Evaluation of biosurfactants for crude oil contaminated soil washing. Chemosphere 2004; 57:1139-1150.
22. Sutcliff IC. Cell envelope composition and organisation in the genus Rhodococcus. Anton Leeuw Int J G 1998; 74:49-58.
23. Van Hamme JD, Ward OP. Physical and metabolic interactions of Pseudomonas sp. Strain JA5-B45 and Rhodococcus sp. Strain F9-D79 during growth on crude oil and effect of a chemical surfactant on them. Appl Environ Microbiol 2001; 67:4874-4879.
24. Franzetti A, Bestetti G, Caredda P et al. Surface-active compounds and their role in bacterial access to hydrocarbons in Gordonia strains. FEMS Microbiol Ecol 2008; 63:238-248.
25. Rosenberg E, Gottlieb A, Rosenberg M. Inhibition of bacterial adherence to hydrocarbons and epithelial cells by emulsan. Infect Immun 1983; 39:1024-1028.
26. Mulligan CN, Yong RN, Gibbs BF. An evaluation of technologies for the heavy metal remediation of dredged sediments. J Hazard Mater 2001; 85:145-163.
27. Christofi N, Ivshina IB. Microbial surfactants and their use in field studies of soil remediation. J Appl Microbiol 2002; 93:915-929.
28. Mulligan CN. Environmental applications for biosurfactants. Environ Pollut 2005; 133:183-198.
29. Banat IM, Makkar RS, Cameotra SS. Potential commercial applications of microbial surfactants. Appl Microbiol Biotechnol 2000; 53:495-508.
30. Kourkoutas Y, Banat IM. Biosurfactant production and application. In: Pandey AP, ed. The Concise Encyclopedia of Bioresource Technology. Philadelphia: Haworth Reference Press, 2004:505-515.
31. Singh A, Van Hamme JD, Ward OP. Surfactants in microbiology and biotechnology: Part 2. Application aspects. Biotechnol Adv 2007; 25:99-121.
32. Barkay T, Navon-Venezia S, Ron EZ et al. Enhancement of solubilization and biodegradation of polyaromatic hydrocarbons by the bioemulsifier Alasan. Appl Environ Microbiol 1999; 65:2697-2702.
33. Beal R, Betts WB. Role of rhamnolipid biosurfactants in the uptake and mineralization of hexadecane in Pseudomonas aeruginosa. J Appl Microbiol 2000; 89:158-68.
34. Maier RM, Soberón-Chávez G. Pseudomonas aeruginosa rhamnolipids: biosynthesis and potential applications. Appl Microbiol Biotechnol 2000; 54:625-633.

35. Noordman WH, Janssen DB. Rhamnolipid stimulates uptake of hydrophobic compounds by Pseudomonas aeruginosa. Appl Environ Microbiol 2002; 68:4502-4508.

36. Rahman KSM, Rahman, TJ, Kourkoutoas Y et al. Enhanced bioremediation of n-alkane in petroleum sludge using bacterial consortium amended with rhamnolipid and micronutrients. Bioresour Technol 2003; 90:159-168.

37. Mata-Sandoval JC, Karns J, Torrents A. Influence of rhamnolipids and triton X-100 on the biodegradation of three pesticides in aqueous phase and soil slurries. J Agric Food Chem 2001; 49:3296-3303.

38. Awasthi N, Kumar A, Makkar R et al. Enhanced biodegradation of endosulfan, a chlorinated pesticide in presence of a biosurfactant. J Environ Sci Health 1999; B34:793-803.

39. Colores GM, Macur RE, Ward DM et al. Molecular analysis of surfactant-driven microbial population shifts in hydrocarbon-contaminated soil. Appl Environ Microbiol 2000; 66:2959-2964.

40. Bramwell DP, Laha S. Effects of surfactant addition on the biomineralization and microbial toxicity of phenanthrene. Biodegradation 2000; 11:263-277.

41. Billingsley KA, Backus SM, Ward OP. Effect of surfactant solubilization on biodegradation of polychlorinated biphenyl congeners by Pseudomonas LB400. Appl Microbiol Biotechnol 1999; 52:255-260.

42. Goudar C, Strevett K, Grego J. Competitive substrate biodegradation during surfactant-enhanced remediation. J Environ Eng 1999; 125:1142-1148.

43. Franzetti A, Di Gennaro P, Bestetti G et al. Selection of surfactants for enhancing diesel-hydrocarbons contaminated media bioremediation. J Hazard Mater 2008; 252:1309-1319.

44. Shreve GS, Inguva S, Gunnan S. Rhamnolipid biosurfactant enhancement of hexadecane biodegradation by Pseudomonas aeruginosa. Mol Mar Biol Biotechnol 1995; 4:331-337.

45. Zhang Y, Miller RM. Enhanced octadecane dispersion and biodegradation by a Pseudomonas rhamnolipid surfactant (biosurfactant). Appl Environ Microbiol 1992; 58:3276-3282.

46. Al-Tahhan RA, Sandrin TR, Bodour AA et al. Rhamnolipid-induced removal of lipopolysaccharide from Pseudomonas aeruginosa: Effect on cell surface properties and interaction with hydrophobic substrates. Appl Environ Microbiol 2000; 66:3262-3268.

47. Zhong H, Zeng GM, Yuan XZ et al. Adsorption of dirhamnolipid on four microorganisms and the effect on cell surface hydrophobicity. Appl Microbiol Biotechnol 2007; 77:447-455.

48. Chen P, Pickard MA, Gray MR. Surfactant inhibition of bacterial growth on solid anthracene. Biodegradation 2000; 11:341-347.

49. Weber WJ Jr, Huang W, Le Boeuf EJ. Geosorbent organic matter and its relationship to the binding and sequestration of organic contaminants. Colloids Surf A 1999; 151:167-179.

50. Fortin J, Jury WA, Anderson MA. Enhanced removal of trapped non-aqueous phase liquids from saturated soil using surfactant solutions. J Contam Hydrol 1997; 24:247-267.

51. Mulder H, Wassink GR, Breure AM et al. Effect of non-ionic surfactants on naphthalene dissolution and biodegradation. Biotechnol Bioeng 1998; 60:397-407.

52. Bai GY, Brusseau ML, Miller RM. Biosurfactant-enhanced removal of residual hydrocarbon from soil. J Contam Hydrol 1997; 25:157-170.

53. Edwards DA, Adeel Z, Luthy RG. Distribution of non-ionic surfactant and phenanthrene in a sediment/aqueous system. Environ Sci Technol 1994; 28:1550-1560.

54. Noordman WH, Wachter JH, de Boer GJ et al. The enhancement by surfactants of hexadecane degradation by Pseudomonas aeruginosa varies with substrate availability. J Biotechnol 2002; 94:195-212.

55. Ron EZ, Rosenberg E. Biosurfactants and oil bioremediation. Curr Opin Biotechnol 2002; 13:249-252

56. Lee M, Kang H, Do W. Application of non-ionic surfactant-enhanced in situ flushing to a diesel contaminated site. Water Res 2005; 39:139-46.

57. Urum K, Pekdemir T, Gopur M. Optimum conditions for washing of crude oil-contaminated soil with biosurfactant solutions. T I Chem Eng-Lond 2003; 81B:203-209.

58. Harvey S, Elashi I, Val des JJ et al. Enhanced removal of exxon valdez spilled oil from alaskan gravel by a microbial surfactant. Biotechnology 1990; 8:228-230.

59. Van Dyke MI, Couture P, Brauer et al. Pseudomonas aeruginosa UG2 rhamnolipid biosurfactants: structural characterization and their use in removing hydrophobic compounds from soil. Can J Microbiol 1993; 39:1071-1078.

60. Vipulanandan C, Ren X. Enhanced solubility and biodegradation of naphthalene with biosurfactant. J Environ Eng 2000; 126:629-634.

61. Cameotra SS, Bollag JM. Biosurfactant-enhanced bioremediation of polycyclic aromatic hydrocarbons. Crit Rev Environ Sci Technol 2003; 30:111-126.

62. Chu W. Remediation of contaminated soils by surfactant-aided soil washing. Pract Period Hazard Toxic Radioact Waste Manage 2003; 7:19-24.

63. Saichek RE, Reddy KR. Effects of system variables on surfactant enhanced electrokinetic removal of polycyclic aromatic hydrocarbons from clayey soils. Environ Technol 2003; 24:503-515.

64. Miller RM. Biosurfactant-facilitated remediation of metal-contaminated soils. Environ Health Perspect 1995; 103 Suppl 1:59-62.
65. Tan H, Champion JT, Artiola JF et al. Complexation of cadmium by a rhamnolipid biosurfactant. Environ Sci Technol 1994; 28:2402-2406.
66. Ochoa-Loza FJ, Artiola JF, Maier RM. Stability constants for the complexation of various metals with a rhamnolipid biosurfactant. J Environ Qual 2001; 30:479-485.
67. Mulligan CN, Yong RN. The use of biosurfactants in the removal of metals from oil-contaminated soil. In: Yong RN, ed. Contaminated Ground: Fate of Pollutants and Remediation. London: Thomas Telford Publishers, 1997:461-466.
68. Maslin P, Maier RM. Rhamnolipid-enhanced mineralization of phenanthrene in organic-metal cocon-taminated soils. Biorem J 2000; 4:295-308.
69. Gutnick DL, Bach H. Engineering bacterial biopolymers for the biosorption of heavy metals; new products and novel formulations. Appl Microbiol Biotechnol 2000; 54:451-460.
70. Bodour AA, Maier RM. Application of a modified drop- collapse technique for surfactant quantification and screening of biosurfactant-producing microorganisms. J Microbiol Methods 1998; 32:273-280.
71. Chen CY, Baker SC, Darton RC. The application of a high throughput analysis method for the screening of potential biosurfactants from natural sources. J Microbiol Methods 2007; 70:503-510.
72. Torsvik V, Øvreås L, Thingstad TF. Prokaryotic diversity-magnitude, dynamics and controlling factors. Science 2002; 296:1064-1066.
73. Keller M, Zengler K. Tapping into microbial diversity. Nat Rev Microbiol 2004; 2:141-50.

CHAPTER 10

Possibilities and Challenges for Biosurfactants Use in Petroleum Industry

Amedea Perfumo, Ivo Rancich and Ibrahim M. Banat*

Abstract

Biosurfactants are a group of microbial molecules identified by their unique capabilities to interact with hydrocarbons. Emulsification and de-emulsification, dispersion, foaming, wetting and coating are some of the numerous surface activities that biosurfactants can achieve when applied within systems such as immiscible liquid/liquid (e.g., oil/water), solid/liquid (e.g., rock/oil and rock/water) and gas/liquid. Therefore, the possibilities of exploiting these bioproducts in oil-related sciences are vast and made petroleum industry their largest possible market at present. The role of biosurfactants in enhancing oil recovery from reservoirs is certainly the best known; however they can be effectively applied in many other fields from transportation of crude oil in pipeline to the clean-up of oil storage tanks and even manufacturing of fine petrochemicals. When properly used, biosurfactants are comparable to traditional chemical analogues in terms of performances and offer advantages with regard to environment protection/conservation.

This chapter aims at providing an up-to-date overview of biosurfactant roles, applications and possible future uses related to petroleum industry.

Introduction

Petroleum has been driving the modern world for the past 100 years; however the high-quality and easily extractable light crude oils are limited. The ultimate recoverable resources are estimated at between 2-4 trillion barrels,[1] which poses two major issues. Firstly, the high priority need for maximizing the efficiency over all the stages of processing in the current petroleum industry. For example, less than half of the crude oil content of any reservoir can be actually extracted by the current techniques and improvements are sought after. Secondly, the challenge of utilizing heavy crude oils, bitumen and tar sand that are abundant in many parts of the world and which may represent the hydrocarbon-based energy of the future. Such poor-quality cruds being extremely viscous with densities higher than water, some solid at ambient temperature and additionally rich in sulphur and metals, are in need of novel technologies for upgrading. Traditional methods for production, transportation and refining are not suitable for such heavy oils and need to be improved.

In the above reasons, biotechnology may find a special niche within the related research areas as important links between microbiological and biotechnological research and petroleum industry have been built up in the recent years with regard to several areas of interest such as biocorrosion and biofouling, degradation of hydrocarbons within oil reservoirs, enzymes and biocatalysts for

*Corresponding Author: Ibrahim M. Banat—School of Biomedical Sciences, University of Ulster, Coleraine, County Londonderry, BT52 1SA, Northern Ireland, UK. Email: im.banat@ulster.ac.uk

Biosurfactants, edited by Ramkrishna Sen. ©2010 Landes Bioscience and Springer Science+Business Media.

petroleum upgrading. Biosurfactants and bioemulsifiers are a novel group of molecules and among the most powerful and versatile bioproducts that the modern microbial biotechnology can offer. In this chapter we discuss some roles and applications of these microbial compounds in oil-related sciences, presenting the processes that exploit commercially available biosurfactant technologies and highlighting those in which they may be potentially applied and have a greater impact on in the near future. Recent laboratory-scale researches along with field trials and patents will be described. Where possible information about technical aspects of the marketed systems will be included.

Surfactants and Biosurfactants in Petroleum Industry

Surfactants are molecules with two functional groups, namely a hydrophilic or polar end and a hydrophobic or nonpolar chain. Due to the affinity towards both polar and nonpolar phases, surfactants present in a mixed system (e.g., oil/water) move from the bulk phase to preferably adsorb at the surface or interface where they cause remarkable changes in surface and interfacial tensions, viscosity, wettability, charge and elasticity.[2]

Most surfactants currently in use are of petrochemical origin and therefore face the increasing environmental awareness and tightening of regulations in this regard. Microorganisms have long been known to be able to produce a variety of surface active compounds that display properties and activities comparable to those of synthetic surfactants. Numerous research describing biosurfactants produced by bacteria, yeasts and fungi have been carried out over the past years and many reviews covering various aspects of the topic are available in literature (see refs. 3-6).

Biosurfactants can potentially replace chemical analogue compounds, even offering additional advantages in all the aspects of petroleum processing including: 1- Extraction, 2- Transportation, 3- Upgrading and refining and 4- Petrochemical manufacturing.

Microbial Enhanced Oil Recovery

Classical oil production technologies involving 'primary' and 'secondary' can only partially recover the oil present in the field, with an efficiency estimated at 30-40% of the overall amount of oil available. Such efficiencies are expected to decrease during the gradual depletion of light crude reservoirs leaving the viscous crude oils. This requires the development of the 'tertiary' processes which aim at enhancing oil recovery (EOR).[7] Among these, microbially enhanced oil recovery (MEOR) exploiting microbial activities and metabolites, is at present gaining increased attention due to some advantages such as:

- Natural products are generally harmless and less detrimental to the environment;
- Microbial processes do not require large thermal consumption of energy;
- Costs of microbial products are not affected by crude oil price and can be produced using inexpensive raw-substrates or even waste materials;
- Microbial products/activities can be stimulated in situ within the reservoir, potentially allowing both tailor-made and cost-effective treatments.

Several metabolites are of interest for applications in MEOR including gas (e.g., carbon dioxide, methane and hydrogen), acids (e.g., acetate and butyrate), solvents (e.g., acetone, n-butanol and ethanol), biomass for selective plugging and biosurfactants/biopolymers.[8] Biosurfactants in particular have several benefits enhancing oil displacement and movement through oil-bearing rocks by means of three main mechanisms: (i) reduction of interfacial tension between oil-rocks and oil-brine; (ii) modification of the wettability of porous media; (iii) emulsification of crude oil. In addition, biosurfactant production contributes to the metabolism of viscous oils by microorganisms that release lighter hydrocarbon fractions thus making the oil even more fluid. The strategies investigated so far for MEOR involving biosurfactants include:

- Injection of ex situ produced biosurfactants into the reservoirs;
- Injection of laboratory-selected biosurfactant-producing microorganisms into the reservoirs;
- Stimulation of indigenous microbial population to produce biosurfactants in situ through supplying suitable nutrients.

Injection of Ex Situ Produced Biosurfactants into Oil Reservoirs

Biosurfactants can be produced in industrial-scale through fermentation technologies. However, the cost for the final product is still high for applications in this specific area. Several reasons are implicated and include costs for activity and maintenance of bioreactor apparatus, product extraction and purification, production of biosurfactants at generally low yields (1-10 g/l) by natural bacteria, reduced fermentation efficiency due to foaming and other metabolic-associated problems. Thus, while this option is not yet economically sustainable, experimental evidences supported the efficacy of the flooding technique in which biosurfactants replaced or assisted conventional chemical surfactants.

Lichenysin is one of the most powerful biosurfactants ever characterized. It is synthesized by *Bacillus licheniformis* JF-2 (ATCC 39307), isolated from well injection water[9] and recently reclassified as *B. mojavensis*.[10] Lichenysin, even at low concentrations (10-60 mg/l), is able to reduce interfacial tension to ultra low values (less than 10^{-2} mN/m) required to release the trapped oil. In addition, it is not affected by temperature ($\leq$140°C), pH (from 6 to 10), salinity (up to 10% w/v NaCl) and calcium concentrations ($\leq$340 mg/l $CaCl_2$).[11] It has been tested in core flooding experiments in a partially purified form and showed that, when included into the formulation of a flooding solution containing 2, 3-butanediol and 1g/l of partially hydrolyzed polyacrilamide (PHPA), residual oil was recovered from sandstone cores at up to 40%, compared to 10% recovered by the fluid containing chemical surfactants only.[12]

Similar results of improved flooding performance were obtained with rhamnolipid biosurfactants. In particular, it was observed that in the presence of rhamnolipids the adsorption of the surfactant alkylbenzene sulfonate (ORS) to sandstone was reduced by 25-30% and consequently its loss decreased. Thus, the oil recovered increased 7% when biosurfactants were added to the flooding solution. It was suggested that rhamnolipids acted as sacrificial agents by adsorbing preferably to oil sands thus both altering the wettability of porous media and making the chemical surfactant more available for displacement activity.[13]

Even more effective than low-molecular weight biosurfactants are the higher mass bioemulsifiers and biopolymers. For example, emulsan by *Acinetobacter venetianus* RAG-1 (ATCC 31012) used at a concentration of 0.1 mg/ml removed 89% of crude oil pre-adsorbed to limestone samples and up to 98% when used at 0.5 mg/ml.[14]

Injection of Laboratory-Selected Biosurfactant-Producing Microorganisms into Oil Reservoirs

Most studies focuses on the possibility of introducing biosurfactant-producing bacteria along with nutrients into the oil wells to allow their growth and activity. However to be suitable for this MEOR strategy, bacteria are required to thrive and be metabolically active at the extreme conditions typical of petroleum reservoirs.[15] Although extremophilic microorganisms have been isolated from different environments, native strains from oil reservoirs would be optimal candidates. The use of exogenous strains is disadvantageous due to competition with indigenous bacteria.

Most of biosurfactant-producing bacteria so far described and tested for in situ MEOR applications belong to *Bacillus* genus that commonly includes thermo- and halotolerant, facultative anaerobic strains. Among them, *B. mojavensis* JF-2 has been extensively investigated. This strain can grow while producing lichenysin under both aerobic and anaerobic conditions and at relatively high temperature (40°C),[16] which makes it a good candidate for in situ activity. Various processes exploiting JF-2 strain for oil recovery applications have been proposed including injection into oil-bearing formations alone[17] or as part of a microbial consortium.[18] An increase of 14% in oil production was observed after flooding with *B. mojavensis* JF-2 and the presence of living cells in the production fluids were detected 6 weeks after injection.[19,20]

Most other biosurfactant-producing microorganisms are not suitable for MEOR applications due to reservoir conditions. However, some thermotolerant *Pseudomonas aeruginosa* strains have been isolated from injection waters and found effective in displacing trapped oil both in laboratory tests and within low-temperature reservoirs.[21,22] Rhamnolipid biosurfactants produced by this species are very active compounds, with a critical micelle concentration (CMC) of 70 mg/liter, stable at high temperatures up to 90°C, best performing at lower pH and only slightly affected by salinity and calcium ions. The use of *P. aeruginosa* for in situ MEOR techniques is however limited for several reasons: (i) it is classified as risk-group 2 organism with restriction and regulation on its handling and dispersion into the environment; (ii) rhamnolipid synthesis is controlled by a complicated quorum-sensing system related to environmental stimuli; (iii) it is typically an aerobic mesophile that could not be actively growing under reservoir conditions. The possibility to overcome such limitations by engineering microorganisms in order to produce rhamnolipids in situ has been suggested and cloning biosynthetic genes into host organisms was attempted with limited success.[23-25]

Synthesis of biosurfactants under anaerobic conditions is of particular interest for application of MEOR processes, though most biosurfactant-producing microorganisms are strictly aerobic or facultative anaerobes. Few strictly anaerobic bacteria have been so far characterised as biosurfactant-producers. *Anaerophaga thermohalophila* strain Fru22[T] (DSM 12881[T]) for example, is a strictly anaerobic bacterium able to grow at elevated temperature (50°C) and high salinity (7.5% w/v NaCl) while producing a surface active compound preliminary characterized as a low-molecular weight lipopeptide (<12 kDa) which may include sugar moieties. Although no further attempt of investigating oil displacing activity has been reported, on the basis of its unique physiological properties strain Fru22[T] appears to be a good candidate for in situ MEOR.[26]

Mixed microbial consortia can be particularly effective for in situ treatments as they offer a broader range of activities and products in comparison with single species. A recently patent "MMMAP" (Multi-strain Mixed Microbial Application) consisting of thermophilic, barophilic, acidophilic and anaerobic strains belonging to *Thermoanaerobacterium* sp., *Thermotoga* sp. and *Thermococcus* sp. isolated from oil well water is claimed to be active in producing biosurfactants, fatty acids, alchools, methane and carbon dioxide at in situ temperature up to 90°C. Its injection into wells supplemented with specific nutrients resulted in 3-fold increased oil recovery.[27]

Stimulation of Indigenous Biosurfactant-Producing Microorganisms within Oil Reservoirs

The third strategy of MEOR is based on the concept that oil reservoirs are inhabited by indigenous microbial communities able to grow or survive under extreme conditions. Knowledge of such microbial ecosystems is still limited due to obvious difficulties in collecting representative samples as well as carrying out in situ analyses. Therefore whether indigenous microorganisms are native or contaminants exogenously introduced through water flooding, drilling or other oil well operations is still to be confirmed as well as their metabolism and activities established.[15]

Technologies involving injection of nutrient solutions (e.g., carbon substrates and minerals) into the oil well to stimulate the resident microbial communities have long been known and are available on a commercial basis. Benefits such as enhanced oil recovery, reduced oil viscosity and prolonged well lifetime are generally claimed, though a scientific monitoring of in situ activities is difficult and untreated controls are impossible to include. For example, in recent field trials, Youssef et al[28] provided direct proof that the presence of biosurfactant-producing bacteria in a nutrient-stimulated oil well was likely due to exogenous contamination and therefore could not be maintained over the duration of the treatment. As a result, in the wells treated with only nutrients no significant surface activities were detected.

MEOR Field Trials

The real potential of biosurfactants in MEOR applications can however be fully assessed only in field-scale. Several yet sporadic trials have been carried out during the past years and tentatively reviewed.[29-31] The real impact of biosurfactant-based MEOR techniques however has never been estimated because of lack of both quantitative information regarding microbial processes in situ and consistency in data collection and processing. Only recently a small field-scale MEOR experiment provided for the first time data of in situ metabolism and activities. Molecular techniques combined with traditional methods showed that *Bacillus* strains injected into oil wells maintained activity, consuming the glucose and nutrients supplied and releasing CO_2 and fermentation products including a lipopeptide biosurfactant leading to an increased production estimated as one barrel of oil/day over 7 weeks after the treatment.[28]

Crude Oil Transportation in Pipeline

Crude oil often needs to be transported over long distances from the extraction fields to the refineries. One of the major factors affecting pipelining is oil viscosity that slows the flow. Heavy oils in particular are characterised by viscosities ranging from 1000 cP to more than 100,000 cP at 25°C and cannot be transported through conventional pipelining systems that optimally requires viscosities of <200 cP. Heating or diluting with solvents were the traditional methods applied to reduce oil viscosity. However, a promising technology consisting of producing a stable oil-in-water emulsion that facilitates oil motility has been recently developed and introduced new routes to the application of the bioemulsifier-type of biosurfactants which have been found particularly suitable for this application. They are high-molecular weight surfactants characterised by different properties compared to glycolipids and lipopeptides. They are not effective in reducing interfacial tensions, but have excellent capability to stabilize oil-in-water emulsions. Due to the high number of reactive groups in the molecule, bioemulsifiers bind tightly to oil droplets and form an effective barrier that prevents drop coalescence. Among the bioemulsifiers, emulsan (Fig. 1) and its analogs synthesised by *A. venetianus* RAG-1, are certainly the most powerful, yet others such as alasan and biodipersan produced by different *Acinetobacter* strains have been extensively studied.[32]

Emulsan was applied in a field trial for pipeline transportation of a Boscan heavy crude oil of viscosity of about 200,000 cP. The bioemulsifier was used at a surfactant-oil ratio of 1:500 and produced a 70% w/w oil-in-water stable emulsion named hydrocabosol with viscosity reduced to 70 cP which was pumped through 380 miles over 64 hours. It was estimated that under optimal conditions the emulsion could have been transported for 26,000 miles.[33] Once transported to the refinery, hydrocarbosols can be either de-emulsified and utilized directly without de-watering or treated with specific enzymes called emulsanes to depolymerise the bioemulsifier thus breaking the emulsion before use.[34] To our knowledge there are no commercial applications of bioemulsifiers yet. Low-molecular weight biosurfactants can also be effective emulsifying agents. Rhamnolipids produced by *P. aeruginosa* strain USB-CS1 for example were able to emulsify a viscous crude oil to give an emulsion with viscosity reduced to less than 500 cP and stable for 14 days.[35]

In the case of waxy crude oils, their transportation is generally affected by the problem of paraffin precipitation that can cause numerous negative consequences from reduction and eventually block of the internal diameter of pipes to changes in the oil composition. Traditional techniques for treating wax included thermal, mechanical and chemical methods but all they failed to be fully successful as energy consuming, detrimental to the pipes and highly toxic respectively. Thus, over the past decade microbial treatments became an increasing valuable alternative.[36] Many bacteria are known to be able to grow on paraffinic hydrocarbons while producing biosurfactants that act as dispersing and solubilizing agents and make the paraffinic fractions more available for the up-take by cells. In this way not only wax deposits can be dissolved and prevented but also heavy crude oil fractions can be degraded by bacteria to lighter fractions.

Bacteria capable of degrading *n*-paraffins belong predominantly to *Pseudomonas* and *Bacillus* species and a mixed consortium was found particularly effective in the treatment of two paraffinic oils by Lazar et al.[37] Laboratory pilot tests were carried out by using a flow equipment containing ten liters of paraffinic oil to simulate a pipeline system. Bacterial consortium supplemented with brine and essential microelements (nitrogen and phosphorous) was circulated along with the oil for 5 days alternating flowing and stationary periods. Microbial activity was monitored and bio-surfactant production was detected all through the experiment. As a result, the authors reported a decrease of total paraffin content up to 10% and consequently of the freezing points up to 7-9°C. The viscosities also resulted much lowered especially at low temperatures.

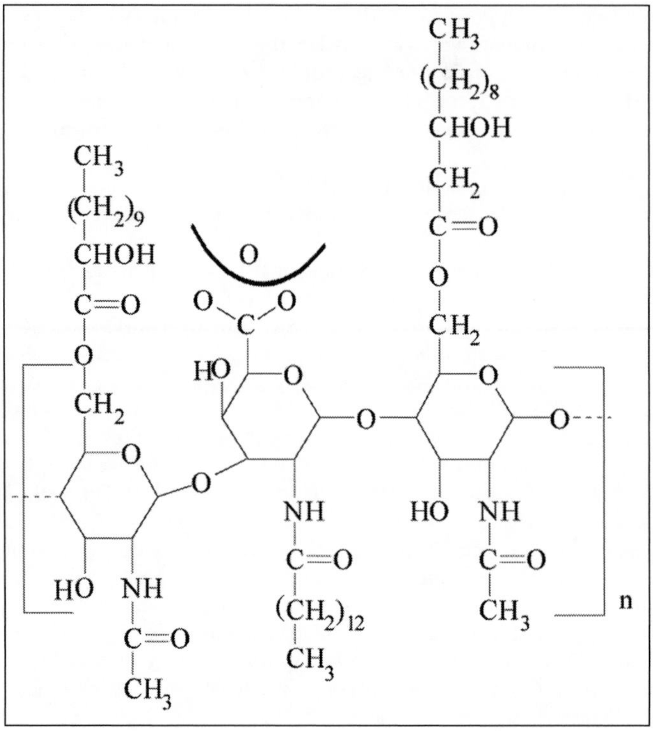

Figure 1. Structure of emulsan bioemulsifier produced by *A. venetianus* RAG-1. It is composed of a backbone of a repeating trisaccharide motif bound to fatty acid chains. Redrawn from reference 3.

Biological solutions to paraffin control problem find nowadays concrete application. Several commercial bioproducts have been formulated over the past few years and are currently available in the market. Micro-Bac International for example (Round Rock, TX) is manufacturer of a wide product line containing a proprietary combination of natural microorganisms able to control paraffins of chain length ranging from C_{16} up to C_{60} through the production of biosurfactants and other metabolites.

Clean-Up of Oil Containers/Storage Tanks

Large amounts of crude oil are daily moved and distributed to refineries with oil tankers, barges, tank cars and trucks, thus increasing the problem of the clean-up and maintenance of the containers.

A process for cleaning tanks used in oil transportation and storage by means of microbial bioemulsifiers was proposed for the first time in 1981 in a patent by Gutnick and Rosenberg.[38] The process included: (i) a washing phase with an aqueous solution of emulsan derivatives (α- and β-emulsans) produced by *A. venetianus* ATCC 31012 where an oil-in-water emulsion was induced by vigorous agitation into the tank; (ii) removal of such emulsion from the clean tank and (iii) recovering of the hydrocarbon residues by breaking the emulsion by physical or chemical methods. However, this potential application remained limited to this report as we are not aware of further development into a commercially available technology.

In 1991, Banat et al[39] described the application of microbial biosurfactants for the clean-up of oil storage tanks. Sludge and oil deposits normally accumulate at the bottom and on the walls of storage tanks thus requiring periodical cleaning operations. Traditional methods are generally manual,

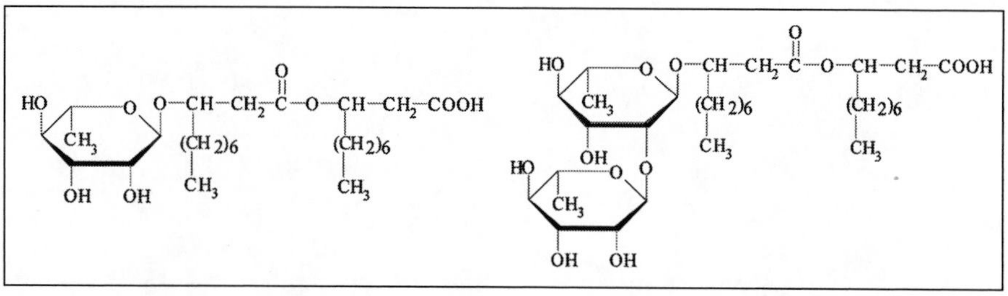

Figure 2. Structure of mono- and di-rhamnolipid produced by *P. aeruginosa* species. The predominant compounds are composed of one or two rhamnose units linked to two units of β-hydroxy-decanoic acid. Some minor congeners are also synthesised as part of a mixture.

hazardous, time-consuming and expensive. Biosurfactants can effectively drive the cleaning activity as demonstrated in a field trial conducted at the Kuwait Oil Company. Two tonnes of rhamnolipid (Fig. 2) biosurfactant-containing culture broth were produced, sterilised and added to an oil sludge tank along with fresh crude oil and water and circulated continuously for 5 days at ambient temperature of 40-50°C. The oil sludge was effectively lifted and mobilised from the bottom of the tank and solubilised within the emulsion formed. The treatment recovered 91% of hydrocarbons in the sludge. The value of the recovered crude covered the cost of the cleaning operation.

Since then, long and accurate researches and experiments carried out over the years lead to a substantial improvement of such technique and the development of the BioRecoil® process patented in 2004 by Idrabel Italia (Italy) and Jeneil Biosurfactant Company (USA).[40]

The process consists of three main steps:

i. **Feasibility study.** Data collection, tank survey, evaluation of sludge composition and concentration, laboratory tests as well as risk assessment, environmental impact and cost analysis are initially carried out in order to set-up the optimal working conditions and design a tailor-made treatment.

ii. **Oil tank treatment.** A mixture composed of water, biosurfactant and fluidizing agent is circulated onto the tank until obtaining an uniform emulsion (Fig. 3a,b). Rhamnolipid biosurfactants are preferably used to this end as capable of efficiently dispersing heavy hydrocarbon fractions by means of both micro- and macro-emulsions, with consequent reduction of the sludge viscosity. When the circulation is stopped, the emulsion breaks and separates in an upper phase containing hydrocarbons and a lower phase containing water, while inorganic residual matter and sand sink to the bottom (Fig. 3c). The hydrocarbon fraction is recovered, analysed and, according to its specific characteristics, transferred to other storage tanks or alternatively to refining plants to be processed.

iii. **Disposal of wastes and residues.** The treatment ends with the safe disposal of the wastes (Fig. 3d). The water used in the process or extracted from the sludge, is sent to the waste-water facilities of the refinery and analysed for oil content, organic content (e.g., COD) and temperature before being discharged or reused. The inorganic phase that remains at the bottom of the tank and that is mainly composed of sediments, metal residues, sand or gravel is in practice the only material that needs to be disposed.

This process can offer numerous benefits including recovery of oil (generally >90%) and reduction of material to be disposed of (<5%), safer in situ operations, use of natural biosurfactant products hence high environmental compatibility and reduction in the tank downtime and risk of damage.

Formulation of Petrochemicals

A totally unexplored area for potential applications of biosurfactants is the formulation of petrochemical products. Biotechnological alternatives to the existing bulk petroleum-derived products have generally failed for various reasons and mostly for not satisfying economic criteria.

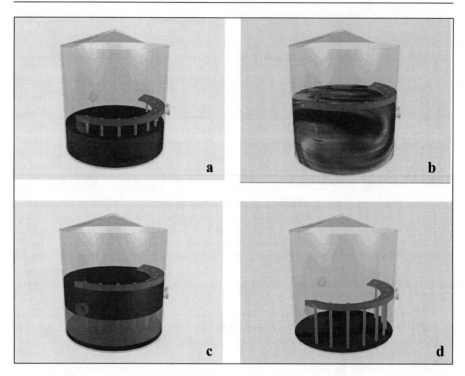

Figure 3. BioRecoil® process for the clean-up of oil storage tanks. Before the treatment, aged oil and residues are deposited at the bottom and on the walls of the tank (a). A rhamnolip-id-containing solution is circulated and oil is mobilized and entirely emulsified (b). To end the treatment, emulsion separates in a hydrocarbon-containing upper phase and a lower water phase (c); the former is recovered, while the latter is discharged or reused in the refinery plant. Inorganic materials are safely disposed (d) and a final make-up of the tank can be applied if necessary. Courtesy of Idrabel Italia.

However, those market niches where environmental concern is a major factor might look at biotechnological solutions with increasing interest in the near future. One such area includes the manufacturing of emulsified fuels.

Diesel fuel blended with water has been known since the early 1900s and is currently applied especially in Europe for public transport fleets, marine engines, locomotives but also heat facilities in industrial and institutional complexes. The advantages of diesel emulsions are:

- Improved combustion efficiency due to the microexplotions of water particles;
- Reduction of emission of hazardous pollutants such as nitrogen oxides (≤25%), carbon oxide (≤5%), black smoke (≤80%) and particulate matter (≤60%);
- Reduction of diesel consumption.

An additional aspect is that such fuels are easily applicable without need of engine modification.

Emulsified fuels are technically water-in-diesel emulsions with a typical content of water of 10-20% (v/v). They are prepared using specific surfactant packages along with a variety of additives (e.g., detergents, lubricity enhancers, antifoaming agents, ignition improvers, antirust agents and metal deactivators). Surfactants are expected to stabilize the emulsion and ensure that the finely dispersed water droplets remain in suspension within the diesel fuel (Fig. 4). Non-ionic surfactants such as alcohol ethoxylates, fatty acids ethoxylates and sugar esters of fatty acids are currently the most used.[41,42]

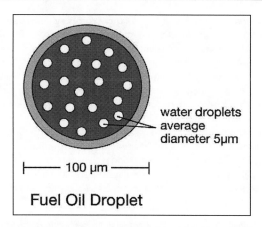

Figure 4. Typical aspect of a drop of emulsified diesel with dispersed microdroplets of water. Surfactants control the water droplets size and prevent their coalescence.

We investigated the possibility to replace traditional chemical compounds with microbial biosurfactants to formulate fuel or diesel emulsions. Preliminary experiments (unpublished data) were carried out in collaboration with Idrabel Italia (Genoa, Italy), in which rhamnolipid mixture produced by *P. aeruginosa* AP02-1 were used in order to prepare a water-in-diesel emulsion consisting of 15% water and 85% diesel (v/v). Five major parameters were evaluated: stability, density (optimally 0.76 to 0.79 g/cm³ at 15°C), viscosity (optimally 2 to 4.5 mm²/s at 40°C), water and sulphur content (optimally less than 2 mg/kg). Among them, emulsion stability was the most relevant factor as phase separation should not occur over 4 months. Stability depends on many factors both physicochemical (e.g., temperature, energy supply, order of mixing the components) and distinctively related to the surfactant properties. Biosurfactant potential candidate was required to satisfy the following basic criteria:
- The molecule should contain only carbon, hydrogen and oxygen and be free of sulphur and nitrogen atoms. The absence of aromatic rings is further requisite;
- The hydrophilic-lipophilic balance (HLB) should be in the range of 3-6;
- It should be used in a very pure form. This may limit the potential use of biosurfactants from microorganisms due to the difficulties of achieving high-grade purification;
- It should have a very low critical micelle concentration (CMC);
- It should burn readily without release of soot.

We produced several diesel emulsions generally satisfying some of the test factors (density, viscosity and sulphur content); however they lacked in stability and had inadequate consistency. An excess of air content likely due to an inappropriate mixing was the main cause of the destabilization of the phase equilibrium. It is important to note however that rhamnolipid may not have been a suitable choice of biosurfactant in order to achieve a stable emulsion. One of the longer chain heteropolysaccharides and proteins emulsifying-type biosurfactants may have been a better candidate. Although further investigations will be needed, to the best of our knowledge this aspect of biosurfactant applications has not been reported before.

Conclusion and Future Perspectives

During the past 20 years microbial biosurfactants and bioemulsifiers have been extensively investigated and their potential in most fields of the petroleum industry highlighted by the large number of related patents. Only few however had successful commercialization mainly due to the well-known problem of the high production costs. Several other aspects should be taken into consideration to realise their potentials. Though many different types of biosurfactants have been described from a variety of microorganisms, the literature focused predominantly on *Bacillus* sp.,

Pseudomonas and *Acinetobacter* sp. A number of other promising genera are known and should be closely examined. For example, *Rhodococcus* sp. produces trehalose lipid-type biosurfactants mainly during the growth in presence of hydrocarbons but limited efforts to evaluate their potential utility in petroleum industry have been carried out. More attention should also be directed towards extremophilic and hyper-extremophilic biosurfactant-producing microorganisms to allow use in oil field conditions. Although the biotechnological importance of such microbial groups is well-documented with regards to enzymes (extremozymes) in particular, lack of information about production of bioactive compounds remains.

Further progress is expected to be achieved when more advanced methods are developed and applied. Molecular techniques and in particular gene expression monitoring would significantly contribute to the detection and control of activities and processes in situ and in real time. To this end the current knowledge of biosurfactant genes is still insufficient and needs to be explored with the aim of gaining better control of the production technologies and improvement of products yields.

References

1. Hall C, Tharakan P, Hallock J et al. Hydrocarbons and the evolution of human culture. Nature 2003; 426:318-322.
2. Kanicky JR, Lopez-Montilla JC, Pandey S et al. Surface chemistry in the petroleum industry. In: Holmberg K, ed. Handbook of Applied Surface and Colloid Chemistry. John Wiley and Sons Ltd, 2001:251-267.
3. Desai J, Banat IM. Microbial production of surfactants and their commercial potential. Microbiol Mol Biol Rev 1997; 61:47-64.
4. Banat IM, Makkar RS, Cameotra SS. Potential commercial applications of microbial surfactants. Appl Microbiol Biotechnol 2000; 53:495-508.
5. Van Hamme JD, Singh A, Ward OP. Physiological aspects. Part 1 in a series of papers devoted to surfactants in microbiology and biotechnology. Biotechnol Adv 2006; 24:604-620.
6. Singh A, Van Hamme JD, Ward OP. Surfactants in microbiology and biotechnology: Part 2. Application aspects. Biotechnol Adv 2007; 25:99-121.
7. Planckaert M. Oil reservoirs and oil production. In: Ollivier B, Magot M, eds. Petroleum Microbiology. Washington DC: ASM Press, 2005:3-19.
8. Van Hamme JD, Singh A, Ward OP. Recent advances in petroleum microbiology. Microbiol Mol Biol Rev 2003; 67:503-549.
9. Jenneman GE, McInerney MJ, Knapp RM et al. A halotolerant, biosurfactant-producing bacillus species potentially useful for enhanced oil recovery. Dev Ind Microbiol 1983; 24:485-492.
10. Folmsbee M, Duncan K, Han SO et al. Re-identification of the halotolerant, biosurfactant-producing bacillus licheniformis strain JF-2 as Bacillus mojavensis JF-2. Syst Appl Microbiol 2006; 29:645-649.
11. McInerney MJ, Javaheri M, Nagle DP Jr. Properties of the biosurfactant produced by bacillus licheniformis strain JF-2. J Ind Microbiol 1990; 5:95-101.
12. McInerney MJ, Maudgalya SK, Knapp R et al. Development of biosurfactant-mediated oil recovery in model porous systems and computer simulations of biosurfactant-mediated oil recovery. Topical report accessed January 2008 from http://www.osti.gov/bridge/servlets/purl/834170-BP4QI4/native/834170.pdf
13. Daoshan L, Shouliang L, Yi L et al. The effect of biosurfactant on the interfacial tension and adsorption loss of surfactant in ASP flooding. Colloids and Surfaces A: Physicochem Eng Aspects 2004; 244:53-60.
14. Gutnick D, Rosenberg E, Belsky I et al. ψ-emulsans. US Patent 4,380,504 1983.
15. Magot M. Indigenous microbial communities in oil fields. In: Ollivier B, Magot M, eds. Petroleum Microbiology. Washington DC: ASM Press, 2005:21-33.
16. Javaheri M, Jenneman GE, McInerney MJ et al. Anaerobic production of a biosurfactant by bacillus licheniformis JF-2. Appl Environ Microbiol 1985; 50:698-700.
17. McInerney MJ, Jenneman GE, Knapp RM et al. Biosurfactant and enhanced oil recovery. US Patent 4,522,261, 1985.
18. Bryant RS. Microbial enhanced oil recovery and compositions therefor. US Patent 4,905,761, 1990.
19. Bryant RS, Burchfield TE, Dennis DM et al. Microbial-enhanced waterflooding: Mink unit project. SPE Reservoir Eng 1990; 5:9-13.
20. Bryant RS, Stepp AK, Bertus KM et al. Microbial-enhanced waterflooding field pilots. Dev Petrol Sci 1993; 39:289-306.
21. Rocha C, San-Blas F, San-Blas G et al. Biosurfactant production by two isolates of pseudomonas aeruginosa. World J Microbiol Biotechnol 1992; 8:125-128.
22. Li Q, Kang C, Wang H et al. Application of microbial enhanced oil recovery technique to daqing oilfield. Biochem Eng J 2002; 11:197-199.

23. Cabrera-Valladares N, Richardson AP, Olvera C et al. Monorhamnolipids and 3-(3-hydroxyalkanoylo xy)alkanoic acids (HAAs) production using escherichia coli as a heterologous host. Appl Microbiol Biotechnol 2006; 73:187-194.
24. Ochsner UA, Koch AK, Fiechter A et al. Isolation and characterization of a regulatory gene affecting rhamnolipid biosurfactant synthesis in pseudomonas aeruginosa. J Bacteriol 1994; 176:2044-2054.
25. Wang Q, Fang X, Bai B et al. Engineering bacteria for production of rhamnolipid as an agent for enhanced oil recovery. Biotechnol Bioeng 2007; 98:842-853.
26. Denger K, Warthmann R, Ludwig W et al. Anaerophaga thermohalophila gen nov, sp nov, a moderately thermohalophilic, strictly anaerobic fermentative bacterium. Int J Syst Evol Microbiol 2002; 52:173-178.
27. Lal B, Reddy MRV, Agnihotri A et al. Process for enhanced recovery of crude oil from oil wells using novel microbial consortium. US Patent 20070092930, 2007.
28. Youssef N, Simpson DR, Duncan KE et al. In situ biosurfactant production by bacillus strains injected into a limestone petroleum reservoir. Appl Environ Microbiol 2007; 73:1239-1247.
29. Banat IM. Biosurfactant production and possible uses in microbial enhanced oil recovery and oil pollution remediation—a review. Bioresour Technol 1995; 51:1-12.
30. Bryant R. Potential use of microorganisms in petroleum recovery technology. Proc Okla Acad Sci 1987; 67:97-104.
31. McInerney MJ, Nagle DP, Knapp RM. Microbially enhanced oil recovery: past, present and future. In: Ollivier B, Magot M, eds. Petroleum Microbiology. Washington DC: ASM Press, 2005:215-237.
32. Gutnick DL, Shabtai Y. Exopolysaccharide bioemulsifiers. In: Kosaric N, Cairns WL, Gray NCC, eds. Biosurfactants and Biotechnology. New York: Marcel Dekker Inc, 1987:211-246.
33. Hayes ME, Hrebenar KR, Murphy PL et al. Bioemulsifier-stabilized hydrocarbosols. US Patent 4,943,390, 1990.
34. Hayes ME, Hrebenar KR, Murphy PL et al. Combustion of viscous hydrocarbons. US Patent 4,684,372, 1987.
35. Rocha CA, Gonzalez D, Iturralde ML et al. Production of oily emulsions mediated by microbial tenso-active agent. US Patent 6,060,287, 2000.
36. Etoumi A. Microbial treatment of waxy crude oils for mitigation of wax precipitation. J Pet Sci Eng 2007; 55:111-121.
37. Lazar I, Voicu A, Nicolescu C et al. The use of naturally occurring selectively isolated bacteria for inhibiting paraffin deposition. J Pet Sci Eng 1999; 22:161-169.
38. Gutnick D, Rosenberg E. Cleaning oil-contaminated vessels with α-emulsans. US Patent 4,276,094, 1981.
39. Banat IM, Samarath N, Murad M et al. Biosurfactant production and use in oil tank clean-up. World J Microbiol Biotechnol 1991; 7:80-84.
40. Pesce L. A biotechnological method for the regeneration of hydrocarbons from dregs and muds, on the basis of biosurfactants. European Patent EP1427547, 2004.
41. Clark RH, Morley C, Stevenson PA. Diesel fuel compositions. US Patent 7,229,481, 2007.
42. Lif A, Holmberg K. Water-in-diesel emulsions and related systems. Adv Colloid Interface Sci 2006; 123-126:231-239.

Bacterial Biosurfactants, and Their Role in Microbial Enhanced Oil Recovery (MEOR)

J.M. Khire*

Abstract

Surfactants are chemically synthesized surface-active compounds widely used for large number of applications in various industries. During last few years there is increase demand of biological surface-active compounds or biosurfactants which are produced by large number of microorganisms as they exert biodegradability, low toxicity and widespread application compared to chemical surfactants. They can be used as emulsifiers, de-emulsifiers, wetting agents, spreading agents, foaming agents, functional food ingredients and detergents. Various experiments at laboratory scale on sand-pack columns and field trials have successfully indicated effectiveness of biosurfactants in microbial enhanced oil recovery (MEOR).

Introduction

There are large number of reports of various chemicals, produced synthetically or occurring naturally, showing the properties of surfactant which show specific and preferential interaction at surfaces and interfaces between fluid phases having different degrees of polarity and hydrogen bonding e.g., oil and water or air and water interfaces.[1] This is the result of the presence of both hydrophobic and hydrophilic moieties at the surface of these molecules which results in their orientation at the interface and is known as surfactants. Surfactants are very versatile and have found uses in as detergents lowering the interfacial tension, emulsifiers, dispersants, deemulsifiers, wetting agents, foam retardants, stabilizers, gelling agents etc.[2-5] Chemical surfactants are generally produced as by-products of the petrochemical industry and consist primarily of alkylbenzene sulfonates, alkyl phenol ethoxylates, synthetic fatty alcohols and their derivatives. These products are believed to account for 70-75% of the surfactant consumption in the industrialized countries. The current worldwide production of surfactants is around 12.5 M tones per year, worth around US $28 bn and growing by about 500,000 tones/y. Around 60% of surfactant production is used in household detergents, 30% in industrial and technical applications, 7% in industrial and institutional cleaning and 6% in personal care.[6]

Although chemical surfactants are both inexpensive and efficient, they have adverse effect on the environment causing pollution. The potential advantages of biosurfactant include biodegradability resulting in lower levels of pollution, low toxicity, biocompatibility and digestibility which allows their application in cosmetics, pharmaceuticals and as functional food additives, can be produced from cheap raw materials which are available in large quantities. Similarly they show selectivity

*J.M. Khire—NCIM Resource Center, Division of Biochemical Sciences, National Chemical Laboratory, Pune 411 008, India. Email: jmkhire@yahoo.com

Biosurfactants, edited by Ramkrishna Sen. ©2010 Landes Bioscience and Springer Science+Business Media.

Table 1. Major types of biosurfactants produced by bacteria

Bacteria	Biosurfactant Type
Aeromonas sp	Glycolipid[13,14]
Bacillus subtilis	Lipopeptide[15]
B. subtilis ATCC 21332 LB5a	Lipopeptide[16]
Bacillus subtilis A8-8	Lipopepetide[17]
Bacillus subtilis	Lipopeptide[4]
Bacillus sp	Lipopolysaccharide[18]
Klebsiella oxitoca	Lipopolysaccharide[19]
Pantoea sp	Glycolipid[20]
Ps. aeruginosa NCIMB 40044	Rhamnolipid[21]
Ps. aeruginosa AT10	Rhamnolipid[22]
Ps. aeruginosa strain BS2	Rhamnolipid[22]
Ps. aeruginosa DS10-129	Rhamnolipids[23]
Ps. aeruginosa LB1	Rhamnolipid[24]
Ps. aeruginosa	Glycolipid[25]
Ps. aeruginosa HR	Glycolipid[26]
Ps. fluorescens HW 6	Glycolipid[27]
Ps. aeruginosa S2	Rhamnolipid[28]
Ps. aeruginosa RB 28	Rhamnolipid[29]
Pseudoxanthomonas kaohsiungensis sp nov[30]	—
Pseudomonas sp DSM 2874	Rhamnolipids[31]
Pseudomonas XD-1	Liopeptide[32] Glycopeptide
Streptococcus thermophilus A	Glycolipid[33]

and specificity towards hydrocarbon substrates. Their compatibility with chemical product generally leads to novel formulations. Earlier work on biosurfactants mainly focused on the properties, biosynthesis and chemistry which have been reviewed by many workers.[7-10] However, during the last few years significant work has been reported on biosurfactant production by new strains, hyper secretary mutant, lab scale and field trials for microbial enhanced oil recovery which forms the subject matter of the present chapter.

Biosurfactant Producing Bacteria

Large number of microorganisms especially bacteria are reported to produce biosurfactants[4,7,11] however the chemical nature of biosurfactant is dependent on the producing species.[12] Table 2 summarizes few recently reported biosurfactant producing bacteria.

Selection of Biosurfactant Producer

One of the simplest criterions for the primary isolation of biosurfactant producing bacteria is to look for haemolysis on blood agar[34,35] and an emulsification index value (E-24).[36] In rapid 'drop-collapse' method for screening rhamnolipid biosurfactant by microorganisms the microwell plate with polystyrene platform having small wells was used. If the culture broth contained biosurfactant, the droplets of the broth in the oil-coated wells collapsed.[37] In axisysmmetric drop shape analysis profile (ADSA-P) method suspension of biosurfactant producing organism was placed on solid surface coated with fluoroethylene-propylene and the profile of the droplet was determined with contour monitor and surface tension was measured.[38] The indicator methylene blue was used to form colored complex in case of determination of bacterial peptidolipid biosurfactant.[39] Very specific and sensitive reverse phase HPLC method with C18 column was used for the analysis of a biosurfactant produced by *Bacillus licheniformis* JF-2.[40] Enzyme-linked immunosorbent assay (ELISA)[41] was used for detection of lipopeptide biosurfactant from *B. lichenifirmis* JK-2. The method was very sensitive (as low as 0.01 mg dm^{-3}) and capable of handling large number of samples simultaneously. In case of surfactin[42] production from *Bacillus subtilis* genetic locus (sfp) plays major role. They demonstrated the utility of using PCR of the sfp gene as a tool of identifying *Bacillus* sp that produce surfactin along with hemolysis zone assay, quantification by HPLC and NMR in parallel to ensure that the PCR provided correct results.

Factors Affecting Production of Biosurfactants

The fermentation process is the key factor which governs the overall economics of biosurfactant production as the raw materials account for about 10-30% of the overall cost of biosurfactant production. Their production is either

1. Growth-associated as in case of production of rhamnolipid by *Pseudomonas aeruginosa*[43] and probiotic bacteria (*Lactobacillus lactis* 53 and *Streptococcus thermophilus* A).[44]

2. Growth limiting conditions as in case of biosurfactant production by *Pseudomonas aeruginosa* strain BS2 in synthetic medium supplied with distillery and whey wastes a crystalline biosurfactant was produced after the onset of nitrogen-limiting conditions.[45] Low phosphate concentration stimulated bioemulsifier production in *Pseudomonas aeruginosa* during cultivation on ethanol.[46] During rhamnolipid production by *Pseudomonas aeruginosa* the iron conc. in the medium plays important role. Thus threefold increase in production of biosurfactant was found when cells were shifted from medium containing 36 μM iron to medium containing 18 μM iron without change in biomass yield.[47]

3. Resting cells: Pilot plant production of rhamnolipid biosurfactant by resting cells of *Pseudomonas aeruginosa* resulted in the reduction of cost of product recovery as the growth and the product formation phases can be separated.[48] The resting cells of *Pseudozyma antartica* T-34 has been reported[49] to produce mannosylerythritol lipids (12 g/lit) by feeding the cells on glucose only.

4. Precursor supplement: Addition of certain precursors in the fermentation medium causes both qualitative and quantitative increase in biosurfactant production. Thus increase in production of rhamnolipid biosurfactant in *Pseudomonas aeruginosa* by 3-(3-hydroxy-alkanoyloxy) alkanoic acid has been reported.[50] Use of soybean waste frying oil as the substrate for production of biosurfactant by *Pseudomonas aeruginosa* mutant EBN-8 in the presence or absence of rhamnolipid precursor, under fed batch conditions produce 9.3 g rhamnolipid/lit with the addition of precursor.[51]

Factors Affecting Biosurfactant Production

The type, quality and quantity of biosurfactant production of bacteria are influenced by the carbon source,[52] nitrogen source and ratio of C/N.[53] The trace elements also play crucial role in biosurfactant production. The appropriate supplementation of iron[54-56] and manganese[57] resulted in substantial enhancement in surfactin production. Iron concentration also markedly affected rhamnolipid production from *Pseudomonas aeruginosa*.[1] During surfactin production by *Bacillus licheniformis* JF-2, three-fold increase in yield of biosurfactant was found by decreasing 50% of the phosphate content in the medium.[40] The two times increase in the production of surfactin (3.34 g/l) production by *Bacillus licheniformis* ATCC 21332 was reported[58] by statistical experimental design (Taguchi method) in which interactive correlations of selective metal ions (Mg^{2+}, K^{2+}, Mn^{2+}

and Fe^{2+}) was studied. Surfactin like biosurfactant was reported[59] from *Bacillus subtilis* MTCC 2423 in which sucrose and potassium nitrate were the best carbon and nitrogen source. Similarly the addition of various metal ions (Mg^{2+}, Ca^{2+}, Fe^{2+} and trace elements) increased the two fold yield of biosurfactant when they were added together rather than individual. Amino acids such as aspartic acid, aspargine, glutamic acid, valine and lysine increased the yield of biosurfactant by about 60%.

Among water-insoluble substrates the vegetable oils and oil wastes were used as cheap raw material. e.g., rapseed oil was used for lipopeptide biosurfactant[31] production by *Pseudomonas* sp DSM 2874. Similarly sunflower and soybean oils were used for the production of rhamnolipids by *Pseudomonas aeruginosa* DS 10-129,[23] lipopeptide by *Serratia marcescens* sophorolipid[60] biosurfactants. The palm oil is used as carbon source for biosurfactant production by *Pseudomonas aeruginosa* A41.[61] Even vegetable oil refinery waste (COD = 20 g/l) supplemented with sodium nitrate has been reported[62] for improved production of biosurfactant by *Pseudomonas aeruginosa* mutant strain. The whey produced in dairy industries was most cheap and viable substrate for production of rhamnolipid type biosurfactant by *Pseudomonas aeruginosa* strain BS2,[63] *Lactobacillus lactis* 53 and *Streptococcus thermophilus*.[64] Similarly starchy substrates such as potato process effluent has been reported as substrate for production of lipopeptide biosusurfactant by *Bacillus subtilis*.[15,65-67] The cassava flour wastewater was reported as substrate for lipopeptide biosurfactant by *Bacillus subtilis* ATCC 21332 and *Bacillus subtilis* LB5a.[16,68,69] The clarified blackstrap molasses was used as a sole carbon and energy source with or without auxiliary synthetic nitrogen source for rhamnolipid production by *Pseudomonas aeruginosa* EBN-8 mutant.[70] Various agriculture residues like barley bran, corn shoots and Eucalyptus globus chips were used as raw material for biosurfactant production by *Lactobacillus pentosus* for simultaneous production of lactic acid and biosurfactant.[71] Recently statistical optimization fermentation medium for production of biosurfactant from *Bacillus licheniformis* K51 has been reported[72] in which important medium ingredients were identified by initial screening method of Plackett-Burman which was followed by Box-Behnken response method in which further optimization of medium ingredients was carried out. Thus the relative biosurfactant yield as critical micelle dilution (CMD) was increased from 10x to 105x, which is ten times higher than the nonoptimized rich medium.

Biosurfactant Production by Extremophiles

Although there are various reports on mesophilic microorganisms producing biosurfactants or bioemulsifiers, reports of thermophilic organisms secreting these surface-active compounds are rare.[73] Microorganisms growing above 50°C are generally considered thermophiles. Main advantage of use of thermophiles for biosurfactant production is due to faster reaction rates, reduced risk of contamination, reduced viscosity of growth, higher solubility of molecules in the fermentation medium and elimination of pathogens due to higher incubation temperature.[74,75] Both Gram-positive and Gram-negative thermophiles has been reported from thermal and nonthermal environments. Large number of thermophilic bacteria that can utilize hydrocarbon as their sole source of carbon and energy.[76] From oil-field injection water novel strain of *Bacillus licheniformis* JF-2 was isolated[77] which was growing in medium with NaCl conc. up to 10%, at temp up to 50°C and in the pH range 4.6-9.0 secreting biosurfactant, lichenysin under anaerobic conditions. Among thermophilic halophiles bioemulsifier was isolated from *Methanobacterium thermoautotrophicum*[78] which was growing up to 80°C and active over a wide range of pH (5-10) at very high salt conc. (up to 200 g/l).

In our laboratory, after screening more than 30 different bacterial isolates from hot water spring for their capability to synthesize biosurfactant under thermophilic conditions, we reported novel biosurfactant production by strain of *Bacillus stearothermophilus* VR-8.[79] Emulsification activity produced by this strain was stable over a wide pH (2-8) range as compared to liposan[80] which was active in a narrow pH range of 2-5. It was also 100% stable at 80°C for 30 min and 60% at 90 and 100°C as compared to liposan which was reported to be stable only up to 70°C. At a 5% NaCl conc. only an 8% loss of activity occurred, compared to total loss of emulsification activity in the presence of salt conc. above 5% in the case of *Candida tropicalis* and *Debaromyces polymorphus*.[81]

Very few reports are available in the literature for biosurfactant production from psychrophiles. Novel biosurfactant from antartica strain *Arthrobacter protophormiae*[82] was produced during growth of an organism on an immiscible carbon source, n-hexadecane; it reduced the surface tension of the medium from 68 nNm^{-1} to 30.60 nNm^{-1} and exhibited good emulsification activity. The biosurfactnt was thermostable and pH-stable. The strain was able to produce biosurfactant up to a NaCl conc. of 10% and was able to recover 90% of the oil from sand pack column.

Recovery of Biosurfactant

One of the most important steps in production of biosurfactant is fast, efficient and cheap recovery process which amount to around approximately 60% of the total production cost. Generally the steps of recovery of biosurfactant depend upon the end use of the product. Thus the biosurfactant required for the MEOR does not necessarily be extra pure as required in pharmaceutical preparation especially in cosmetics and medicine.

The most common biosurfactant recovery methods are either extraction with solvents (e.g., chloroform-methnaol, dichloromethane-methanol, butanol, ethyl acetate, pentene, hexane, acetic acid, ether) or acid precipitation. However, there are reports of the use of ammonium sulfate precipitation, crystallization centrifugation, adsorption, foam precipitation etc. Various processes employed for the recovery of biosurfactants are shown in Table 2. Precipitation of biosurfactant by ammonium sulphate has been reported for biosurfactant from *Arthrobacter*[83] and *Acinetobacter calcoaceticus*[84] which does not require much infra-structure and used for recovery of crude biosurfactant. Partially purified lipopeptide biosurfactant from *Bacillus subtilis* A8-8 was obtained by HCl precipitation, methanol treatment and silica-gel chromatography.[17] The biosurfactant from *Bacillus coagulans* was isolated from fermented broth by acid precipitation followed by neutralization and lyophilization.[85] The biosurfactant from *Pseudomonas aeruginosa* EBN-8 was isolated from the supernatant by acid precipitation followed by solvent extraction (70) while acetone was used to precipitate biosurfactant from *Pseudomonas* PG-1.[86] The use of methyl tertiary butyl ether was reported for the extraction of biosurfactant from *Rhodococcus*.[87] Membrane ultrafiltration is

Table 2. Downstream processes for recovery of biosurfactants

Recovery Process	Biosurfactant Source
Batch process	
Ammonium sulphate precipitation	*Arthrobacter RAG-1*[83] *Acinetobacter calcoaceticus*[84]
Acid precipitation	*Bacillus subtilis*[17] *Bacillus coagulans*[85]
Solvent precipitation	
Methanol	*Bacillus subtilis*[17]
Acetone	*Pseudomonas* PG-1[86]
Methyl tertiary butyl ether	*Rhodococcus*[87]
Continuous process	
Ultrafiltration	*Bacillus subtilis*[88]
Assymetrical flow field-flow fractionation (AsFlFFF)	*Pseudomonas* sp[91]
Foam fractionationation	*Bacillus subtilis*[89]
Wood based activated carbon	*Pseudomonas aeruginosa* BS2[90]
Adsorption and elution on Ion exchange chromatography	*Pseudomonas aeruginosa*[48]

fast, one-step recovery process with high level purity but requires special ultrafiltration units with porous polymer membrane with specific cut-off molecular weight which was reported for purification of lipopeptide biosurfactant from *Bacillus subtilis*.[88] For charged biosurfactant, rhamnolipid, from *Pseudomonas aeruginosa* ion-exchange chromatography is used to adsorb biosurfactant on ion-exchange resin and then eluted with appropriate buffer.[48] Foam fractionation requires specially designed bioreactors which facilitates foam recovery during fermentation and was reported for the first time during continuous surfactin production.[89] The biosurfactant recovery methods including solvent extraction, precipitation, crystallization, centrifugation and foam fractionation cannot be used when distillery wastewater was used as the nutrient for biosurfactant production by *Pseudomonas aeruginosa* BS2, because these methods imparts colour to the biosurfactant. The biosurfactant obtained was nonesthetic in appearance with lowered surface-active properties. Hence they used new down streaming technique using wood-based activated carbon. In this method WAC (1%) was equilibrated for 90 min in the pH range 5-10 at 40°C to achieve 99.5% adsorption efficiency and eluted with acetone with 89% recovery of biosurfactant. The recovery process was continuous as the WAC can be reused for three consecutive cycles.[90] Purification of biosurfactant from *Pseudomonas* sp G11 by asymmetrical flow field-flow fractionation (AsFlFFF) using pure water as the carrier has been reported.[91]

Biosurfactant Production by Biotransformation

During past few years there are several reports of production of biosurfactants through the biotransformation route. For this microbial surfactants are produced by fermentation to obtain various hydrophobic and hydrophilic moieties of biosurfactants which are then joined by enzymatic treatment to produce commercial surfactants. Compared to chemical synthesis these enzymatic methods have several advantages such as low energy requirement, minimal thermal degradation, high biodegradability and high regioselectivity. There are various reports of this easy transformation using selected yeast strains to upgrade oil quality by desaturating or saturating the components of fatty acids.[92-94] The conversion of oleic acid to recinoleic acid by soil bacterium BMD-120 and conversion of soybean lecithin to a new biosurfactant by phospholipase D from *Streptococcus chromofuscus* has been reported.[95] The major disadvantage of applying enzymes for the production of surfactants is high enzyme costs and difficulty in solubilizing both hydrophilic and hydrophobic substrates in the reaction media. But these problems can be solved by using immobilized enzymes and enhancement in enzyme stability and activity by genetic engineering. Similarly recent advances in multiple-phase enzymatic reaction systems and supercritical fluid techniques will help to solve the problem of low substrate solubility. Similarly advances in metabolic engineering and the development of novel fermentation techniques such as self-cycling fermentation[96,97] will help in enhancing the productivity of biosurfactants.

Improved Strains for Biosurfactant Production

One of the most important factors for economical production of biosurfactant is use of mutant strain which may be hyper secretary or recombinant which can grow on cheap raw material supported with efficient recovery process.

The *Pseudomonas putida* PCL1445 produces two cyclic lipopeptide biosurfactants, putisolvins I and II. Studies on the regulation of putisolvin production indicate that dnak, together with the dnaj and grpE heat shock genes were involved in the possible regulation (directly or indirectly) of putisolvin biosynthesis at the transcription level.[98] A gamma ray induced mutant viz. *B. subtilis* AB01335-1M4 and *B. subtilis* AB02238-1R2 showed 5 and 3 times more surfactin production, respectively, compared to parent strains when grown on minimal medium.[99] Isolation of facultative anaerobic strain which could produce biosurfactant with crude oil as carbon source and reduce surface tension from 16.36 mN/m to 6.49 mN/m has been reported.[100] They isolated the mutant of this strain by both UV and EMS which could further reduce the surface tension by 32.8%.

Biosurfactants and Microbial Enhance Oil Recovery (MEOR)

The majority of the world's energy comes from nonrenewable fossil fuel source. The crude oil produced from these resources by currently used methods leads to only 8-30% recovery of the total oil present in the reservoir.[101] MEOR is the use of microorganisms to retrieve additional oil from existing wells, thereby enhancing the petroleum production of an oil reservoir. In this technique, selected natural microorganisms are introduced into oil wells to produce metabolic products including biosurfactant or bioemulsifier which are considered to be useful for the release of trapped oil.

Types of MEOR

MEOR is used in the third phase of oil recovery from well, known as tertiary oil recovery. Recovering oil usually requires three stages.

Stage 1: Primary recovery: 12-15% of the oil in the well is recovered without the need to introduce other substances into the well.

Stage 2: Secondary recovery: The oil well is flooded with water or other substances to drive out an additional 15 to 20% more oil from the well

Stage 3: Tertiary recovery: This stage may be accomplished through different methods, including MEOR, to additionally recover up to 11% more oil from the well.

The Science of MEOR

The microorganisms used in MEOR can be applied to a single oil well or to an entire oil reservoir. They need certain conditions to survive, so nutrients and oxygen are often introduced into the well at the same time. MEOR also requires that water to be present. Microorganisms grow between the oil and the well's rock surface to enhance oil recovery by the following methods.

Reduction of oil viscosity: Oil is a thick fluid that it does not flow easily. Microorganims help break down the molecular structure of crude oil, making it more fluid and easier to recover from the well.

Production of carbon dioxide gas: As a by-product of metabolism, microorganisms produce carbon dioxide gas. Over time, this gas accumulates and displaces the oil in the well, driving it up and out of ground.

Production of biomass: When microorganisms metabolize the nutrients they need for survival, they produce organic biomass as a by-product. This biomass accumulates between the oil and the rock surface of the well, physically displacing the oil and making it easier to recover from the well.

Selective plugging: Some microorganisms secrete slimy substances called exopolysaccharides to protect themselves from drying out or falling prey to other organisms. This substance helps bacteria plug the pores found in the rocks of the well so that oil may move past rock surfaces more easily. Blocking rock pores to facilitate the movement of oil is known as selective plugging.

Production of biosurfactants: Microorganisms produce bioactive compounds called biosurfactants when they breakdown the oil. These biosurfactants act like slippery detergents, helping the oil move more freely away from rocks and crevices so that it may travel more easily out of the well.

The selection of microbes and subsurface environment of the reservoir plays very important role in the MEOR.[102] Thus *Pseudomonas aeruginosa* (P-1) isolated from crude oil contaminated water for biosurfactant production and showed its successful application under laboratory test and pilot plant for enhanced oil recovery from Daquing oilfield, China.[103] They used metabolic products (PIMP) of 10% could enhance the oil recovery in the model reservoir by 11.2% and also decrease injection pressure by 40.1%. PIMP which served as biosurfactant, could reduce the crude oil viscosity by 38.5%. In the pilot tests, about 80% of wells used showed a significant increase in crude oil production after PIMP injection and shut-in for about 1 month. The pilot tests also revealed that PIMP could prolong cycle of oil well washing so that the total oil production was increased.

Naturally fractured oil reservoirs represent over 20% of the world's oil reserves.[104] However, relatively little success has been achieved in increasing oil production from these complex reservoirs.[105] The in situ MEOR in fractured porous media has been demonstrated[106] by using etched-glass micromodels having different fracture angle orientation along with nonfractured model to compare the efficiency of MEOR in fractured and nonfractured porous media. They used surfactin producer *Bacillus subtilis* and dextran producer *Leuconostoc mesenteroides* for this experiment. Their results show that higher oil recovery efficiency can be achieved by using biosurfactant-producing bacterium in fractured porous media. Biopolymer producing (dextran) *Leuconostoc mesenteroides* does not help to increase oil recovery due to matrix-fracture plugging effect. The increase in oil recovery was related to reduction in viscosity and interfacial tension by surfactin production by *Bacillus subtilis.*

The MEOR in a high temperature (73°C) reservoir, Dagang oilfield in China has been reported.[107] They have isolated three microbial strains viz. *Arthrobacter* sp (A02), *Pseudomonas* sp (P15) and *Bacillus* sp (B24) from the reservoir sample. The strains A02 and P15 demonstrated a good capacity in degradation of oil and B24 was more effective in reduction of interfacial tension of oil and formation brine due to its production of biosurfactant from fermentation of crude oil. When these organisms were inoculated with nutrients into all the 7 production wells in the unit the oil production steadily increased. After 6 months of inoculation about 8700 t of additional oil was obtained compared with the predicated oil production by water flooding alone.

First time well-documented MEOR has been reported recently.[108] They showed that in situ biosurfactant production by *Bacillus* strains injected into Viola limestone petroleum reservoir sufficient to mobilize the oil. For this they have selected five wells. Two wells received an inoculum (a mixture of *Bacillus* strain RS-1 and *Bacillus subtilis* subsp *spizizenii* NRRL B-23049) and nutrients (glucose, sodium nitrate and trace metals), two wells received just nutrients and one well received only formation water. Results showed that inoculated organisms grow profusely and produced lipopeptide biosurfactant about 90 mg/liter which was approximately nine times higher than the amount required to mobilize entrapped oil from sandstone cores. Carbon dioxide, acetate, lactate, ethanol and 2, 3-butanediol were detected in the produced fluids of the inoculated wells while only carbon dioxide and ethanol were detected in the produced fluids of the nutrient-only-treated wells. Technical data of modeling in situ MEOR indicate growth rates (0.06 = 0.01 h^{-1}), carbon balances (107% ± 34%), biosurfactant production rates (0.02 ± 0.0001 h^{-1}) and biosurfactant yields (0.015 ± 0.001 mol biosurfactant/mol glucose) which clearly demonstrate the technical feasibility of microbial processes for oil recovery.

Successful utilization of stratal microflora has been reported for enhanced oil recovery[109] in the high-temperature horizons of the Kongdian bed (60°C) of the Dagang oil field (China). They have pumped water-air mixture and nitrogen and phosphorus mineral salts into the oil stratum through injection oil wells in order to stimulate the activity of the stratal microflora which produces oil-releasing metabolites. They observed the cell numbers of thermophilic hydrocarbon-oxidizing, fermentative, sulfate-reducing and methanogenic microorganisms increased 10-10,000 fold. The rates of methanogenesis and sulfate reduction increased in the near-bottom zone of the injection wells and of some production wells. The microbial growth was associated with the accumulation of bicarbonate ions, volatile fatty acids and biosurfactants in the formation waters, as well as of CH_4 and CO_2 both in the gas phase and oil. As a result the water content in the production liquid from the trial site decreased and the oil content increased. This allowed the recovery of more than 14,000 tons of additional oil over 3.5 years.

Conclusion and Future Perspectives

Large number of biosurfactant producing organisms has been reported during last few years with novel properties. Their effectiveness in MEOR has been clearly demonstrated. Efforts were also being made to enhance the yield of biosurfactants by isolating hyper secretary mutants and recombinant strains and efficient recovery methods to compete with chemical surfactants. But still combined efforts are needed among microbiologists, petroleum and reservoir engineers and geologist to revolutionize the process of MEOR.

References

1. Desai JD, Banat IM. Microbial production of surfactants and their commercial potential. Microbial Mol Biol Rev 1997; 61:47-64.
2. Lin SC. Biosurfactants: Recent advances. J Chem Tech Biotechnol 1996; 66:109-120.
3. Makkar RS, Cameotra SS. An update on the use of unconventional substrates for biosurfactant production and their new applications. Appl Microbiol Biotechnol 2002; 58:428-434.
4. Mukherjee S, Das P, Sen R. Towards commercial production of microbial surfactants. Trends in Biotechnol 2006; 24:509-515.
5. Singh A, Hamme V, Jonathan D et al. Surfactants in microbiology and biotechnology: part 2. Application aspects. Biotechnol Adv 2007; 25:99-121.
6. Edsar C. Focus on surfactants. Latest Market Analysis 2006; 5:1-2.
7. Cooper DG. Biosurfactants. Microbiol Sci 1986; 3:32-38.
8. Desai JD. Microbial surfactants; evaluation, types and future applications. J Sci Ind Res 1987; 46:440-449.
9. Rosenberg E. Microbial surfactants. Crit Rev Biotechnol 1986; 3:109-132.
10. Syldatk C, Wagner F. Production of biosurfactants. In: Kosaric N, Cairns WL, Gray NCC, eds, Biosurfactants and Biotechnology. New York: Marcel Dekker, Inc., 1987:89-120.
11. Banat IM, Makkar RS, Cameotra SS. Potential commercial applications of microbial surfactants. Appl Microbiol Biotechnol 2000; 53:495-508.
12. Maier RM. Biosurfactants: Evolution and diversity in bacteria. Adv Appl Microbiol 2003; 52:101-121.
13. Cui Z, Liu W, Qi Y et al. Isolation of biosurfactant producing bacteria and characteristics of the biosurfactant. Bing Turang (Nanjing, China) 2004; 36:644-647.
14. Ilori MO, Amobi CJ, Odocha AC. Factors affecting biosurfactant production by oil degrading aeromonas sp isolated from a tropical environment. Chemosphere 2005; 61:985-992.
15. Noah KS, Fox SL, Bruhn DF et al. Development of continuous surfactin production from potato effluent by bacillus subtilis in an airlift reactor. Appl Biochem Biotechnol 2002; 98-100:803-813.
16. Nitschke M, Pastore GM. Biosurfactant production by B. subtilis using cassava-processing effluent. Appl Bichem Biotechnol 2004; 112:163-172.
17. Lee SC, Yoo JS, Kim SH et al. Production and characterization of lipopeptide biosurfactant from bacillus subtilis A8-8. J Microbiol Biotechnol 2006; 16:716-723.
18. Kim JS, Song H, Chung N et al. Optimization of production conditions of biosurfactant from bacillus sp and its purification. Eungyong Sangmyong Hwahakhoeji 2005; 48:109-114.
19. Kim P, Kim JH. Characterization of a novel lipopolysaccharide biosurfactant from klebsiella oxitoca. Biotechnol Bioprocess Eng 2005; 10:494-499.
20. Vasileva TE, Gesheva V. Biosurfactant production by antartica facultative anaerobe pantoea sp during growth on hydrocarbons. Current Microbiol 2007; 54:136-141.
21. Haba E, Espuny MJ, Busquets M et al. Screening and production of rhamnolipids by pseudomonas aeruginosa 47T2 NCIB 40044 from waste frying oils. J Appl Microbiol 2000; 88:379-387.
22. Abalos A, Pinazo A, Infante MR et al. Physicochemical and antimicrobial properties of new rhamnolipids produced by pseudomonas aeruginosa AT10 from soyabean oil refinery wastes. Langmuir 2001; 17:1367-71.
23. Rahman KSM, Rahman TJ, McClean S et al. Rhamnolipid biosurfactant production by strains of pseudomonas aeruginosa using low-cost raw materials. Bitechnol Prog 2002; 18:1277-81.
24. Nitschke M, Costa SGVAO, Haddad R et al. Oil wastes as unconventional substrates for rhamnolipids by pseudomonas aeruginosa LB1. Bitechnol Prog 2005; 21:1562-66.
25. Rashedi H, Jamshidi E, Assadi M. Isolation and production of biosurfactant from pseudomonas aeruginosa from iranian southern wells soil. Int J Enviorn Sci Technol 2005; 2:121-127.
26. Rashedi H, Mazaheri AM, Jamshidi E et al. Optimization of the production of biosurfactant by pseudomonas aeruginosa HR isolated from an iranian southern oil well. Iranian J Chem and Chemical Eng 2006; 25:25-30.
27. Vasileva TE, Galabova D, Stoimenova E et al. Production and properties of biosurfactants from newly isolated pseudomonas fluorescens HW-6 growing on hexadecane. J Biosciences 2006; 61:553-559.
28. Chen SY, Lu WB, Wei YH et al. Improved production of biosurfactant with newly isolated pseudomonas aeruginosa S2. Biotechnol Prog 2007; 23:661-666.
29. Sifour M, Al-Jilawi MH, Aziz GM. Emulsification properties of biosurfactant produced from pseudomonas aeruginosa RB 28. Pakistan J Biological Sci 2007; 10:1331-35.
30. Chang JS, Chou CL, Lin GH et al. Pseudoxanthomonas kaohsiungensis, sp nov., a novel bacterium isolated from oil-polluted site produces extracellular surface activity. Systematic and Applied Microbiology 2005; 28:137-144.

31. Trummler K, Effenberger F, Syldatk C. An integrated microbial/enzymatic process for production of rhamnolipids and l-(+)-rhamnose from rapeseed oil with pseudomonas sp DSM 2874. Eur J Lipid Sci Tech 2003; 105:563-71.
32. Yin H, Xie D, Peng H et al. Study on the pseudomonas XD-1 releasing biosurfactants. Huanjing Kexue Xuebao 2005; 25:220-225.
33. Rodrigues LR, Teixeira JA, van der Mei HC et al. Isoaltion and partial characterization of a biosurfactant produced by streptococcus thermophilus A. Colloids and Syrfaces, B: Biointerfaces 2006; 53:105-112.
34. Rodrigues L, Moldes A, Teixeria J et al. Kinetic study of fermentative biosurfactant production by lactobacillus strains. Biochem Eng J 2006; 28:109-116.
35. Rashedi H, Mazaheri A, Mahnaz J et al. Optimization of the production of biosurfactant by pseudomonas aeruginosa HR isolated from an iranian southern oil well. Iranian J Chem Chemical Eng 2006; 25:25-30.
36. Cooper DG, Goldenberg BG. Surface active agents from two bacillus species. Appl Enviorn Microbiol 1987; 53:224-229.
37. Tugrul T, Cansunar E. Detecting surfactant-producing microorganisms by the drop-collapse test. World J Microbiol Biotechnol 2005; 21:851-853.
38. Van der Vegt W, Vander Mei HC, Noordmans J et al. Assesment of bacterial biosurfactant production through axisymmetric drop shape analysis by profile. Appl Microbiol Biotech 1991; 35:766-770.
39. Shulga AN, Karpenko EV, Eliseev SA et al. The method for determination of anionogenic bacterial surface-active peptidolipids. Microbiol Journal 1993; 55:85-88.
40. Lin SC, Sharma MM, Georgiou G. Production and deactivation of biosurfactant by bacillus licheniformis JF-2. Biotechnology Prog 1993; 9:138-145.
41. Lin SC, Minton MA, Sharma MA et al. Structural and immunological characterization of a biosurfactant produced by bacillus licheniformis JF-2. Appl Enviorn Microbiol 1994; 60:31-38.
42. Heieh FC, Li MC, Lin TC. Rapid detection and characterization of surfactin-producing bacillus subtilis and closely related species based on PCR. Current Microbiol 2004; 49:186-191.
43. Rashedi H, Mazaherri A, Jamshidi E et al. Production of rhamnolipids by pseudomonas aeruginosa growing on carbon sources. Int J Enviorn Sc Technol 2006; 3:297-303.
44. Rodrigues L, Teixeria J, Oliveira R et al. Response surface optimization of the medium components for the production of biosurfactants by probiotic bacteria. Process Biochem 2006; 41:1-10.
45. Dubey K, Juwarkar A. Distillery and curd whey wastes as viable alternative sources for biosurfactant production. World J Microbiol Biotechnol 2001; 17:61-69.
46. Mulligan CN, Mahmourides G, Gibbs BF. The influence of phosphate metabolism on biosurfactant production by Pseudomonas aeruginosa. J Biotechnol 1989; 12:199-210.
47. Guerra-Santos IH, Kappeli O, Fiechter A. Pseudomonas aeruginosa biosurfactant production in continuous culture with glucose as carbon source. Appl Enviorn Microbiol 1984; 48:301-305.
48. Reiling HE, Wyass UT, Guerra-Santos LH et al. Pilot plant production of rhamnolipid biosurfactant by pseudomonas aeruginosa. Appl Enviorn Microbiol 1986; 51:985-989.
49. Morita T, Konishi M, Fukuoka T et al. Physiological differences in the formation of the glycolipid biosurfactants, mannosylerythritol lipids, between pseudozyma antartica and pseudozyma aphidis. Appl Microbiol Biotechnol 2007; 74:307-315.
50. Deziel E, Lepine F, Milot S et al. rhlA is required for the production of a novel biosurfactant promoting swarming motility in pseudomonas aeruginosa: 3-(3-hydroxyalkanoyloxy)alkanoic acids (HAAs), the precursors of rhamnolipids. Microbiol 2003; 149:2005-13.
51. Raza Z, Khan MS, Khalid ZM et al. Production kinetics and tensioactive characteristics of biosurfactant from a pseudomonas aeruginosa mutant grown on waste frying oils. Biotechnol Lett 2006; 28:1623-31.
52. Wei YH, Chou CL, Chang JS. Rhamnolipid production by indigeneous pseudomonas aeruginosa J4 originating from petrochemical wastewater. Biochemical Engineering J 2005; 27:146-154.
53. Wu JY, Yeh KL, Lu WB et al. Rhamnolipid production with indigenous pseudomonas aeruginosa EM 1 isolated from oil-contaminated site. Bioresource Technol 2008; 99:1157-64.
54. Wei YH, Chu IM. Enhancement of surfactin production in iron-enriched media by bacillus subtilis ATCC 21332. Enz Microb Technol 1998; 22:724-728.
55. Wei YH, Wang LF, Chang JS et al. Identification of induced acidification in iron-enriched cultures of bacillus subtilis during biosurfactant fermentation. J Biosci Bioeng 2003; 96:174-178.
56. Wei YH, Wang LF, Chang JS. Optimizing iron supplement strategies for ehanced surfactin production with bacillus subtilis. Biotechnol Progress 2004; 20:979-983.
57. Wei YH, Chu IM. Mn^{2+} imprives production of surfactin by bacillus subtilis. Biotechnol Lett 2002; 24:479-482.

58. Wei YH, Lai CC, Chang JS. Using taguchi experimental design methods to optimize trace element composition for enhanced surfactin production by bacillus subtilis ATCC 21332. Process Biochem 2007; 42:40-45.

59. Makkar RS, Cameotra. Effects of various nutritional supplements on biosurfactant production by a strain of bacillus subtilis at 45°C. J Surfactants Detergents 2006; 5:11-17.

60. Ferraz C, De Araujo AA, Pastore GM. The influence of vegetable oils on biosurfactant production by serratia marcescens. Appl Biochem Biotechnol 2002; 98-100:841-847.

61. Thaniyavarn S, Pinphanichkarn P, Leepipatpiboon N et al. Biosurfactant production by pseudomonas aeruginosa A41 using palm oil as carbon source. J General and Applied Microbiol 2006; 52:215-222.

62. Raza ZA, Rehman A, Khan MS et al. Improved production of biosurfactant by a pseudomonas aeruginosa mutant using vegetable oil refinery wastes. Biodegradation 2007; 18:115-121.

63. Dubey K, Juwarkar A. Determination of genetic basis for biosurfactant production in distillery and curd whey wastes utilizing pseudomonas aeruginosa strain BS2. Indian J Biotechnol 2004; 3:74-81.

64. Rodrigues LR, Teixeira JA, Oliveira R. Low-cost fermentative medium for biosurfactant production by probiotic bacteria. Biochemical Engineering Journal 2006; 32:135-142.

65. Thompson DN, Fox SL, Bala G. Biosurfactants from potato process effluents. Appl Biochem Biotechnol 2000; 84-86:917-930.

66. Thompson DN, Fox SL, Bala GA. The effect of pretreatments on surfactin. Biotechnol 2001; 91-93:487-501.

67. Noah KS, Bruhn DF, Bala GA. Surfactin production from potato process effluent by bacillus subtilis chemostat. Appl Biochem Biotechnol 2005; 122:465-473.

68. Nitschke M, Pastore G. Production and properties of a surfactant obtained from bacillus subtilis grown on cassava wastewater. Bioresource Technol 2006; 97:335-341.

69. Nitschke M, Pastore G. Cassava flour wastewater as a substate for biosurfactant production. Appl Biochem Biotechnol 2003; 106:295-302.

70. Raza ZA, Khan MS, Khalid ZM. Physicochemical and surface-active properties of biosurfactant produced using molasses by a Pseudomonas aeruginosa mutant. J Enviornmental Science and Health, Part A: Toxic/Hazardous Substances and Enviornmental Engineering 2007; 42:73-80.

71. Moldes AB, Torrado AM, Barral MT et al. Evaluation of biosurfactant production from various agricultural residues by lactobacillus pentosus. J Agric Food Chem 2007; 55:4481-86.

72. Joshi S, Yadav S, Nerurkar A et al. Statistical optimization of medium components for the production of biosurfactant by bacillus licheniformis K51. J Microbiol Biotechnol 2007; 17:313-319.

73. Banat IM. The isolation of a thermophilic biosurfactant producing bacillus sp. Biotechnol Lett 1993; 15:591-94.

74. Sharp RJ, Munster B. Thermophiles. In: Herbert RA, Codd GA, eds. Microbes in Extreme Environments. London: Academic Press, 1986.

75. Weigel J, Ljungdaht LG. Importance of thermophilic bacteria in biotechnology. CRC Rev Biotechnol 1986; 3:39-108.

76. Philips WE, Perry JJ. Thermomisrobium fosteri sp nov. A hydrocarbon utilizing obligate thermophile. Int J Syst Bacteriol 1976; 26:220-225.

77. Jenneman GE, McInerney MJ, Knapp RM et al. A halotolerant biosurfactant producing bacillus species potentially useful for enhanced oil recovery. Dev Ind Microbiol 1983; 24:485-492.

78. Trebbau de Acevado G, McInerney MJ. Emulsifying activity in thermophilic and extremely thermophilic microorganisms. J Ind Microbiol 1996; 16:1-7.

79. Gurjar M, Khire JM, Khan MI. Bioemulsifier production by bacillus stearothermophilus VR-8 isolate. Lett Appl Microbiol 1995; 21:83-86.

80. Cirigliano MC, Carman GM. Isolation of bioemulsifier from candida lipolytica. Appl Environ Microbiol 1984; 48:747-750.

81. Singh M, Desai JP. Hydrocarbon emulsification by candida tropicalis and debaromyces polymirphus. Indian J Expt Biol 1989; 27:224-226.

82. Pruthi V, Cameotra SS. Production, properties of a biosurfactant synthesized by arthrobacter protophormiae- an antartica strain. World J Microbiol Biotechnol 1997; 13:137-139.

83. Zukerberg A, Diver A, Peeri D et al. Emulsifier of arthrobacter RAG-1: chemical and physical properties. Appl Environ Microbiol 1979; 37:414-420.

84. Rosenberg E, Rubinovitz C, Gottlieb A et al. Production of biodispersan by acinetobacter calcoacticus A2. Appl Environ Microbiol 1988; 54:317-322.

85. Huszcza E, Burczyk B. Biosurfactant from bacillus coagulas. J Surfactants Detergents 2003; 6:61-64.

86. Chameotra SS, Singh HD. Purification and characterization of alkane solubilizing factor produced by pseudomonas PG-1. J Ferment Bioeng 1990; 69:341-344.

87. Kuyukina MS, Ivshina IB, Philip JC et al. Recovery of rhodococcus biosurfactants using methyl tertiary butyl ether extraction. J Microbiol Methods 2001; 46:149-156.

88. Lin SC, Jiang HJ. Recovery and purification of the lipopeptide biosurfactant of bacillus subtilis by ultrafiltration. Biotechnol Techniques 1997; 11:413-416.

89. Chen CY, Baker SC, Darton RC. Continuous production of biosurfactant with foam fractionation. J Chemical Technology and Biotechnology 2006; 81:1915-22.

90. Dubey KV, Juwarkar AA. Adsorption-desorption process using wood-based activated carbon for recovery of biosurfactant from fermented distillery wastewater. Biotechnol Progress 2005; 21:860-867.

91. Cho SK, Shim SH, Park KR et al. Purification and characterization of biosurfactant produced by pseudomonas sp G11 by assymetrical flow field-flow fractionation (AsFlFFF). Anal Bioanalytical Chemistry 2006; 386:2027-33.

92. Haferburg D, Hommel R, Claus R et al. Extra-cellular microbial lipids as biosurfactants. Adv Biochem Eng Biotechnol 1986; 33:53-93.

93. Montel D, Ratomahenina R, Glazy P. A study of the influence of the growth media on the fatty acids composition in Candida lipolytica. Biotechnol Lett 1985; 7:733-736.

94. Ratledge C. Lipid biotechnology: a wonderland for the microbial physiologist. J Am Oil Chem Soc 1987; 64:1647-56.

95. Yamane T. Enzyme technology for the lipid industry: an engineering overview. J Am Oil Chem Soc 1987; 64:1657-62.

96. Brown WA, Cooper DG. Self-cycling fermentation applied to acinetobacter calcoaceticus RAG-1. Appl Enviorn Microbiol 1991; 57:2901-06.

97. Zenaitis MG, Cooper DG. Antibiotic production by streptomyces aureofaciens using self-cycling fermentation. Biotechnol Bioeng 1994; 44:1331-36.

98. Dubern JF, Lagendijk EL, Lugtenberg BJ et al. The heat shock genes dnaK, dnaJ and grpE are involved in regulation of putisolvin biosynthesis in Pseudomonas putida PCL1445. J Bacteriol 2005; 187:5967-76.

99. Bashandy As, Abu Shady HM, Aziz NH et al. Enhanced production and properties of a surfactant by a gamma ray induced mutant of bacillus subtilis. Egyptian J Biotechnol 2005; 20:290-303.

100. Liu Q, Li Q. Breeding of biosurfactant producing strain. Weishengwuxue Zazhi 2005; 25:54-56.

101. Khire JM, Khan MI. Microbially enhanced oil recovery (MEOR). Part 1. Importance and mechanism of MEOR. Enz Microbiol Technol 1994; 16:170-172.

102. Khire JM, Khan MI. Microbially enhanced oil recovery (MEOR). Part 2. Microbes and subsurface environment for MEOR. Enz Microbiol Technol 1994; 16:258-259.

103. Li Q, Kang C, Wang H et al. Application of microbial enhanced oil recovery technique to daqing oilfield. Biochemical Engineering Journal 2002; 11:197-199.

104. Saidi AM. Simulation of naturally fractured reservoirs. SPE symposium on reservoir simulations, San Francisco, California, USA. 1983. SPE Paper 12270.

105. Delshad M, Asakawa K, Pope GA et al. Simulation of chemical and microbial enhanced oil recovery methods. DEO/SPE Improved oil recovery symposium, Tulsa, Oklahoma, USA. 2002. SPE paper 36746.

106. Soudmand-asli A, Ayatollahi SS, Mohabatkar H et al. The in situ microbial enhanced oil recovery in fractured porous media. J Petroleum Science and Engineering 2007; 58:161-172.

107. Jinfeng L, Lijun M, Bozhong M et al. The field pilot of microbial enhanced oil recovery in a high temperature petroleum reservoir. J Petroleum Science Engineering 2005; 48:265-271.

108. Youssef N, Simpson DR, Duncan KE et al. In situ biosurfactant production by bacillus strains injected into a limestone petroleum reservoir. Appl Environ Microbiol 2007; 73:1239-47.

109. Nazina TN, Griror'yan AA, Feng Q et al. Microbiological and production characteristics of the high temperature kongdian petroleum reservoir revealed during field trial of biotechnology for the enhancement of oil recovery. Microbiology 2007; 76:297-309.

Chapter 12

Molecular Engineering Aspects for the Production of New and Modified Biosurfactants

Alexander Koglin, Volker Doetsch and Frank Bernhard*

Abstract

Biosurfactants are of considerable industrial value as their high tenside activity in combination with their biocompatibility makes them attractive for many applications. In particular members of the lipopeptide family of biosurfactants contain significant potentials for the pharmaceutical industry due to their intrinsic antibiotic characteristics. The high frequency of lipopeptide (LP) production in common soil microorganisms in combination with the enormous structural diversity of the synthesized biosurfactants has created an abundant natural pool of compounds with potentially interesting properties. Unfortunately, the bioactivity of lipopetides against pathogenic microorganisms is often associated with problematic side effects that restrict or even prevent medically relevant applications. The accumulated knowledge of lipopetide biosynthesis and their frequent structural variations caused by natural genetic rearrangements has therefore motivated numerous approaches in order to manipulate biosurfactant composition and production mechanisms. This chapter will give an overview on current engineering strategies that aim to obtain lipopeptide biosurfactants with redesigned structures and optimized properties.

Introduction

Biosurfactants comprise a heterogenous group of low molecular weight microbial amphiphilic polymers that combine structural features of conventional surfactants with a variety of biological activities. They are usually water-soluble with a relatively low critical micellar concentration in the order of 10^{-5} M. Producers are a wide range of bacteria and lower fungi, while biosurfactants from higher eukaryotes remain the exception. Microbial biosurfactants can roughly be grouped into the classes of heteropolysaccharides, lipids and peptides as well as any mixtures thereof like lipopeptides, glycolipids or protein-lipid-carbohydrate compounds. Their environmentally friendly nature based on high biodegradability and biocompatibility, that is often associated with less toxicity if compared with synthetic surfactants, becomes more and more appreciated in particular as ecological concerns increasingly gain importance. The general capability to emulsify hydrocarbons play important roles in soil remediation by solubilization of poorly soluble organic contaminants like oil spills or pesticides. Mixtures of biosurfactants with chelating agents, organic solvents and others are used for the bioremediation of metal contaminated land sites.[1] An interesting perspective is the microbial enhanced oil and bitumen recovery from natural

*Corresponding Author: Frank Bernhard—Centre for Biomolecular Magnetic Resonance, Goethe-University of Frankfurt/Main, Institute for Biophysical Chemistry, Max-von-Laue-Str. 9, D-60438 Frankfurt/Main, Germany. Email: fbern@bpc.uni-frankfurt.de

Biosurfactants, edited by Ramkrishna Sen. ©2010 Landes Bioscience and Springer Science+Business Media.

deposits by lowering interfacial tension at the oil-rock interface. Biosurfactants are further used in tank oil cleaning, as ingredients in laundry detergents and for reducing viscosity in heavy oils, thus facilitating transportation and pipelining.

An application with promising perspectives for future developments is the biological control of pathogens with biosurfactants and their use as antibiotics in therapeutic treatments of infections as antibacterial, antifungal or antiviral drugs.[2,3] Biosurfactants represent interesting alternatives to chemical drugs and pesticides for combating human and crop diseases. Immunomodulation, antitumor effects and specific inhibition of enzymes are some already described bioactivities. Precoating medical insertion materials like implants or catheters with biosurfactants can help to prevent adhesion of microbes and biofilm formation.

Surface activity and bioactive performance are often not optimal for specific applications and still contain a high potential for improvements. However, the scaffolds of biosurfactants are often too complex to become efficiently amenable to chemical synthesis or modification, in particular under economic aspects. The continuous demand to decrease production costs and to generate compounds with improved properties for extended applications has therefore initiated biosurfactant engineering projects based on a variety of biotechnological, molecular or genetic approaches. Directed and combinatorial strategies have been attempted to generate arrays of modified products in particular of lipopeptide derivatives. Optimized and even artificial biosurfactants could be synthesized in future by rational design, while production cost could be minimized by increasing the overall production yields, by improving the secretion of synthesized biosurfactants and by reducing the biosynthetic heterogeneity for better streamlined purification processes. We will provide an overview on progress that has been achieved in lipopeptide engineering. Based on recent insights in the dynamics and new structural features of lipopeptide synthetases, we will further emphasis on engineering strategies that might become considered in the near future.

Lipopetides as Targets for Engineering

Lipopeptides (LPs) are one major class of biosurfactants that was mostly in focus of recent engineering approaches due to the particular interest in their high surface activities and antibiotic potentials. Their immense natural diversity and versatility in functions provide a robust platform for combinatorial rearrangement strategies. Basic prerequisite for the design of molecular engineering approaches is the thorough understanding of the general biosynthetic machineries including the posttranslational processing and transportation pathways of a selected biosurfactant. In addition, detailed knowledge of its three-dimensional structure would be essential. The hydrophobic parts of LPs are generally composed of long-chain fatty acids, hydroxyl fatty acids or α-alkyl-β-hydroxy fatty acids while the hydrophilic moieties contain amino acids and derivatives thereof, in addition to other compounds such as carboxylic acids or alcohols. Bacteria and filamentous fungi are the main producers of LPs. Their relatively low complexity, the availability of complete genome sequences in many cases and the possibility to cultivate the producers in large scales by routine fermenter techniques and at reasonable costs considerably support molecular engineering approaches.

LPs are synthesized by large nonribosomal peptide synthetase (NRPS) systems via a thioemplate mechanism (Fig. 1). Bacterial NRPSs are usually composed of multiple subunits and organized in operons. The biosynthetic pathway of LP production, in particular the synthesis of the peptide moiety, is well-understood and a series of excellent reviews have been published.[4-7] An interesting feature of NRPS systems is their modular design where the individual modules act as building blocks for the incorporation of the single amino acid components in the final LP product (Fig. 1). These modules act as the minimal biosynthetic active units of NRPS systems and they are constructed of three basic domains. The amino acid adenylation domain (A-domain) recognizes and generates the activated amino acid substrates by ATP hydrolysis and the N-terminal condensation domain (C-domain) catalyses the actual peptide bond formation by a condensation reaction between two activated substrates. The thiolation domain (T-domain) located C-terminally of the A-domain serves as shuttling unit which transfers the activated substrates and the growing peptide chain tethered as thioesters to a covalently bound

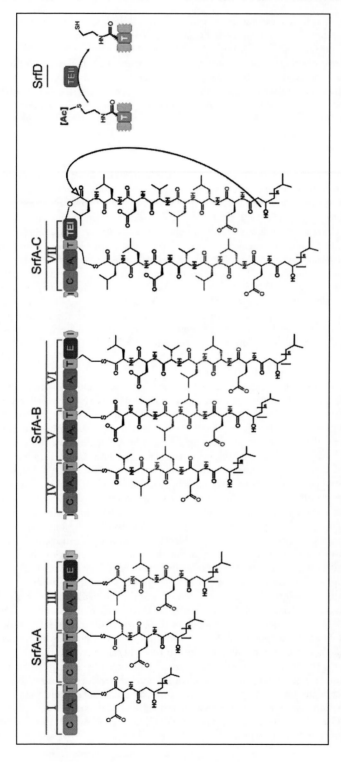

Figure 1. Modular design of NRPS systems. Schematic view of the surfactin synthetase system comprising the three subunits SrfA-A, SrfA-B and SrfA-C and the accessory protein SrfD encoding for the thioesterase II. The modules I-VII of the Srf subunits are indicated. Each module consists of the domains C (condensation), A (adenylation) and T (thiolation). Different substrate specificities of the A-domains are indicated by colour. The modules III and VI contain in addition an E (epimerization) domain. The module VII contains the terminal TEI domain which releases the final peptide product. The growing peptide chain of surfactin catalysed by the individual modules is illustrated. The TEII enzyme regenerates misacylated T-domains. A color version of this image is available at www.landesbioscience.com/curie.

4'-phosphopantetheine (4'-PP) cofactor from the upstream catalytic domains to the downstream C-domains. These core catalytic domains of a minimal NRPS module are arranged in the sequence of C-A-T giving a total molecular weight of approx. 120 kDa. A full length assembly line containing several modules can therefore easily reach the mega-Dalton range. Individual modules can furthermore be supplemented with additional domains catalyzing the specific modification of activated amino acids linked to the T-domains. Epimerization from the L- to the D-configuration as well as N-methylation can be catalyzed by such integrated enzymatic domains and these modifications are often important for the bioactivity of the corresponding LPs.

Native NRPS systems are continuously subject of vigorous natural rearrangements. Deletions, insertions and replacements of complete catalytic units as well as the combination of different enzyme systems in covalently linked assembly lines are frequently observed and characteristic features.[8] A remarkable heterogeneity in LP structure and production has therefore already been evolved by nature. Rearrangements of NRPS systems and structural redesigns appear therefore to be natural mechanisms in order to constantly expand the diversity of microbial produced LPs. These features implicate molecular engineering approaches for the directed reprogramming of NRPS systems resulting in the rational design and tuning of LP structures in order to generate new therapeutics or to obtain better suitable bioactivities. The individual modules, enzymatic domains and subunits of NRPS systems can be considered as a pool of relatively independent building blocks that could be specifically arranged for the production of desired compounds. Sequence alignments of NRPS modules clearly identified highly conserved sequence motifs of the distinct enzymatic domains and less conserved linker regions where natural rearrangements preferentially occur.[9] The already existing and rapidly increasing collection of natural NRPS sequences provides therefore a sound basis for the design of engineering strategies.

Common Strategies for the Engineering of Biosurfactants

The individual choice of an engineering strategy depends on the anticipated goals of the project and on the desired requirements of the final product. General motivations and aspects for engineering projects can be (I) the modulation of the bioactivity of LPs according to specific requirements, (II) the elimination of residues causing nondesired side effects in particular in medical applications, (III) the general optimization of emulsifying, solubilization and foaming properties, (IV) the modification of the chemical stability in order to accelerate decomposition after environmental applications and to improve the biocompatibility of the compound, (V) a restricted variability in the pathways for the LP biosynthesis in order to enhance the productivity of compounds of primary interest, (VI) reducing the production costs by increasing production yields, product recovery and by streamlining expression processes that facilitate less complex purification protocols and (VII) improving the fitness of surfactant producers in order to make them competitive against indigenous microorganisms. Microbial organisms often produce a set of related LPs and the composition of their production profile can be influenced by abiotic and nutritional culture conditions. Biosurfactant production can thus already be modulated by the fermentation conditions and by feeding of specific precursors.[10,11]

General molecular engineering strategies for the production of newly designed LPs are illustrated in Figure 2 as exemplified with the surfactin biosynthetic operon comprising seven modules organized in the three subunits SrfA-A, SrfA-B and SrfA-C. Structural targets for LP engineering can be type and sequence of amino acid residues in the peptide backbone as well as the nature, length and branching of the fatty acid chain moiety. Engineering approaches can in principle target on: (1) Deletion of modifying domains such as epimerization domains. This could result in the incorporation of L-amino acids into the LP product instead of the D-derivatives. (2) Complete modules could be deleted from the NRPS system resulting in the production of shorter LPs. (3) Terminal communication domains required for the recognition and specific interaction of subunits could be exchanged resulting in altered sequences of LP synthesis. (4) Exchange of A-domains or (5) of complete modules responsible for the selection of substrates could result into incorporation of new compounds. (6) The exchange of NRPS

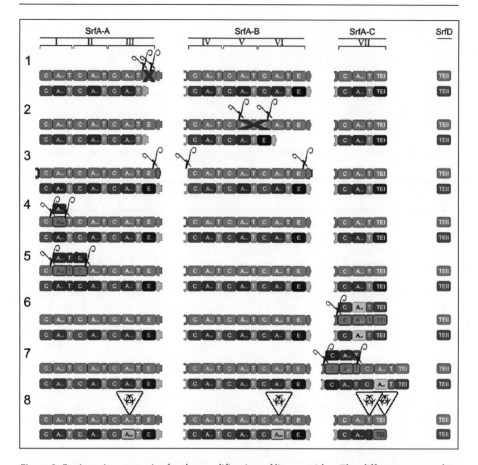

Figure 2. Engineering strategies for the modification of lipopeptides. The different approaches are exemplified with the surfactin synthetase cluster comprising the three subunits SrfA-A, SrfA-B and SrfA-C and the associated SrfD protein. Structures of the NRPS system before and after engineering are illustrated. 1) Deletion of modifying E-domains; 2) Excision of complete modules; 3) Manipulation of terminal COM-domains for the interaction of subunits; 4) Swapping of A-domains; 5) Swapping of complete modules; 6) Exchange of complete subunits; 7) Insertion of complete modules; 8) Site directed mutagenesis in order to modify substrate specificities. The individual domains of the modules are indicated. C: Condensation domain; A: Adenylation domain; T: Thiolation domains; E: Epimerization domain; TEI: Thioesterase I; TEII: Thioesterase II. Colours of the A-domains indicate different substrate specificities. A color version of this image is available at www.landesbioscience.com/curie.

subunits with e.g., corresponding subunits of related systems could alter the composition of parts of the LP product. (7) The insertion of new modules could result in the production of extended LPs. (8) Specific directed mutagenesis could be used to modify the enzymatic activity of distinct domains such as the substrate specificity of A-domains or of the terminal thioesterase I (TEI)-domain responsible for cyclization and release of the LP. However, it should be considered that all these approaches affect the structure of the NRPS and the impacts on folding pathways and protein interactions as well as on kinetics and coordination of enzymatic reactions can not be predicted.

Additional options for the structural tailoring of biosurfactants are to manipulate precursor pathways or modifying enzymes that act posttranslationally on the synthesized compounds, e.g., by attachment of specific residues. The LP syringomycin for example is chlorinated on a threonine residue and hydroxylated on an aspartic acid residue after peptide biosynthesis.[12] An outstanding feature of NRPS systems is the incorporation of unusual compounds. These can be primary metabolites like ornithine or substances having their own biosynthetic pathways. Feeding modified precursors or manipulation of specific precursor pathways can thus result in new products.[13] The N-terminal fatty acid moiety determines to a large extent the biological properties of LPs. Mutation of external enzymes involved in selection and activation of the fatty acid can result in the formation of LPs with modified fatty acid chains.[14] Increases in yield of natural LPs can be obtained by general engineering approaches of the producer strains. Modifying the regulatory regions involved in biosurfactant expression by up-mutations may be considered. Straight forward would be to replace weak endogenous promoters with strong promoters that can even be better controlled by stable inducers. Specific producer strains like spore-forming microbes could be selected as ideal candidates to become developed as biopesticides for the direct application to contaminated land sites. The high resistance against dryness of *Bacillus* spores would be in particular beneficial for formulations into stable products.

Complex combinatorial platforms that comprise a set of different approaches like enzymatic module swapping, complete protein subunit exchanges, modification of accessory tailoring enzymes, or manipulation of precursor structures are often employed.[6,15] The common strategy for molecular engineering approaches is to modify the desired parts of the cloned biosynthetic pathways by standard techniques in *E. coli*, to transfer the modified genetic elements into the producer strain and to obtain stably engineered producer strains by recombination. Alternatively, modified partial or even complete biosurfactant assembly lines could be transferred and expressed in trans from suitable vectors into corresponding deletion mutants. This strategy is independent from recombination events that are often difficult to select. Essential prerequisites are that the producer organisms are susceptible for basic genetic manipulations and that corresponding vectors, efficient gene transfer and selection techniques as well as cultivation protocols have already been developed. While this might be the case for many bacterial producers, it still represents a major bottleneck for the engineering of filamentous fungi and higher eukaryotic organisms.

Surfactin and Daptomycin as Case Studies for Applied Lipopetide Engineering

One of the most potent biosurfactants is the heptalipopeptide surfactin produced by *Bacillus subtilis*. Concentrations as low as 0.005% already reduce the surface tension below 30 mN/m. Surfactin consists of a loop of seven amino acids in the chiral sequence LLDLLDL that is modified by attachment of a β-hydroxy fatty acid containing 12-15 carbons (Fig. 3A).[16] It folds into a β-sheet structure with a horse-saddle conformation. The acyl chain enables the rapid penetration of cellular membranes and confers surfactin a broad antibacterial and antiviral activity. As the membrane disintegration property is nonspecific, it will be associated with cytotoxic and haemolytic side-effects upon clinical applications. Nevertheless, potential applications already exist in the curing of mycoplasma infected cell cultures as at lower biosurfactant concentrations, the more sensitive mycoplasma membranes are preferentially penetrated. Its property as biotensid makes surfactin furthermore effective in remediation of oil or heavy metal contaminated soils or water. The solubility and surface-active properties of surfactin depend on the nature and orientation of the individual residues. The presence of two negatively charged amino acid residues in surfactin, aspartate and glutamate, facilitate the binding of heavy metals.[17]

The three surfactin synthetase subunits SrfA-A, SrfA-B and SrfA-C (Fig. 1) provide seven modules for the incorporation of the seven amino acid residues of the surfactin peptide moiety. Surfactin synthesis starts with the loading of an activated β-hydroxyl fatty acid to the C-domain of module 1 of SrfA-A, probably with help of the associated protein SrfTEII representing a thioesterase Type II enzyme also responsible for the editing and recycling of mis-acylated T-domains.[18,19] A Type I thioesterase integrated at the C-terminus of SrfA-C catalyzes the lactone bond formation between the carboxyl group of the final amino acid residue (L-Leu) and the β-hydroxyl group of

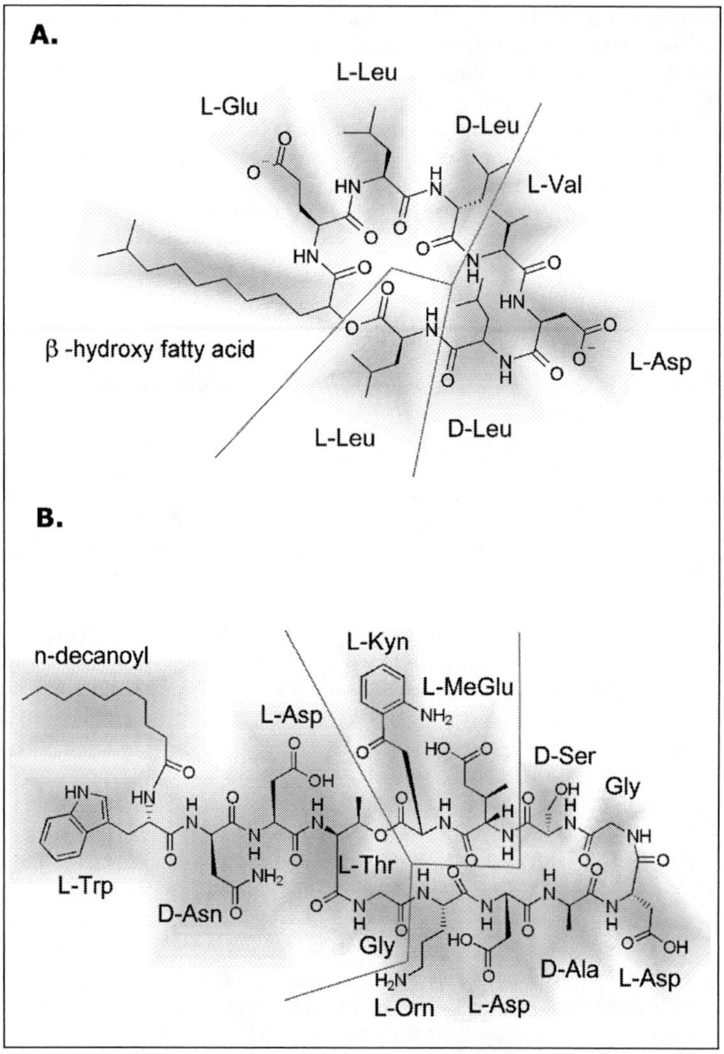

Figure 3. Structures of lipopeptides. A) Surfactin. B) Daptomycin. Residues incorporated by the individual subunits of the NRPS systems are separated by lines.

the fatty acid to form mature surfactin. Beside the generalized organization of a standard module for NRPSs, the surfactin synthetase is carrying additional catalytic functions. Two epimerization domains are located at the C-terminal ends of the SrfA-A and SrfA-B subunits adjacent to the C-domains of module 3 and module 6. The epimerization domains are responsible for balancing the population of the D- and L-stereoisomer of cognate amino acids at the α-position to a 50/50 ratio. The epimerization reaction is carried out after condensation of the activated amino acid residue to the growing peptide chain. Only the D-stereoisomer is recognized by the subsequent biosynthetic system and incorporated during the biosynthesis of surfactin. The mechanism of discrimination between L-Leu and D-Leu by the subsequent domains in the case of surfactin has not been analysed yet. The in trans acting enzyme phosphopantetheine transferase Sfp is responsible for the modification of the T-domains with the 4′-PP cofactor.

The peptide moiety of surfactin follows the classical NRPS paradigm and engineering approaches resemble therefore those generally designed for NRPSs and also polyketide synthases, that show a strikingly similar architecture.[20] Signature sequences determining the pockets for substrate specificity within A-domains have been postulated and indicate amino acid positions interesting for directed mutagenesis approaches.[21] In fact, corresponding point mutations introduced in related NRPS systems successfully altered substrate specificities.[21] Shortened surfactin derivatives have been constructed by translocation of the terminal TEI enzyme catalysing peptide release from the seventh module to the fourth or fifth, respectively.[22] Rearranged or chimeric surfactin synthetases as well as enlargements or reductions of the peptide backbone were generated by fusion, swapping, deletion or insertion approaches. The terminal leucine activating module of SrfAC was modified by exchanging the A-T domains against several corresponding regions from the gramicidin S and the δ-(α-aminoadipoyl)-cysteinyl-D-valine synthetase systems.[23] Accordingly, A-T domains from the second and fifth module were exchanged.[24] In some cases, the resulting surfactin derivatives were produced, although always at significant lower levels. However, the incorporation of ornithine specific A-T domains in the second module of SrfA-A obviously resulted in global conformational alterations of the surfactin structure, presumably resulting in premature cyclization or in the formation of branched derivatives. It has become evident that the choice of fusion points is extremely critical for the resulting hybrid enzyme. As the precise boundaries between individual domains or modules are difficult to determine, highly conserved signature motifs within the C-, A-, or T-domains could serve as general and easy to identify fixed fusion points. A systematic evaluation of the suitability of such motifs for the recombination of surfactin synthetase domains revealed few conserved sequence motifs in a hinge region of A-domains and at the N-terminus of C-domains as potentially effective boundaries for the construction of hybrid enzymes.[25,26] In contrast, fusions at arbitrary sequences or at other conserved motifs resulted in partially or completely inactive hybrid enzymes.

Daptomycin is a member of the A21978C family of acidic lipodepsipeptides produced by *S. roseosporus* (Fig. 3B) and the complete NRPS cluster is encoded by the three subunits DptA, DptBC and DptD.[15,27] Daptomycin is the active compound of the antibiotic Cubicin and marketed in the United States for the treatment of skin infections caused by Gram-positive pathogens. Its 13 amino acid core is cyclized by an intramolecular ester bond at position Thr4 to form a 10-residue ring in addition to a 3-residue side chain (Fig. 3B). Two nonproteinogenic amino acids, ornithine and kynurenine, are found in position 6 and 13, respectively. Several strategies have been applied to generate modified daptomycin derivatives with altered properties.[28-30] (I) Hybrid NRPS systems were created by exchanging the gene encoding for the terminal third subunit DptD with the terminal subunits of two related NRPS cluster from *Streptomyces sp.*[28] Favourable for the successful exchange was the very similar preference of the first modules in the two replacement subunits as well as in DptD for 3-methyl-Glu. These mixed NRPS systems resulted in the replacement of the terminal nonproteinogenic amino acid kynurenine usually incorporated by DptD with Trp and Ile/Val now incorporated by the second modules of the replacement subunits. (II) The modification of individual residues could be altered by elimination of the modifying enzymes. The deletion of the Glu12-methyltransferase gene resulted in L-Glu12-daptomycin. (III) Module exchanges at intradomain linkers of Ala8 resulted in D-Ser8, D-Asn8 or D-Lys8 and at Ser11 in D-Ala or D-Asn. Most of the derivatives retained in vitro antibacterial activities similar to that of daptomycin and some showed even an improved activity pattern. These combined engineering strategies generated libraries of novel daptomycin lipopeptides which were produced in substantial amounts of up to 250 mgs per litre of fermentation.[28,29]

Problems and Considerations for Biosurfactant Engineering

A basic intrinsic problem for many engineering approaches that focus on the construction of hybrid enzymes is the fact that the enzymatic units of NRPS systems are not completely autonomous. Substrates and intermediate products have to be passed to and accepted by adjacent domains. The efficient production of new or altered peptides needs to rely on close cooperation and interaction between modified and original parts of the NRPS system. Spatial domain arrangements and the formation of protein interfaces must not be disturbed. Often unclear remains what confines enzymatic units like modules or domains and how can the exact borders be identified. Origin and location of donor domains selected for swapping experiments might impact their function. A key question addresses the specificity of the enzymatic reactions. Besides selection of the amino acid constituents by the A-domains, potential specificities of peptide bond formation, amino acid modification, peptide transfer or peptide cleavage have to be considered. The acceptance of the newly designed LP by the recombined assembly line might be restricted. Modifying domains might prefer distinct characteristics of amino acids. The recently reported relatively low substrate specificity of some epimerization domains adds a promising perspective to that question.[31]

A rather nonspecific target selection could be described for the NRPS associated enzyme Srf TEII.[18] This crucial repair enzyme regenerates functional 4'-PP cofactors of holo-T-domains. The thiol function of the 4'-PP cofactor is essential for its function to transfer tethered substrates covalently bound as thioesters from one catalytic active domain to the next. Mispriming of 4'-PP cofactors by acetyl- and short-chain acyl- residues interrupts the biosynthetic system. Due to the large variety of acyl modifications and due to the fact that the Srf TEII has to be able to interact with all seven 4'-PP cofactor-modified T-domains of the entire surfactin assembly line, the Srf TEII has to be—in contrast to TEI at the end of the last module—rather nonspecific. The structures of the Srf TEII and its active complex in comparison with TEI enzymes show how modulation of the conserved thioesterase fold is used to change the function of the enzyme from one that recognizes relatively specifically the final product of an assembly line to one with a shallow but easily accessible active site that provides a rather unspecific but indispensable repair function.[18,32]

Any change in biosurfactant structure might cause significant problems for the physiology of producer strains. Although much knowledge has accumulated on the biosynthesis of LPs, only few is known on their secretion mechanisms and metabolic routes inside the cell. Compounds with altered bioactivities could become toxic to the producer or they might have negative side effects to other cellular processes. Export systems might not efficiently recognize modified LP structures or they could become overloaded by increased biosurfactant synthesis resulting in intracellular product accumulation. Manipulation of precursor or posttranslational modification pathways could affect also other biosynthetic systems with consequences that are difficult to predict. Co-engineering of associated pathways and enzymes might therefore be necessary in order to establish stable and efficient producer cell lines for modified or newly designed biosurfactants.

Future Aspects for Lipopeptide Engineering as Revealed by Recent Structural Details

During the last couple of years several structures of isolated domains[33-37] proteins,[18,38] functional complexes[18,32,39,40] and just recently, the first crystal structure of a full length module of NRPS systems[41] and structures of related full length fatty acid synthase clusters[42,43] have been reported. Interestingly, most of the reported structures demonstrate a particular structural flexibility or restricted dynamics. Well-defined interaction surfaces or at least specific residues are elucidated to be involved in the recognition between proteins or domains. Unfortunately, this inherent interdomain mobility is hampering crystallization or the crystallized molecules may even not represent the active domain orientation.

So called communication (COM) domains have been identified in NRPS assembly lines and they are described as less ordered pairs of helices responsible for the communication in stable interactions between NRPS subunits. COM domains are sequentially isolated, almost completely unravelled peptide sequences of 15-20 amino acid residues in length located on corresponding sites of the full length subunits.[44-46] The analysis of the NRPS system for the biosynthesis of tyrocidine revealed that COM-domains direct the docking of the individual subunits and thus ensure the correct assembly of the biosynthetic NRPS cluster.[45,46] This observation is interesting in order to understand how multi-subunit enzyme clusters can interact in general and how assembly lines of secondary metabolites can be structurally organized. The interaction between the two not natively interacting subunits TycA and TycC of the tyrocidin biosynthetic cluster could be enforced by interchanging the corresponding COM sequences. A similar result was found for the surfactin synthetase.[46] Furthermore, subunits of two complete different NRPS assembly lines could be mixed by using matching pairs of COM domains.[33,46]

The importance of protein-protein interactions and of an efficient communication within engineered NRPSs is increasingly recognized. Specific protein contacts modulate the necessary temporary association of functional enzymatic units as well as the communication between domains and modules that directs the timing and dynamics of LP product formation. The often observed low biochemical activity of the newly designed nonnative assembly lines might therefore indicate that probably still unknown processes involved in the three-dimensional assembly and structural orientation of NRPS systems are not fully restored. When larger units of NRPSs have to be rearranged by domain or module swapping or by the construction of hybrid systems, lack of an efficient communication of the newly inserted enzymatic unit with the rest of the assembly line could constitute a major bottleneck for the efficient production of modified LPs. Interfaces for the recognition and interaction of domains, modules, subunits and accessory modifying enzymes have to be conserved or restored upon molecular engineering approaches.

Changes in enzyme activity or different interaction events of a protein often require a switch in structural components. Natural product assembly lines like NRPS systems must be dynamic entities in order to ensure progress of the biosynthetic process. Particularly two conceptual models are mainly discussed in order to describe those conformational changes, the induced fit mechanism where the binding of effectors induce a modification of the protein structure and the shift of a pre-existing equilibrium of different protein conformers.[36,47] A native protein can therefore exist as an ensemble of potentially partial overlapping conformational sub-states that could differ at ligand binding sites or interaction surfaces. Binding partners can specifically select their cognate conformation thus biasing the preformed equilibrium towards the binding state. A slow conformational exchange of domains in NPRS systems is observed in several clusters including the surfactin synthetase.[18,34] The observed exchanges are usually in a time range of $100 \, s^{-1}$ and slower and they can be described as distinct movements of either single secondary structural elements or of even entire domains by high-resolution NMR spectroscopy. Structural mobility was so far described for T-domains as well as for associated thioesterase enzymes responsible for maintaining full activity of NRPS systems and for releasing the final product.[18,34,36] This conformational exchange is discussed as an important driving force for the selective interaction with other cognate domains of the NRPS system. The dynamics of the central T-domains could act as pacemaker that directs the kinetics of peptide synthesis. The underlying structural mechanisms that control this conformational exchange are just about to emerge. It is furthermore not known how general the observed dynamics of T-domains are and whether different time ranges are involved in order to modulate the kinetics of the biosynthesis process of the entire assembly line. At the moment, it is also not clear how specific those interactions are and how stringent protein-protein recognition process within NRPS systems will be controlled. However, these mechanisms will certainly become important for engineering approaches that result in larger impacts of the NRPS structure like manipulations of entire domains, modules or subunits.

Conclusion

Experimental tools as well as large pools of sequenced NRPS systems are available providing a basic platform for engineering strategies. The first successful reports on the engineering and high level production of LPs are encouraging that the routine de novo design of compounds might become feasible in future. The current amount of information from intramodule and intersubunit protein-protein interactions and substrate recognition is still too limited to draw general conclusions for the more efficient engineering of LPs. However, the presently available data already demonstrate how the internal dynamic of a protein structure can contribute to the specificity of protein-protein interactions as well as to the mechanisms of substrate recognition. They further suggest that the timing of structural exchange processes could also contribute to the interaction between domains or isolated proteins. Future structures of full length modules or even subunits will allow gaining more detailed insight in the NRPS architecture while dynamic movements and structural exchanges are difficult to assess. More details on the specificity of the protein-protein interaction and substrate recognitions are needed, even on isolated domains, to gain insights into these processes and to allow a specific and efficient modification of isolated domains and even full length assembly lines.

Acknowledgements

The work was financially supported by the Deutsche Forschungsgemeinschaft (DFG grants BE19-11 and MA811-19/1 and by a HF5PO grant to AK).

References

1. Mulligan CN. Environmental applications for biosurfactants. Environ Pollution 2005; 133:183-98.
2. Ongena M, Jacques P. Bacillus lipopeptides: Versatile weapons for plant disease biocontrol. Trends in Microbiol 2007; 16:115-25.
3. Rodrigues L, Banat IM, Teixeira J et al. Biosurfactants: Potential applications in medicine. J Antimicrob Agents 2006; 57:609-18.
4. Doekel S, Marahiel MA. Biosynthesis of natural products on modular peptide synthetases. Metabolic Engin 2001; 3:64-77.
5. Marahiel MA, Stachelhaus T, Mootz HD. Modular peptide synthetases involved in nonribosomal peptide synthesis. Chem Rev 1997; 97:2651-74.
6. Mootz HD, Marahiel MA. Design and application of multimodular peptide synthetases. Curr Opin Biotechnol 1999; 10:341-8.
7. Schwarzer D, Finking R, Marahiel MA. Nonribosomal pepides: From genes to products. Nat Prod Rep 2003; 20:275-87.
8. Duitman EH, Hamoen LW, Rembold M et al. The mycosubtilin synthetase of bacillus subtilis ATCC6633: A multifunctional hybrid between a peptide synthetase, an amino transferase and a fatty acid synthase. Proc Natl Acad Sci USA 1999; 96:13294-9.
9. Mootz HD, Marahiel MA. Biosynthetic systems for nonribosomal peptide antibiotic assembly. Curr Opin Chem Biol 1997; 1:543-51.
10 Pryor SW, Gibson DM, Hay AG et al. Optmization of spore and antifungal lipopeptide production during the solid-state fermentation of bacillus subtilis. Appl Biochem Biotechnol 2007; 143:63-79.
11 Huber FM, Pieper RL, Tietz AJ. The formation of daptomycin by supplying decanoic acid to strepto-myces roseosporus cultures producing the antibiotic complex A21978C. J Biotechnol 1988; 7:283-92.
12. Guenzi E, Galli G, Grgurina I et al. Characterization of the syringomycin synthetase gene cluster. A link betweem prokaryotic and eukaryotic peptide synthetases. J Biol Chem 1998; 273:32857-63.
13. Amir-Heidari B, Thirlway J, Micklefield J. Auxotrophic-precursor directed biosynthesis of nonribosomal lipopeptides with modified tryptophan residues. Org Biomol Chem 2008; 6:975-8.
14. Powell A, Borg M, Amir-Heidari B et al. Engineered biosynthesis of nonribosomal lipopeptides with modified fatty acid side chains. J Am Chem Soc 2007; 129:15182-91.
15. Baltz RH. Molecular engineering approaches to peptide, polyketide and other antibiotics. Nat Biotechnol 2006; 24:1533-40.
16. Bonmatin JM, Labbé H, Grangemard I et al. Production, isolation and characterization of [Leu4]- and [Ile4] surfactins from bacillus subtilis. Letts Peptide Sci 1995; 1:41-7.
17. Mulligan CN, Yong RN, Gibbs BF et al. Metal removal from contaminated soil and sediments by the biosurfactant surfactin. Environ Sci Technol 1999; 33:3812-20.
18. Koglin A, Löhr F, Bernhard F et al. Structural basis for the selectivity of the external thioesterase of the surfactin synthetase. Nature 2008; 454:907-11.
19. Steller S, Sokoll A, Wilde C et al. Initiation of surfactin biosynthesis and the role of the SrfD-thioesterase protein. Biochemistry 2004; 43:11331-43.
20. Cane DE, Walsh CT. The parallel and convergent universes of polyketide synthases and nonribosomal peptide synthetases. Chem Biol 1999; 319-25.
21. Stachelhaus T, Mootz HD, Marahiel MA The specificity code of adenylation domains in nonribosomal peptide synthetases. Chem Biol 1999; 6:493-505.
22. De Ferra F, Rodriguez F, Tortora O et al. Engineering of peptide synthetases. Key role of the thioesterase-like domain for efficient production of recombinant peptides. J Biol Chem 1997; 272:25304-9.

23. Stachelhaus T, Schneider A, Marahiel MA. Rational design of peptide antibiotics by targeted replacement of bacterial and fungal domains. Science 1995; 269:69-72.
24. Schneider A, Stachelhaus T, Marahiel MA. Targeted alteration of the substrate specificity of peptide synthetases by rational module swapping. Mol Gen Genet 1998; 257:308-18.
25. Elsner A, Engert H, Saenger W et al. Substrate specificity of hybrid modules from peptide synthetases. J Biol Chem 1997; 272:4814-9.
26. Symmank H, Saenger W, Bernhard F. Analysis of engineered multifunctional peptide synthetases: Enzymatic characterization of surfactin synthetase domains in hybrid bimodular systems. J Biol Chem 1999; 274:21581-8.
27 Baltz RH, Miao V, Wrigley SK. Natural products to drugs: Daptomycin and related lipopeptide antibiotics. Nat Prod Rep 2005; 22:717-41.
28. Miao V, Coeffet-Le Gal MF, Nguyen K et al. Genetic engineering in streptomyces roseosporus to produce hybrid lipopeptide antibiotics. Chem Biol 2006; 13:269-76.
29. Nguyen KT, Ritz D, Gu JQ et al. Combinatorial biosynthesis of novel antibiotics related to daptomycin. Proc Natl Acad Sci USA 2006; 103:17462-7.
30. Coeffet-Le Gal MF, Thurson I, Rich P et al. Complementation of daptomycin dptA and dptD deletion mutants in trans and production of hybrid lipopeptide antibiotics. Microbiology 2006; 152:2993-3001.
31. Stein DB, Linne U, Marahiel MA. Utility of epimerization domains for the redesign of nonribosomal peptide synthetases. FEBS J 2005; 272:4506-20.
32. Frueh DP, Arthanari H, Koglin A et al. Dynamic thiolation-thioesterase structure of a nonribosomal peptide synthetase. Nature 2008; 454:903-6.
33. Wu N, Cane DE, Khosla C. Quantitative analysis of the relative contributions of donor acyl carrier proteins, acceptor ketosynthases and linker regions to intermodular transfer of intermediates in hybrid polyketide synthases. Biochemistry 2002; 41:5056-66.
34. Bruner SD, Weber T, Kohli RM et al. Structural basis for the cyclization of the lipopeptide antibiotic surfactin by the thioesterase domain SrfTE. Structure 2002; 10:301-10.
35. Samel SA, Wagner B, Marahiel MA et al. The thioesterase domain of the fengycin biosynthesis cluster: a structural base for the macrocyclization of a nonribosomal lipopeptide. J Mol Biol 2006; 359:876-89.
36. Koglin A, Mofid MR, Löhr F et al. Conformational switches modulate protein interactions in peptide antibiotic synthetases. Science 2006; 312:273-6.
37. Alekseyev VY, Liu CW, Cane DE et al. Solution structure and proposed domain domain recognition interface of an acyl carrier protein domain from a modular polyketide synthase. Protein Sci 2007; 16:2093-107.
38. Johnson MA, Peti W, Herrmann T et al. Solution structure of Asl1650, an acyl carrier protein from anabaena sp. PCC 7120 with a variant phosphopantetheinylation-site sequence. Protein Sci 2006; 15:1030-41.
39. Drake EJ, Nicolai DA, Gulick AM. Structure of the EntB multidomain nonribosomal peptide synthetase and functional analysis of its interaction with the EntE adenylation domain. Chem Biol 2006; 4:409-19.
40. Samel SA, Schoenafinger G, Knappe TA et al. Structural and functional insights into a peptide bond-forming bidomain from a nonribosomal peptide synthetase. Structure 2007; 15:781-92.
41. Tanovic A, Samel SA, Essen LO et al. Crystal structure of the termination module of a nonribosomal peptide synthetase. Science 2008; 321:659-63.
42. Jenni S, Leibundgut M, Boehringer D et al. Structure of fungal fatty acid synthase and implications for iterative substrate shuttling. Science 2007; 316:254-61.
43. Leibundgut M, Jenni S, Frick C et al. Structural basis for substrate delivery by acyl carrier protein in the yeast fatty acid synthase. Science 2007; 316:288-90.
44. Hahn M, Stachelhaus T. Selective interaction between nonribosomal peptide synthetases is facilitated by short communication-mediating domains. Proc Natl Acad Sci USA 2004; 101:15585-90.
45. Hahn M, Stachelhaus T. Harnessing the potential of communication-mediating domains for the biocombinatorial synthesis of nonribosomal peptides. Proc Natl Acad Sci USA 2006; 103:275-80.
46. Chiocchini C, Linne U, Stachelhaus T. In vivo biocombinatorial synthesis of lipopeptides by COM domain-mediated reprogramming of the surfactin biosynthetic complex. Chem Biol 2006; 13:899-908.
47. Eisenmesser EZ, Millet O, Labeikovsky W et al. Intrinsic dynamics of an enzyme underlies catalysis. Nature 2005; 438:117-21.

CHAPTER 13

Rhamnolipid Surfactants:
Alternative Substrates, New Strategies

Maria Benincasa, AnaMª Marqués, Aurora Pinazo and Angels Manresa*

Abstract

This chapter concentrates on the various possibilities of using alternative substrates and new strategies. Such strategies include an integrated production system to reduce the environmental impact and an attempt to minimize residues, which reinforces socio-economic and region-structural development. Additionally, we offer an overview of the physicochemical and biological properties of rhamnolipid surfactants associated with the applications of these molecules in different circumstances.

Introduction

For many years efforts have been made to find alternative surfactants to those that are traditionally synthesized and as a result biosurfactants have emerged as an increasingly popular competitor. The growth of these biosurfactants has become even more achievable given the current trends towards eco-efficiency. The likelihood that products derived from renewable resources will be successful increases if they can be shown to have a quality and price comparable to that of their synthetic counterparts.[1-3] There are several features that make biosurfactants commercially promising: their effectiveness at high salinity and within a wide pH range and the fact that they offer new possibilities for industrial applications. Their most important advantage is probably their ecological applicability, they are biodegradable and they are produced by a variety of microorganisms that occur naturally in soils.

As Van Hamme[4] pointed out, a wide variety of microorganisms that occur naturally in soils produce biosurfactants. In terms of the problems associated with interphase contact, there are many different types of low molecular weight surfactants[5,6] that offer solutions. These include glycolipids, lipopeptides, flavolipids, proteins, sulphonolipids, hetero-glycolipids lipo-polysaccharides, fatty acids, conronmycolyc acids, phospholipids and high molecular weight products, such as liposan or emulsan. To date, several glycolipid surfactants have been characterized. The hydrophobic moiety is a hydroxyl or α-alkyl-β-hydroxy-fatty acid of different carbon chain length, the hydrophilic moiety includes: sophorose in the sophorolipids of *Torulopsis*,[7] celobiose in the surfactants produced by *Ustilago maydis*[8] and mannosylerithryol which is the polar head of the biosurfactants accumulated by different strains of *Candida antarctica*.[9] Within the prokaryote microorganisms few genera produce surface active glycolipids, such as those produced by *Rhodococcus*,[10,11] or the well-known rhamnolipids produced by *Pseudomonas*.[5,12] This chapter thus attempts to address various possible scenarios of using alternative substrates and novel production strategies to minimize wastes and residues.

*Corresponding Author: Angels Manresa—Laboratori de Microbiologia, Facultat de Farmàcia, Universitat de Barcelona, Joan XXIII s/n 08028 Barcelona, Spain. Email: amanresa@ub.edu

Biosurfactants, edited by Ramkrishna Sen. ©2010 Landes Bioscience and Springer Science+Business Media.

Substrates

Despite the advantages and potential applicability of these biological compounds, their success depends upon economic processes and the use of low-cost raw material. Such material accounts for 10-30% of the final product.[13] Therefore, the use of inexpensive substrates like agro-industrial by-products or waste may represent an interesting and achievable strategy. However, much effort is still needed to achieve the level of competitiveness of their chemical counterparts. The selection of waste substrates involves the complicated search for a waste or by-product with the right nutrient balance to support optimal growth and production. The nature and composition of such complex substrates should be evaluated for each microorganism. It is difficult to create guidelines for optimal biosurfactant production due to the large metabolic diversity of surfactant-producing microorganisms.

In 1988, with the aim of exploiting lactic-whey from local industry, Kock et al[14] used the genetically engineered lactose-using *Pseudomonas aeruginosa* strain to produce rhamnolipids. Despite the efforts to produce rhamnolipids from lactose-whey, or corn step liquor from the cane-sugar industry, production was very low.[14,15] A variety of cheap raw materials have recently been shown to support rhamnolipid production. For example, glycerol, a sub-product form the oil and fat industry, has been suggested as a substrate that could produce approximately 3-4 g/L of rhamnolipids (calculated in terms of rhamnose).[16] Another example is the use of soy molasses to produce sophoroselipids from *Candida bombicola*.[17] However, water-soluble substrates have a low production yield.

Various attempts have been made to exploit agroindustrial residues: Mercadé et al[18] reported that *Pseudomonas aeruginosa* 47T2 could grow and produce rhamnolipids when cultivated with olive oil mill effluent (OOME). The black water from olive oil production is acidic (pH 3-4.5) and is a major pollutant (TOC:80.000 mg/L) in the agro-industrial industry in Mediterranean countries. This substrate is rich in carbohydrates (2-8% w/w) and is made up of 1% w/w fatty acids (mainly oleic acid), other organic acids, minerals and vitamins. The yield was 14 g of rhamnolipid per kg of OOME. Waste frying oil (WFO) has great potential for microbial growth and transformation: of the thirty-six strains screened, nine *Pseudomonas* strains showed satisfactory growth and surface activity properties. This decreased the surface tension of the medium to 34-36 mN. Other genera such as *Rhodoccocus* and *Candida* also produced glycolipids from waste frying oil.[19] Recently, Ali Raza et al[20,21] reported a feed batch process with waste soybean frying oil for rhamnolipid production (9.3 g rhamolipid/L) with a production yield of 2.7 g/L.

The application of LC-MS has shown that the composition of rhamnolipids depends upon the nature of the substrate. The surfactant produced is a mixture of rhamnolipid homologues of mono-rhamnosidyl (R_1), or di-rhamnosidyl (R_2) residues, with a variety of alkyl-chains, which depend on the composition of the substrate supply in the culture (Table 1). Nevertheless, the main homologues produced (regardless of the substrate or strain) are L-rhamnosyl-β-hydroxydecanoyl-β-hydroxydecanoate ($R_1C_{10}C_{10}$) and L-rhamnosyl L-rhamnosyl-β-hydroxydecanoyl-β-hydroxydecanoate ($R_2C_{10}C_{10}$).[22-28]

Abalos et al (2001)[22] identified a mixture of up to seven rhamnolipid homologues, using the strain *P. aeruginosa* AT10 when cultivated on soybean oil refinery wastes. Optimization of the culture medium, applying the full factorial central composite rotational design and the response surface methodology, increased production from 3.6 to 16.5 g/L of rhamnolipids.[29] The LC-MS analysis of the product showed that the different homologues containing either one or two rhamnose residues and varying contents of saturated or unsaturated alkyl-chains chains appeared during the incubation time (Fig. 1), $R_1C_{10}C_{10}$ being the major component (85%).[25] When sunflower-soapstock (vegetable oil refinery waste) was used as the substrate, *P. aeruginosa* LBI, gave a mixture of six rhamnolipid homologues (Table 2). In that study, most of the rhamnolipid was produced by the time cell growth had ceased. Product yield increased from 5.33 to 12.5 g/L after 48 hours of incubation. The final production was 15.6 g/L, with 63.4% of substrate conversion.[23]

Table 1. Chemical composition of the rhamnolipids produced by P. aeruginosa *from different substrates*

RLs	Mw	[M-H]⁻	RGLA Soy[22]*	WFO[37]	Sunflower Soapstock[23]	Soapstock and VINHAÇA**
$R_2C_{10}C_{10}$	650	649	31.9	35.20	28.9	22
$R_1C_{10}C_{10}$	504	503	25.2	23.29	23.4	54,4
$R_1C_{10}C_{10}$	504	503	25.2	23.29	23.4	-
$R_1C_{10}C_{12:1}$	530	529	7.1	10.21	7.9	-
$R_2C_{10}C_{12:1}$	676	675	6.7	6.59	23.0	3,9
$R_2C_{10}C_{10}$	650	649	31.9	35.20	28.9	-
$R_2C_{10}C_{12:1}$	676	675	6.7	6.59	23.0	-
$R_2C_{10}C_{12}$	678	677	12.9	12.05	11.3	-
$R_1C_{10}C_{12}$	532	531	2.8	10.19	5.5	3,9
$R_1C_{10}C_8$	476	475	-	1.26	-	-
$R_2C_{10}C_8$	622	621	-	1.18	-	
$R_2 C_{12}C_{12:1}$	706	705				0,6
$R_1C_{12:2}$	358	357	6.4	-	-	-
$R_1C_{8:2}$	302	301	6.8	-	-	-
$R_2C_8C_{12}$	652	651	-	-	-	9,3

*From references, **unpublished information.

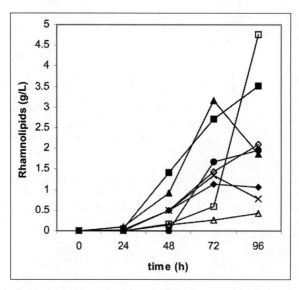

Figure 1. Time course of rhamnolipid homologues accumulation in a submerged culture of P. aeruginosa AT10 incubated in aerated mineral medium with free fatty acids from soybean at 30°C. Rha-C8:2 (●); R1-C10-C12:1(◆);R2-C10-C12:1 (◊); R1-C10-C10 (■); R2-C10-C10 (□); R1-C12:2 (×); R1-C10-C12 (▽); R2-C10-C12 (▲). From reference 25.

Table 2. Surface properties of $R_2C_{10}C_{10}$ and rhamnolipid mixtures (M_6, M_7) in water at 20°C

Compound	CMC ($\times 10^2$ mg/L)	γ_{cmc} (mN/m)	pC_{20}	Γ_m ($\times 10^7$ mg/cm^2)
$R_2C_{10}C_{10}$	1.1	28.8	0.93	1.04
M_6	2.3	27.3	0.09	1.16
M_7	1.5	26.8	0.42	1.23

From reference 22.

Integrated Systems

There are various approaches to reducing the cost of a biotechnological process: one approach is to obtain several products in the same process. However, this often affects the productivity of the accumulated products. Examples of such a process include the simultaneous accumulation of polyhydroxyalkanoates and rhamnolipids[30] or rhamnolipids and lipases.[19,31] Other integrated processes follow different strategies. Early in the 1980s Kosaric planned an integrated process involving a municipal water treatment plant. In this strategy several goals were achieved: the anaerobic process produced methane, which could be used as biogas and CO_2, which was used as a substrate for microbial-lipid accumulation and autotroph microorganisms. The second step was the conversion of this lipid into biosurfactants.[32]

The sunflower-oil refining process gives two main waste products: a greasy alkaline (pH 10-12) substance, called soapstock and acidic water (pH 2.6). Previous studies[23] demonstrated that soapstock was an efficient substrate for rhamnolipid production by *Pseudomonas aeruginosa* LBI. However, besides water for dilution, large quantities of acid had to be added to achieve the physiological pH needed for growth (pH 6.8). Thus, Benincasa and Accorsini[33] proposed the use of soapstock and wastewater from sunflower oil processing as an integrated system for rhamnolipid production. This new culture medium only required the addition of acidic wastewater and varying amounts of $NaNO_3$ as a nitrogen source. When C/N was 8/1, cell growth lasted 48 hours, during which time rhamnolipid accumulated to 7.3 g/L. Although most of the rhamnolipids reported are $R_1C_{10}C_{10}$ and R_2C_{10}, the final rhamnolipid composition depends not only on the production strain, but also on the nature of the carbon substrate.

Another integrated system designed for rhamnolipid production involves soapstock as the main carbon source and vinasse, from sugar-cane ethanol production. The current need for an alternative energy source to reduce the petroleum dependence of transportation systems led to the adaptation of the sugar-cane industry for ethanol production. In the ethanol process, 10 L of vinasse (distillation process wastewater) is produced for every litre of product. This large volume of wastewater represents a significant environmental problem for the ethanol industry. As stated above, soapstock is an important substrate in rhamnolipid production. However, besides the water for dilution, it requires large amounts of acid to achieve the optimum pH for microbial growth. Vinasse has a pH of around 3.5 and it contains nutrients such as phosphorus and potassium. The addition of $NaNO_3$ (4.6 g/L) is essential since both residues are poor in nitrogen. Maximum biosurfactant concentration (6.5 g/L) was achieved after 48 hours of cultivation. The volumetric production (Q_P) was 0.15 g/L.h. However, productivity was lower than that of other refinery wastes, such as carbon sources in a mineral medium used by *Pseudomonas* sp.[20] It is important to highlight that this medium significantly reduced the production costs and helped to minimize the environmental problem associated with wastewater discharge, since the COD (Chemical oxygen demand) of the substrate had been reduced by 94% at the end of the fermentation. In contrast to previous studies[3,25] where rhamnolipid concentration increased significantly during the stationary growth phase, the biosurfactant production in this integrated system was growth associated. This behavior is related to the fact that vinasse is rich in readily metabolisable carbon source, such as sugars (8 g/L), which led to an increase in production during the early stages. Similar behavior was observed by Patel and Desai,[34] when they cultivated *P. aeruginosa* GS3 on sugar-cane molasses. Another factor that may contribute to this production pattern is the high C/N ratio in the culture medium, which was 14.5/1. The integrated process of soapstock and vinasse produced (Table 1) a mixture of six rhamnolipid homologues (RL_{LBIM9}). The major proportion of the mixture corresponded to $R_2C_{10}C_{10}$ (54.4%) and $R_1C_{10}C_{10}$ (22%). These are the typical rhamnolipids usually found in mixtures produced by *Pseudomonas* sp.[12,26] Comparing the homologues obtained in the integrated process using soapstock and oil refinery wastewater, five homologues were identical ($R_2C_{10}C_{10}$, $R_2C_{10}C_{12}$, $R_2C_{10}C_{12}$, $R_1C_{10}C_{10}$, $R_1C_{10}C_{12:1}$, $R_1C_{10}C_{12}$), whereas homologues containing C_8 and $C_{12}C_{12}$ (R_1C_8: 2.6%; $R_2C_{12:1}C_{12}$ and $R_2C_{12}C_{12:1}$: 0.60%) were obtained only when vinasse was used as a substrate. The integrated process development for biosurfactant production might be an interesting strategy, not only economically, but environmentally.

Physicochemical Properties

Rhamnolipid Solutions

Some basic physicochemical properties that characterise rhamnolipid solutions depend on the hydrophile-lipophile balance in the compound molecule. Some of these properties are surface tension, critical micellar concentration (cmc) and interfacial tension. Properties like the formation of emulsions and microemulsions, wetting solid surfaces, the effect of electrolytes on the surface behaviour and rhamnolipid interactions with keratin can be described in terms of the basic properties. Other properties, such as the influence of pH on the aggregation and the formation of thin liquid films, depend on the protonation degree of the carboxyl group in the polar head. In the sections that follow, both categories of properties are reviewed.

Rhamnolipids produced from oily waste substrate by *P. aeruginosa* result in a mixture of rhamnolipid homologues. The properties of this mixture depend upon the amount of each homologue present, which is determined by the specific bacterial strain applied, culture conditions and medium composition. In general, rhamnolipids reduce the surface tension of water from 72.3 mN/m to approximately 30 mN/m. The interfacial tension of water/oil systems is reduced from 43 mN/m to less than 1 mN/m.[35]

Several authors have studied the physicochemical properties of rhamnolipid mixtures obtained from different waste sources and bacterial strains. Abalos et al[22] used soybean waste as a carbon source; one pure homologue ($R_2C_{10}C_{10}$) and two different mixtures (M_6, M_7) were obtained after purification. Surface tension as a function of increasing concentrations of $R_2C_{10}C_{10}$, M_6 and M_7 was measured. For all the concentrations tested the surface tension decreased gradually with increasing concentration of surfactant before reaching a constant value. The break point in the surface tension was taken as the cmc. The maximum adsorption Γ_{max} at the interface was calculated using the Gibbs adsorption isotherm. Values of cmc, γ_{cmc} and Γ_m are given in Table 2.

The cmc of pure surfactant $R_2C_{10}C_{10}$ was 1.1×10^2 mg/L, which is consistent with other values reported for pure rhamnolipids.[35] The cmc for the M_6 mixture was 2.3×10^2 mg/L, which is clearly different from that of the pure compound. The rational for this value is as follows: firstly, the high hydrophilic character of the molecules in the mixture directly affects micellisation, resulting in higher cmc values. Secondly, assuming that the unsaturated rhamnolipid molecules in M_6 are involved in micellisation, the presence of insaturations affects the conformation of the molecules in the micelles. This therefore alters both the aggregation number and the cmc values. To measure the rhamnolipids efficiently, Abalos et al[22] calculated the pC_{20}, as defined by Rosen.[36] The resulting values are given in Table 2 and indicate that the most efficient compound was $R_2C_{10}C_{10}$.

When waste frying oils were used as a carbon source, a mixture of eleven rhamnolipid homologues with some unsaturated fatty acid were obtained.[37] Unsaturated $C_{12:1}$ and $C_{14:1}$ hydrophobic chains were present in the mixture at up to 18.95%. Surface tension measurements yielded a cmc value of 108 mg/L and a γ_{min} of 32.8 mN/m. The cmc was larger than that of the mixture in which all the hydrophobic chains were saturated.[38,39] This indicates a possible correlation between the degree of unsaturation and the cmc. The carbon source used by Benicasa et al[23] was a soapstock.

The resulting rhamnolipid mixture contained 31% of unsaturated fatty acids; it had a cmc of 120 mg/L, a surface tension of 24 mN/m and an interfacial tension of 1.31 mN/m. Various waste frying oils were recently evaluated as possible substrates for rhamnolipid production in the presence or absence of a rhamnolipid precursor.[21] The surface tension of the cell-free culture broth (CFCB) was 29.1 mN/m and the interfacial tension against n-hexadecane was lower than 1 mN/m.

A mixture of rhamnolipid surfactants, obtained from corn oil rich in $R_2C_{10}C_{12}$ and $R_2C_{10}C_{12:1}$ species,[38] had a cmc of 37 mg/L and a surface tension of 36 mN/m, compared to the species with a high content of $R_2C_{10}C_{10}$, which had a cmc of 53 mg/L and a surface tension of 31 mN/m. The authors suggested that the presence of longer fatty acid chains increased the hydrophobicity of the molecules and so there was a tendency to aggregate as micelles at concentrations lower than those at which species rich in C_{10} chains aggregate.

Emulsions and Microemulsions

Rhamnolipid surfactants emulsify hydrocarbons and, in general, stabilise emulsions. Haba et al[37] tested the ability of rhamnolipids to emulsify oils used in a number of industries such as the cosmetic, agrochemical, or bioremediation industries. Table 3 illustrates the stability of some oil-in water emulsions where pure rhamnolipid compounds were added.

Linseed oil formed a strong, stable emulsion, whereas isopropyl palmitate formed a weak emulsion, which collapsed within a week. Unstable emulsions were formed with C_{12}-C_{14} n-alkanes and mineral oil, whereas stable emulsions were obtained with crude oil. No emulsion was formed when either almond oil or toluene was added.

Similar emulsion tests were carried out with a mixture of rhamnolipids produced from soap-stock and vinasse (Table 4): all the oils tested formed emulsions. The most stable emulsions were obtained using petroleum oil, isopropyl palmitate and almond oil. Emulsions formed with mineral oil, toluene and linseed oil were moderately stable. In general, emulsions formed with rhamnolipid mixtures formed easily and their stability was higher than those formed with pure rhamnolipids. Xie et al[40] studied the influence of alcohols on the phase behaviour of microemulsions formed by R_1 and R_2 rhamnolipid biosurfactants. Xie et al[40] concluded that increasing the chain length of the linear alcohol reduced the range within which the two-phase microemulsions were formed.

Table 3. Stability of the o/w emulsions for rhamnolipids with some organic compounds

Substrat	RL:Substratet:H$_2$O	%E$_{24}$	%E$_{168}$
Linseed oil	0.10:0.56:0.34	90	90
Almond oil	0.10:0.56:0.34	-	-
i-Propilpalmitate	0.10:0.56:0.34	30	-
	0.05:0.75:0.20	30	-
Crude oil	0.10:0.50:0.40	66.6	40
	0.10:0.15:0.75	77.7	70
	0.15:0.31:0.54	62.5	40
Kerosene	0.15:0.31:0.54	80	-
	0.05:0.45:0.50	50	-
Toluene	0.15:0.31:0.54	-	-
n-Alkanes (C$_{12-14}$)	0.15:0.31:0.54	60	-
Mineral oil	0.15:0.31:0.54	50	-

From reference 37.

Table 4. Emulsification index (E24) shown by the rhamnolipid mixture against hydrocarbon sources of rhamnolipids produced in the integrated system sunflower soapstock-vinasse

Hydrocarbon Source	E24 (%)
Petroleum crude oil	75 ± 0.3
Benzene	60 ± 1.5
Kerosene	50 ± 0.2
Mineral oil	42 ± 0.7
Toluene	33 ± 0.6
Isopropyl plamitate	73 ± 0.3
Castor oil	67 ± 0.2
Linseed oil	28 ± 0.4
Almond oil	83 ± 0.4
Unpublished information	

Moreover, when n-butanol was used, the phase existence range of single-phase microemulsion was wider than the others. Thus, when rhamnolipids are used to form microemulsions, the results are similar to, or even better than, those yielded by other surfactants.[41-43]

Wetting Properties

Surfactants in aqueous solutions tend to be adsorbed by solid surfaces, which alter the adhesion tension of the surface. This behaviour may cause partial or complete wetting of the surface by the aqueous surfactant solution. This is the basis of many industrial and biological processes. Rhamnolipid surfactants have been used for this purpose. Ishigami et al[44] carried out one of the earliest studies in this area. They modified polymer surfaces with sodium salt and methyl ester of rhamnolipid B. Surfaces treated with methyl ester showed a larger wetting action than the surfaces treated with sodium salt. More recently, the wetting properties of rhamnolipids R_1 and R_2 and their mixtures were studied by advancing the contact angles of sessile drops. For a comparison of wetting performance, sodium dodecyl sulphate (SDS) was chosen as the commercial reference.[45] A hydrophilic glass surface, a hydrophobic polymer, polyethylene terephthalate (PET) and a gold surface were used as solid surfaces. At low surfactant concentration similar contact angles were obtained with rhamnolipids and SDS for the three surfaces tested, but the wetting ability of rhamnolipids increased with concentration. SDS and rhamnolipids gave similar rhamnolipid concentrations, which were one order of magnitude lower than those of SDS. Surface tension data were also included in the studies and were related to the contact angles by adhesion tension calculations. Compared to SDS, the rhamnolipid solutions rendered lower adhesion tension profiles for all surfaces.

Effect of Electrolytes

The addition of an electrolyte to a surfactant solution causes a decrease in the repulsive forces between similar charges.[36] Thus, for ionic surfactants in general, the surface activity increases with added electrolyte and both micelle formation and micellar growth are enhanced.

The effect of NaCl on the surface and bulk properties of rhamnolipid structures was investigated by Helvaci and Özdemir.[46] The presence of NaCl in the bulk phase was reported to shield the carboxylate groups of the rhamnolipid molecules, causing them to behave like non-ionic surface active agents. For the more hydrophobic R_1 molecules the effect of reduced repulsive interactions in terms of the compaction of the monolayer was strong: the surface tension and the cmc values were reduced and the surface concentration and coefficient elasticity were increased.

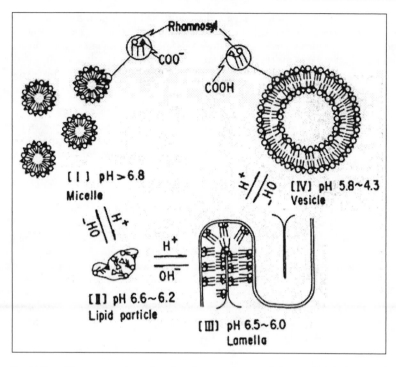

Figure 2. pH-Sensitive conversion of molecular aggregates of rhamnolipids. From reference 48, with permission.

Effect of pH on Aggregation Morphology

Rhamnolipid B andits precursor rhamnolipd A, under weakly acidic conditions within a narrow pH range of about 5-7, reversibly altered the morphologies of their molecular aggregates from vesicles to lamella, then to lipid particles and finally to micelles[47] (Fig. 2). Moreover, the pH dependent conversion of molecular aggregates of rhamnolipids may be associated with the biological functions inside and outside the bacterial membrane under weakly alkaline or neutral conditions in the hydrocarbon-assimilating bacterium. When growing in acidic conditions, the bacterial cell membrane seems to be protected by rhamnolipids.[44]

To further study how pH affects the morphology of rhamnolipids, Champion et al[48] used cryo-transmission electron microscopy to examine the morphology of vitrified, frozen hydrated suspensions of rhamnolipid over a pH range between 5.5 and 8. They determined the effect of 0.8 mM octane, which is a model alkane and 0.5 mM cadmium, which is a model of heavy metal; as pH increased, the morphology changed from lamellar to vesicular and then to micellar.[48] According to Israelachvili,[49] these changes may be attributed to the molecular structure and charge of the rhamnolipid. Considering that the pKa reported[47] for rhamnolipid was 5.6, the negative charge of the polar head of the rhamnolipid would increase when the pH increases from 5.5 to 8 and thus the repulsion between the adjacent polar heads would also increase and increase the head diameter. This would explain the observed progression in morphology from bilayer sheets to vesicles to micelles.

The behaviour of rhamnolipids as emulsifiers is determined by the way molecules pack at the interface. Packing, in turn, depends on the polar head charge, which is determined by the pH of the medium. To determine how R_1 and R_2 behave as emulsifiers, Özdemir et al[45] measured the surface and interfacial tensions of pure R_1 and R_2 solutions at two pH values. The pH values were chosen based on their potential applications, using decane and hexadecane as oil phases. Results revealed that both R_1 and R_2 form compact phases at the surface beginning from very low concentrations. R_1 is more surface active at concentrations below the cmc and is independent of the bulk phase pH. Nevertheless, neither the value of cmc nor the minimum surface tension at cmc was significantly affected by the type of rhamnolipid. They depended only upon the solution pH; there are significant interactive forces between the undissociated rhamnolipid molecules at pH 5, which increase the compaction at the surface monolayer.

Foam Film

Foam consists of a high-volume fraction of gas dispersed in a liquid. The macroscopic properties of foam depend on the properties of the individual particles and on the interaction between them. In general, a fluid dispersion can have different particle size, composition and thus different surface tension.

Cohen et al[50] applied the free thin liquid foam (foam film) method to study the interaction of rhamnolipid thin liquid foams by measuring the surface forces in each of the two interfaces present in the foam. The equilibrium film thickness was measured as a function of the electrolyte concentration. Film thickness gradually decreased from approximately 100 to 5 nm and three different types of film were found: common films thicker than 30 nm, common black films ranging from 6 to 20 nm in thickness and 5 nm thick Newton black foam films. At a later stage, disjoint pressure isotherms were measured. Measurements corroborated the common film type and demonstrated the presence of an aqueous core in the common films and common black films. Measurements also confirmed the bilayer structure of the Newton black films. The experimental studies revealed that surface forces play an important role in the stability of the common films. Nonsurface forces led to an additional positive component of the disjoining pressure and became operative in the region of the thinner common black films and Newton black films.

Applications

Biosurfactants and Petroleum

The pollution of water and soil with oil products is a frequent occurrence that has increased with the rise of industrial activity: more than 5.6 million of tons of oil has been released into the environment by oil spills since 1970.[51] Diesel oil spills from pipeline ruptures, tank failures, storage problems and transportation accidents are the most frequent causes of soil and water oil pollution (Lee et al, 2006). For example, the Prestige oil spill of 660,000 tons of a Russian heavy fuel (type M-100) in November 2002 affected more than 800 km of the north-western Spanish coast.[52]

Many microorganisms have been reported to degrade fuel and diesel oil in different habitats or conditions. Surfactant activity and hydrophobicity favour the interaction between the microorganism and the insoluble substrate, overcoming the diffusion limitation during the substrate transport to the cell. In recent years, many studies have examined the ability of new surfactants to accelerate oil-product degradation in both laboratory and field conditions.[53] Biosurfactants have recently received much more attention as an environmentally friendly alternative to conventional chemically synthetic surfactants.[28]

Rhamnolipids produced by *Pseudomonas aeruginosa* AT10 were investigated for their potential to enhance bioavailability and thus the biodegradation of crude oil by a microbial consortium in a liquid medium. The addition of rhamnolipids accelerated the biodegradation of total petroleum hydrocarbons from 32% to 61% after 10 days of incubation. When the addition of the biosurfactant increased, the result was more apparent in the group of targeted isoprenoids; biodegradation increased from 16% to 70%. Furthermore, the biodegradation of some alkylated PAHs increased from 9% to 44%.[54] There are two possible mechanisms for enhancing biodegradation: to increase the solubility of the substrate, which facilitates its uptake by microbial cells, or the interaction with the cell surface, which increases the hydrophobicity of the surface and allows hydrophobic substrates to associate more easily. Results indicate that in situ biosurfactant production not only increased emulsification of the oil but also promoted the adhesion of the hydrocarbon to the cell surfaces of other bacteria. The emulsification (solubilisation) of hydrocarbons with surfactants favours the influx of hydrophobic organic pollutants from soil and water to microbial cells and thereby also favours their degradation. This is crucial for rapid biotechnological environmental purification.[53]

Biosurfactants have also been tested in enhanced oil recovery and in the transportation of crude oils. They were shown to be effective in the reduction of several factors; they reduced the interfacial tension of oil and water in situ, the viscosity of the oil, the removal of water from emulsions prior to processing and the release of bitumen from tar sands.[55] Low concentration of rhamnolipids produced by *P. aeruginosa* PA1 can also be effectively used for paraffinic or aromatic oil removal in contaminated sandy soils.[56]

BioSurfactants and Heavy Metals

The rapid increase in industrial activity has gradually redistributed many toxic metals from the Earth's crust to the environment increasing the chances of human exposure.[57] The movement of metals in soils is limited by soil texture, structure and organic matter content. Additionally, metal toxicity hinders microbial degradation and only some redox transformations or methylations can lead to solubilisation or increase the solubility or volatility.

The traditional treatment of contaminated soils has disadvantages in that it cannot completely remove hazardous contaminants. Other methods such as soil washing are slow, although, the kinetics can be enhanced by using an agent that promotes desorption of the soil bound metals and facilitates their transport through the soil matrix. Thus, a surfactant that would be an ideal complexing agent in mobilising metals must be soluble in water, chemically stable under environmental conditions, not strongly bound to soil particles and have a high affinity for complexing metals.[57] Surfactants can be added to washing water to assist in the solubilisation, dispersal and desorption of contaminants from excavated soils or sediments in a washing unit. The cleaned soil would then be returned to the original site.[58,59]

The anionic rhamnolipids carry a negative charge. Thus, when the molecule encounters a cationic metal that carries a positive charge, an ionic bond is formed. This bond is stronger than the bond between the metal and the soil. The polar head groups of micelles can bind metals, making them more soluble in water. Micelles help recover the metals from the soil surfaces and move them into solution, making them easier to recover by flushing.[60] Rhamnolipids have been used to extract copper from mine ores; with 2% rhamnolipid, 28% of copper was extracted from a mining residue.[61] Rhamnolipids were also investigated[62] for their potential to recover Cd (II) from kaolin, a representative soil component. Results obtained by Asei et al[60] indicated that the soil-washing process with added rhamnolipids was successful in remediating low permeable clayey soil. Rhamnolipids have also been used to extract heavy metals (copper, zinc and nickel) from sediments by a continuous flow configuration. The removal was up to 37% of Cu, 13% of Zn and 27% of Ni when rhamnolipids without additives were applied. Adding 1% NaOH to 0.5% rhamnolipid enhanced the removal of copper fourfold compared with the use of 0.5% rhamnolipid alone.[57,65] Juwarkar et al[57] used rhamnolipid biosurfactant on column experiments to remove Cd and Pb; di-rhamnolipid removed not only the leachable or available fraction of Cd and Pb, but also the bound metals. In comparison, tap water only removed the mobile fraction. Additionally, the microbial population of the contaminated soil was increased after using the biosurfactant technology and revealed no toxic effect.

Rhamnolipids and Antimicrobial Activity

Although most biosurfactants are considered to be secondary metabolites, some may play essential roles in the survival of biosurfactant-producing microorganisms acting as biocide agents.[66]

The antibacterial effects of various rhamnolipids are described in the literature; Abalos et al[22] identified seven rhamnolipids in cultures of *P. aeruginosa* AT10 from soybean oil refinery wastes and showed inhibitory activity against the bacteria *Escherichia coli, Micrococcus luteus, Alcaligenes faecalis* (32 µg/ml), *Serratia marcescens, Mycobacterium phlei* (16 µg/ml) and *Staphylococcus epidermidis* (8 µg/ml). Furthermore, they exhibited excellent antifungal properties against *Aspergillus niger* (16 µl/ml) *Chaetonium globosum, Penicillium crysogenum, Aerobacidium pullulans* (32 µg/ml) and phytopathogenic *Botrytis cinerea* and *Rhizoctonia solani* (18 µg/ml). Benincasa et al[23] also reported rhamnolipid from *P. aeruginosa* LBI as having good antimicrobial behaviour against bacteria (*S. aureus, S. faecalis* and *P. aeruginosa*) and as being active against phytopathogenic fungal species. In 2005 Yilmaz and Sidal[67] reported antimicrobial activity of rhamnolipds for beta-hemolytic *Streptococcus* sp. They reported the lowest activity of rhamnolipds in *P. aeruginosa*. The addition of rhamnolipids to irrigation lines resulted in a 100% control of zoosporic plant pathogens in recirculating systems where pants were hydroponically cultivated.[68]

Biosurfactants in Food, Cosmetics and Pharmaceuticals

In the past five decades, biosurfactants have attracted a great deal of attention as potential alternatives to chemical surfactants, especially in food, cosmetics and pharmaceuticals. Industrial processes frequently involve extreme conditions including high pressures or temperatures, alkaline and acidic conditions and ionic concentrations, but much biosurfactant activity is not affected. In particular, biosurfactants from extremophile microorganisms could be of commercial interest due to their unique properties.[66]

Owing to their association with emulsion formation and stabilisation, foaming, wetting, solubilising activities,[70] biosurfactants could be exploited in food processing and formulation. Such complex systems have minimal stability, which may be improved by additives such as surfactants.[69] High-molecular-mass biosurfactants are good emulsifiers and are useful for making oil/water emulsions for pharmaceutical, cosmetics and food products. In dairy products the addition of emulsifiers improves texture and consistency. This quality is of special interest for low-fat products.[6] Despite the advantages of biosurfactants, few reports are available regarding their use in food products and food processing.[66] Biosurfactants are not yet used in food processing on a large scale due to the numerous regulations set by governmental agencies for new food ingredients and the lengthy approval process. Nevertheless, an increasing number of patents are being issued on biosurfactants[68-70] demonstrating the current interest in using these microbial-derived products in cosmetics, pharmaceuticals and foodstuffs.

Although few data are available in the literature regarding the toxicity of microbial surfactants,[13] they are generally considered low or nontoxic products and are therefore appropriate for use in products for human consumption. The increase in consumer awareness of adverse allergic effects caused by artificial products has stimulated the development of alternative ingredients such as biosurfactants. For this reason, was studied the cellular toxicity of *P. aeruginosa* 47T2 rhamnolipid with keratinocyte and fibroblast cultures and compared to SDS.[71] The result (Fig. 3) showed that 47T2 rhamnolipid was less toxic to keratinocites than SDS, whereas on

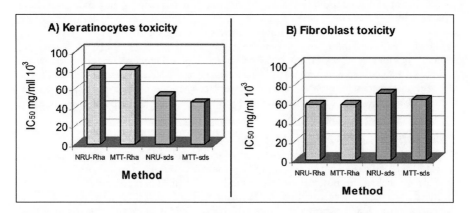

Figure 3. Comparative cytotoxicity of rhamnolipids from P. aeruginosa 47T2 vs SDS in keratinocytes (A) and fibroblasts (B) as detected with neutral red uptake NRU and MTT assays. Results are expressed as IC50 (the dose inhibiting viability to 50%). Unpublished information.

fibroblast, toxicity was higher with biosurfactant than with SDS. Stipcevic et al[72] demonstrated that di-rhamnolipid BAC-3 (50 µl/ml) in the presence of serum and under certain conditions that favour keratinocyte differentiation, the proliferation of fibroblasts was inhibited and the proliferation of keratinocytes stimulated. These results support the efficacy of BAC-3 shown in skin treatment and wound healing. Furthermore, Thanomsub et al[73] reported that di-rhamnolipid a from *P. aeruginosa* B189 showed strong antiproliferative activity in a human breast cancer cell line (MCF-7) at minimum inhibitory concentration (MIC) at 6.25 µg/ml. In contrast, rhamnolipid b showed MIC against insect cell line C6/36 at 50 µg/ml. Despite the advantages of biosurfactants, few reports are available regarding their use in food products and food processing.[69]

To avoid adverse reactions like skin or eye irritation, the concentrations of ingredients used in commercial formulations must be carefully controlled. To predict the effect of rhamnolipids on skin and hair, experiments were conducted to asses the interactions of these surfactants with keratin and *stratum corneum*. Özdemir[45] investigated the adsorption characteristics of keratin-rhamnolipid (RL-Keratin) and keratin-SDS (SDS-Keratin) at the air/liquid interface. Tests were conducted at pH 6.2 and 5.0 and revealed weaker interactions for RL-Keratin than for SDS-Keratin.

Food processors do not yet use biosurfactants on a large scale due to the many regulations regarding the approval of new food ingredients required by governmental agencies, which is a particularly long process. Nevertheless, an increasing number of patents have been issued on biosurfactants[74-76] demonstrating the current interest in using these microbial-derived products in cosmetics, pharmaceuticals and foodstuffs.

Despite their potential, only a few studies examine applications in the biomedical field such as the compilation by Rodrigues et al.[63] Among the main activities described are antimicrobial, antiviral, antitumor, anti-adhesive and cell differentiation induction. Some are suitable alternatives to synthetic medicines and antimicrobial agents and may be used as safe and effective therapeutic agents in the future. Possible applications as emulsifiers for drug transport to the infection site, such as agents supplementing the pulmonary surfactant or adjuvants for vaccines have also been suggested.

The high production costs could be compensated by the requirement of a small amount of biosurfactant with higher efficacy.[77] Moreover, these molecules can be tailor-made to suit different applications by changing the growth substrate or growth conditions. Additionally, the toxicological aspects of a new biosurfactant should be emphasized in order to certify the safety of these compounds for use in the cosmetic and especially pharmaceutical and food industries.[66,69]

Various programs are now underway all over the world aimed at constructing a sustainable society. Among such programs is the introduction of green technology, which is one of the most important challenges. Considering the current social and technological circumstances, the use of biosurfactants, which are environmentally friendly and highly functional materials, is an attractive option.

Conclusion

This chapter primarily deals with the possibilities and prospects of using various cheaper alternative substrates and new strategies for the production of rhamnolipid biosurfactants. The nature and structure of a biosurfactant molecule can be tailored for a particular application by changing the carbon substrate. An integrated production system towards enhancing product yield, reducing adverse environmental impact and effectively utilizing agro-industrial residues that adequately addresses socio-economic development issues. The chapter also attempts to offer an overview of the physicochemical and biological properties of rhamnolipidic biosurfactants for their potential commercial, environmental and biomedical applications.

Acknowledgements
The financial support of the Comissió Interdepartamental de Recerca i Tecnologia CIRIT project (2005GR00143) and the Comisión Interministerial de Ciencia y Tecnologia (CICYT), project (CTQ2007-60749/PPQ) and (CTQ2004-07771-C02-01/PPQ) is gratefully acknowledged.

References

1. Makkar RS, Cameotra SS. An update on the use of unconventional substrates for biosurfactant production and their new applications. Biotechnology 2002; 58:428-434.
2. Mukherjee SDP, Sen R. Towards commercial production of microbial surfactants. Trends Biotechnol 2006; 24:509-515.
3. Nitsche M, Siddhartha GAO, Contiero J. Ramnolipid surfactants: an update on the general aspects of these remarcable biomolecules. Biotechnol Progress 2005; 21:1593-1600.
4. Van Hamme JD, Singh A, Ward OP. Physiological aspects. Part 1 in a series of papers devoted to surfactants in microbiology and biotechnology. Biotechnol Adv 2006; 24:604-620.
5. Lang S. Biological amphiphiles (microbial surfactants). Curr Opinion Colloid Surf Sci 2002; 7:12-20.
6. Rosenberg E, Ron E. High- and low- molecular- mass microbial surfactants. Applied Microbiol and Biotechnol 1999; 52:154-162.
7. Hommel K, Ratkedge C. Biosynthetic mechanisms of low molecular weight surfactant s and their precursor molecules. In: Kosaric N ed. Biosurfactants Production and Applications. New York: Marcel Dekker, 1993:3-65.
8. Fiechter A. Biosurfactants: moving towards industrial application. Trends Biotechnol 1992; 10:208-217.
9. Kitamoto D, Yanagishita H, Shinbo T et al. Surface active properties antimicrobial activities of mannosylerythritol lipids as biosurfactants produced by Candida antarctica. J Biotechnol 1993; 29:91-96.
10. Espuny MJ, Egido S, Mercadé ME et al. Characterization of trehalose tetraester produced by a waste lube oil degrder Rhodococcus sp. 51T7. Toxicol Environm Chem 1995; 48:83-88.
11. Ristau E, Wagner F. Formation of novel trehalose lipids from Rhodococcus erythropolis under growth limiting conditions. Biotechnol Lett 1983; 5:95-100.
12. Lang S, Wullbrandt D. Rhamnose lipids- biosynthesis, microbial production and application potential. Appl Microbiol Biotechnol 1999; 51:22-32.
13. Rodrigues L, Teixeira J, Oliveira R et al. Response surface optimization of the medium components for the production of biosurfactants by probiotic bacteria. Process Biochemistry 2006; 41:1-10.
14. Koch AK, Reiser J, Käppeli O et al. Genetic construction of lactose-utilizing stains of Pseudomonas aeruginosa and their application in biosurfactant production. Bio/Technology 1988; 1335-1339.
15. Dubey K, Juwarkar A. Distellery and curd whey wastes as viable alternative sources for biosurfactant production. Wold J Microbiol Biotechnol 2001; 17:61-69.
16. Santa Anna LM, Sebastian GV, Menezas EP et al. Production of biosurfactants from Pseudomonas aeruginosa PA1 isolated in oil environments. Brazilian J Chem Eng 2002; 159-166.
17. Solaiman D, Ashby RD, Zerkowski JA et al. Simplified soy molasses-based medium for reduced-cost production of sophorolipids by Candida bombicola. Biotechnology Lett 2007; 29:1341-1347.
18. Mercadé ME, Manresa A, Robert M et al. Olive oil mill effluent (OOME). New substrate for biosurfactant production. Bioresource Technol 1993; 43:1-6.
19. Haba E, Espuny MJ, Busquets M et al. Screening and production of rhamnolipids by Pseudomonas aeruginosa 47T2 NCIB 40044 from waste frying oils. J Appl Microbiol 2000; 88:379-387.
20. Ali Raza Z, Rehman A, Saleem Khan M et al. Improved production of biosurfactant by a Pseudomonas aeruginosa mutant using vegetable oil refinery wastes. Biodegradation 2006; 18:115-121.
21. Ali Raza Z, Saleem Khan M, Khalid ZM et al. Production kinetics and tensioactive characteristics of biosurfactant from Pseudomonas aeruginosa mutant grown on waste frying oils. Biotechnol Lett 2006; 28:1623-1631.
22. Abalos A, Pinazo A, Infante R et al. Physico chemical and antimicrobial properties of new rhamnolipids produced by Pseudomonas aeruginosa AT10 from soybean oil refinery wastes. Langmuir 2001; 17:1367-1371.
23. Benincasa M, Abalos A, Oliveira I et al. Chemical structure, surface properties and biological activitires of the biosurfactatn produced by Pseudomonas aeruginosa LBI. Antonie van Leeuwenhoek 2004; 85:1-8.
24. Déziel E, Lépine F, Dennie D et al. Liquid chromatography/mass spectrometry analysis of mixture of rhamnolipids produced by Pseudomonas aeruginosa strain 57RP grown on mannitol or napthalene. Biochim et Biophys Acta 1999; 1440:244-252.
25. Haba E, Abalos A, Jáuregui O et al. Use of liquid chromatography-mass spectroscopy for studuing the compositin and properties of rhamnolipids produced by different strains of Pseudomonas aeruginosa. J Surf Det 2003; 6:155-161.
26. Monteiro SA, Sassaki GL, LM dS et al. Molecular and structural characterization of the biosurfactatn produced by Pseudomonas aeruginosa DAUPE 614. Chem Phys Lipids 2007; 147:1-13.
27. Perfumo A BIM, Canganella F, Marchant R. Rhamnolipid production by a novel thermophilic hydrocarbon-degrading Pseudomonas aeruginosa AP02-1. Appl Microbiol Biotechnol 2006; 72:132-138.

28. Wei YH, Chou CL, Chang JS. Rhamnolipid production by indigenous Pseudomonas aeruginosa J4 originating from petrochemical wastewater. Biochem Eng J 2005; 27:146-154.
29. Abalos A, Maximo F, Manresa A et al. Utilization of response surface methodology to optimize the culture media for the production of rhamnolipids by Pseudomonas aeruginosa AT10. J Chem Technol Biotechnol 2001; 77:777-784.
30. Rehm B, Mitsky T, Steinbüchel A. Role of fatty acid de novo synthesis in polyhydroxyakanoic acid (PHA) and rhamnolipid synthesis in Pseudomonads: Establishment of the transacylase (PhaG)-mediated pathway for PHA biosynthesis in E. coli. Appl Environ Microbiol 2001; 67:3102-3109.
31. Haba E, Bresco O, Ferrer C et al. Isolation of lipase-secreting bacteria by deplying used frying oil as selective substrate. Enz Microbial Technol 2000; 26:40-44.
32. Kosaric N, Cairns WL, Gray NCC et al. The role of nitrogen in multiorganism strategies for biosurfactant production. JAOCS 1984; 61:1735-1743.
33. Benincasa M, Accorsini FB. Pseudomonas aeruginosa LBI production as an integrated process using the wastes from sunflower-oil refining as a substrate. Bioresource Technol 2008; 99:3843-3849.
34. Patel RM, Desai AJ. Biosurfactant production by Pseudomonas aeruginosa GS3 from molasses. Lett Appl Microbiol 1997; 25:91-94.
35. Parra JL, Guinea J, Manresa A et al. Chemical characterization and physicochemical behavior of bio-surfactants. JAOCS 1989; 66:141-145.
36. Rosen MJ. Surfactants and Interfacial Phenomena. New Jersey: Jonh Wiley, 2004.
37. Haba E, Pinazo A, Jauregui O et al. Physicochemical characterization and antimicrobial properties of rhamnolipids produced by Pseudomonas aeruginosa 47T2 NCBIM 40044. Biotechnology Bioeng 2003; 81:316-322.
38. Mata-Sandoval J, Karns J, Torrents A. High-performance liquid chromatography method for the characterization of rhamnolipids mixture produce by Pseudomonas aeruginosa UG2 on corn oil. J of Chromatography 1999; 864:211-220.
39. Syldatk C, Lang S, Wagner F. Chemical and physical characterization of four interfacial-active rhamno-lipids from Pseudomonas sp. DSM 2874 Grown on n- Alkanes. Z Naturforsch 1985; 40c:51-60.
40. Xie Y, Li Y, Ye R. Effect of alchols on the phase behavior of microemulsions formed by a biosurfac-tant-rhamnolipid. J Dispersion Science and Technology 2005; 26:455.
41. Garti N, Binyamin H, Aserin A. Stabilization of water-in-oil emulsions by submicrocristalin alpha- form fat particles. JAOCS 1998; 75:1825-1831.
42. Richard C. The salinity-requeriment diagram-A useful tool in chemical floding research and develop-ment. Soc Pet Eng J 1982; 22:259-270.
43. Rodríguez C, ADP. Effect of ionic surfactants on the phase behavior and structure of sucrose ester/water/oil systems. J Colloid Interface Sci 2003; 262:500.
44. Ishigami Y, Gama Y, Ishii F et al. Colloid chemical effect of polar head moieties of a rhamnolipid-type biosurfctant. Langmuir 1993; 9:1634-1636.
45. Özdemir G, Malayglu U. Wetting characteristics of aqueous rhamnolipids solutions. Colloids Surf 2004; 39:1-7.
46. Helvaci SS, P S, Özdemir G. Effect of electrolytes on the surface behavior of rhamnolipids R1 an R2. Colloids Surf B 2004; 35:225-233.
47. Champion JT, GJC HL, Retterer J et al. Electrón microscopy of rhamnolipid (biosurfactant) morphol-ogy: Effects of pH, cadmium and octane. J Colloid and Interface Science 1995; 170:569-574.
48. Ishigami Y, Gama Y, Nagahora H et al. The pH sensitive conversion of molecular aggregates of rham-nolipid biosurfactant. Chem Lett 1987; 275:763-766.
49. Israelachvili JN, MDJ, Ninham BW. Theory of self-assembly of hydrocarbon amphiphiles into micelles and bilayers. J Chem Soc Faraday Trans II 1976; 72:1525-1568.
50. Cohen R, Ozdemir G, Exerowa D. Free thin liquid films (foam films) from rhamnolipids: type of the film and stability. Colloids and Surfaces 2003; 29:197-204.
51. Batista SB, Mounteer AH, Amourin FR et al. Isolation and characterization of biosurfactant/bioemulsifi-er-producing bacteria from petroleum contaminated sites. Bioresource Technology 2006; 97:868-875.
52. Diez S, Sabaté J, Viñas M et al. The prestige oil spill. I. Biodegradation of a heavy fuel oil under simu-lated conditions. Environmental Toxicology and Chemistry 2005; 24:2203-2217.
53. Karpenko EV, Vil'danova-Martsishin RI, Shchegelova NS et al. The prospects of using bacteria of the genus Rhodococcus and microbial surfactants for the degradation of oil pollutants. Applied Biochemistry and Microbiology 2006; 42:175-179.
54. Abalos A, Viñas M, Sabaté M et al. Enhance biodegradtion of Casablanca crude oil by a microbial consortium in presence of a rhamnolipid produced by Pseudomonas aeruginosa AT10. Biodegradation 2004; 15:249-260.
55. CN M, Young RN, Gibbs BF. Environmental applications for biosurfactants. Environmental pollution 2005; 133:183-198.

56. Santa Anna LM, Soriano AU, Gomes AC et al. Use of biosurfactant in the removal of oil from contaminated sandy soil. J Chem Technol Biotechnol 2007; 82:687-691.
57. Juwarkar AA, Nair A, Dubey KV et al. Biosurfactant technology for remediation of cadmium and lead contamination soils. Chemosphere 2007; 68:1996-2002.
58. Christofi N, Ivshina IB. Microbial surfactants and their use in field syudies of soil remediation. J Appl Microbiol 2002; 93:915-929.
59. Mulligan CN, Young RN, Gibbs BF. Heavy metal removal from sediments by biosurfactants. J Hazardous Materials 2001; 85:111-125.
60. Asçi Y, Nurbas M, Sag Açikel Y. Sorption of Cd (II) onto kaolin as soil component and desorption of Cd (II) from kaolin using rhamnolipid biosurfactant. J Hazardous Materials 2007; B139:50-56.
61. Dahrazma B, Mulligan CN. Investigation of the removal of heavy metals from sediments using rhamnolipid in a continous flow configutation. Chemosphere 2007; 69:705-711.
62. Dahrozma B, Mulligan CN. Extraction of cooper from a low grade ore by rhamnolipids. Prac. Period Hazard. Toxic Rad. Waste Manag. ASCE 2004; 8:166-172.
63. Rodrigues L, Banat IM, Teixeira J et al. Biosurfactants: potential applications in medicine. J Antimicrob Chemother 2006; 57:609-618..
64. Yilmaz ES, Sidal U. Investigation of antimicrobial effect of a Pseudomonas originting surfactant. Biology 2005; 60:723-725.
65. Nielsen CJ, Ferrin DM, Stanghellini ME. Efficacy of biosurfactants in the management of Phytophthora capsicion pepper in recirculating hydroponic systems. Can J Plant Pathol. 2006; 28:450-460.
66. Nitschke M, Costa SGVAO. Biosurfactants in food industry. Food Sci Technol 2007; 18:252-259.
67. Banat I, Makkar R, Cameotra S. Potential commercial applications of microbial surfactants. Appl Microbiol Biotechnol 2000; 53:495-508.
68. Han SG, Kim JC, Kim YS. Cosmetics composition comprising sophorolipids. KR20044033376-A.
69. Imura T, Kitamoto D, Fukuoka T et al. Emulsifier or solubilizer for cosmetics, pharmaceuticals, foodstuffs and fuels, contains self-assembly of biosurfactant. JP2007181789-A.
70. Kitagawa M, M S, Yamamoto S et al. Skin care cosmetic for treating dermatological disorders such as rough skin, acne, eczema, asteatosis and senile xerosis, contains biosurfactants as main ingredients. WO20077060956-A1.
71. Sanchez L, Mitjans M, Infante MR et al. Assesment of the potential skin irritation of lysine-derivative anionic surfactatns using mouse fibroblast and human keratinocytes as an alternative to animal water testing. Pharmaceutical Research 2004; 21:1637-1641.
72. Stipcevic T, Piljac T. Di-rhamnolipid from Pseudomonas aeruginosa displais different effects on human keratinocyte and fibroblast cultures. J Dermatol Sci 2005; 40:141-143.
73. Thanomsub B, Pumeechockchai W, Limtrakul A et al. Chemical structures and biological activities of rhamnolipids produced by Pseudomonas aeruginosa B189 isolated from milk factory waste. Bioresource Technology 2006; 97:2457.
74. Özdemir G, Sezgin ÖE. Keratin-rhamnolipids and keratin-sodium dodecyl sulphate interactions at the air/interface. Colloids Surf B 2006; 52:1-7.
75. Cameotra SS, Makkar RS. Recent applications of biosurfactants as biological and immunological molecules. Curr Opinion Microbiol 2004; 7:262-266.

CHAPTER 14

Selected Microbial Glycolipids:
Production, Modification and Characterization

Olof Palme, Anja Moszyk, Dimitri Iphöfer and Siegmund Lang*

Abstract

This chapter deals with two types of biosurfactants that are not in the spotlight of general research: glycoglycerolipids and oligosaccharide lipids. The main focus is on glycolglyc-erolipids from marine bacteria like *Microbacterium* spec. DSM 12583, *Micrococcus luteus* (Hel 12/2) and *Bacillus pumilus* strain AAS3 and on oligosaccharide lipids from *Tsukamurella* spec. DSM 44370 and *Nocardia corynebacteroides* SM1. General and special structures, microbial producers, production conditions and chemo-enzymatic modifications as well as properties are outlined.

Introduction

Biosurfactants have long since been in focus of international research for their interesting properties. As surface active compounds they can replace chemically synthesized surfactants, involving benefits such as production from renewable resources, low toxicity and good biodegradability (Mukherjee et al[1]). Besides usual surfactant applications in cleaning or remediation (van Bogaert et al[2], Whang et al[3]), they offer quite many biological activities, making them interesting issues of pharmaceutical research (Stipcevic et al,[4] Hardin et al,[5] Rodrigues et al[6]).

There are three types of biosurfactants that should be mentioned here for their importance in research over the years: Rhamnolipids from *Pseudomonas aeruginosa*, Mannosylerythritolipids from *Pseudozyma aphidis* and Sophorolipids from *Candida bombicola*. They were discovered in 1949, 1956 and 1961, respectively and have ever since been targets of major research interest (e.g., Nitschke et al,[7] Fukuoka et al[8]).

Nevertheless, this article deals with different kinds of biosurfactants, which have not been in spotlight recently: Glycoglycerolipids and Oligosaccharide Lipids. Both are diverse classes of glycolipids, ranging from membrane compounds of eukaryotic cells and thermophilic bacteria to microbial secondary metabolites. Their production has been reported to be in a range of about 100 mg to 10 g, which makes them interesting candidates for different practical applications. Recent progress in research concerning glycoglycerolipids and oligosaccharide lipids shall be the topic of the following chapters.

Glycoglycerolipids

General Information

Glycoglycerolipids are abundant membrane constituents of plants and bacteria and can also be produced by chemical synthesis. In general they are composed of carbohydrate unit(s), a

*Corresponding Author: Siegmund Lang—Technical University of Braunschweig, Institute of Biochemistry and Biotechnology, Biotechnology Group, Spielmannstr. 7, D-38106 Braunschweig, Germany. Email: s.lang@tu-bs.de

Biosurfactants, edited by Ramkrishna Sen. ©2010 Landes Bioscience and Springer Science+Business Media.

glycerol moiety and a variety of short or long chained saturated or unsaturated fatty acids. As for glycoglycerolipids of natural origin, both our group (Lang and Trowitzsch-Kienast,[9] Lang[10]) and, in particular Hölzl and Dörmann,[11] presented very interesting overviews. In the latter review, the structures, their biosynthesis pathways and possible functions have been summarized in a comprehensive manner. In brief, as for chloroplasts of plants the monogalactosyldiacylglycerol (MGDG) and digalactosyldiacylglycerol (DGDG; with αGal(1→6)βGal linkage) and additionally, sulfoquinovosyldiacylglycerol (SQDG) are dominant and seem indispensable for maximal efficiency of photosynthesis. Galactolipids are also crucial for growth under normal and phosphate limiting conditions. Among the photosynthetic bacteria the anoxygenic ones contain a large variety of phospho- and glycoglycerolipids in their membranes. A number of studies suggest that these compounds play a specific role in anoxygenic photosynthesis. As for nonphotosynthetic bacteria, galactolipids with a head group structure related to plant and cyanobacterial MGD and DGD are absent. In general, those glycoglycerolipids are mostly composed of one or two sugars or sugar derivatives (e.g., glucose, galactose, mannose, glucuronic acid) bound to diacylglycerol. The head group diversity is further increased by the variety of different glycosidic linkages. The carbohydrates occur in α- or β-anomeric configuration and are connected in (1→2), (1→3), (1→4) or (1→6) linkage. Compared to this high diversity, the hydrophobic part is rather simple with a preponderance of saturated or monounsaturated fatty acids. However, the degree of structural variability of glycoglycerolipids found in the phyla *Firmicutes, Actinobacteria, Proteobacteria, Deinococcus-Thermus, Thermotogae and Spirochaetes* surpasses that in photosynthetic bacteria.

Considering the number of additional studies on glycoglycerolipids (GGL) published recently, we would like to distinguish as follows: 1. GGL from eukaryotic cells, 2. GGL from prokaryotic cells and 3. GGL from a synthetical route.

Glycoglycerolipids from Eukaryotic Cells

Terasaki and Itabashi[12] found the well-known MGDG and DGDG in *Cladosiphon okamuranus* and, additionally, a galactolipase activity responsible for hydrolyzing the acyl groups of above glycoglycerolipids. The initially observed large amount of free fatty acids (45% of the total lipids; e.g., 16:3n-3, 18:3n-3) in this brown alga could be confirmed by proof for the corresponding enzyme. The authors claim that this is the first report on the presence of acyl-hydrolase activity in seaweeds.

As for the glycoglycerolipids of the sea alga *Laminaria japonica*, Lee et al[13] performed studies on some physico-chemical properties and their ability to become incorporated into immunostimulating complexes (ISCOMs), used as a delivery system for microbial and tumor antigens in vesicular form. ISCOM modification by embedding glycolipids such as MGDG, DGDG and sulfoquinovosyldiacylglycerol (SQDG), instead of the phospholipid component in vesicles, showed a drastic increase of the used antigen presentation efficiency of ISCOMs to immunocompetent cells.

Using commercially available plant galactoglycerlipids Popova and Hincha[14] investigated the effects of the sugar head group on the phase behaviour of phospholipid model membranes in the dry state. They showed that all additives decreased T_m, the gel to liquid-crystalline phase transition temperature, of the dry phosphatidylcholine bilayers. Nevertheless, DGDG was much more effective than DLPC (1,2-dilinolenoyl-sn-glycero-3-phosphatidylcholine) or Gal (galactose). diGal had a similar effect as DGDG, pointing to the sugar head group and not to the lipid unsaturation, with the strongest influence on membrane phase behaviour. However, the degree of unsaturation in the fatty acyl chains of DLPC leads to a larger spacing in the model membranes, even in the absence of sugar and thus allows the sugars easier access (Rog et al[15]).

From the cultured marine dinoflagellate *Amphidinium carterae*, Wu et al[16] isolated a new unsaturated glycoglycerolipid, (2S)-1,2-O-6,9,12,15-dioctadecatetraenoyl-3-O-[α-D-galactopyranosyl-(1′′′′→6′′′)-O-β -D-galactopyranosyl]-glycerol. It has been isolated together with two known saturated ones, (2S)-1,2-distearoyl-3-O-(6-sulpho-a-D-quinovopyranosyl)-glycerol and (2S)-1-stearoyl-3-O-(6-sulpho-a-D-quinovopyranosyl)-glycerol. Their structures were elucidated on the basis of chemical and spectral data (e.g., 1H- or 13C-NMR).

Glycoglycerolipids from Prokaryotic Cells

After growing the thermophilic bacterium *Meiothermus taiwanensis* at 55°C aerobically, Yang et al[17] isolated and determined the structure of the main glycoglycerolipid to be α-Gal(1-6)-β-Gal(1-6)-β-GalNAcyl(1,2)-α-Glc(1,1)-glycerol diester, where N-acyl is a C17:0 or hydroxy C17:0 fatty acid and the glycerol esters were mainly iso- and anteisobranched C15:0 and C17:0. The fatty acids were examined by gas chromatography coupled with mass spectrometry (GC-MS) analysis of their methyl esters derived from methanolysis, whereas the structure of the carbohydrate moiety was elucidated by MS/MS and NMR spectroscopic analyses. The authors claim that this is the first complete glycolipid structure from thermophilic bacteria.

The relative amounts of the polar lipids and nonpolar waxes in chlorosomes isolated from *Chlorobium tepidum* (green sulfur bacterium) have been determined by Sørensen et al.[18] The main component of the polar lipid fraction of chlorosomes was identified as rhamnosyldiacylglycerol, which together with monogalactosyl-diacylglycerol comprises more than 55% of the lipid species on a molar basis. Together with phospholipids and aminoglycosphingolipid, these components presumably form a lipid monolayer surrounding. Thus the observed lipid distribution can be used to compare the polar lipid content with the surface area of chlorosomes.

Mycoplasmae are wall-less, parasitic, Gram-positive bacteria and the smallest organisms capable of self-replication. They are pathogens infecting a broad spectrum of diverse hosts such as animals, plants and humans, where they cause several invasive or chronic diseases. For instance, it is suggested that *Mycoplasma fermentans* is involved in triggering the development of AIDS in HIV-positive individuals, acting as a cofactor in pathogenesis. Although little is known about the molecular mechanisms underlying *M. fermentans* pathogenicity, it is reasonable to assume that the interactions with host cells are mediated by components of its plasma membrane. In this context, Brandenburg et al[19] report on the comprehensive physico-chemical characterization and biological activity of a certain glycoglycerolipid, 6'-O-(3''-phosphocholine- 2''-amino- 1''-phospho- 1'', 3''-propanediol) -a-D-glucopyranosyl- (1'-3)- 1,2-diacyl-sn-glycerol (MfG1-II), from this strain. Compared to LPS (lipopolysaccharide from deep rough mutant *Salmonella minnesota*), the β↔α gel-to-liquid crystalline phase transition behaviour of the hydrocarbon chains exhibits high similarity between the two glycolipids. A lipopolysaccharide-binding protein (LBP)-mediated incorporation into negatively charged liposomes was observed for both compounds. The determination of the supramolecular aggregate structure confirmed the existence of a mixed unilamellar and cubic structure for MfG1-II, similar to that observed for the lipid A moiety of LPS. Additionally, the biological data indicated that MfG1-II was able to induce cytokines such as tumor necrosis factor-α (TNF-α) in human mononuclear cells, although to a significantly lower degree than LPS, while the effect was higher than that of other bacterial activators like glycosphingolipid from *Spingomonas paucimobilis*. Furthermore, it could be shown that inflammatory response in primary rat astrocytes such as activation of protein kinase C, secretion of nitric oxid and prostaglandine E2 is triggered by MfG1-II, too.

Another organism of this group is *Acholeplasma laidlawii*. Glycoglycerolipids derived from the membranes of this bacterium bind to human cell lines. In addition, the 3-O-[2'-O-(α-D-glucopyranosyl)-6'-O-acyl-α-glucopyranosyl]-1,2-di-O-acyl-sn-glycerol (GAGDG) augments the HIV-1 infection through binding both lymphoid cells and HIV-1 virus. This glycoglycerolipid shows the highest binding efficiency to HIV-1 (Shimizu et al[20]). In connection with these findings, the acyl chain at the C_6' position of glucose may play an important role for binding ability. Thus the variation of the acyl chain at C_6' shows that the branching forms of acyl chains with C14 or C16 are necessary for efficiently capturing HIV-1.

Glycoglycerolipids from Synthetical Route

Recently, the potential of glycoglycerolipids for cancer chemoprevention has been observed. Antitumor-promoting effects could be shown by glycoglycerol- or glycoglycerlipid-mediated inhibition of the tumor-promoting activity caused by the tumor promotor 12-O-tetradecanoylphorbol-13- acetate (TPA), by using a short-term in vitro assay for Epstein-Barr virus early antigen (EBV-EA) activation. Colombo et al[21] claimed that their research

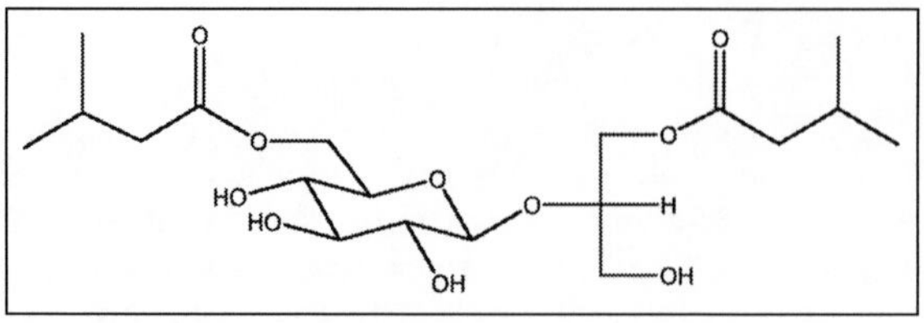

Figure 1. 1-O-(3-Methylbutanoyl)-2-O-[6-O-(3-methylbutanoyl)-β-*D*-galactopyranosyl]-sn-glycerol (modified according to Colombo D. et al[22]).

groups have thoroughly explored the structure-antitumor-promoting activity relationships of some glycoglycerolipid analogues with the aim of obtaining new active cancer chemopreventive agents which are structurally related to the natural compounds. In all chemically synthesized compounds, the ester function was replaced by different metabolically more stable groups like ether, alkyl or ketone. The only example of these occurring naturally is the abundant ether bond in *Archaebacteria*. The studies show that the ester function replacement caused a loss in activity that was rather small compared to the effect caused by the acyl chain length. In that case, a strong reduction of the inhibitory effect on EBV activation was evidenced when compounds with acyl chains very short (C2) or longer (C12-C18) than C10 were tested. When investigated in an in vivo two-stage carcinogenesis test, two of the alkyl derivatives exhibited remarkable inhibitory effects on mouse skin tumor promotion.

In additional studies on altering the acyl chain, Colombo et al[22] could show that branched acyl chains enhance the in vitro antitumor-promoting activity whereas aliphatic or aromatic rings display a negative effect. The most potent product is shown in Figure 1.

Selected Glycoglycerolipids from Prokaryotes

Molecular Structures

The marine bacterium *Microbacterium* spec. DSM 12583, isolated from the Mediterranean sponge *Halichondria panicea*, is able to form a glucosylmannosyl-glycerolipid (GGL 2), 1-O-acyl-3-[α-glucopyranosyl-(1-3)-(6-O-acyl-α-mannopyranosyl)] glycerol, when grown on a complex medium with glycerol. Its molecular structure could be elucidated and is shown in Figure 2. It consists of a constant carbohydrate and a variable fatty acid moiety.

Another marine strain, *Micrococcus luteus* (Hel 12/2), was isolated from the North Sea. This bacterium produces a dimannosyl-glycerolipid (GGL 5), Mannopyranosyl(1α-3)-6-acylman-nopyranosyl(1α-1)-3-acylglycerol on artificial seawater supplemented with glucose (20 g/L), yeast extract (3.5 g/L), peptone (3.5 g/L) and suitable nitrogen/phosphate sources. Its molecular structure is shown in Figure 2 as well and shows the same composition of a constant carbohydrate and a variable fatty acid moiety.

A third marine bacterium, *Bacillus pumilus* strain AAS3, could be isolated from the Mediterranean sponge *Acanthella acuta* and synthesizes a diglucosyl-glycerolipid (GGL 11), 1,2-O-diacyl -3-[β-glucopyranosyl-(1-6)-β-glucopyranosyl)]glycerol, when grown on artificial seawater supplemented with glucose (20 g/L), yeast extract (10 g/L) and suitable nitrogen/phosphate sources. Figure 2 shows its chemical structure. Like both other glycolipids it is made from a constant carbohydrate and a variable fatty acid moiety.

Production, Downstream Processing and Analysis

Glucosylmannosyl-Glycerolipid from Microbacterium Spec. DSM 12583

Submerse cultivations of *Microbacterium* spec. DSM 12583 were performed with artificial seawater medium containing all important salts and trace elements. Glucose and glycerol served as energy and carbon sources. Glucose was the first substrate where the glucosylmannosyl-glycerolipid production with *Microbacterium* spec. DSM 12583 was reported (Wicke et al[23]). After medium

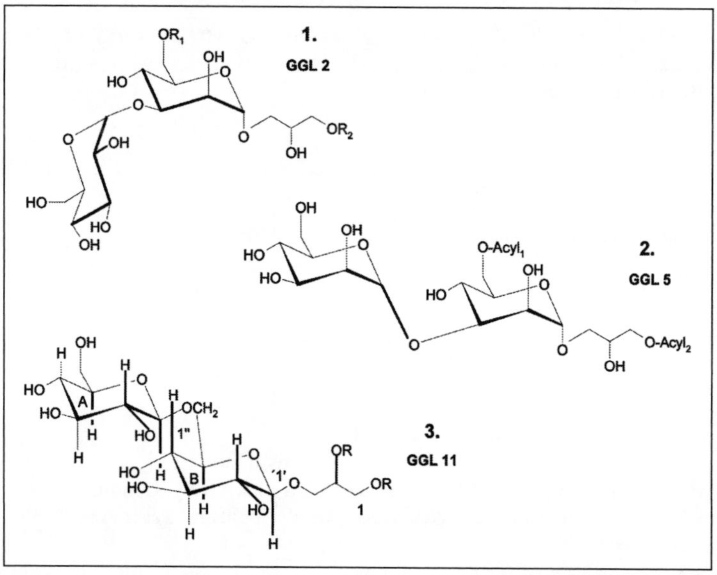

Figure 2. 1) GGL 2 produced by *Microbacterium* spec. DSM 12583 complex medium with glycerol—R = anteiso-C15:0 and -C17:0, but also iso-C16:0; 2) GGL 5 produced by *Micrococcus luteus* (Hel 12/2) grown on artificial seawater supplemented with glucose (20 g/L), yeast extract (3.5 g/L), peptone (3.5 g/L) and suitable nitrogen/phosphate sources, and 3) GGL 11 produced by *Bacillus pumilus* strain AAS3 grown on artificial seawater supplemented with glucose (20 g/L), yeast extract (10 g/L) and suitable nitrogen/phosphate sources—R = anteiso-C15:0 and -C17:0, but also traces of iso-C16:0.

variation experiments, glycerol was determined as a carbon source with higher production capability (Lang et al[24]).

Bioreactor fermentations were performed at a stirring rate of 500 rpm, temperature of 30°C, pH adjusted at 6.5 and aeration rate of 0.4 L/(L·min). Besides glycerol, the medium contained 3.5 g/L peptone and 3.5 g/L yeast extract as carbon and energy sources.

After cultivation, the product was obtained by extraction with a mixture of CH_2Cl_2/CH_3OH (2/1, v/v). After extraction, the cell residues were separated from the organic phase. Freeze-drying reduced the dichloride methane/methanol phase containing the glycoglycerolipids. There were four different cell-associated glycoglycerolipids produced, which were isolated by chromatography on silica gel columns. The main compound was GGL 2.

The glucosylmannosyl-glycerolipid concentrations were determined via thin-layer chromatography (TLC, stationary phase: silica gel plates, mobile phase: $CHCl_3/CH_3OH/H_2O$ (65/15/2, v/v/v), detection reagent anisaldehyde/sulphuric acid/acetic acid) coupled with densitometry.

The glucosylmannosyl-glycerolipid is formed dependent on bacterial growth and is catabolized very fast after reaching the stationary phase.

In bioreactor experiments, the results shown in Table 1 could be obtained.

In recent studies, an HPLC-based analysis method was developed to determine the glucosylmannosyl-glycerolipid concentration. Therefore the HPLC-system was calibrated by using purified GGL 2 in different concentrations which was isolated from cell extracts using MPLC. A silica gel column was used as stationary phase. The mobile phase was a mixture of $CHCl_3/CH_3OH/H_2O$ (65/15/2) with a flow rate of 0.5 mL/min. Detection was performed with an ultraviolet detector at $\lambda = 240$ nm.

Figure 3 shows the chromatogram of the crude extract from *Microbacterium* spec. DSM 12583.

Table 1. *Cultivation results of* **Microbacterium** *spec. DSM 12583 in 10 L bioreactor on artificial seawater medium + 20 g/L glycerol as carbon source (30°C, 500 rpm, 0.4 L/(L min), pH-value 6.5)*

Parameter	Results
Reactor operating time [h]	54
Biomass$_{max}$ [g/L]	14.0
GGL 2$_{max}$ [mg/L]	522.0
P_V [mg/[L·h]]	11.8
μ_{max} [1/h]	0.137
$Y_{P/X}$ [mg/g]	46.0
$Y_{P/S}$ [mg/g]	30.1

By using 10 g/L glycerol and 15 g/L complex components (10 g/L peptone and 5 g/L yeast extract) as carbon source, a yield of the glucosylmannosyl-glycerolipid of 789 mg/L was achieved in bioreactor scale. With a maximum of nearly 14 g/L biomass, a specific production of 57 mg/g biomass or 32 mg/g carbon source (peptone, yeast extract, glycerol) was obtained, respectively.

Compared to earlier values, an increase by the factor 1.5 of the glucosylmannosyl-glycerolipid concentration could be achieved. In addition, the previous method of TLC with consequent densitometry for the determination of GGL 2 concentrations was replaced by an HPLC method.

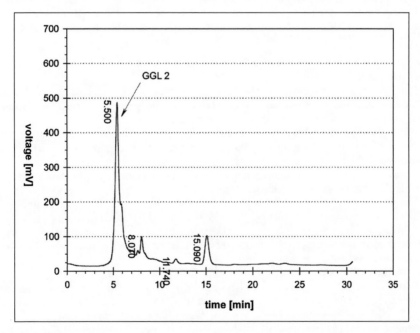

Figure 3. Chromatogram of crude extract from *Microbacterium* spec. DSM 12583. Silica gel column as stationary phase, CHCl$_3$/CH$_3$OH/H$_2$O (65/15/2, v/v/v), pump rate 0.5 mL/min, measuring time 30 min, room temperature, detection with UV (λ = 240 nm).

Table 2. Cultivation conditions for **Micrococcus luteus** *(Hel 12/2)* **in 10 L bioreactor on** *artificial seawater medium*

Parameter	Conditions
Working volume [L]	8
Temperature [°C]	30
pH-Value	Unregulated
Revolutions per minute	500
Aeration [L/[L·min]]	0.4
C-Source	20 g/L glucose
N-Source	5.0 g/L NaNO$_3$
P-Source	0.89 g/L Na$_2$HPO$_4$
Yeast extract [g/L]	3.5
Bacto Peptone [g/L]	3.5

Dimannosyl-Glycerolipid from Micrococcus Luteus *(Hel 12/2)*

Cultivations with *Micrococcus luteus* (Hel 12/2) were done in artificial seawater medium containing yeast extract and peptone. Main energy and carbon source was glucose. Detailed cultivation conditions are shown in Table 2.

The product was obtained by extraction with a mixture of CH$_2$Cl$_2$/CH$_3$OH (2/1, v/v). After separating the different product molecules via MPLC, single glycoglycerolipid concentrations were determined via TLC (stationary phase: silica gel plates, mobile phase: CHCl$_3$/CH$_3$OH/H$_2$O (65/15/2, v/v/v), detection reagent anisaldehyde/sulphuric acid/acetic acid) coupled with densitometry.

This dimannosyl-glycerolipid is produced dependent on bacterial growth as well. After reaching the stationary phase it is decomposed very quickly.

Table 3 summarizes the results obtained in bioreactor cultivation experiments producing this glycoglycerolipid.

Medium variation experiments showed that adding Na$_2$HPO$_4$ as phosphate source had a positive effect on bacterial growth. Furthermore, the addition of only small amounts of glucose yields higher amounts of the glycoglycerolipid.

Diglucosyl-Glycerolipid from Bacillus pumilus *Strain AAS3*

The strain *Bacillus pumilus* strain AAS3 was grown in artificial seawater media containing yeast extract. Main energy and carbon source was glucose.

Table 3. Cultivation results of **Micrococcus luteus** *(Hel 12/2)* **in 10 L bioreactor on** *artificial seawater medium*

Parameter	Results
Reactor operating time [h]	56
Biomass$_{max}$ [g/L]	16.5
GGL 5$_{max}$ [mg/L]	182.5
P$_V$ [mg/[L·h]]	5.49
μ_{max} [1/h]	0.12
Y$_{P/X}$ [mg/g]	11.0
Y$_{P/S}$ [mg/g]	10.7

Table 4. *Cultivation results of* Bacillus pumilus *strain AAS3 in 50 L bioreactor on artificial seawater medium 20 g/L glucose 10 g/L yeast extract (30˚C, pH 7.5, 500 rpm, 0.4 L/(L·min))*

Parameter	Results
Reactor operating time [h]	20
Biomass$_{max}$ [g/L]	10.5
GGL 11$_{max}$ [mg/L]	91.0
P_V [mg/[L·h]]	8.27
$_{max}$ [1/h]	0.55
$Y_{P/X}$ [mg/g]	8.7
$Y_{P/S}$ [mg/g]	5.1

The glycoglycerolipid was purified by extraction with methanol. Quantitative measurements were performed by TLC/Densitometer CD 60 with silica gel 60 as stationary phase, CHCl$_3$/CH$_3$OH/H$_2$O (65/15/2, v/v/v) as solvent system and α-naphthol/sulphuric acid as detecting reagent at 580 nm.

Table 4 gives an overview of the results obtained in bioreactor cultivations using *Bacillus pumilus* strain AAS3.

When grown on marine broth containing peptone and yeast extract as carbon and nitrogen sources, a maximum yield for the diglucosyl-glycerolipid of only 30 mg/L was achieved. Compared with the maximum yield achieved in artificial seawater medium, the yield could be increased to 90 mg/L.

Chemo-Enzymatic Modification of Glycoglycerolipids

The glycoglycerolipid from *Microbacterium* spec. DSM 12583 could be hydrolysed enzymatically using lipase from *Candida antarctica* (Novozyme Lipase 435). This site-specific enzymatic hydrolysis removed the fatty acids completely, yielding the glycoglycero-moiety (Fig. 4).

The enzymatic hydrolysis of the glucosylmannosyl-glycerolipid was performed in two steps. First, the fatty acid on the glycerol residue was cleaved. Afterwards the ester bond at the sugar was split. By using Novozyme Lipase 435 it was possible to produce glucosylmannosyl-glycerol (GG 2) as well as the intermediate GGL 2a. Under optimised conditions (50°C, tert. amyl alcohol (H$_2$O < 1%) and the addition of 0.9% (v/v) water) a yield of 90% was achieved. Comparable results could be obtained in the works of Ramm et al.[25] In this work the diglucosyl-glycerolipid could be enzymatically hydrolysed with a lipase. Differently to the enzymatic hydrolysis of glucosylmannosyl-glycerolipid the working temperature was lower (40°C). At this temperature, only the intermediate GGL 2a was produced. By using immobilized lipase, both products of the enzymatic hydrolysis (GGL 2a, GG 2) could be produced and isolated easily.

For the enzymatic hydrolysis it was exceptional that the reaction was performable in organic solvents with low water content (< 1%). Experiments at similar conditions are mentioned in Inada[26] and Haas et al.[27] There, immobilized lipase was used for the hydrolysis of Phosphatidylcholin. Best yields could be achieved in the organic solvents butyl alcohol or tert. amyl alcohol.

Like the glucosylmannosyl-glycerolipid from *Microbacterium* spec. DSM 12583, the diglucosyl-glycerolipid from *Bacillus pumilus* strain AAS3 could be hydrolysed enzymatically using lipase from *Candida antarctica* (Novozyme Lipase 435). The result of this site-specific enzymatic hydrolysis is GG 11. By the enzymatic acylation of GG 11 with 4-pentenoic acid the main product GGL 12 (doubled acylated glycoglycerolipid), the byproduct GGL 13 (ternary acylated) and the intermediate product GGL 14 (mono-acylated) were produced (Fig. 5). The yield of GGL 12 was 88%.

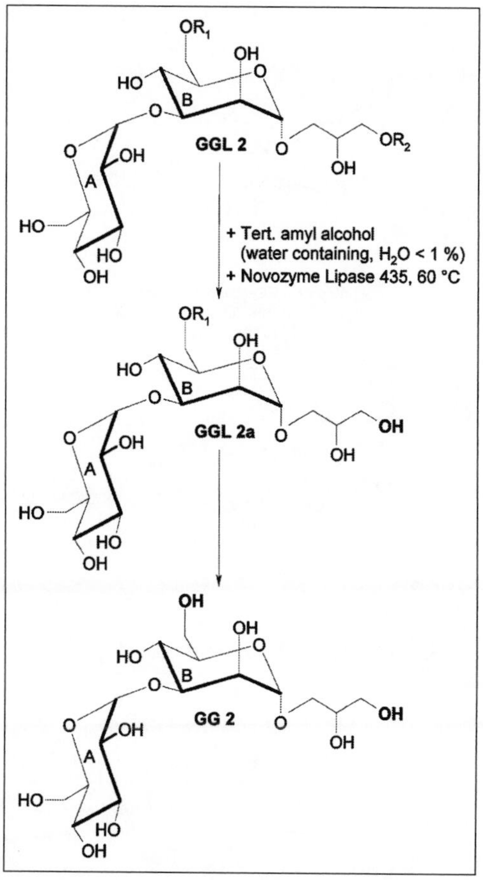

Figure 4. Enzymatic conversion of glycogylerolipids from *Microbacterim* spec. DSM 12583 with a lipase (Novozyme Lipase 435) to produce first GGL 2a and than GG 2.

Oligosaccharide Lipids

General Information

Acylated oligosaccharides are common structures in pro- and eukaryotic cell surfaces and thus play important roles in cell-cell interaction. In the following, the important role of these molecules shall be illustrated by some examples that do not make any claim to be complete. Eukaryotic sphingolipids, which consist of sphingosine, fatty acids and oligosaccharides, are important components of cell membranes (Lockhoff[28]). Lipooligosaccharides are as well part of the outer membrane of Gram-negative bacteria, where they play an important role in their survival and their interaction with the environment (Alexander and Rietschel[29]). Examples of prokaryotic lipooligosaccharides are the virulence factors of the humanpathogenic bacteria *Neisseria meningitidis* (Zughaier et al[30]) and *Campylobacter jejuni* (Dzieciatkowska et al[31]). Complex oligo- and polysaccharide lipids can often be found in Gram-negative bacteria of environments containing aliphatic and aromatic hydrocarbons (Leone et al[32]). Finally, thermophilic and halophilic bacteria as well form complex glyco- and glycoglycero-lipids as membrane components, which are essential for the thermal stability and biological functions of the bacteria in extreme environments (Yang et al[17], Silipo et al[33], Pask-Hughes and Shaw[34]).

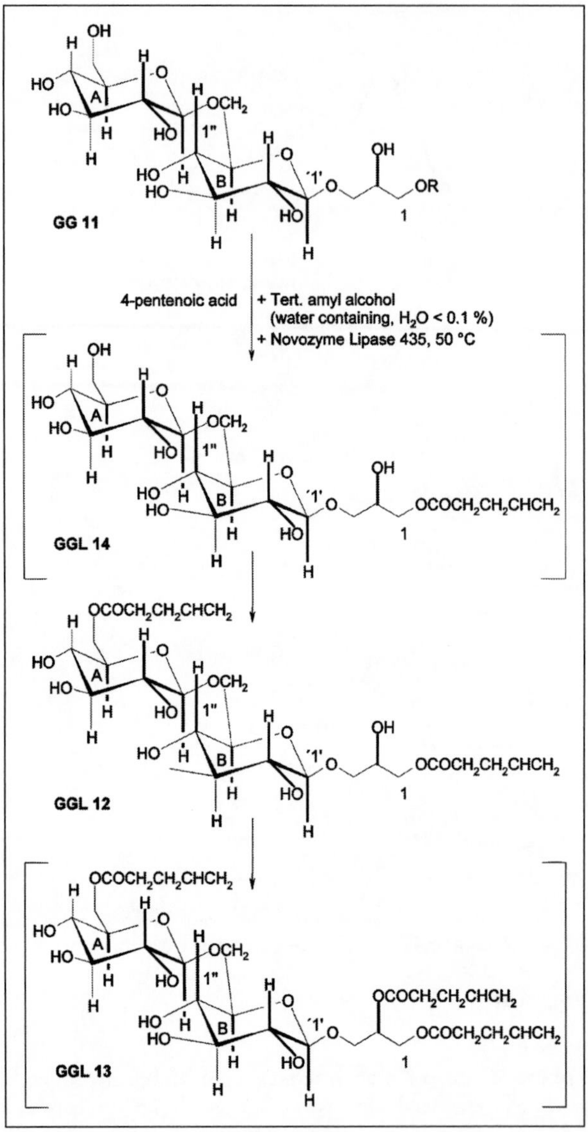

Figure 5. Enzymatic conversion of glycogylerolipids from *Bacillus pumilus* strain AAS3 with a lipase (Novozyme Lipase 435) to produce GGL 12, structure verifications for GGL 13 and GGL 14 were not performed, determination by R_F-values of TLC.

Nevertheless, this chapter wants to focus on bacterial oligosaccharide lipids that consist of acylated oligosaccharides containing more than two carbohydrate molecules and are formed and secreted in larger amounts as secondary metabolites. One of them is an acylated trisaccharide formed of three glucose molecules in a Gram-positive actinomycete, which is produced in the presence of hexadecane as carbon source (Esch et al[35]). It bears structural resemblances with respect to its acylation pattern and carbon hydrate backbone to a pentasaccharide lipid from *Nocardia corynebacteroides* (Powalla et al[36]), which is produced on n-alkanes as well. A completely different structure can be found in a Gram-negative bacterium of the genus *Tsukamurella* grown on plant oils (Vollbrecht et al[37]). We will put our focus on the two latter oligosaccharide lipids from *Nocardia corynebacteroides* and *Tsukamurella* spec. because both of them are not only structurally well-characterized but there are also detailed data concerning their physico-chemical properties, microbial production and, in case of the *Tsukamurella*-glycolipids, chemo-enzymatic modification.

Selected Oligosaccharide Lipids

Molecular Structures

The soil-bacterium *Tsukamurella* spec. DSM 44370 produces a mixture of di-, tri- and tetrasaccharide lipids when grown on plant oils such as sunflower or calendula oil. Their molecular structures could be elucidated and are shown in Figure 6. In contrast to most other microbial glycolipids that consist of a constant carbohydrate and a variable fatty acid moiety, the *Tsukamurella* spec. product is a mixture of molecules containing different sugar moieties.

Another strain derived from soil samples, *Nocardia corynebacteroides* SM1, produces a mixture of di- and pentasaccharide lipids when grown on n-alkanes with chain lengths between C14 to C16. The disaccharide lipids are trehalose-containing corynomycolates known from other bacteria as well (e.g., *Rhodococcus erythropolis* DSM 43215, Kim et al[38]). Figure 6 displays the structure of the pentasaccharide lipids. The exact position of one acylic residue could not be determined by NMR without destroying the hydrocarbon backbone.

Finally, a Gram-positive actinomycete growing on n-hexadecane secretes a family of anionic glycolipid surfactant homologues. The major homologue could be elucidated and its structure is shown in Figure 6. It resembles the pentasaccharide lipid from *Nocardia corynebacteroides* SM1 with respect to the kind of carbohydrates and their arrangement, differing in the number. The acylation positions of the trisaccharide lipid are acylated in the pentasaccharide lipid as well, while the acyle components differ a lot: the pentasaccharide lipid mostly contains short fatty acids, while trisaccharide lipid consists of uncommon acyloxyacyl structures, 3-hexanoyloxyoctanoate and 3-hexanoyloxydecanoate, as well.

Production, Downstream Processing and Analysis

Oligosaccharide Lipids from Tsukamurella *Spec. DSM 44370*

Submerse cultivations of *Tsukamurella* spec. were performed in mineral media containing all important salts and trace elements, where nitrogen- and phosphate amount are of special importance. Plant oils served as energy and carbon source, but also as antifoam agent. Although sunflower oil was the first substrate where glycolipid production with *Tsukamurella* spec. was reported, it is known that product formation also takes place on various other oily substrates (Vollbrecht et al[39], Langer et al[40]). Among others, calendula and rapeseed oil, as unusual substrates, were used as carbon sources to test their potential for improving product formation or modifying its composition. Calendula oil is a triglyceride consisting of about 60% of calendula acid, which is octadec-8, 10-trans,12-cis-trienic acid. Rapeseed oil contains about 60% of erucic acid (C22:1), so both are significantly different to sunflower oil, which contains about 80% of oleic acid (C18:1). Bioreactor fermentations were performed with a stirring rate of 550 rpm, temperature of 30°C and aeration rate of 0.4 L/(L·min). The medium contained 1.78 g/L K_2HPO_4 and 7.44 g/L $(NH_4)_2SO_4$.

After cultivation, the product was obtained by several extraction steps starting with MTBE extraction. This crude extract was dissolved in Methanol/Water and extracted with cyclohexane to separate product (aqueous phase) and residual oil substrate (hydrophobic phase). The methanol/water phase containing the glycolipids was reduced by freeze-drying.

Glycolipid content and composition were measured by HPLC with a stationary phase of Nucleosil 120-5C18 and a gradient system of H_2O/CH_3OH as mobile phase. Detection was performed with an evaporative light scattering detector.

Table 5 shows results of fermentations performed with sunflower, rapeseed and calendula oil as carbon sources.

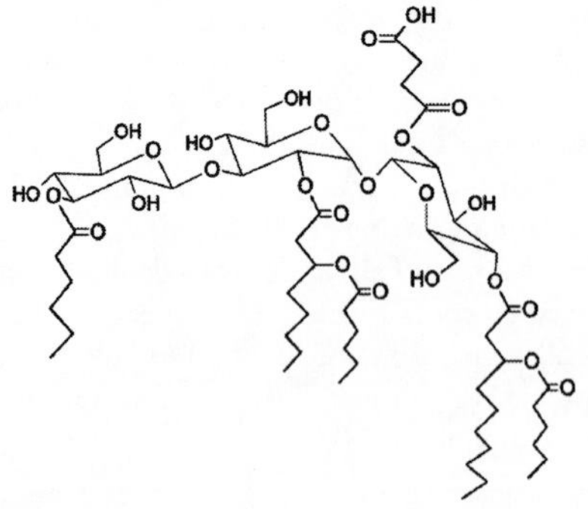

Figure 6. 1) Molecular structures of the glycolipids GL 1, GL 1B, GL 2 and GL 3 produced by *Tsukamurella* spec. GL 1: R = H, GL 1B: R = octadecanoic acid. A, B, C and D: order for the sugar moieties (according to Vollbrecht et al[37]). 2) Possible structures of the pentasaccharide lipid from *Nocardia corynebacteroides* SM1 grown on n-alkanes (C14-C15). R = CH3COO (2x), CH3CH2COO and CH3(CH2)2COO (3x), CH3(CH2)6COO (2x), HOOC(CH2)2COO (1x), (R) = position cannot be elucidated definitely (according to Powalla et al[36]). 3) Molecular structure of the major glycolipid isolated from an actinomycete grown on n-hexadecane (according to Esch et al[35]).

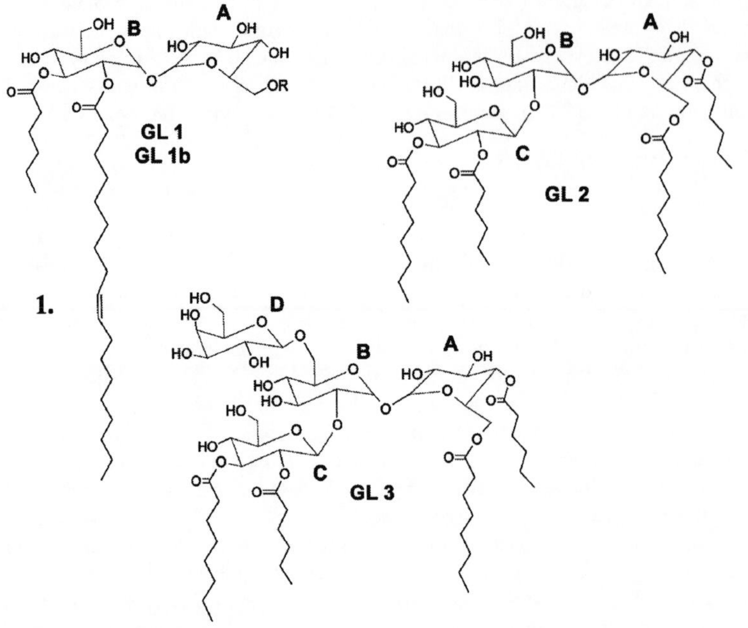

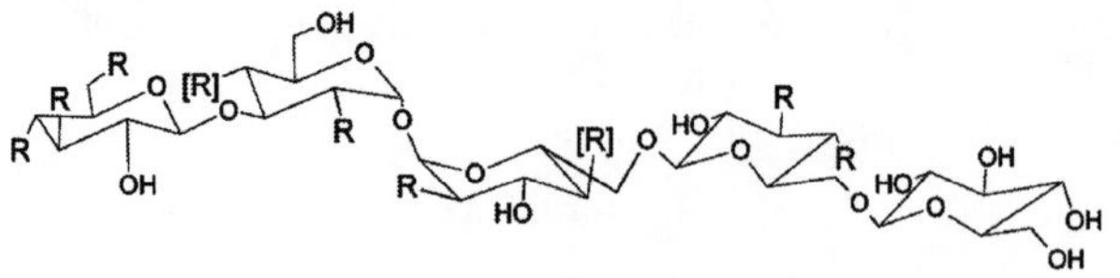

Table 5. *Comparison of typical parameters from bioreactor cultivations with* Tsukamurella *spec. using sunflower, rapeseed and calendula oil as carbon sources. All parameters were determined at the end of the respective cultivation, except where stated*

Parameter	Sunflower Oil	Rapeseed Oil	Calendula Oil
Cultivation volume [L]	20	20	5
Start concentration of carbon source [g/L]	190	200	120
Cultivation time [h]	140	140	190
Biomass [g/L]	40	39	50
Substrate consumption [g/L]	130	110	100
Volumetric productivity [g/[L·h]]	0.16	0.09	0.07
$Y_{P/X}$	0.56	0.33	0.28
$Y_{P/S}$	0.17	0.12	0.14
Product concentration [g/L]	22.5	13	14
GL 1 [%][a]	33	33	15
GL 2 [%]	33	33	24
GL 3 [%]	33	33	61

[a]The exact composition of the longest fatty acid chain at C2 is probably dependent on the oil used.

Obviously, the highest product amounts are obtained using sunflower oil as substrate, but the highest biomass production takes place in the fermentation with calendula oil. The results also illustrate that differences in the composition of the glycolipidic products depends on the substrate used, for cultivation with calendula oil clearly promotes the formation of one glycolipid, GL 3. The growth behaviour of *Tsukamurella* spec. in bioreactor cultivations is the typical one for bacteria in batch cultivation: a start with a lag-phase, followed by exponential growth until ammonium and phosphate are consumed and finally a stationary phase until the end of the cultivation. Glycolipids are mainly produced under ammonium- and phosphate-limiting conditions after growth has finished. Not only is the amount of products of interest but also their composition. By separating the different product molecules via HPLC, the single glycolipid concentrations were determined. It is remarkable that cultivation with calendula oil leads to a significantly different product species ratio with GL 3 accounting for more than 60% of the whole product.

Pentasaccharide Lipids from Nocardia corynebacteroides *SM1*

Cultivations with *Nocardia corynebacteroides* were performed in salt media containing yeast extract. Main energy and carbon sources were n-alkanes of chain lengths C10-C18, technical n-alkane mixtures, different sugars and ethanol.

The product was obtained by extraction with ethyl acetate. Quantification was performed by TLC (stationary phase: Chromarods SII, mobile phase: $CHCl_3/CH_3OH/H_2O$, detection reagent anisaldehyde/sulphuric acid/acetic acid) coupled with a flame ionisation detector.

Bacterial growth as well as product formation only took place when alkanes of chain lengths C12-C16 or mixtures of these were used as carbon sources. Neither shorter-chained alkanes nor hydrophilic carbon sources promoted growth of *Nocardia corynebacteroides*. The best glycolipid concentrations were obtained using n-tetradecane, yielding 2.9 g/L, but also n-pentadecane and n-hexadecane were successful substrates yielding values of 2.8 and 2.7 g/L glycolipid, respectively.

Medium variation experiments showed that n-alkanes as carbon sources, nitrate as nitrogen source and small amounts of yeast extract yielded the highest amounts of pentasaccharide lipid products. Product formation only took place under nitrogen-limited conditions.

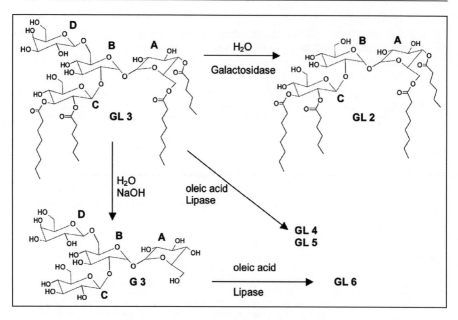

Figure 7. Overview of chemo-enzymatic conversions with oligosaccharide lipid GL 3 from *Tsukamurella* spec. First, it was possible to produce GL 2 with a β-Galactosidase by removing sugar moiety D. Second, GL 3 could be directly acylated at the C_6-positions of C and D with a lipase to give GL 4 (acylation at C) and GL 5 (acylation at C and D). Third, it could be deacylated chemically to give G 3 and then reacylated at C_4/C_6 of A and C_2/C_3 of C to afford GL 6. A, B, C and D: order for the sugar moieties.

Chemo-Enzymatic Modification of Oligosaccharide Lipids from *Tsukamurella* spec

The oligosaccharide lipids from *Tsukamurella* could be deacylated chemically by boiling in NaOH. This hydrolysis removed the fatty acids completely, yielding the carbohydrate backbone. Additionally, site-specific enzymatic acylations could be performed with lipase from *Candida antarctica* (Novozyme Lipase 435). Native GL 3 could rather easily be acylated with oleic acid at the C_6-positions of sugar moieties C and D and afforded 90% GL 4 (acylation at C_6-position of moiety D) and GL 5 (acylations at C_6-positions of moieties C and D) under optimised conditions. Both products were difficult to isolate, however as they were sensitive to traces of acids and increased temperature. Compared to the four native acylation positions in GL 3, the additional acylation positions (or the fatty acid chain length) appear to be unfavourable energetically.

In keeping with this the lipase-catalyzed acylation of G 3, the sugar backbone of GL 3, with oleic acid resulted in one major glycolipid, GL 6 and two side products. GL 6 resembles native GL 3 both in the extent of acylation and the position of the four substituents. As there are no naturally occurring molecules with higher or lower acylation levels, this state seems to be the energetically most favoured.

The most effective enzymatic conversion that was performed with GL 3 was the release of one galactose molecule using β-galactosidase from *Aspergillus oryzae*. This yielded GL 2, one of the natural *Tsukamurella* oligosaccharide lipids. Figure 7 gives an impression of possible chemo-enzymatic modifications of *Tsukamurella* oligosaccharide lipids.

Physico-Chemical and Bioactive Properties

As glycolipids are characteristic amphiphiles, they all show surface active properties. These can be quantified by two values, the critical micelle concentration and the lowering of surface

Table 6. *Surface activity characteristics at 25° C of glycoglycerolipids from* Microbacterium *spec. (GGL 2),* Bacillus pumilus *strain AAS3 (GGL 11 and derivative GGL 12), oligosaccharide lipids from* Tsukamurella *spec. (GL 1-3, derivative GL 4) and pentasaccharide lipid from* Nocardia corynebacteroides *compared to the commercially available biosurfactant* APG 1200 Plantaren®

Glycolipid	cmc [mg/L]	σ_{cmc} [mN/m]
GGL 2	200	33
GGL 11	50	29
GGL 12	250	40
GL 1	10	35
GL 2	100	23
GL 3	100	24
GL 4	200	23
Pentasaccharide lipid	30	26
APG 1200 Plantaren®	20	27

tension of water, which under standard conditions has a value of 72 mN/m. Table 6 shows the characteristic values of glycoglycerolipids from *Microbacterium* spec. DSM 12583 and from *Bacillus pumilus* strain AAS3 as well as their derivatives, from *Tsukamurella* spec. glycolipids and their derivatives, the pentasaccharide lipids from *Nocardia corynebacteroides* and those of the commercially available alkylpolyglycoside *APG 1200 Plantaren*® (Cognis, Düsseldorf, Germany) for comparison.

Regarding the surface activities, the pentasaccharide lipid from *Nocardia corynebacteroides* performs nearly as well as the commercial product *APG 1200 Plantaren*®, which reduces the surface tension of water to 27 mN/m. Most of the glycolipids from *Tsukamurella* spec., with exception of GL 1, perform better than this, lowering the surface tension to a value of 23 or 24 mN/m. GL 4 did not perform as well as GL 2 or GL 3. Although it could reduce the surface tension of water to 23 mN/m like GL 2, it does it at a cmc of 200 mg/L instead of 100 mg/L measured for GL 2. The only glycoglycerolipid performing nearly as well as this is the Diglucosyl-glycerolipid from *Bacillus pumilus* strain AAS3, GGL 11. It reduces the surface tension of water to 29 mN/m at a rather low cmc of 50 mg/L. The other glycoglycerolipids GGL 2 and GGL 12 generally perform poorer with respect to their surface activity.

Besides their physico-chemical properties, antimicrobial effects of glycolipids have often been reported, while only few studies describe their antitumor-promoting activities. The glycoglyc-erolipids from *Microbacterium* spec. DSM 12583, *Micrococcus luteus* (Hel 12/2) and *Bacillus pumilus* strain AAS3 and their derivatives as well as the natural *Tsukamurella* spec. products and their derivatives were tested in this respect. It was found out that the native glycoglycerolipids GGL 2, GGL 5 and GGL 11 and particularly the free glycoglycerol moieties GG 2 and GG 11 as well as the native oligosaccharide lipids GL 1 and GL 3 and their derivative G 3 showed effective inhibition of the 12-*O*-tetradecanoylphorbol-13-acetate (TPA) induced activation of Epstein-Barr virus early antigen (Table 7). For instance, 32 nmol ($1.1 \cdot 10^{-2}$ mg/mL in DMSO; 1000% ratio to TPA) of GG 11 gave a 97.5% inhibition of TPA-induced activation of EBV-EA, leaving a residual activation of 2.5%. In this regard, glycoglycerolipids GGL 2, GGL 5 and GGL 11 show comparable responses as other products like synthetic galactoglycerolipids with branched and unsaturated acyl chains (Colombo et al,[41] Colombo et al,[21] Colombo et al,[42]) natural azaphilones and uncommon amino acids from red-mold rice (Akihisa et al[43]) or natural lupane- and oleanane-type triterpenoids (Fukuda et al[44]). In this context, the 97.4% and 97.5% inhibition at 10^3 mol ratio/TPA of G 3 and GG 11, respectively, make them potential antitumor-promotion therapeutics.

Table 7. Antitumor-promoting activities of glycoglycerolipids and oligosaccharide lipids: Inhibition of TPA-induced activation of Epstein-Barr virus early antigen (EBV-EA)

Compound	% To Control (% Viability of Raji-Cells)[a]			
	1000	500	100	10
GGL 2	15.2 (70)	60.7	87.7	100.0
GGL 5	9.1 (70)	41.5	84.1	95.7
GGL 11	16.5 (80)	59.7	84.1	100.0
GGL 12	15.2 (60)	51.4	79.4	100.0
GG 2	7.1 (60)	42.0	71.6	93.8
GG 11	2.5 (70)	38.5	74.3	91.7
GL 1	9.2 (60)	46.4	74.0	100.0
GL 2	24.1 (80)	62.5	86.3	100.0
GL 3	10.5 (60)	47.0	76.4	100.0
GL 4	11.7 (70)	59.4	80.3	100.0
G 3	2.6 (60)	40.9	69.5	89.5

[a]Values are EBV-EA activation (%) in the presence of different concentrations of the test compound (mol ratio/TPA), relative to the control (100%). Activation was attained by treatment with 32 pmol TPA.

Conclusion

This chapter thus focuses more on the recent progress made in the R&D of two new varieties of lipidic biosurfactants, namely, Glycoglycerolipids and Oligosaccharide lipids. Both are diverse classes of glycolipids, mainly ranging from membrane components of eukaryotic cells and thermophilic bacteria to secondary metabolites of microbial origin. Their ease of production by chemical and biochemical routes makes them interesting candidates for various important practical implications. As biosurfactants have interesting features with respect to their surfactant and bioactive properties, they are getting more and more into focus of research and application interest. Besides the better known classes of biosurfactants, glycoglycerolipids and oligosaccharide lipids and their derivatives exhibit interesting characteristics, especially with respect to their antitumour-promoting capabilities. Their unusual carbohydrate patterns make them good candidates for active agents as they are able to interact with glycosylated surface structures of biological membranes.

References

1. Mukherjee S, Das P, Sen R. Towards commercial production of microbial surfactants. Trends Biotechnol 2006; 24(11):509-515.
2. Van Bogaert IN, Saerens K, De Muynck C et al. Microbial production and application of sophorolipids. Appl Microbiol Biotechnol 2007; 76(1):23-34.
3. Whang LM, Liu PW, Ma CC et al. Application of biosurfactants, rhamnolipid and surfactin, for enhanced biodegradation of diesel-contaminated water and soil. J Hazard Mater 2008; 151(1):155-163.
4. Stipcevic T, Piljac A, Piljac G. Enhanced healing of full-thickness burn wounds using di-rhamnolipid. Burns 2006; 32(1):24-34.
5. Hardin R, Pierre J, Schulze R et al. Sophorolipids improve sepsis survival: effects of dosing and derivatives. J Surg Res 2007; 142(2):314-319.
6. Rodrigues L, Banat IM, Teixeira J et al. Biosurfactants: potential applications in medicine. J Antimicrob Chemother 2006; 57(4):609-618.
7. Nitschke M, Costa SG, Contiero J. Rhamnolipid surfactants: an update on the general aspects of these remarkable biomolecules. Biotechnol Prog 2005; 21(6):1593-1600.
8. Fukuoka T, Morita T, Konishi M et al. Characterization of new glycolipid biosurfactants, tri-acylated mannosylerythritol lipids, produced by Pseudozyma yeasts. Biotechnol Lett 2007; 29(7):1111-1118.

9. Lang S, Trowitzsch-Kienast W. In: Biotenside. Stuttgart, Leipzig, Wiesbaden: B.G. Teubner GmbH, 2002.

10. Lang S. Surfactants produced by microorganisms. In: Holmberg K, ed. Novel Surfactants—Preparation, Applications and Biodegradability, 2nd ed. New York, Basel: Marcel Dekker Inc, 2003:279-315.

11. Hölzl G, Dörmann P. Structure and function of glycoglycerolipids in plants and bacteria. Prog Lipid Res 2007; 46:225-243.

12. Terasaki M, Itabashi Y. Glycolipid acyl hydrolase activity in the brown alga Cladosiphon okamuranus Tokida. Biosci Biotechnol Biochem 2003; 67(9):1986-1989.

13. Lee IA, Popov AM, Sanina NM et al. Morphological and immunological characterization of immuno-stimulatory complexes based on glycoglycerolipids from Laminaria japonica. Acta Biochim Pol 2004; 51(1):263-272.

14. Popova AV, Hincha DK. Effects of the sugar headgroup of a glycoglycerolipid on the phase behavior of phospholipid model membranes in the dry state. Glycobiology 2005; 15(11):1150-1155.

15. Rog T, Murzyn K, Gurbiel R et al. Effects of phospholipid unsaturation on the bilayer nonpolar region: a molecular simulation study. J Lipid Res 2004; 45:326-336.

16. Wu J, Long L, Song Y et al. A new unsaturated glycoglycerolipid from a cultured marine dinoflagellate Amphidinium carterae. Chem Pharm Bull 2005; 53(3):330-332.

17. Yang FL, Lu CP, Chen CS et al. Structural determination of the polar glycoglycerolipids from thermophilic bacteria Meiothermus taiwanensis. Eur J Biochem 2004; 271:4545-4551.

18. Sørensen PG, Cox RP, Miller M. Chlorosome lipids from Chlorobium tepidum: characterization and quantification of polar lipids and wax esters. Photosynth Res 2008; 95:191-196.

19. Brandenburg K, Wagner F, Müller M et al. Physicochemical characterization and biological activity of a glycoglycerolipid from Mycoplasma fermentans. J Biochem 2003; 270:3271-3279.

20. Shimizu T, Arai S, Imai H et al. Glycoglycerolipid from the membranes of Acholeplasma laidlawii binds to human immunodeficiency virus-1 (HIV-1) and accelerates its entry into cells. Curr Microbiol 2004; 48:182-188.

21. Colombo D, Compostella F, Ronchettia F et al. Inhibitory effect of stabilized analogues of glyco-glycerolipids on Epstein-Barr virus activation and mouse skin tumor promotion. Cancer Lett 2002; 186:37-41.

22. Colombo D, Frachini L, Toma L. Cyclic and branched acyl chain galactoglycerolipids and their effect on antitumor-promoting activity. Eur J Med Chem 2006; 41:1456-1463.

23. Wicke C, Hüners M, Wray V et al. Production and structure elucidation of glycoglycerolipids from a marine sponge-associated microbacterium species. J Nat Prod 2000; 63:621-626.

24. Lang S, Beil W, Tokuda H et al. Improved production of bioactive glucosylmannosyl-glycerolipid by sponge-associated Microbacterium species. Mar Biotechnol 2004; 6:152-156.

25. Ramm W, Schatton W, Wagner-Döbler I et al. Diglucosyl-glycerolipids from the marine sponge-associated Bacillus pumilus strain AAS3: their production, enzymatic modification and properties. Appl Microbiol Biotechnol 2004; 64:497-504.

26. Inada Y. Manufacture of glycerophosphorylcholine from phosphatidylcholine with modified lipase. Japanese Patent 1996; JP 63105685 A2 880510.

27. Haas MJ, Cichowicz DJ, Phillips J et al. The hydrolysis of phosphatidylcholine by an immobilized lipases: optimization of hydrolysis in organic solvents. J Am Oil Chem Soc 1993; 70:111-117.

28. Lockhoff O. Glycolipide als Immunmodulatoren—Synthesen und Eigenschaften. Angew Chem 1991; 103:1639-1649.

29. Alexander C, Rietschel ET. Bacterial lipopolysaccharides and innate immunity. J. Endotoxin 2001; 7:167-202.

30. Zughaier SM, Lindner B, Howe J et al. Physicochemical characterization and biological activity of lipooligosaccharides and lipid A from Neisseria meningitidis. J Endotoxin Res 2007; 13(6):343-357.

31. Dzieciatkowska M, Brochu D, Belkum AV et al. Mass spectrometric analysis of intact lipooligosac-charide: direct evidence for O-acetylated sialic acids and discovery of O-linked glycine expressed by Campylobacter jejuni. Biochemistry 2007; 46(50):14704-14714.

32. Leone S, Izzo V, Silipo A et al. A novel type of highly negatively charged lipooligosaccharide from Pseudomonas stutzeri OX1 possessing two 4,6-O-(1-carboxy)-ethylidene residues in the outer core region. Eur J Biochem 2004; 271(13):2691-2704.

33. Silipo A, Lanzetta R, Parrilli M et al. The complete structure of the core carbohydrate backbone from the LPS of marine halophilic bacterium Pseudoalteromonas carrageenovora type strain IAM 12662T. Carbohydr Res 2005; 340(8):1475-1482.

34. Pask-Hughes RA, Shaw N. Glycolipids from some extreme thermophilic bacteria belonging to the genus Thermus. J Bacteriol 1982; 149:54-58.

35. Esch SW, Morton MD, Williams TD et al. A novel trisaccharide glycolipid biosurfactant containing trehalose bears ester-linked hexanoate, succinate and acyloxyacyl moieties: NMR and MS characterization of the underivatized structure. Carbohydr Res 1999; 319(1-4):112-123.

36. Powalla M, Lang S, Wray V. Penta- and disaccharide lipid formation by Nocardia corynebacteroides grown on n-alkanes. Appl Microbiol Biotechnol 1989; 31:473-479.

37. Vollbrecht E, Heckmann R, Wray V et al. Production and structure elucidation of di- and oligosaccharide lipids (biosurfactants) from Tsukamurella sp. nov. Appl Microbiol Biotechnol 1998; 50:530-537.

38. Kim JS, Powalla M, Lang S et al. Microbial glycolipid production under nitrogen limitation and resting cell conditions. J Biotechnol 1990; 13(4):257-266.

39. Vollbrecht E, Rau U, Lang S. Microbial conversion of vegetable oils into surface-active di-, tri- and tetrasaccharide lipids (biosurfactants) by the bacterial strain Tsukamurella spec. Fett/Lipid 1999; 101:389-394.

40. Langer O, Palme O, Wray V et al. Production and modification of bioactive biosurfactants. Proc Biochem 2006; 41(10): 2138-2145.

41. Colombo D, Scala A, Taino IM et al. 1-O-, 2-O- and 3-O-β-glycosyl-sn-glycerols: structure-antitumor-promoting activity relationship. Bioorg Medicinal Chem Letters 1996; 6:1187-1190.

42. Colombo D, Franchini L, Toma L et al. Antitumor-promoting activity of simple models of galacto-glycerolipids with branched and unsaturated acyl chains. Eur J Medicinal Chem 2005; 40:69-74.

43. Akihisa T, Tokuda H, Yasukawa K et al. Azaphilones, furanoisophtalides and amino acids from the extracts of Monascus pilosus-fermented rice (red-mold rice) and their chemopreventive effects. J Agric Food Chem 2005; 53:562-565.

44. Fukuda Y, Sakai K, Matsunaga S et al. Cancer chemopreventive activity of lupane- and oleanane-type triterpenoids from the cones of Liquidamber styraciflua. Chem Biodivers 2005; 2:421-8.

CHAPTER 15

Production of Microbial Biosurfactants by Solid-State Cultivation

Nadia Krieger,* Doumit Camilios Neto and David Alexander Mitchell

Abstract

In recent years biosurfactants have attracted attention because of their low toxicity, biodegradability and ecological acceptability. However, their use is currently extremely limited due to their high cost in relation to that of chemical surfactants. Solid-state cultivation represents an alternative technology for biosurfactant production that can bring two important advantages: firstly, it allows the use of inexpensive substrates and, secondly, it avoids the problem of foaming that complicates submerged cultivation processes for biosurfactant production. In this chapter we show that, despite its potential, to date relatively little attention has been given to solid-state cultivation for biosurfactant production. We also note that this cultivation technique brings its own challenges, such as the selection of a bioreactor type that will allow adequate heat removal, of substrates with appropriate physico-chemical properties and of methods for monitoring of the cultivation process and recovering the biosurfactants from the fermented solid. With suitable efforts in research, solid-state cultivation can be used for large-scale production of biosurfactants.

Introduction

Surfactants are amphipathic molecules that reduce the surface tension at oil-water or air-water interfaces. They have applications in many areas, including environmental protection, petroleum production and cosmetics. The great majority of surfactants used in these applications and available on the market are produced by chemical synthesis routes. There is currently interest in replacing these chemical surfactants with surfactants of biological origin, the so-called "biosurfactants", which usually are of lower toxicity and more easily biodegradable.[1-5]

Biosurfactants have their best potential market in applications in which it is necessary to disperse tensioactive agents in the environment, for example, in the cleaning of spills of oils and other hydrophobic compounds and in the enhancement of recovery of oil from reservoirs. Beyond this, they can be used to improve the quality of oil, in the synthesis of new polymers, as additives to cosmetics and in the synthesis of bioplastics.[6-8] However, despite their potential, the use of biosurfactants in these applications is currently extremely limited, the major reason being that the cost of production of biosurfactants is very high in relation to the cost of production of chemical surfactants. As a result, there are no commercial large-scale processes for biosurfactant production.[9] It will be necessary to reduce production costs significantly before biosurfactants can find widespread use.

Most research into the production of biosurfactants has been undertaken using submerged cultivation of the producing microorganism. However, this production method creates serious problems with foam formation. Solid-state cultivation is an alternative method for the production of microbiological products that has the potential to avoid these problems. However, there has

*Corresponding Author: Nadia Krieger—Chemistry Department, Federal University of Parana, PO Box 19081, Curitiba 81531-990, PR Brazil. Email: nkrieger@ufpr.br

Biosurfactants, edited by Ramkrishna Sen. ©2010 Landes Bioscience and Springer Science+Business Media.

been relatively little research into the production of biosurfactants by solid-state cultivation and, further, this cultivation technique has its own challenges.

In this chapter we explore the potential advantages that solid-state cultivation technology can bring to the production of biosurfactants. We show that a relatively small amount of work has been done in this area and outline future investigations that will need to be undertaken.

Microbial Biosurfactants That It Would Be Interesting to Produce at Large Scale

A variety of microorganisms can produce biosurfactants. Biosurfactants are generally produced as a mixture of compounds of the same chemical group ("congeners" or "chemical homologues"). The composition of the mixture depends on the strain of microorganism and on the conditions under which it is cultivated and may affect the physicochemical properties of the biosurfactant.

According to Zajic and Seffens,[10] biosurfactants can be classified in five major groups: (1) glycolipids; (2) lipopolysaccharides; (3) lipopeptides; (4) phospholipids; (5) fatty acids and neutral lipids. Each group of biosurfactants presents distinct physicochemical properties and specific physiological functions, the majority being constituted by different hydrophilic and hydrophobic moieties. Most biosurfactants are anionic or neutral, but some are cationic, as is the case of those that contain amino-groups. The hydrophobic moiety can be formed by long-chain fatty acids, hydroxy-fatty acids or by α-alkyl-β-hydroxy-fatty acids, while the hydrophilic portion of the molecule is composed of carbohydrates, amino acids, cyclic peptides, phosphate, carboxylic acids or alcohols.[11]

To date most interest in developing processes for the production of microbial biosurfactants has focused on glycolipids and lipopeptides. In the case of glycolipids, there have been studies into the production of rhamnolipids by *Pseudomonas aeruginosa*, of sophorolipids by *Candida bombicola* and of mannosylerythritol lipids by *Pseudozyma* (previously *Candida*) *antarctica*.[6] In the case of lipopeptides, there has been interest in the use of strains of *Bacillus* to produce molecules like surfactin, iturin and fengycin.[6] Since these biosurfactants (at least the general family types) have been covered in other chapters of this book, we will not discuss their properties in any detail. The important point, which will be relevant in terms of the solid-state cultivation production technology, is that they are produced by unicellular, aerobic organisms.

Production of Biosurfactants by Classical Submerged Cultivation Is Problematic

The great majority of studies into the production of biosurfactants uses submerged cultivation. This is also the case in the few small scale production processes that exist, such as the production of the lipopeptide biosurfactant of *Bacillus subtilis,* Surfactin (Sigma-Aldrich Co.).

The microorganisms typically used for the production of biosurfactants are aerobic organisms. Therefore submerged cultivation processes are conducted with forced aeration and agitation. However, this creates a serious problem when the biosurfactant starts to be produced because large quantities of foam are produced.[12-14] This foaming has several deleterious effects. Firstly, there is a tendency for the microorganism to accumulate within the foam, thereby removing cells from the culture medium.[13,14] Secondly, the presence of the foam reduces the efficiency of gas transfer between the gas and liquid phases in the bioreactor, reducing the rates of supply of oxygen to the liquid and removal of carbon dioxide from it. Thirdly, the foaming is typically so severe that the foam tends to leave the headspace through any available orifice. This not only represents a loss of cells from the system but also greatly increases the risk of contamination of the bioreactor.

Two main strategies have been used to combat the problem of foaming during the production of biosurfactants in submerged cultivation: the addition of antifoaming agents and mechanical breakage of the foam. However, neither solution is particulary attractive. The addition of anti-foaming agents brings three disadvantages:[13,14] Firstly, the most efficient antifoaming agents are organic mixtures based on polypropylene or polymers derived from silicone and these are relatively expensive. Secondly, antifoaming agents decrease the efficiency of oxygen and carbon dioxide transfer between the gas and liquid phases and may even be toxic to the microorganism. Thirdly, antifoaming agents represent a "chemical contaminant" that must be later separated from the biosurfactant during downstream processing.

Mechanical devices for breaking the foam may be internal or external to the bioreactor. Internal devices include foam-breakers in the headspace of the bioreactor (typically mounted on the agitator shaft). However, such foam breakers are not effective when large quantities of foam are produced, as is the case in biosurfactant production processes. It is therefore necessary to install external devices in which the foam is collapsed. The cells and medium removed by the foam can then be recycled back to the bioreactor. However, such systems must operate aseptically and make the construction and operation of the bioreactor significantly more expensive.[13,15,16]

Solid-State Cultivation as an Alternative Cultivation Technique with Potential for Biosurfactant Production

In the face of the problems with biosurfactant production in submerged cultivation, solid-state cultivation is an interesting alternative.

Solid-state cultivation involves the growth of microorganisms on moist organic solid particles, within beds in which there is a continuous gas phase between the particles.[17] The majority of water in the system is absorbed within the solid particles. There is relatively little free liquid water in the interparticle spaces, being limited to a thin film on the surface of the particles and possibly a few small droplets. This "architecture" of the system in solid-state cultivation avoids the foaming problem that plagues submerged cultivation processes for biosurfactant production. Even though in some bioreactors air is blown forcefully through the bed, since the air passes through the interparticle spaces and is not sparged through a liquid containing biosurfactant, foam does not form in the first place.

The difference in system architecture also has an important consequence for the design of large-scale bioreactors. Typically the major consideration in the design of bioreactors for aerobic submerged cultivation processes is the maintenance of sufficiently high rates of gas-to-liquid mass transfer, in order to maintain an acceptably high dissolved oxygen concentration. In the case of solid-state cultivation processes the major consideration is the maintenance of sufficiently high rates of heat removal, in order to maintain the temperature of the substrate bed as close as possible to the optimal temperature for growth and product formation. However, in other respects, solid-state cultivation processes are similar to submerged cultivation processes. In other words, there is a need for upstream processes, including the production of a suitable inoculum and substrate preparation, and downstream processes, including product recovery, purification and waste disposal.

What Is the State of the Art of Biosurfactant Production in Solid-State Cultivation?

Despite the potential advantages that solid-state cultivation has for the production of biosurfactants, there has been relatively little effort to develop processes. The earliest work was done by Ohno et al.[18-22] In fact, their aim was not actually to produce biosurfactant, but rather to produce compounds with antibiotic activity against phytopathogens: They isolated strains of *Bacillus subtilis* that produced the cyclic lipopeptides iturin A and surfactin, these cyclic peptides having both antibiotic activity and surfactant properties. The majority of their studies were undertaken in Erlenmeyer flasks, although they did undertake one study in which in which 3 kg of *okara* (a residue of the manufacture of tofu) was placed in an 8-litre jar. This jar was placed in a waterbath and "air was supplied through silicon-rubber tubing connected to a compressor".[22] No more detail is presented than this, so it is not possible to determine whether the bed would have been aerated effectively. In fact it is not even made clear whether the tubing was placed in such a manner that the air was forced to cross the bed in order to leave the jar. In any case, temperature control in this "jar bioreactor" was very poor: despite the fact that the waterbath was maintained at 23°C, the temperature within the jar rose to 45°C. In fact, it should be noted that *okara* does not have properties that suit it well to the realization of large-scale solid-state cultivation processes in bioreactors. It has quite a small particle size and a tendency to form a paste at high water contents.

Later, Veenadig et al[12] studied the production of surfactants by *Bacillus subtilis* cultivated on wheat bran. In these studies they did not identify the particular biosurfactant produced, nor did they use specific analytical methods like HPLC. Rather, they analyzed the performance of their cultivations in terms of the emulsifying activity and the reduction in surface tension provoked by samples removed during the cultivation. The packed bed was a stainless steel column of 15 cm diameter and 34.5 cm height. Samples from the packed-bed were removed from a sampling orifice at 17 cm bed height. Note that since gradients are typical of packed-bed bioreactors, these samples did not give a clear picture about what was happening in the bioreactor as a whole. In one study they investigated the effect of the aeration rate used during the cultivation, over the range of 10 to 20 L/min. The surface tension measured when samples removed from the bed were added to water was lower for the higher air flow rates. In other words, the samples corresponding to the higher air flow rates provoked greater reductions in surface tension. Pure water has a surface tension of 72 dynes/cm. Samples removed at the beginning of the cultivations reduced the surface tension to around 55 dynes/cm. For the aeration rate of 10 L/min, the samples removed during the cultivation were not able to reduce the surface tension to values below 50 dynes/cm. On the other hand, a sample removed at 55 h from the packed bed operated with an aeration rate of 20 L/min was able to reduce the surface tension to a value as low as 24 dynes/cm. Veenadig et al[12] also evaluated the performance of flask cultivations. Over the first 30 h the surface tensions obtained with samples removed from the flasks were quite similar to these obtained in the packed bed with an aeration rate at 20 L/min (the surface tension measured when the samples were added to water fell from an initial value of 55 dynes/cm to values of around 35 dynes/cm for the 30 h sample). Longer cultivation times did not lead to lower surface tensions.

More recently, Das and Mukherjee[23] studied the production of lipopeptide biosurfactants by two thermophilic strains of *Bacillus subtilis*. The substrate used was waste potato peels, which were washed, blanched (80°C), dried, ground, redried and then autoclaved. Both submerged cultivation and solid-state cultivation were studied; in both cases the experiments were done in Erlenmeyer flasks. In the case of submerged cultivation the potato peel was added at a concentration of 2% (m/v) to a mineral salt medium. In the case of solid-state cultivation 2 mL of this mineral salt medium was added per 5 g of ground potato peels. The comparison between submerged and solid-state cultivation was undertaken on the basis of the amount of biosurfactant produced per gram of dry solids. On this basis the levels of biosurfactant produced were reasonably similar in the two systems, for the better-producing strain being 80 mg per gram of dry solids for submerged cultivation and 67 mg per gram of dry solids for solid-state cultivation. These values were increased to 102 and 92 mg per gram of dry solids, respectively, when glucose was added to the mineral salts medium (at a level of 0.5% m/v).

In our own work we have produced rhamnolipids by *Pseudomonas aeruginosa* in solid-state cultivation.[24] In this case sugar cane bagasse was used as a support material and was impregnated with a solution containing mineral salts and glycerol. Cultures were undertaken in Erlenmeyer flasks. Rhamnolipids were extracted from the fermented solid and quantified in terms of the amount of rhamnose produced. The performance of the solid-state cultivation was compared with that of a submerged culture done in Erlenmeyer flasks (note that the bacterium was also cultivated within a bioreactor but, as soon as rhamnolipid production started, the foaming problem was so severe that all the liquid was lost from the bioreactor in a short space of time). The comparison was done on the basis of the amount of rhamnolipids produced per volume of nutrient solution. In the case of submerged culture, this was the total volume of nutrient solution in the flask. In the case of solid-state cultivation, this was the amount of nutrient solution added to the sugar cane bagasse. Production was similar in both systems, reaching 1.6 g of rhamnose per litre at 144 h, corresponding to a level of 8.0 g per kg of dry fermented substrate.[25] We are undertaking further studies with the aim of improving the productivity of the solid-state cultivation system.

What Challenges Do We Face in the Production of Biosurfactants by Solid-State Cultivation?

From the previous section, it is clear that much remains to be done in the development of solid-state cultivation systems for the production of biosurfactants. Many different issues will need to be addressed. Some of the most important ones are discussed in the following subsections. The discussion presented in these subsections is quite concise. Anyone with an interest in developing a large-scale solid-state cultivation system and who does not have an in-depth understanding of the technology is strongly advised to read the book of solid-state cultivation bioreactors of Mitchell et al.[17]

Bioreactor Selection

What will be the best type of bioreactor to use for the production of biosurfactants? Mitchell et al[17] discuss in depth the various types of bioreactors available for solid-state cultivation but, in a simple analysis, we might consider the following "typical" bioreactors:

   i. Tray or bag systems. In these bioreactors a relatively thin layer of substrate is contained within a tray or a plastic bag. Each tray or bag contains several kilograms of substrate. A large number of trays and bags is placed in a room and conditioned air is circulated around the tray but is not blown forcefully through the bed. The substrate may be left untouched or may be mixed daily by hand. Note that laboratory studies in Erlenmeyer flasks, such as those undertaken by Das and Mukherjee[23] and Krieger et al,[24] correspond to this kind of system.

   ii. Rotating drums. In these bioreactors a horizontal drum is filled to about 20 to 30% of its volume with the substrate and then rotated continuously to agitate the bed. Conditioned air is blown into the headspace of the drum but is not forced through the bed itself.

   iii. Packed-beds. In these bioreactors the substrate sits on a perforated base plate in a column. Air is blown forcefully through the bed. Typically the bed is not agitated; however, it is possible to have infrequent mixing. Note that while the bed is static significant temperature and moisture gradients can occur within it[17] and that this can lead to significant gradients in growth and product formation. However, the few authors who have studied biosurfactant production in packed-bed bioreactors have not addressed this issue.[12,26]

   iv. Agitated and aerated bioreactors. These bioreactors may be of various different designs but are characterized by the fact that agitation is continuous or frequent and that air is blown forcefully through the bed.

The major considerations in choosing a bioreactor for a particular process are the capital and operating costs and the effectiveness of heat removal and moisture control while minimizing damage to the microorganism. We can expect heat removal to be a significant challenge: Bacteria tend to grow reasonably fast, so we can expect high rates of production of waste metabolic heat. In bioreactors other than tray/bag bioreactors the air stream plays a major role in heat removal, since at large scale removal of heat from solid beds to water jackets or cooling coils is not efficient. Therefore we can expect that aeration rates will be determined by cooling requirements and not by oxygen requirements. In other words, the aeration rates required for cooling will be more than sufficient to provide oxygen to the particle surface.[17]

We might expect processes for biosurfactant production to be quite large (for example, based on our own results, 100 metric tons of rhamnolipid biosurfactant would require of the order of 10000 metric tons of fermented substrate). Although it is not impossible to operate tray systems at this scale, it would probably be more cost effective to use other bioreactor types. Note that the majority of solid-state cultivation processes involve filamentous fungi and the damage caused to fungal hyphae when a bed is mixed is often an important consideration in selecting a bioreactor and operating mode. In the case of biosurfactants, the most interesting processes involve bacteria, which are much less susceptible to mechanical damage in an agitated bed of solids. In this case, it is quite probable that "agitated and aerated bioreactors" will be the most appropriate, as these allow the most efficient heat removal, facilitate the addition of water (it can be sprayed as a fine mist onto the bed surface during agitation) and maintain relatively homogeneous conditions throughout the bed.

What Will Be the Best Substrate to Use?

Will it be possible to use oil-rich meals as the solid substrates? If so, this could reduce substrate costs significantly. However, it needs to be demonstrated whether high yields will be obtained on such substrates or not. The strategy of simply absorbing a nutrient medium used in liquid culture onto a solid support, the strategy used by Krieger et al,[24] should also be considered.

Note that it will not be sufficient to prove that a particular substrate (and the method of preparing it, such as chopping or grinding etc.) promotes high yields in laboratory scale studies. It will also be important to ensure that any such substrate is "well-behaved" within a bioreactor. This means that:

- The substrate is not so sticky that it will produce a cohesive mass when it is agitated within a bioreactor. If this happens, then the bed will lack interparticle spaces for the flow of air (which is important for supplying oxygen). In the case of biosurfactants this is an important consideration, since oils or glycerol will quite often be present in the substrate in order to act as an inducer of biosurfactant production and can increase the cohesiveness of the particles.
- The substrate at the bottom of the bed will not compact under the weight of overlying substrate. If this happens, the interparticle spaces in this region will disappear.
- The particle size is not so fine that it provokes high pressure drops when air is blown forcefully through the bed.

Note that it is not sufficient to characterize the original substrate. The properties of the substrate can change significantly during the cultivation.

Downstream Processing

It is interesting to consider whether the solid might be used directly in some applications at the end of the process. For example, it is conceivable that the solids could be mixed in with soil during bioremediation treatments. In this case all that would be necessary would be to dry the solids.

For those processes in which it is desired to extract the biosurfactant from the solids, it will be necessary to determine the most efficient extraction method. Several issues need to be addressed. Firstly, what extraction method should be used? Krieger et al[24] extracted the rhamnolipid biosurfactant of *Pseudomonas aeruginosa* with water and then undertook a liquid-liquid extraction into chloroform. Possibly liquid extraction is the most feasible method, but work still needs to be done to determine the best solvent system. Secondly, in what mode should an extraction system be operated? Will batch extraction be sufficiently efficient, or will it be necessary to use a counter-current extraction system? Obviously at large scale it will be necessary to recover and recycle the solvent. Note that these issues have received some attention for other products of solid-state cultivation processes, such as enzymes, but not for biosurfactants.[27] Supercritical fluid extraction is also a possibility. It has been studied for recovery of other types of products from the solids at the end of solid-state cultivation processes, but has not been studied for the recovery of biosurfactants.

In the case that the biosurfactant is extracted from the solids, it is important to consider what will be done with the residual solids. In our laboratory we have used sugar cane bagasse in up to four sequential cultivations, without significant loss of process productivity. However, this strategy may have worked due to the fact that the function of the bagasse is to provide an inert solid support. It might not be successful when the nutrients for growth are provided by the original solid substrate.

Note that there is another potential use for the residual solids. The addition of biosurfactants has been shown to enhance the production of some enzymes in solid-state cultivation.[28] Possibly solids from which the biosurfactant has been extracted could be used as a substrate or at least a solid support (with the addition of an impregnating nutrient solution) for a subsequent process for enzyme production.

Monitoring of the Cultivation Process

There are some important issues to be addressed as to how to monitor a solid-state cultivation process for the production of biosurfactant.

Determination of microbial growth in solid-state cultivation systems is not straightforward. This is especially the case in processes involving filamentous fungi, since the fungal hyphae typically penetrate into the substrate, forming a tight association between the biomass and residual substrate, making it impossible to separate and determine the dry mass of biomass. In biosurfactant-producing processes that involve bacteria, there is the possibility of dislodging the bacteria from the solids and trying to determine their amount or number in some manner. However, at best this is likely to give only a coarse indication of growth, since recovery of cells is likely to be partial and solid matter may also be extracted from the residual solid substrate. Note that for the purpose of deciding how to design and operate the bioreactor it is probably more important to characterize the oxygen uptake kinetics than to put a lot of effort into measuring the biomass itself.[17] This is because heat production is directly related with oxygen consumption and heat removal is one of the major factors guiding bioreactor design and operation.

Various methods can be used to monitor biosurfactant production during the process. It is of course possible to remove reasonably large samples and extract the biosurfactant in the same manner as one would in a preparative process. However, it will probably also be possible to develop HPLC methods to monitor the levels of biosurfactants, although this may be complicated by the fact that some biosurfactants are not pure compounds but rather mixtures of congeners. Some authors have monitored the process by adding samples of the fermented solids to water and determining the reduction of surface tension. However, this is an extremely coarse method that does not give a real indication of the amount of biosurfactant. The surface tension measured in these assays tends to fall sharply to a certain value (which corresponds to the surface tension at the critical micellar concentration of the biosurfactant) early in the process and then to remain constant at this value despite the fact that the real biosurfactant level, as measured by some other method, is still increasing significantly.

Conclusion

Solid-state cultivation is an interesting technique for the production of biosurfactants and might make commercial production processes economically viable. However, there is an urgent need to undertake the studies to improve production and to demonstrate the feasibility of processes at pilot scale.

Acknowledgements

Nadia Krieger and David Mitchell thank CNPq, a Brazilian agency of the advancement of science and technology, for research scholarships. Doumit Camilios Neto thanks CAPES, a Brazilian agency for the capacitation of researchers, for a doctoral scholarship. The authors are grateful to CNPq and the company Corn Products Brazil for financing their work in the area of biosurfactants.

References

1. Karanth NGK, Deo PG, Veenanadig NK. Microbial production of biosurfactants and their Importance. Curr Sci 1999; 77:116-126.
2. Makkar RS, Cameotra SS. An update on the use of unconventional substrates for biosurfactant production and their new applications. App Microbiol Biotechnol 2002; 58:428-434.
3. Nitschke M, Costa SGVAO, Contiero J. Rhamnolipid surfactants: Na update on the general aspects of these remarkable biomolecules. Biotechnol Progr 2005; 21:1593-1600.
4. Nitschke M, Costa SGVAO, Haddad R et al. Oil waste as unconventional substrate for rhamnolipid biosurfactant production by Pseudomonas aeruginosa LBI. Biotechnol Progr 2005; 21:1562-1566.
5. Costa SGVAO, Nitschke M, Haddad R et al. Production of Pseudomonas aeruginosa LBI rhamnolipids following growth on Brazilian native oils. Process Biochem 2006; 41:483-488.
6. Lang S. Biological amphiphiles (microbial biosurfactants). Curr Opin Colloid Interface Sci 2002; 7:12-20.

7. Batista SB. Bactérias de ambientes contaminados com petróleo ou derivados produtoras de surfactantes e emulsificantes. Dissertation, Universidade Federal de Viçosa 2002;1-32.
8. Kosaric N, Cairns WL, Gray NCC. Introduction: Biotechnology and the surfactant industry. In: Kosaric N, Cairns WL, eds. Biosurfactants and Biotechnology. New York: M Dekker, 1987:163-181.
9. Mukherjee S, Das P, Sen R. Towards commercial production of microbial surfactants. Trends Biotechnol 2006; 24:509-515.
10. Zajic JE, Seffens W. Biosurfactants. Crit Revi Biotechnol 1984; 1:87-107.
11. Jacobucci DFC. Estudo da influência de biosurfactantes na biorremediação de efluentes oleosos. Dissertation, Universidade Estadual de Campinas 2000;1-117.
12. Veenanadig NK, Gowthaman MK, Karanth NGK. Scale up studies for the production of biosurfactant in packed column bioreactor. Bioprocess Eng 2000; 22:95-99.
13. Lee BS, Kim EK. Lipopeptide production from Bacillus sp. GB16 using a novel oxygenation method. Enzyme Microb Technol 2004; 35:639-647.
14. Yeh MS, Wei TH, Chang JS. Bioreactor design for enhanced carrier-assisted surfactin production with Bacillus subtilis. Process Biochem 2006; 41:1799-1805.
15. Deshpande NS, Barigou M. Performance characteristics of novel mechanical foam breakers in a stirred tank reactor. J Chem Tech Biotechnol 1999; 74:979-987.
16. Vadar-Sukan F. Foaming: Consequences, prevention and destruction. Biotechnol Adv 1998; 16:913-948.
17. Mitchell DA, Krieger N, Berovic M. Solid-state fermentation bioreactors: Fundamentals of design and operation. Heidelberg: Springer 2006:1-450.
18. Ohno A, Ano T, Shoda M. Production of antifungal antibiotic, iturin in a solid state fermentation by Bacillus subtilis NB22 using wheat bran as a substrate. Biotechnol Lett 1992; 14:817-822.
19. Ohno A, Ano T, Shoda M. Production of the antifungal peptide antibiotic, iturin by Bacillus subtilis NB22 in solid state fermentation. J Ferment Bioeng 1993; 75:23-27.
20. Ohno A, Ano T, Shoda M. Production of a Lipopeptide Antibiotic, Surfactin, by Recombinant Bacillus subtilis in solid state fermentation. Biotechnol Bioeng 1995; 47:209-214.
21. Ohno A, Ano T, Shoda M. Effect of temperature on production of lipopeptide antibiotics, iturin A and surfactin by a dual producer, Bacillus subtilis RB14, in solid-stage fermentation. J Ferment Bioeng 1995; 80:517-519.
22. Ohno A, Ano T, Shoda M. Use of soybean curd residue, okara, for the solid state substrate in the production of a lipopeptide antibiotic, Iturin A, by Bacillus subtilis NB22 Process Biochem 1996; 31:801-806.
23. Das K, Mukherjee AK. Comparison of lipopeptide biosurfactants production by bacillus subtilis strains in submerged and solid state fermentation systems using a cheap carbon some industrial applications of biosurfactants. Process Biochem 2007; 42:1191-1199.
24. Krieger N, Mitchell DA, Camilios Neto D et al. Inventors; Universidade federal do paraná (UFPR), assignee. Produção de ramnolipídeos por fermentação em estado sólido. Patent 2007:PI0701366-3.
25. Meira JA. Produção de biosurfactantes por fermentação no estado sólido e desenvolvimento de aplicações para tratamento de solos contaminados por hidrocarbonetos. Dissertation, Universidade Federal do Paraná 2007;1-94.
26. Martins VG, Kalil SJ, Bertolin TE et al. Solid state biosurfactant production in a fixed-bed column bioreactor. Z Naturforsch C 2006; 61:721-726.
27. Lonsane BK, Kriahnaiah MM. Product leaching and downstream processing. In: Doelle HW, Mitchell DA, Rolz CE, eds. Solid State Cultivation. London: Elsevier, 1992:147-171.
28. Kristensen JB, Börjesson J, Bruun MH et al. Use of surface active additives in enzymatic hydrolysis of wheat straw lignocelluloses. Enzyme Microb Technol 2007; 40:888-895.

CHAPTER 16

Rhamnolipid Biosurfactants:
Production and Their Potential in Environmental Biotechnology

Orathai Pornsunthorntawee, Panya Wongpanit and Ratana Rujiravanit*

Abstract

Certain species of *Pseudomonas* are able to produce and excrete a heterogeneous mixture of biosurfactants with a glycolipid structure. These are known as rhamnolipids. In the biosynthetic process, rhamnolipid production is governed by both the genetic regulatory system and central metabolic pathways involving fatty acid synthesis, activated sugars and enzymes. These surface-active compounds can be produced from various types of low-cost substrates, such as carbohydrates, vegetable oils and even industrial wastes, leading to a good potential for commercial exploitation. By controlling environmental factors and growth conditions, high rhamnolipid production yields can be achieved. Rhamnolipids provide good physicochemical properties in terms of surface activities, stabilities and emulsification activities. Moreover, these surface-active compounds exhibit antimicrobial activities against both phytopathogenic fungi and bacteria. Due to an increase in concerns about environmental protection and the distinguishing properties of the rhamnolipids, it seems that rhamnolipids meet the criteria for several industrial and environmental applications, such as environmental remediation and biological control. Rhamnolipids have already been commercially produced, making them more economically competitive with synthetic surfactants. In the near future, rhamnolipids may be commercially successful biosurfactants.

Introduction

Surfactants, or surface active agents, can be classified into two main groups: synthetic surfactants and biosurfactants. Synthetic surfactants are produced by organic chemical reactions, while biosurfactants are produced by biological processes, being excreted extracellularly by microorganisms such as bacteria, fungi and yeast. When compared to synthetic surfactants, biosurfactants have several advantages, including high biodegradability, low toxicity, low irritancy and compatibility with human skin.[1,2] Due to these superior characteristics, biosurfactants have shown potential use in petroleum, petrochemical, food, cosmetics and pharmaceutical industries.[3] Nowadays, an increase in concerns about environmental protection has led to the consideration of biosurfactants as alternatives to synthetic surfactants and the development of cost-effective bioprocesses for the biosurfactant production is of great interest.[4-9] By the year 2010, it is predicted that biosurfactants will perhaps capture about 10% of the surfactant market, reaching US$ 200 million in sales.[10]

Synthetic surfactants are usually categorized according to the nature of their polar head group; however, biosurfactants are commonly differentiated based on the types of biosurfactant-producing microbial species and the nature of their chemical structures. Major classes of biosurfactants include

*Corresponding Author: Ratana Rujiravanit—The Petroleum and Petrochemical College, Chulalongkorn University, Bangkok 10330, Thailand. Email: ratana.r@chula.ac.th

Biosurfactants, edited by Ramkrishna Sen. ©2010 Landes Bioscience and Springer Science+Business Media.

lipopeptides and lipoproteins, glycolipids, phospholipids and polymeric surfactants.[11] Most of these compounds are either non-ionic or anionic. Only a few are cationic, such as those containing amine groups. Normally, the hydrophobic parts of biosurfactant molecules contain long-chain fatty acids, hydroxyl fatty acids, or α-alkyl-β-hydroxy fatty acids, while the hydrophilic parts can be carbohydrates, carboxylic acids, amino acids, cyclic peptides, phosphates, or alcohols.[12] The critical micelle concentrations (CMCs) of biosurfactants are found to be in the range of 1-200 mg/l and their molecular weights generally range from 500 to 1500 amu.[13]

One of the most common biosurfactants that has been isolated and studied is the glycolipids, which are composed of carbohydrates in combination with long-chain aliphatic acids or hydroxyl aliphatic acids. From the point of view of surfactant properties, one of the best examples of glycolipids is rhamnolipids produced by certain species of *Pseudomonas*.[2] In general, rhamnolipids— rhamnose-containing glycolipid biosurfactants—are excreted as a heterogeneous mixture of several homologues. With the use of modern analytical methods, such as liquid chromatography (LC) and mass spectrometry (MS), the chemical structure of each homologue in the mixture can be elucidated. Rhamnolipids show good physicochemical properties and biological activities. Although these surface-active compounds have potential use in several applications, most of the research has been focused on environmental remediation. Rhamnolipids can be produced from various types of low-cost substrates and high production yields can be achieved by controlling environmental factors and growth conditions. Therefore, rhamnolipids represent one of the most effective biosurfactants for commercial exploitation.

Chemical Structures and Properties of Rhamnolipid Biosurfactants

Pseudomonas strains, Gram-negative bacteria, have been reported to excrete rhamnolipids beginning in 1949.[14] Although there are many types of rhamnolipid species, all of them possess similar chemical structures.[15] Normally, rhamnolipids contain a hydrophilic head formed by one or two rhamnose molecules and a hydrophobic tail that contains one or two fatty acid chains.[16] Figure 1 shows the four general chemical structures of rhamnolipids produced by certain species of *Pseudomonas*. The two major types of rhamnolipids are L-rhamnosyl-3-hydroxydecanoyl-3-hydroxydecanoate, or monorhamnolipid (Rha–C_{10}–C_{10}) and L-rhamnosyl-L-rhamnosyl-3-hydroxydecanoyl-3-hydroxydecanoate, or dirhamnolipid (Rha–Rha–C_{10}–C_{10}); however, most of the biosurfactants produced by *Pseudomonas aeruginosa* strains are dirhamnolipid.[17,18] Only a few reports show that monorhamnolipid is the predominant component.[19,20] The difference in types and proportion of rhamnolipids in the mixture might result from the age of the culture, bacterial strains,[21] specific culture conditions and substrate composition.[22]

To fractionate and characterize the types of rhamnolipids in the mixture, a number of analytical methods can be used. In the past, high performance liquid chromatography (HPLC)

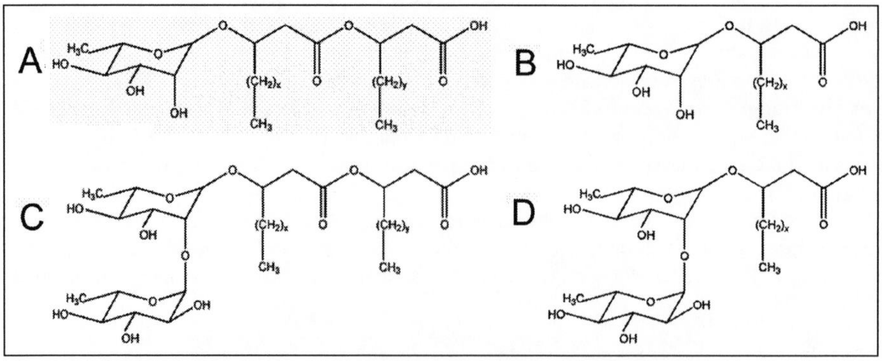

Figure 1. The four general chemical structures of rhamnolipid biosurfactants produced by certain species of *Pseudomonas*.

equipped with a photodiode array detector or UV detector[23-25] and gas chromatography/ mass spectrometry (GC/MS)[25,26] were the most widely-used techniques; however, they are time-consuming and do not provide reliable quantification analysis. Recently, HPLC equipped with an evaporative light scattering detector (ELSD)[27,28] and liquid chromatography/mass spectrometry (LC/MS)[21,29-31] were developed as efficient techniques for the analysis of the rhamnolipid species. To identify the chemical structures of rhamnolipids, Fourier transform infrared (FT-IR) spectroscopy[32] and nuclear magnetic resonance (NMR) analysis[8,32,33] were also performed. Today, nearly 30 rhamnolipid species, which differ in fatty acid chain composition and rhamnose moieties, have been reported.

Rhamnolipids exhibit free carboxylic groups and act as anions when the pH is above 4.0.[10] These surface-active compounds are soluble in methanol, chloroform, ethyl ether and an alkaline aqueous solution.[13] Rhamnolipids reduce the surface tension of pure water from 72 to below 30 mN/m, with a CMC in the range of 5-200 mg/l, depending on the components in the mixture.[34] The presence of longer fatty acid chains probably increases hydrophobicity of the molecules, leading to the formation of the micellar structure at lower concentration.[25] Table 1 summarizes the rhamnolipid compositions and surface activities of the biosurfactants produced by some *Pseudomonas* strains. It has also been found that rhamnolipids are able to retain their surface activities even under extreme conditions of temperature and pH.[32]

Table 1. *Rhamnolipid compositions and surface activities of biosurfactants produced by different* **Pseudomonas** *strains**

Strain	Chemical Structure		ST (mN/m)	CMC (mg/l)	Ref.
AT10	Rha-C_{10}-C_{10}	Rha-$C_{8:2}$	26.8	120.0	6
	Rha-C_{10}-C_{12}	Rha-Rha-C_{10}-C_{10}			
	Rha-$C_{12:1}$-C_{10}	Rha-Rha-C_{10}-C_{12}			
	Rha-$C_{12:2}$				
SP4	Rha-C_{10}-C_{10}	Rha-C_{12}-C_{10}	29.0	200.0	32
	Rha-C_{10}-C_8	Rha-Rha-C_{10}-C_8			
	Rha-C_8-C_{10}	Rha-Rha-C_8-C_{10}			
	Rha-C_{10}-$C_{12:1}$	Rha-Rha-C_{10}-$C_{14:1}$			
	Rha-$C_{12:1}$-C_{10}	Rha-Rha-$C_{12:1}$-C_{12}			
	Rha-C_{10}-C_{12}				
DAUPE 614	Rha-C_{10}-C_{10}	Rha-Rha-C_{10}-C_{10}	27.3	13.9	33
	Rha-C_{10}-C_8	Rha-Rha-C_{10}-C_8			
	Rha-C_8-C_{10}	Rha-Rha-C_8-C_{10}			
	Rha-C_{10}-$C_{12:1}$	Rha-Rha-C_{10}-$C_{12:1}$			
	Rha-C_{12}-C_{10}	Rha-Rha-C_{12}-C_{10}			
	Rha-C_{10}-C_{12}	Rha-Rha-C_{10}-C_{12}			
LBI	Rha-C_{10}-C_{10}	Rha-Rha-C_{10}	23.0	120.0	36
	Rha-C_{10}-$C_{12:1}$	Rha-Rha-C_{10}-$C_{12:1}$			
	Rha-C_{10}-C_{12}				

*ST: surface tension; CMC: critical micelle concentration.

Another topic of interest related to the physicochemical properties of rhamnolipids is their emulsification activity. From the reported works, rhamnolipids produced from different *Pseudomonas* strains can effectively emulsify and stabilize emulsions with various types of hydrocarbons and oils. Wei et al found that the biosurfactant produced by *Pseudomonas aeruginosa* J4 achieved a maximum emulsion index of 70 and 78% for diesel and kerosene, respectively.[8] Benincasa et al also reported that the biosurfactant produced by *Pseudomonas aeruginosa* LBI could form stable emulsions with *i*-propyl palmitate, castor oil, almond oil, crude oil, kerosene and benzene for 21 days, suggesting potential applications of the excreted rhamnolipids in the pharmaceutical and cosmetic industries and environmetal pollution treatment.[31] Pornsunthorntawee et al found that the biosurfactant produced by *Pseudomonas aeruginosa* SP4 was able to emulsify various types of vegetable oils, including palm oil, soybean oil, coconut oil and olive oil, indicating its potential use as an emulsifying agent in the food industry.[32] Stable emulsions of *n*-alkanes and aromatic compounds have also been reported; however, the emulsification activity of rhamnolipids was found to depend on the carbon sources used in the biosurfactant production.[35]

Besides their good physicochemical properties, rhamnolipids provide interesting biological activities, including antimicrobial activity against phytopathogenic fungi species and bacteria. Abalos et al reported that rhamnolipids produced by *Pseudomonas aeruginosa* AT10 showed antifungal properties against *Gliocadium virens*, *Penicillium chrysogeum*, *Aspergillus niger*, *Chaetonium globosum*, *Aureobasidium pullulans*, *Rhizotecnia solani* and *Botrytis cinerea*.[6] The biosurfactant produced by *Pseudomonas aeruginosa* LBI was found to be active against various phytopathogenic fungi species, such as *Penicillium funiculosum* and *Alternaria alternate*.[31] Stipcevic et al found that dirhamnolipid showed differential effects on human keratinocyte and fibroblast cultures, leading to the enhancement of the burn-wound healing process.[37,38] Thanomsub et al reported that rhamnolipids produced by *Pseudomonas aeruginosa* B189 displayed significant antiproliferative activity against the human breast cancer cell line MCF-7 and the insect cell line C6/36, showing potential application as anticancer drugs or agrochemicals.[26]

Biosynthesis of Rhamnolipid Biosurfactants

When cultivated in a liquid medium, *Pseudomonas* strains excrete mainly two types of rhamnolipids: mono-rhamnolipid and di-rhamnolipid. In the biosynthetic pathway of these two surface-active compounds, the rhamnosyl moiety and the fatty acid moiety are produced by de novo synthesis.[10] The donor of the rhamnosyl moiety is activated sugar, known as deoxy-thymidine-diphospho-L-rhamnose (dTDP-L-rhamnnose).[39,40] To produce a rhamnosyl donor, D-glucose-1-phosphate is firstly synthesized by the specific reaction catalyzed by the AlgC enzyme. The production of dTDP-L-rhamnnose, which involves four sequential reactions catalyzed by the enzymes encoded by the *rml* genes, subsequently occurs.[41] The synthesis of the fatty acid moiety of rhamnolipids is governed by the RhlG enzyme, which is responsible for draining the fatty acid precursors of rhamnolipids from the general fatty acid synthetic pathway at the level of the ketoacyl reduction.[42] The biosynthesis of rhamnolipids proceeds by two sequential reactions catalyzed by the two specific rhamnosyltranferases—Rt 1 and Rt 2. The Rt 1 enzyme contains two polypeptides encoded by the *rhlA* and *rhlB* genes,[41] while the Rt 2 enzyme is encoded by the *rhlC* gene.[43] In both reactions, dTDP-L-rhamnnose acts as the rhamnosyl donor. The respective recipient in the first reaction is the fatty acid moiety of rhamnolipids, while that in the second reaction is monorhamnolipid, yielding dirhamnolipid as a product.[39-41] Due to the fact that the rhamnolipid biosynthesis also involves a complex genetic regulatory system, the construction of strains with enhanced rhamnolipid production is much more difficult.[41] Figure 2 shows the biosynthetic pathway of rhamnolipids.

Production of Rhamnolipid Biosurfactants

For the production of microbial metabolites on a large scale, it is important to know the regulation mechanisms of the chosen microorganism. In general, biosurfactant production can be

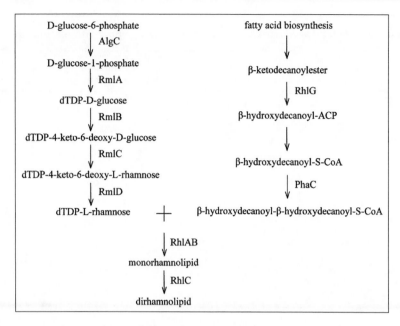

Figure 2. Biosynthetic pathway of rhamnolipid biosurfactants and the involved enzymes.

induced by hydrocarbons or water-insoluble substrates. The production of microbial metabolites is governed by several factors: the nature of the carbon source; the concentrations of nitrogen and ions in the media; culture conditions like pH, temperature, agitation rate and oxygen availability; the nature of the selected microorganism; and, the adopted fermentation strategies.[10] Therefore, all of these factors should be considered in the establishment of a rhamnolipid production process in order to achieve high rhamnolipid production yields.

The *Pseudomonas* species are able to utilize both water-soluble carbon sources (such as glycerol, glucose, mannitol and ethanol)[8,20,44] and water-immiscible substrates (like *n*-alkane and vegetable oils)[8,44,45] for the rhamnolipid production. Normally, it seems that the water-immiscible substrates can provide a higher level of rhamnolipid production.[8,44] It was reported that rhamnolipid production by *Pseudomonas aeruginosa* UG2 was about 100-165 mg of rhamnolipid per gram of substrate when hydrophobic substrates such as long chain alcohols and corn oil were used as carbon sources. Compared to hydrophilic substrates, including glucose and succinic acid, only a rhamnolipid production of 12-36 mg/g was obtained.[17] However, Wu et al recently reported a different trend, showing that glucose and glycerol used as carbon sources in the biosurfactant production by *Pseudomonas aeruginosa* EM1 were superior to olive oil and soybean oil in terms of both rhamnolipid yield and productivity. This further suggests that the carbon source preference for the rhamnolipid production depends on the bacterial strain.[46] Table 2 lists rhamnolipid production by some *Pseudomonas* strains using different substrates.

The type of nitrogen source is crucial to cell growth and rhamnolipid production. It was found that sodium nitrate ($NaNO_3$) was the most efficient nitrogen source for the rhamnolipid production by *Pseudomonas aeruginosa* EM1 in terms of rhamnolipid yields; however, using urea and yeast extract, organic compounds, as nitrogen sources provided better cell growth.[46] In fact, it has been reported that the organic nitrogen source can promote cell growth, but it is unfavorable for the production of glycolipid biosurfactant.[50] Chen et al also found that nitrate-based compounds, inorganic nitrogen sources, seemed to be good nitrogen sources for the rhamnolipid production by *Pseudomonas aeruginosa* S2, giving a maximum rhamnolipid concentration of nearly 2,300 mg/l.[51]

Table 2. *Rhamnolipid production by Pseudomonas strains using different substrates*

Strain	Carbon Source	Concentration of Rhamnolipids (g/l)	Ref.
J4	Kerosene	0.7	8
	Diesel	1.3	
	Glucose	1.4-1.5	
	Glycerol	1.4-1.5	
	Grape seed oil	2.0-2.1	
	Sunflower oil	2.0-2.1	
	Olive oil	3.6	
LBI	Buriti oil	2.9	22
	Cupuaçu oil	6.6	
	Babassu oil	6.8	
	Andiroba oil	8.1	
	Passion fruit oil	9.2	
	Brazilian nut oil	9.9	
EM1	Soybean oil	2.6	46
	Olive oil	3.7	
	Glucose	4.9	
	Glycerol	7.5	
PA1	*n*-hexadecane	1.3	47
	Babassu oil	2.0	
	Glycerol	6.9	
DSM2659	Glucose	1.5	48
YPJ-80	Glucose	4.4	49

Culture conditions also play an important role in the rhamnolipid production. Wei et al reported that the rhamnolipid production by *Pseudomonas aeruginosa* J4 increased about 80% when the agitation rate was increased from 50 to 200 rpm. Further increasing the agitation rate decreased the transfer efficiency of oxygen gas into the liquid medium, leading to unsuitable conditions for the biosurfactant production.[8] Chayabutra and Ju found that the rate of rhamnolipid production by *Pseudomonas aeruginosa* ATCC 10145 significantly increased when pH was in the range of 6.5 to 6.7.[30] While Robert et al found that the best temperature for the biosurfactant production by *Pseudomonas aeruginosa* 44T1 was 37°C,[44] it was found that the rhamnolipid production by *Pseudomonas chlororaphis* NRRL B-30761 was best achieved at 23°C.[52]

Based on the kinetics of biosurfactant production, fermentation strategies can be divided into four types: growth-associated production, production under growth-limiting conditions, production with precursor supplementation and production by resting or immobilized cells. For growth-associated production, parallel relationships exist between growth, substrate utilization and biosurfactant production. Production under growth-limiting conditions can be characterized by a sharp increase in the biosurfactant level as a result of a limitation of one or more medium components. In the third fermentation strategy, the biosurfactant precursors are added to the culture medium, resulting in both qualitative and quantitative changes in the biosurfactant product.[3] When using resting or immobilized cells, the microorganism is separated from the culture medium after cultivation under optimal growth conditions and the wet biomass is subsequently used for the biosurfactant production. For rhamnolipid production, the widely-used fermentation strategies are production under growth-limiting conditions and production by resting or immobilized cells.[10]

Many works have demonstrated that the limitation of multivalent ions and nitrogen is able to cause the overproduction of rhamnolipids. It was reported that the rhamnolipid production by *Pseudomonas aeruginosa* DSM2659 was promoted as the iron concentration in the culture media was reduced.[48] Mulligan et al found that an inorganic phosphate-limited medium provided the best yield of rhamnolipid production by *Pseudomonas aeruginosa* ATCC 9027.[53] Matsufuji et al reported that a high production of rhamnolipids was achieved when *Pseudomonas aeruginosa* IFO 3924 was cultivated under nitrogen-limiting conditions at a carbon to nitrogen (C/N) ratio of 18/1.[54] Santa Anna et al found that a C/N ratio of 60/1 caused the overproduction of rhamnolipids by *Pseudomonas aeruginosa* PA1.[47] These results suggest that the effect of C/N ratio on the rhamnolipid production depends on the bacterial strains. Yateem et al also reported that an increase in the nitrogen concentration caused a reduction of the rhamnolipid production by *Pseudomonas aeruginosa* KISR C1, but the bacterial growth was enhanced, leading to an increase in the bacterial number.[55] The fermentation strategy involving production by resting or immobilized cells can be used for the continuous production of rhamnolipids. Jeong et al immobilized *Pseudomonas aeruginosa* BYK-2 (KCTC 18012P) in poly(vinyl alcohol) beads and found that the relative activity of rhamnolipid production was maintained during 15 cycles in a repeated batch culture.[56]

To facilitate the industrial development of rhamnolipid production, one possible method to decrease the production cost is the utilization of alternative low-cost substrates. For rhamnolipid production by *Pseudomonas*, urban and agroindustrial wastes with a high content of carbohydrates or lipids may meet the requirements for use as alternative substrates.[10] Mercadé et al showed that *Pseudomonas aeruginosa* JAMM NCIB 40044 was able to grow on olive oil mill effluent as the sole carbon source.[4] Abalos et al used soybean oil refinery wastes for the rhamnolipid production by *Pseudomonas aeruginosa* AT10.[6] Wastes obtained from sunflower,[36,57] soybean, cottonseed, babassu, palm and corn oil refineries[58] were tested for rhamnolipid production by *Pseudomonas aeruginosa* LBI. The use of these low-cost substrates to generate a valuable product combines waste minimization in vegetable oil processing with economical biosurfactant production, hopefully resulting in a reduction of pollution problems.[36]

Potential Applications of Rhamnolipid Biosurfactants

Rhamnolipids have been shown to have potential use in several applications, but most of the research has focused on environmental remediation. Currently, bioremediation is thought to be as a cost- and performance-effective technology to solve environmental pollution problems. The pollutants can range from polycyclic aromatic hydrocarbons, refined petroleum products, acid mine drainage, pesticides, industrial waste and heavy metals to crude oil.[34] With the use of rhamnolipids, the biodegradation of these pollutants can be significantly enhanced. It has been found that the biodegradation of Casablanca crude oil was accelerated in the presence of rhamnolipids produced by *Pseudomonas aeruginosa* AT10.[59] Zhang et al reported that rhamnolipids increased the solubility of phenanthrene (polycyclic aromatic hydrocarbons) in a test solution, resulting in the enhancement of the phenanthrene biodegradation rate.[60] In addition, rhamnolipids produced by *Pseudomonas aeruginosa* UG2 was found to increase the solubilization of pesticides, resulting in the stimulation of biodegradation rate and extent.[61,62] The enhancement of hexadecane biodegradation by rhamnolipids has also been reported.[63]

Besides their use as a pure culture, rhamnolipids can stimulate the biodegradation of contaminated soil and water. Rahman et al showed that rhamnolipid-containing additives had positive effects on the bioremediation of gasoline-contaminated soil.[64] The potential use of rhamnolipids produced by *Pseudomonas aeruginosa* J4 for the biodegradation of diesel-contaminated water and soil has also been reported.[65] Clifford et al found that rhamnolipids produced by *Pseudomonas aeruginosa* ATCC 9027 significantly improved the solubilization of tetrachloroethylene (PCE), a common ground water pollutant, indicating the potential use of the tested biosurfactant in surfactant-enhanced aquifer remediation (SEAR) applications.[66] Cassidy et al also suggested that rhamnolipids might be applied in intrinsic bioremediation using in situ rhamnolipid production at an abandoned petroleum refinery.[67]

In some cases, biodegradation processes are too slow or infeasible, so it is necessary to remove the contaminants from the environment.[41] Urum et al investigated the removal of crude oil from soil in air sparging assisted stirred tank reactors using two surfactants, sodium dodecyl sulfate (SDS) and rhamnolipids. The results indicated that rhamnolipids removed oil from the contaminated soil sample comparable to the tested synthetic surfactant.[68] Bai et al reported that monorhamnolipid produced by *Pseudomonas aeruginosa* ATCC 9027 displayed efficiency in the removal of residual hexadecane from soil higher than three synthetic surfactants: SDS, polyoxyethylene and sorbitan monooleate.[69] Noordman et al showed that rhamnolipids produced by *Pseudomonas aeruginosa* UG2 effectively removed phenanthrene from soil.[70] Mulligan and Wang found that rhamnolipid foam effectively removed inorganic heavy metal, including cadmium and nickel, from a contaminated soil sample.[71] The removal of copper,[72] zinc and lead[73] by rhamnolipids has also been reported.

In soil remediation applications, one of the important considerations is the size of the surfactant microstructures. Because contaminants are often found in very small soil pores, the movement of surfactant molecules through the soil can be easily limited by the pore size. Therefore, the size of the rhamnolipid microstructures should be studied closely for their effective use. It was previously reported that rhamnolipids could form various types of microstructures in an aqueous media (including lamellar sheets, vesicles and micelles), depending on concentration and pH.[16,74] The sizes of these rhamnolipid microstructures ranged from less than 50 nm to larger than 1 μm, while the smaller-sized soil pores was in the range of 2 μm-0.2 mm. Thus, the appropriate size of rhamnolipid microstructure could be achieved by controlling the concentration and pH.

Conclusion and Future Perspectives

Although economic considerations limit the expansion of the biosurfactant market, rhamnolipids have recently been produced on a large scale by Jeneil Biosurfactants Corporation. The development of cost-effective bioprocesses for rhamnolipid production could perhaps lead to the widespread use of these surface-active compounds. Because of the distinguishing characteristics of rhamnolipids, several industrial applications, especially environmental remediation, may be realized in the near future. It is also interesting to study the contribution of each rhamnolipid component to the properties of the biosurfactant produced by the *Pseudomonas* in order to obtain a biosurfactant with the desired properties for specific purposes. Moreover, future research focusing on the structural modification of rhamnolipids would probably enlarge the potential use of these surface-active compounds. Knowledge of the biological activities of rhamnolipids is another key factor in introducing these surface-active compounds in high value-added exploitation, such as in cosmetics and in the pharmaceutical industry as anticancer drugs. In addition, the formation of rhamnolipid vesicles may perhaps meet the criteria for drug delivery applications. Rhamnolipids may be commercially successful biosurfactants in the near future.

References
1. Banat IM, Makkar RS, Cameotra SS. Potential commercial applications of microbial surfactants. Appl Environ Microb 2000; 53:495-508.
2. Cameotra SS, Makkar RS. Recent applications of biosurfactants as biological and immunological molecules. Curr Opin Microbiol 2004; 7:262-266.
3. Desai JD, Banat IM. Microbial production of surfactants and their commercial potential. Microbiol Mol Biol Rev 1997; 61:47-64.
4. Mercadé ME, Manresa MA, Robert M et al. Olive oil mill effluent (OOME). New substrates for biosurfactant production. Bioresour Technol 1993; 43:1-6.

5. Fox SL, Bala GA. Production of surfactant from Bacillus subtilis ATCC 21332 using potato substrates. Bioresour Technol 2000; 75:235-240.

6. Abalos A, Pinazo A, Infante MR et al. Physicochemical and antimicrobial properties of new rhamnolipids produced by Pseudomonas aeruginosa AT10 from soybean oil refinery wastes. Langmuir 2001; 17:1367-1371.

7. Nitschke M, Ferraz C, Pastore GM. Selection of microorganisms for biosurfactant production using agroindustrial wastes. Braz J Microbiol 2004; 35:81-85.

8. Wei YH, Chou CL, Chang JS. Rhamnolipid production by indigeneous Pseudomonas aeruginosa J4 originating from petrochemical wastewater. Biochem Eng J 2005; 27:146-154.

9. Nitschke M, Pastore GM. Production and properties of a surfactant obtained from Bacillus subtilis grown on cassava wastewater. Bioresour Technol 2006; 97:336-341.

10. Nitschke M, Costa SGVAO, Contiero J. Rhamnolipid surfactants: an update on the general aspects of these remarkable biomolecules. Biotechnol Prog 2005; 21:1593-1600.

11. Healy MG, Devine CM, Murphy R. Microbial production of biosurfactants. Resour Conserv Recycl 1996; 18:41-57.

12. Mulligan CN, Yong RN, Gibbs BF. Surfactant-enhanced remediation of contaminated soil: a review. Eng Geol 2001; 60:371-380.

13. Lang S, Wagner F. Structure and properties of biosurfactants. In: Kosaric N, Cairns WL, Gray NCC, eds. Biosurfactants and Biotechnology. New York: Marcel Dekker, 1987:21-45.

14. Jarvis FG, Johnson MJ. A glyco-lipid produced by Pseudomonas aeruginosa. J Am Chem Soc 1949; 71:4124-4126.

15. Torrens JL, Herman DC, Miller-Maier RM. Biosurfactant (rhamnolipid) sorption and the impact on rhamnolipid-facilitated removal of cadmium from various soils under saturated flow conditions. Environ Sci Technol 1998; 32:776-781.

16. Sánchez M, Aranda FJ, Espuny MJ et al. Aggregation behaviour of a dirhamnolipid biosurfactant secreted by Pseudomonas aeruginosa in aqueous media. J Colloid Interface Sci 2007; 307:246-253.

17. Mata-Sandoval JC, Karns J, Torrent A. Effect of nutritional and environmental conditions on the production and composition of rhamnolipids by P. aeruginosa UG2. Microbiol Res 2001; 155:249-256.

18. Rahman KSM, Rahman TJ, McClean S et al. Rhamnolipid biosurfactant production by strains of Pseudomonas aeruginosa using low-cost raw materials. Biotechnol Prog 2002; 18:1277-1281.

19. Arino S, Marchal R, Vandecasteele JP. Identification and production of a rhamnolipid biosurfactant by a Pseudomonas species. Appl Environ Microbiol 1996; 45:162-168.

20. Sim L, Ward OP, Li ZY. Production and characterization of a biosurfactant isolated from Pseudomonas aeruginosa UW-1. J Ind Microbiol Biotechnol 1997; 19:232-238.

21. Déziel E, Lépine F, Dennie D et al. Liquid chromatography/mass spectrometry analysis of mixtures of rhamnolipids produced by Pseudomonas aeruginosa strain 57RP grown on mannitol or naphthalene. Biochim Biophys Acta 1999; 1440:244-252.

22. Costa SGVAO, Nitschke M, Haddad R et al. Production of Pseudomonas aeruginosa LBI rhamnolipids following growth on Brazilian native oils. Process Biochem 2006; 41:483-488.

23. Rendell NB, Taylor GW, Somerville M et al. Characterisation of Pseudomonas rhamnolipids. Biochim Biophys Acta 1990; 1045:189-193.

24. Schenk T, Schuphan I, Schmidt B. High-performance liquid chromatograph determination of the rhamnolipids produced by Pseudomonas aeruginosa. J Chromatogr A 1995; 693:7-13.

25. Mata-Sandoval JC, Karns J, Torrent A. High-performance liquid chromatography method for the characterization of rhamnolipid mixtures produced by Pseudomonas aeruginosa UG2 corn oil. J Chromatogr A 1999; 864:211-220.

26. Thanomsub B, Pumeechockchai W, Limtrakul A et al. Chemical structures and biological activities of rhamnolipids produced by Pseudomonas aeruginosa B189 isolated from milk factory waste. Bioresour Technol 2006; 97:2457-2461.

27. Noordman WH, Brusseau ML, Jassen DB. Adsorption of a multicomponent rhamnolipid surfactant to soil. Environ Sci Technol 2000; 34:832-838.

28. Trummler K, Effenberger F, Syldatk C. An integrated microbial/enzymatic process for production of rhamnolipids and L-(+)-rhamnose from rapeseed oil with Pseudomonas sp. DSM 2874. Eur J Lipid Sci Technol 2003; 105:563-571.

29. Déziel E, Lépine F, Milot S et al. Mass spectrometry monitoring of rhamnolipids from a growing culture of Pseudomonas aeruginosa strain 57RP. Biochim Biophys Acta 2000; 1485:145-152.

30. Chayabutra C, Ju LK. Polyhydroxyalkanoic acids and rhamnolipids are synthesized sequentially in hexadecane fermentation by Pseudomonas aeruginosa ATCC 10145. Biotechnol Prog 2001; 17:419-423.

31. Benincasa M, Abalos M, Oliveira I et al. Chemical structure, surface properties and biological activities of the biosurfactant produced by Pseudomonas aeruginosa LBI from soapstock. Antonio van Leeuwenhoek 2004; 85:1-8.

32. Pornsunthorntawee O, Wongpanit P, Chavadej S et al. Structural and physicochemical characterization of crude biosurfactant produced by Pseudomonas aeruginosa SP4 isolated from petroleum-contaminated soil. Bioresour Technol 2008; 99:1589-1595.

33. Monteiro SA, Sassaki GL, de Souza LM et al. Molecular and structural characterization of the biosurfactant produced by Pseudomonas aeruginosa DAUPE 614. Chem Phys Lipids 2007; 147:1-13.

34. Finnerty WR. Biosurfactants in environmental biotechnology. Curr Opin Biotechnol 1994; 5:291-295.

35. Patel RM, Desai AJ. Biosurfactant production by Pseudomonas aeruginosa GS3 from molasses. Lett Appl Microbiol 1997; 25:91-94.

36. Benincasa M, Accorsini FR. Pseudomonas aeruginosa LBI production as an integrated process using the wastes from sunflower-oil refining as a substrate. Bioresour Technol 2007; doi:10.1016/j.biortech.2008; 99:3843-3849.

37. Stipcevic T, Piljac T, Isseroff RR. Di-rhamnolipid from Pseudomonas aeruginosa displays differential effects on human keratinocyte and fibroblast cultures. J Dermatol Sci 2005; 40:141-143.

38. Stipcevic T, Piljac A, Piljac G. Enhanced healing of full-thickness burn wounds using di-rhamnolipid. Burns 2006; 32:24-34.

39. Burger MM, Glaser L, Burton RM. The enzymatic synthesis of rhamnose-containing glycolipids by extracts of Pseudomonas aeruginosa. J Biol Chem 1963; 238:2595-2602.

40. Burger MM, Glaser L, Burton RM. Formation of rhamnolipids of Pseudomonas aeruginosa. Methods Enzymol 1966; 8:441-445.

41. Maier RM, Soberón-Chavéz G. Pseudomonas aeruginosa rhamnolipids: biosynthesis and potential applications. Appl Microbiol Biotechnol 2000; 54:625-633.

42. Campos-García J, Caro AD, Nájera R et al. The Pseudomonas aeruginosa rhlG gene encodes an NADPH-dependent β-ketoacyl reductase which is specifically involved in rhamnolipid synthesis. J Bacteriol 1998; 180:4442-4451.

43. Rahim R, Olvera C, Graninger M et al. Cloning and functional characterization of the Pseudomonas aeruginosa rhlC gene that encodes rhamnosyltransferase 2, an enzyme responsible for di-rhamnolipid biosynthesis. Mol Microbiol 2001; 40:708-718.

44. Robert M, Mercadé ME, Bosch MP et al. Effect of carbon source on biosurfactant production by Pseudomonas aeruginosa 44T1. Biotechnol Lett 1989; 11:871-874.

45. Syldatk C, Lang S, Matulovic U et al. Production of four interfacial active rhamnolipids from n-alkane or glycerol by resting cells of Pseudomonas species DSM 2874. Z Naturforsch 1985; 40c:61-67.

46. Wu JY, Yeh KL, Lu WB et al. Rhamnolipid production with indigenous Pseudomonas aeruginosa EM1 isolated from oil-contaminated site. Bioresour Technol 2008; 99:1157-1164.

47. Santa Anna LM, Sebastian GV, Menezes EP et al. Production of biosurfactants from Pseudomonas aeruginosa PA1 isolated in oil environments. Braz J Chem Eng 2002; 19:159-166.

48. Guerra-Santos L, Kappeli O, Fiechter A. Pseudomonas aeruginosa biosurfactant production in continuous culture with glucose as sole carbon source. Appl Environ Microbiol 1984; 48:301-305.

49. Lee Y, Lee SY, Yang JW. Production of rhamnolipid biosurfactant by fed-batch culture of Pseudomonas aeruginosa using glucose as a sole carbon source. Biosci Biotechnol Biochem 1999; 63:946-947.

50. Kim HS, Jeon JW, Kim BH et al. Extracellular production of a glycolipid biosurfactant, mannosylerythritol lipid, by Candida sp. SY16 using fed-batch fermentation. Appl Microbiol Biotechnol 2006; 70:391-396.

51. Chen SY, Lu WB, Wei YH et al. Improved production of biosurfactant with newly isolated Pseudomonas aeruginosa S2. Biotechnol Prog 2007; 23:661-666.

52. Gunther IV NW, Nuñez A, Fett W et al. Production of rhamnolipids by Pseudomonas chlororaphis, a nonpathogenic bacterium. Appl Environ Microbiol 2005; 71:2288-2293.

53. Mulligan CN, Mahmourides G, Gibbs BF. The influence of phosphate metabolism on biosurfactant production by Pseudomonas aeruginosa. J Biotechnol 1989; 12:199-210.

54. Matsufuji M, Nakata K, Yoshimoto A. High production of rhamnolipids by Pseudomonas aeruginosa growing on ethanol. Biotechnol Lett 1997; 19:1213-1215.

55. Yateem A, Balba MT, Al-Shayji Y et al. Isolation and characterization of biosurfactant-producing bacteria from oil-contaminated soil. Soil and Sediment Contamination 2002; 11:41-55.

56. Jeong HS, Lim DJ, Hwang SH et al. Rhamnolipid production by Pseudomonas aeruginosa immobilised in polyvinyl alcohol beads. Biotechnol Lett 2004; 26:35-39.

57. Benincasa M, Contiero J, Manresa MA et al. Rhamnolipid production by Pseudomonas aeruginosa LBI growing on soapstock as the sole carbon source. J Food Eng 2002; 54:283-288.

58. Nitscke M, Costa SGVAO, Haddad R et al. Oil wastes as unconventional substrates for rhamnolipid biosurfactant production by Pseudomonas aeruginosa LBI. Biotechnol Prog 2005; 21:1562-1566.

59. Abalos A, Viñas M, Sabaté J et al. Enhanced biodegradation of casablanca crude oil by a microbial consortium in presence of a rhamnolipid produced by Pseudomonas aeruginosa AT10. Biodegradation 2004; 15:249-260.
60. Zhang Y, Maier WJ, Miller RM. Effect of rhamnolipids on the dissolution, bioavailability and biodegradation of phenanthrene. Environ Sci Technol 1997; 31:2211-2217.
61. Mata-Sandoval JC, Karns J, Torrents A. Effect of rhamnolipids produced by Pseudomonas aeruginosa UG2 on the solubilization of pesticides. Environ Sci Technol 2000; 34:4923-4930.
62. Mata-Sandoval JC, Karns J, Torrents A. Influence of rhamnolipids and Triton X-100 on the biodegradation of three pesticides in aqueous phase and soil slurries. J Agric Food Chem 2001; 49:3296-3303.
63. Noordman WH, Wachter JHJ, de Boer GJ et al. The enhancement by surfactants of hexadecane by Pseudomonas aeruginosa varies with substrate availability. J Biotechnol 2002; 94:195-212.
64. Rahman KSM, Banat IM, Thahira J et al. Bioremediation of gasoline contaminated soil by a bacterial consortium amended with poultry litter, coir pith and rhamnolipid biosurfactant. Bioresour Technol 2002; 81:25-32.
65. Whang LM, Liu PWG, Ma CC et al. Application of biosurfactants, rhamnolipid and surfactin, for enhanced biodegradation of diesel-contaminated water and soil. J Hazard Mater 2008; 151:155-163.
66. Clifford JS, Ioannidis MA, Legge RL. Enhanced aqueous solubilization of tetrachloroethylene by a rhamnolipid biosurfactant. J Colloid Interface Sci 2007; 305:361-365.
67. Cassidy DP, Hudak AJ, Werkema DD et al. In situ rhamnolipid production at an abandoned petroleum refinery. Soil and Sediment Contamination 2002; 11:769-787.
68. Urum K, Pekdemir T, Ross D et al. Crude oil contaminated soil washing in air sparging assisted stirred tank reactor using biosurfactants. Chemosphere 2005; 60:334-343.
69. Bai G, Brusseau ML, Miller RM. Biosurfactant-enhanced removal of residual hydrocarbon from soil. J Contain Hydrol 1997; 25:157-170.
70. Noordman WH, Ji W, Brusseau ML et al. Effects of rhamnolipid biosurfactants on removal of phenanthrene from soil. Environ Sci Technol 1998; 32:1806-1812.
71. Mulligan CN, Wang S. Remediation of a heavy metal-contaminated soil by a rhamnolipid foam. Eng Geol 2006; 85:75-81.
72. Mulligan CN, Yong RN, Gibbs BF. Heavy metal removal from sediments by biosurfactants. J Hazard Mater 2001; 85:111-125.
73. Herman DC, Artiola JF, Miller RM. Removal of cadmium, lead and zinc from soil by a rhamnolipid biosurfactant. Environ Sci Technol 1995; 29:2280-2285.
74. Champion JT, Gilkey JC, Lamparski H et al. Electron microscopy of rhamnolipid (biosurfactant) morphology: effects of pH, cadmium and octadecane. J Colloid Interface Sci 1995; 170:569-574.

CHAPTER 17

Biosurfactant's Role in Bioremediation of NAPL and Fermentative Production

Sanket J. Joshi and Anjana J. Desai*

Abstract

Surfactants and biosurfactants are amphipathic molecules with both hydrophilic and hydrophobic moieties that partition preferentially at the interface between fluid phases that have different degrees of polarity and hydrogen bonding which confers excellent detergency, emulsifying, foaming and dispersing traits, making them most versatile process chemicals. One of the major applications of (bio)surfactants is in environmental bioremediation field. Most synthetic organic compounds present in contaminated soils are only weakly soluble or completely insoluble in water, so they exist in the subsurface as separate liquid phase, often referred as a non-aqueous phase liquids (NAPL), which poses as threat to environment. Several studies have revealed the use of surfactants for remediation; however, several factors limit the use of surfactants in environmental remediation, mainly persistence of surfactants or their metabolites and thus potentially pose an environmental concern. Biosurfactants may provide a more cost-effective approach for subsurface remediation when used alone or in combination with synthetic surfactants. There are several advantages of biosurfactants when compared to chemical surfactants, mainly biodegradability, low toxicity, biocompatibility and ability to be synthesized from renewable feedstock. Despite having many commercially attractive properties and clear advantages compared with their synthetic counterparts, biosurfactants have not yet been employed extensively in industry because of their low yields and relatively high production and recovery costs. However, the use of mutants and recombinant hyperproducing microorganisms along with the use of cheaper raw materials and optimal growth and production conditions and more efficient recovery processes, the production of biosurfactant can be made economically feasible. Therefore, future research aiming for high-level production of biosurfactants must be focused towards the development of appropriate combinations of hyperproducing microbial strains, optimized cheaper production media and optimized process conditions, which will lead to economical commercial level biosurfactant production.

Introduction

A surfactant is a substance that, when present at low concentration in a system, has the property of adsorbing onto the surfaces or interfaces of the system and altering to a marked degree the surface or interfacial free energies of those surfaces (or interfaces). Surfactants are amphipathic molecules with both hydrophilic and hydrophobic moieties that partition preferentially at the interface between fluid phases that have different degrees of polarity and hydrogen bonding, such as oil and water or air and water interfaces. Each characteristic they possess confer excellent detergency, emulsifying, foaming and dispersing traits, which makes surfactants most versatile

*Corresponding Author: Anjana J. Desai—Department of Microbiology and Biotechnology Centre, The M.S. University of Baroda, Vadodara 390002, India. Email: desai_aj@yahoo.com

Biosurfactants, edited by Ramkrishna Sen. ©2010 Landes Bioscience and Springer Science+Business Media.

process chemicals. Surfactants are among the most versatile products of the chemical industry appearing in diverse products such as the motor oils, we use in the automobiles, the pharmaceuticals taken when we are ill, the detergents used in cleaning our laundry and our home, the drilling muds used in processing for petroleum and the flotation agents used in benefication of ores. Last decade has seen the extension of surfactant application to high-technology areas as electronic printing, magnetic recording, biotechnology, microelectronics and viral research. World surfactant production in 1999 was 9 million tones, with a value at around 10 billion Euros.[1,2] The largest industrial sectors that uses surfactants is household (61%) followed by industrial processes (25%), personal care (8%) and speciality cleaning (6%).[3]

Many types of surface-active agents are also synthesized by a wide variety of microorganisms. They mostly exhibit the typical amphiphilic character of lipids and are generally extracellular. Unlike chemically synthesized surfactants, which are classified according to the nature of their polar grouping, biosurfactants are categorized mainly by their chemical composition and their microbial origin. In general, their structure includes a hydrophilic moiety consisting of amino acids or peptides, anions or cations; mono-, di-, or polysaccharides; and a hydrophobic moiety consisting of unsaturated or saturated, fatty acids. Accordingly, the major classes of biosurfactants include glycolipids, lipopeptides/lipoproteins, phospholipids and fatty acids, polymeric surfactants and particulate surfactants. The biosurfactant-producing microbes are distributed among a wide variety of genera. The major types of biosurfactants, with their properties and microbial species of origin, the structure, function and physiological role of these biological surface-active agents have been described in several reviews.[4-9]

Bioremediation

One of the major applications of biosurfactants is in environmental bioremediation field, where the biosurfactants can be used in crude or partially purified form.[10] These environmental applications are: bioremediation, soil remediation and flushing: which mainly are emulsification of hydrocarbons; lowering of interfacial tension; metal sequestration, emulsification through adherence to hydrocarbons; dispersion; foaming agent; detergent and soil flushing. Bioremediation is normally seen as a promising cost-effective and performance- effective technology to address numerous environmental pollution problems. Bioremediation involves the acceleration of natural biodegradation processes in contaminated environments by improving the availability of materials (e.g., nutrients and oxygen), conditions (e.g., pH and moisture content) and prevailing microorganisms. These pollutants range from industrial wastes (e.g., polychlorinated biphenyls, trichloroethylene, pentachlorophenol and dioxin), polyaromatic hydrocarbons, refined petroleum products (e.g., jet fuel, gasoline, diesel fuel and the benzene, toluene, ethylbenzene and xylene cluster), acid mine drainage, pesticides, munitions compounds (e.g., trinitrotoluene) and inorganic heavy metals to crude oil. Surfactants (both biosurfactants and synthetic surfactants) are emerging as a technology to enhance the accessibility and bioavailability of hydrophobic chemicals, thereby complementing existing bioremediation methods. However, the use of biosurfactants in remediation experiments is justified on the basis that they are less toxic to the microorganisms performing the biodegradation,[11] diverse with novel chemical structures and characteristics; can be produced from cheap raw materials and the organisms producing these compounds can be modified genetically to overproduce or produce new compounds and have a lower critical micellar concentration (CMC) values as compared to chemical surfactants.[12] Jordan et al[13] proposed that biosurfactants increase the bioavailability of surface-bound nutrients at solid–water interfaces and can be used at low concentrations to enhance bioremediation.

What Are Non-Aqueous Phase Liquids (NAPL)?

Most synthetic organic compounds present in contaminated soils are only weakly soluble or completely insoluble in water. As a result, they exist in the subsurface as separate liquid phase, often referred as a non-aqueous phase liquids (NAPL). NAPL are sparingly soluble in water and they tend to form a separate phase. Oil is a good example of NAPL, as it does not mix with water and forms two separate phases. NAPLs can be lighter than water (LNAPL) or denser than water (DNAPL). Organic liquids that are lighter than water (gasoline, jet fuel, heating oils) are referred to as light non-aqueous phase liquids (LNAPLs). These tend to accumulate above and slightly below the water table.[14] Subsurface contamination by light non-aqueous phase liquids (LNAPL) is a prevalent environmental problem at superfund sites, refineries, pipelines and chemical/industrial facilities.[15] Organic liquids that are heavier than water are referred to as dense non-aqueous phase liquids (DNAPLs). They have the tendency to migrate to considerable depths below the water table. DNAPLs are often a complex mixture of contaminants, but can commonly be classified into two groups: chlorinated solvent DNAPLs such as trichloroethylene (TCE) and tetrachloroethylene (PCE); and polycyclic aromatic hydrocarbons (PAH) such as coal tar and creosote.[16] Polychlorinated biphenyl (PCB) can also be found as a common DNAPL component. The non-aqueous phase liquid cleanup Alliance, established in 2001 includes representatives from the petroleum industry, federal and state government and academia who share an interest in pursuing aggressive technologies for removing large-scale NAPL contamination. Entrapped NAPL pollutants constitute one of the biggest problems in the efforts to bioremediate the sites of aquifers contaminated by such pollutants. The low solubility of these chemicals and their high affinity to solid surface may lead to reduced bioavailability to microbial ecosystems present in soils and sediments that are potentially capable of dissipating these pollutants.[14]

Chemical Surfactants and Bioremediation

It is only last 10-15 years that the use of surfactants in increasing the availability of hydrophobic pollutants in soils and other environments has been widely reported. Previous studies have revealed that surfactants can enhance pollutant desorption and availability. They have been applied in oil washing for secondary oil recovery and to clean oil pipes and oil reservoirs.[12] Remediation of NAPLs by conventional water flushing methods is generally considered to be ineffective, due to low water solubility and mass transfer constraints. Chemical flushing using surfactants can greatly improve NAPL remediation by increasing the apparent solubility of NAPL contaminants. In situ flushing is mostly used to remove synthetic organic contaminants, a type of contaminant not easily removed by conventional methods such as pump and treat. In situ flushing is commonly applied to contaminated sites using surfactants or cosolvents as the primary flushing agents. Surfactants typically consist of a strongly hydrophilic (water loving) group, the "head" of the molecule and a strongly hydrophobic (water fearing) group which is the "tail." The hydrophilic portion causes surfactants to exhibit high solubility in water, while the hydrophobic portion prefers to reside in a hydrophobic phase such as LNAPL or DNAPL. This enables surfactants to enhance the solubility of the contaminant through micellar solubilization, the process by which aggregations of surfactant monomers form a micelle that the NAPL molecule can occupy. The concentration of the surfactant needed to produce this formation is called the critical micelle concentration (CMC). The addition of a surfactant can also be used to enhance the mobility of the contaminant rather than the solubility by reducing the NAPL-water interfacial tension. This reduction results in the decrease of the capillary forces, the forces responsible for the retention of residual and the formation of pooled NAPL, which subsequently results in contaminant mobility.

The majority of work on remediation to enhance the solubility of organic hydrophobic contaminants in soils and other environments has been carried out by chemical surfactants. Chemical surfactants have been shown to remove nonpolar compounds from surfaces but problems can be associated with their use, such as reduced availability of compounds sequestered into micelles, their toxicity and ultimate resistance to biodegradation leading to increased pollution.[17] Several reports suggest synthetic surfactants such as Triton X-100, Tween 80, Afonic 1412-7 (a non-ionic alkyl ethoxylate) and others can enhance the concentration of PAHs in the aqueous phase.[18-20] Studies with non-ionic and anionic surfactant additions have indicated that either they can enhance the biodegradation of soil xenobiotics including phenanthrene, biphenyl and a range of other hydrocarbons or have also been shown to inhibit biodegradation at concentration above their CMC. Actually many synthetic surfactants are known to exert an inhibitory effect on PAH—degrading microorganisms.[12]

Surfactant-enhanced subsurface remediation has been identified as a promising technology for source area treatment, which consists of two general approaches: Solubilization—is the use of surfactants above their critical micelle concentration (CMC) to enhance the solubility of contaminants and thereby decrease the pore volumes of water flushing required for treatment and Mobilization—is the use of surfactant concentrations above the critical microemulsion concentration (CμC) to reduce the interfacial tension (IFT) between NAPL and water phases and mobilize the hydrocarbon as a separate phase. To overcome the capillary forces that entrap the NAPL, large reductions in IFT are necessary. The IFT has to be in an ultra low range (<0.1 mN/m), to release the trapped NAPL and achieve significant mass removal.[21,22] However, several factors limit the use of surfactants in environmental remediation, mainly persistence of surfactants or their metabolites can result in off site migration and thus potentially pose an environmental concern.

Biosurfactants and Bioremediation

Over past few years many reports have shown that biosurfactants can solubilize and mobilize NAPLs adsorbed onto soil constituents.[23-31] Biosurfactants may provide a more cost-effective approach for subsurface remediation when used alone or in combination with synthetic surfactants. As already discussed the critical micelle concentration of many biosurfactants is much lower than synthetic surfactants, suggesting that lower surfactant concentrations can be used, in addition they are less toxic and are biodegradable, which reduces environmental concern. Brusseau et al,[32] have reported, that nearly 22% of residual hexadecane was removed from sand columns by monorhabdolipid acid, at a concentration of 500 mg/l. Mobilization of mixtures of hexane, toluene and kerosene has been reported by using a biodegradable surfactant, dodecylbenzesulphonate, below CMC level, in a lab level column based flow system.[33] Several reports are available for the addition of rhamnolipids above critical micellar concentration (CMC), which enhanced the apparent aqueous solubility of hexadecane, enhanced biodegradation of hexadecane, octadecane, n-paraffins, creosotes and other hydrocarbon mixtures in soil and promoted bioremediation of petroleum sludges.[34-37] Above the CMC, the formation of micelles occurs and hydrocarbons can partition into the hydrophobic micellar core, increasing their apparent aqueous solubility. Table 1 shows few selected studies involving the use of biosurfactants to stimulate hydrophobic organic contaminant biodegradation.

Recently Youssef et al[38] have proposed a hypothesis that mixtures of biosurfactants could be used to achieve the ultra low IFT (<0.1 mN/m) values required for NAPL mobilization. They have shown that, lipopeptide biosurfactants from individual strains or mixtures from different strains, mixtures of lipopeptides and rhamnolipids and mixtures of lipopeptides with synthetic surfactants were tested for their ability to lower interfacial tensions against LNAPL components with different hydrophobicities (toluene, hexane, decane and hexadecane). Their results provided a basis for formulating biosurfactant and synthetic surfactant formulations to achieve ultra low IFT against NAPL components, which will be valuable not only to environmental remediation but also to other applications that rely upon reducing IFT or increasing the solubility of an oil.

Fermentative Production and Recovery of Biosurfactants

Almost all surfactants currently in use, are chemically derived from petroleum; however, interest in microbial surfactants has been steadily increasing in recent years due to their diversity, environment friendly nature, the possibility of their production through fermentation and their potential applications in the environmental protection, crude oil recovery, health care and food-processing industries. There are several advantages of biosurfactants when compared to their chemically synthesized counterparts,[40] such as, high surface and interface activity,[41] temperature, pH and ionic strength tolerance, biodegradability, low toxicity, biocompatibility, digestibility and specificity and ability to be synthesized from renewable feedstock and acceptable production economics.[6,42-44] With environmental compatibility becoming an increasingly important factor in

Table 1. *Studies involving the use of biosurfactants to stimulate hydrophobic contaminant biodegradation[#]*

Compound(s)	Surfactant	Medium
14-16 C alkanes, pristane phenyldecane and Naphthalene	Sophorose lipid	Liquid
Hexachlorobiphenyl	Rhamnolipid	Soil slurries
Octadecane	Rhamnolipid	Soil
Hexachlorobiphenyl	Rhamnolipid Emulsan	Soil
Aliphatic and aromatic	Rhamnolipid	Soil
Phenanthrene	Rhamnolipid	Soil slurries
Metals, phenanthrene and PCBs	Rhamnolipid	Soil
Mixture of alkanes and naphthalene	Rhamnolipid and oleophilic fertilizer	Soil
4,49-dichlorobiphenyl	Rhamnolipid	Soil
Naphthalene	Rhamnolipid	Soil
Naphthalene and phenanthrene	Rhamnolipid	Soil
Naphthalene and methyl naphthalene	Glycolipid and Tween 80	Liquid
Hexadecane and kerosene oil	Crude surfactin	Soil
Phenanthrene and hexadecane	Rhamnolipid	Soil
Phenanthrene, fluoranthene, pyrene and Pentachlorophenol	Rhamnolipid	Soil
Endosulfan	Crude surfactin	Soil
Phenanthrene, fluoranthene and pyrene	Alasan	Liquid
Aliphatic and aromatic hydrocarbons	Crude surfactin	Seawater
Phenanthrene	Sophorolipid	Soil
Phenanthrene and cadmium	Rhamnolipid	Soil
Naphthalene and cadmium	Mono-rhamnolipid	Soil
Toluene, ethyl benzene and butyl benzene	Di-rhamnolipid	Liquid

[#]Adapted from Makkar and Rockne[39]

the selection of industrial chemicals, the use of biosurfactants in environmental applications, such as bioremediation and the dispersion of oil spills, is increasing. In addition, biosurfactants have other uses in the petroleum industry, such as in enhanced oil recovery and transportation of crude oil. Other possible application fields are in the food, cosmetic and pharmaceutical industries. In these industries, most biosurfactants are used as emulsifiers.[6,43-45]

Production of Biosurfactants

It is somewhat difficult to generalize the guidelines for optimal biosurfactant production, as biosurfactants are diverse compounds produced by a variety of microorganisms. However three factors play significant role in biosurfactant production: namely, media constituents—such as carbon and nitrogen sources, the environmental factors and growth conditions such as—pH, temperature, agitation and oxygen availability affect biosurfactant production through their effects on growth.[46] Microorganisms can be divided into three categories based on the type of carbon sources they assimilate for biosurfactant production: those utilizing water-insoluble carbon sources as hydrocarbons, such as *Corynebacterium* sp. and *Arthrobacter* sp.; those utilizing only water-soluble substrates as carbon sources such as *Bacillus* sp.; and those utilizing water-insoluble (hydrocarbons) and water-soluble substrates as carbon sources, such as *Pseudomonas* sp. It is clear that the type or structure and yields of biosurfactant depend on the types of carbon sources utilized by different types of microorganisms used.[47] Also, the production patterns or kinetics of fermentative production by different species are different, which can be grouped into following types: (i) growth-associated production, as observed in rhamnolipid production by some *Pseudomonas* spp.[48,49] and lipopeptide biosurfactant C9-BS by *Bacillus subtilis* C9,[50] (ii) production under growth-limiting conditions, as observed in number of *Pseudomonas* spp.[51-53] and *Bacillus* spp.[54] when the culture reaches the stationary phase of growth due to limitation of nitrogen and/or iron, (iii) production by resting or immobilized cells, as reported for production of rhamnolipid by *Pseudomonas* spp.[55,56] and *P. aeruginosa* CFTR-6,[57] sophorolipid production by *Torulopsis bombicola*[58] and mannosylerythritol production by *Candida antarctica*[59] and (iv) production with precursor supplementation, as reported for the addition of lipophilic compounds to the culture medium of *T. magnolia*,[60] *T. bombicola*[61] resulted in increased biosurfactant yields. Therefore, process development and fermentations have to be optimized on a case by case basis.

Mostly biosurfactant production is carried out by traditional submerged fermentation technology, wherein biosurfactants are released into the broth either at the stationary phase or throughout the exponential phase. The biosurfactant production can be carried out in batch mode or continuous mode at low dilution rates. Lin, et al,[62] has reported the continuous production of lipopeptide biosurfactant by *B. licheniformis* JF-2, using low dilution rates. In addition to the traditional submerged fermentation, other fermentation processes have been employed for the production of biosurfactants: air-lift fermentor, aqueous two-phase fermentations[63,64] and solid state fermentation for the production of surfactin using a recombinant *B. subtilis*[65] have been reported.

Recovery of Biosurfactants

The recovery and concentration of biosurfactants from the fermentation broth can account for a large fraction of the total production costs (up to 60% of the total production cost).[46] Due to economic considerations, use of most of the biosurfactants would have to involve either whole-cell culture broths or other crude and partially purified preparations. Generally most of the environmental applications do not require high degree of product purity as long as the final preparation exhibits the desired properties. Whereas, highly purified biosurfactant without any impurities has to be used for applications in food products or in pharmaceutical preparations.

The optimal recovery processes for biosurfactant varies with the type of fermentation, media components (water-soluble or insoluble media) and the physicochemical properties of the desired biosurfactants, i.e., its ionic charge, water solubility and cellular location (intracellular, extracellular or cell bound).

For large scale or continuous isolation of biosurfactants from the fermentation supernatant, adsorption chromatography on ion-exchange resins, activated carbon, or hydrophobic adsorbents such as Amberlite XAD-2 has been shown to be effective. The most commonly used biosurfactant recovery techniques are listed in Table 2. Extractions with solvents like chloroform-methanol, dichloromethane-methanol, butanol, ethyl acetate, pentane, hexane, acetic acid, ether, etc. are most widely used techniques.[46]

Economical Commercial Production

From the Technical Insights, Hester[67] estimated that biosurfactants would capture 10% of the surfactant market by the year 2010 with sales of $US200 million. However, despite having many commercially attractive properties and clear advantages compared with their synthetic counterparts as discussed above, biosurfactants have not yet been employed extensively in industry because of

Table 2. Commonly used biosurfactant recovery processes

Process	Type (Example) of Biosurfactant
Ammonium sulfate precipitation	Emulsan, bioemulsifier
Acetone precipitation	Bioemulsifier
Acid precipitation	Surfactin, lichenysin
Organic solvent extraction	Trehalolipids, sophorolipids, liposan
Crystallization	Cellobiolipids, glycolipids
Centrifugation	Glycolipids
Adsorption	Rhamnolipids, glycolipids
Foam fractionation	Surfactin
Tangential flow filtration	Mixed biosurfactant
Diafiltration and precipitation	Glycolipids
Membrane ultrafiltration	Glycolipids, surfactin

#Adapted from Desai and Banat[46] and Mukherjee et al.[66]

their low yields and relatively high production (at least 50 times more expensive, depending on the biosurfactant and its purity) and recovery costs.[68] One of the strategy, recently used towards reducing the costs of biosurfactant production, is to select microorganisms capable of producing biosurfactants in high yields and to optimize large-scale fermentation and recovery system conditions.[4] To make the biosurfactant production more economical at commercial level following strategies are utilized: (i) use of random mutagenesis or site directed mutagenesis for development of overproducing mutant or recombinant strains for enhanced biosurfactant yields; (ii) the use of cheaper waste substrates (mainly agroindustrial byproducts); and (iii) development of efficient fermentation processes, either by optimization of the media constituents and culture conditions using statistical means or by optimization of recovery process for maximum biosurfactant production. The first approach, mutagenesis using physical and chemical mutagens have been successfully applied in many instances and hyper-producers have been reported to increase yields several fold, but the use of site directed approach for selection of recombinant hyper-producing strains, has still not been properly tested. Mukherjee et al,[66] have reviewed this aspect for hyperproducers of biosurfactants. They have sited the examples of hyperproducers which showed 2-25 times increase in production of different types of biosurfactants, as well as microorganisms with improved production properties. However, studies for hyperproducing mutants and recombinants represent only laboratory scale studies and the real development and use of mutants and recombinant hyperproducers at scaled up processes has immense hidden potential in terms of yield enhancement and thus economization of the biosurfactant production process, which are yet to be studied. Whereas, other two approaches have been explored to a greater extent and reported to be effective in substantially increasing the production of biosurfactants.[66,68] These two approaches are discussed in some detail.

The Use of Cheaper Waste Substrates
    The choice of inexpensive raw materials is important to the overall economy of the process as they account for 50% of the final production cost and also reduce the expenses with waste treatment. When water-insoluble hydrocarbons are used as the carbon sources, it may be necessary to remove the unutilized hydrocarbons before the extraction of biosurfactants is carried out,[47] which would add up to the cost of biosurfactant production and thus scale up would not be feasible. Thus mainly agroindustrial wastes with high content of carbohydrates, or lipids meet the requirement

Table 3. List of different cheaper raw materials used for the production of biosurfactants by various microorganisms

Raw Material	Microbial Strain	Biosurfactant Type
Waste frying oils	*Pseudomonas aeruginosa* 47T2 NCIB 40044	Rhamnolipids[73]
Oil refinery wastes	Yeast	Glycololipid[74]
Molasses	Mixed culture	_[75]
	Bacillus spp.	Lipopeptide[76]
	Pseudomonas aeruginosa GS3	Rhamnolipids[77]
	Bacillus spp.	Lipopeptides[72]
Starch rich wastes (Potato process effluent)	*Bacillus subtilis* ATCC 21332	Lipopeptides[78]
Cheese whey	Bacillus spp.	Lipopeptides[72]
Lactic whey and distillery wastes	*Pseudomonas aeruginosa* strain BS2	Rhamnolipid[70]
Cassava waste water	*Bacillus subtilis*	Lipopeptide[79]

for use as substrate for biosurfactant production.[69] So far, several renewable substrates from various sources, especially from industrial wastes have been extensively studied for microbial production at an experimental scale. A variety of cheaper raw materials, including oil based wastes, starch rich wastes, dairy wastewater and distillery wastes,[70] molasses and agroindustrial based wastes have been reported to be used as substrates for the biosurfactant production. Dubey and Juwarkar[71] have reported that the effluent from the dairy industries supports good microbial growth and could be used as a cheap raw material for biosurfactant production. Joshi et al[72] have shown biosurfactant production by *Bacillus* spp. using cheese whey and molasses as sole source of nutrition at thermophilic conditions under shaking as well as static conditions. These studies showed that molasses and cheese whey might be comparatively cheaper and better substrates for biosurfactant production at the commercial scale than synthetic media. Moreover, the use of dairy wastewaters provides a strategy for the economical production of biosurfactants and efficient dairy wastewater management. Table 3 shows the list of different cheaper raw materials for the production of biosurfactants by various microorganisms.

Development of Efficient Fermentation Processes

Economy is the bottleneck for every fermentation industry and for economical production of biosurfactant at commercial level efficient fermentation processes are must. This could be achieved either by optimization of the media constituents and culture conditions for maximum biosurfactant production and by optimization of efficient recovery processes for maximum product recovery.

Media and Process Optimization

It has been reported that elements, such as carbon, nitrogen, iron and manganese and the ratio of different elements such as C:N, C:P, C:Fe or C:Mg, are reported to affect the yield of biosurfactants, for example, the addition of iron and manganese to the culture medium was reported to increase the production of biosurfactant by *Bacillus subtilis*,[80] Manresa et al,[49] have reported that production and yield of rhamnolipid by *P. aeruginosa* 44T1 was increased at higher C:N ratio and Vega et al,[81] have reported the biosurfactant production by *P. putida* in combined C/P, C/N$_{inorganic}$, C/Mg ratios with peptone concentrations. Therefore, an economical process demands the optimization of the media components and the process itself. There are a large

Table 4. Use of statistical methods for enhanced biosurfactant production

Microbial Strain	Biosurfactant	Increase in Yield
Bacillus subtilis	Surfactin	1.77 fold[66]
Bacillus licheniformis K51	Lipopeptide	Ten fold[82]
Bacillus licheniformis R2	Lichenysin-A	Four fold[86]
Pseudomonas aeruginosa AT10	Rhamnolipid	Five fold[87]
Bacillus subtilis S499	Lipopeptide	Five times[88]
Lactococcus lactis and *Streptococcus thermophilus*	-	1.6 and 2.1 times[89]
Bacillus subtilis ATCC 21332	Surfactin	Two fold[90]

number of reports on the optimization of C and N sources on the classical method of medium optimization by changing one independent variable while fixing all the others at a fixed level. This is extremely time consuming and expensive for a large number of variables and requires a large number of experiments to determine optimum levels, which are unreliable. Optimizing all the affecting parameters by statistical experimental designs can eliminate these limitations of a single factor optimization process collectively by statistical experimental designs such as response surface methodology (RSM),[82] wherein, initial screening of the ingredients is done to understand the significance of their effect on the product formation and then a few better ingredients are selected for further optimization. These methods have been used by various investigators for enhanced biosurfactant production (Table 4). Sen et al[83-85] have used these methods to determine the optimum media, inoculum and environmental conditions for the enhanced production of surfactin by *Bacillus subtilis*. Joshi et al[82,86] have reported the enhanced production of lichenysin-A by thermophilic *B. licheniformis* K51 and *B. licheniformis* R2 using the statistical optimization procedures. They observed up to four to ten fold increases in the yield of biosurfactant as critical micellar dilution (CMD).

Another issue during the microbial production of lipopeptides is excessive foam which is produced in the bioreactor, when the medium is aerated and agitated. On a smaller scale, it is problematic in operation and process safety, whereas on a larger scale, foaming additionally creates problems for economical viability. Both mechanical and chemical means are available for foam control, wherein mechanical means are preferred over addition of chemical antifoaming agents. As antifoaming agents can cause problems such as, lowering of the mass transfer rate, reaction inhibition, cell toxicity and adverse effect on separation and purification of the products. Several methods have been used to try to enhance the gas-liquid transport and to minimize the adverse effect of foaming without adding antifoaming agents, such as modifying the reactor design, collection of the foam and recycling of the cells under aseptic conditions.[91] It has been also reported that under oxygen limited conditions production of some lipopeptide biosurfactants are enhanced.[54,92] Thus a bioprocess for production of biosurfactant, at limited dissolved oxygen concentration (DO), if available, can minimize the cost of production. Sanket Joshi (PhD Thesis, MSU of Baroda) have reported the production of lichenysin by *B. licheniformis* R2 under uncontrolled DO levels. He observed that if the bioprocess is operated at initial DO saturation at 100% levels and no DO control thereafter, lead to higher yield of lichenysin at early stage (4-6 h) of the batch as compared to controlled DO (30%, 50% and 70%) throughout the batch process. During the batch process the foam was collected aseptically and the cells were recycled to the vessel. The yield in terms of CMD observed was 100X and was maintained throughout the cycle of 72 h (Fig. 1). As shown in Figure 1, the DO dropped to almost zero by 12 hours. The cell free broth of *B. licheniformis* R2 showed ST and CMD as 28 mN/m and 100X respectively.

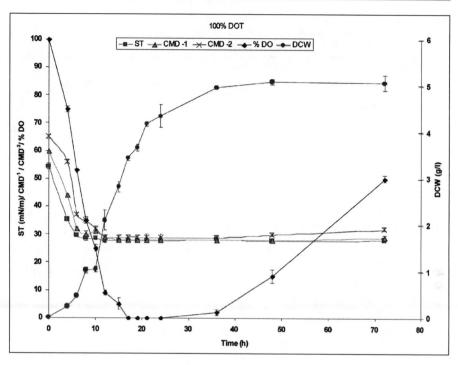

Figure 1. Growth and surface activity (ST, CMD⁻¹ and CMD⁻²) of *B. licheniformis* R2 under initial 100% DO saturation and no further DO control thereafter.

Recovery Processes

One of the important factors which determine the feasibility of a commercial process is the availability of suitable and economical recovery and downstream procedures. The production process is still incomplete without an efficient and economical process for the recovery of the biosurfactants, even after optimum production is achieved using optimal media and culture conditions. As already mentioned, the recovery processes account for 60% of the total production costs. Several conventional methods for the recovery of biosurfactants have been used. Recently few unconventional and interesting recovery methods like adsorbsion to ion exchange resins and membrane ultrafiltration have been reported. These procedures are particularly applicable for large-scale continuous recovery of extracellular biosurfactants from culture broth, a few examples of such biosurfactant recovery strategies are shown in Table 2.

Conclusion

It is accepted that successful commercialization of biosurfactants depends to a great extent on its economical production at a competitive price with chemical counterparts. Till date, it has not been possible to achieve biosurfactant production at a comparable cost to the chemical surfactants, mainly due to their high production costs and low yields.

This limits their commercialization. However, the use of mutants and recombinant hyperproducing microorganisms along with the use of cheaper raw materials and optimal growth and production conditions with more efficient recovery processes can make production of biosurfactant economically feasible. Therefore, future research aiming for high-level production of biosurfactants must be focused towards the development of novel recombinant hyperproducing strains. Appropriate combinations of hyperproducing microbial strains, optimized cheaper production media and optimized process conditions will lead to successful economical commercial level scaled up biosurfactant productions.

References

1. Clapes P, Infante MR. Amino acid-based surfactants: Enzymatic synthesis, properties and potential applications. Biocatal Biotransformation 2002; 20:215-233.
2. Kosaric N. Biosurfactants and their application for soil bioremediation. Food Technol Biotechnol 2001; 39:295-304.
3. Greek BF. Sales of detergents growing despite recession. Chem Eng News 1991; 28:25-52.
4. Desai JD, Desai AJ. Production of biosurfactants. In: N. Kosaric, ed. Biosurfactants: Production, Properties, Applications. New York: Marcel Dekker, Inc., 1993:65-97.
5. Rosenberg E. Microbial surfactants. Crit Rev Biotechnol 1986; 3:109-132.
6. Kosaric N, Gray NCC, Cairns WL. Microbial emulsifiers and de-emulsifiers, In: H.J. Rehm, G. Reed, eds. Biotechnology. Deerfield Beach: Verlag Chemie, 1983; 3:575-592.
7. Banat IM. Biosurfactants production and possible uses in microbial enhanced oil recovery and oil pollution remediation: a review. Bioresource Technol 1995; 51:1-12.
8. Ron EZ, Rosenberg E. Natural roles of biosurfactants. Environ Microbiol 2001; 3:229-236.
9. Hamme VJD, Singh A, Ward OP. Surfactants in microbiology and biotechnology: Part 1. Physiological aspects. Biotech Adv 2006; 24:604-20.
10. Ivshina IB, Kuyukina MS, Ritchkova MI et al. Oleophilic biofertilizer based on a Rhodococcus surfactant complex for the bioremediation of crude oil-contaminated soil. Contaminated Soil, Sediment and Water 2001; 20-24.
11. Banat IM, Makkar RS, Cameotra SS. Potential commercial applications of microbial surfactants. Appl Microbiol Biotechnol 2000; 53:495-508.
12. Christofi N, Ivshina IB. Microbial surfactants and their use in field studies of soil remediation. J Appl Microbiol 2002; 93:915-929.
13. Jordan RN, Nichols EP, Cunningham AB. Role of (bio)surfactant sorption in promoting the bioavailability of nutrients localized at the solid-water interface. Water Science Technol 1999; 39:91-98.
14. Pastewski S, Hallmann E, Medrzycka K. Physiochemical aspects of the application of surfactants and biosurfactants in soil remediation. Environ Eng Sc 2006; 23(4):579-588.
15. Brusseau M, Gierke J, Sabatini D. Field demonstrations of innovative subsurface remediation and characterization technologies: introduction. In: Brusseau ML, Sabatini DA, Gierke JS et al, eds. Innovative Subsurface Remediation Field Testing of Physical, Chemical and Characterization Technologies, 1st ed. Washington, DC: American Chemical Society, 1999:2-5.
16. Fountain JC. Technologies for dense non-aqueous phase liquid source zone remediation: technology evaluation report. Ground-Water Remediation Technologies Analysis Center (GWRTAC). 1998. TE-98-02.
17. Mulligan CN, Yong RN, Gibbs BF. Remediation technologies for metal-contaminated soils and groundwater: an evaluation. Engineering Geology 2001; 60:193-207.
18. Grasso D, Subramaniam K, Pignatello JJ et al. Micellar desorption of polynuclear aromatic hydrocarbons from contaminated soil. Colloids Surf A Physicochem Eng Asp 2001; 194:65-74.
19. Cuypers C, Pancras T, Grotenhuis T et al. The estimation of PAH bioavailability in contaminated sediments using hydroxypropyl-beta-cyclodextrin and Triton X-100 extraction techniques. Chemosphere 2002; 46:1235-1245.
20. Prak DJL, Pritchard PH. Degradation of polycyclic aromatic hydrocarbons dissolved in Tween 80 surfactant solutions by Sphingomonas paucimobilis EPA 505. Canadian J Microbiol 2002; 48:151-158.
21. Sabatini D, Knox R, Harwell J. Emerging technologies in surfactant-enhanced subsurface remediation. In: Sabatini DA, Knox RC, Harwell JH, eds. Surfactant-Enhanced Subsurface Remediation: Emerging Technologies, 1st ed. Washington, DC: American Chemical Society, 1995:1-9.
22. Shiau B, Rouse J, Sabatini D et al. Surfactant selection for optimizing surfactant-enhanced subsurface remediation. In: Sabatini DA, Knox RC, Harwell JH, eds. Surfactantenhanced Subsurface Remediation: Emerging Ttechnologies. Washington, DC: American Chemical Society, 1995:65-79.
23. Zang Y, Miller RM. Enhanced octadecane dispersion and biodegradation by Pseudomonas rhamnolipid surfactant (biosurfactant). Appl Environ Microbiol 1992; 58:3276-3282.
24. Scheibenbogen K, Zytner RG, Lee H et al. Enhanced removal of selected hydrocarbons from soil by Pseudomonas aeruginosa UG2 biosurfactants and some chemical surfactants. J Chem Technol Biotechnol 1994; 59:53-59.
25. Ghosh MM, Yeom IT, Shi Zet al. Surface-enhanced bioremediation of PAH- and PCB-contaminated soil. In: Hinchee RE, Brockman FJ, Vogel CM, ed. Microbial Processes for Remediation, ed. Columbus: Battelle Press, 1995:15-23.
26. Robinson KG, Ghosh MM, Shi Z. Mineralisation enhancement of non-aqueous phase and soil-bound PCB using biosurfactant. Water Sci Technol 1996; 34:303-309.
27. Bai G, Brusseau ML, Miller RM. Biosurfactant enhanced removal of residual hydrocarbon from soil. J Contaminant Hydrology 1997; 25:157-170.

28. Lafrance P, Lapointe M. Mobilisation and cotransport of pyrene in the presence of Pseudomonas aeruginosa UG2 biosurfactants in sandy soil columns. Ground Water Monitoring and Remediation 1998; 18:139-147.
29. Ivshina IB, Kuyukina MS, Philp JC et al. Oil desorption from mineral and organic materials using biosurfactant complexes produced by Rhodococcus species. World J Microbiol Biotechnol 1998; 14:711-717.
30. Park AJ, Cha DK, Holsen M. Enhancing solubilization of sparingly soluble organic compounds by biosurfactants produced by Nocardia erythropolis. Water Environment Research 1998; 70:351-355.
31. Page CA, Bonner JS, Kanga SA et al. Biosurfactant solubilization of PAHs. Environ Eng Sc 1999; 16:465-474.
32. Brusseau ML, Miller RM, Zhang Yet al. Biosurfactant- and cosolvent-enhanced remediation of contaminated media. In: Hinchee RE, Brockman FJ, Vogel CM, ed. Microbial Processes for Remediation. Columbus: Battelle Press, 1995:82-94.
33. Zoller U, Rubin H. Feasibillity of in situ NAPL-contaminated aquifer bioremediation by biodegradable nutrient-surfactant mix. J Environ Sci Health A Tox Hazard Subst Environ Eng 2001; 36(8):1451-1471.
34. Beal R, Betts WB. Role of rhamnolipid biosurfactants in the uptake and mineralization of hexadecane in Pseudomonas aeruginosa. J Appl Microbiol 2000; 89:158-68.
35. Maier RM, Soberon-Chavez G. Pseudomonas aeruginosa rhamnolipids: biosynthesis and potential applications. Appl Microbiol Biotechnol 2000; 54:625-33.
36. Noordman WH, Wachter JJJ, de Boer GJ et al. The enhancement by biosurfactants of hexadecane degradation by Pseudomonas aeruginosa varies with substrate availability. J Biotechnol 2002; 94:195-212.
37. Rahman KSM, Rahman TJ, Kourkoutas Y et al. Enhanced bioremediation of n-alkane in petroleum sludge using bacterial consortium amended with rhamnolipids and micronutrients. Biores Technol 2003; 90:159-168.
38. Youssef NH, Nguyen T, Sabatini DA et al. Basis for formulating biosurfactant mixtures to achieve ultra low interfacial tension values against hydrocarbons J Ind Microbiol Biotechnol 2007; 34:497-507.
39. Makkar RS, Rockne KJ. Comparison of synthetic surfactants and biosurfactants in enhancing biodegradation of polycyclic aromatic hydrocarbons. Environ Toxicol Chem 2003; 22:2280-2292.
40. Nitschke M, Costa SGVAO. Biosurfactants in food industry. Trends in Food Science and Technology 2007; 18:252-259.
41. Finnerty WR. Biosurfactants in environmental biotechnology. Curr Opin Biotechnol 1994; 5:291-295.
42. Ishigami Y. Biosurfactants face increasing interest. Inform 1993; 4:1156-1165.
43. Khire JM, Khan MI. MEOR: importance and mechanism of MEOR. Enz Microbiol Technol 1994a; 16:170-172.
44. Khire JM, Khan MI. MEOR: microbes and the subsurface environment. Enz Microbiol Technol 1994b; 16:258-259.
45. Georgiou G, Lin SC, Sharma MM. Surface-active compounds from microorganisms. Bio/Technol 1992; 10:60-65.
46. Desai JD, Banat IM. Microbial production of surfactants and their commercial potential. Microbiol Mol Biol Rev 1997; 61:47-64.
47. Lin SC. Biosurfactants: Recent Advances. J Chem Tech Biotechnol 1996; 66:109-120.
48. Robert M, Mercade ME, Bosch MP et al. Effect of the carbon source on biosurfactant production by Pseudomonas aeruginosa 44T. Biotechnol Lett 1989; 11:871-874.
49. Manresa MA, Bastida J, Mercade ME et al. Kinetic studies on surfactant production by Pseudomonas aeruginosa 44T1. J Industrial Microbiol 1991; 8:133-136.
50. Kim HS, Yoon BD, Lee CH et al. Production and properties of a lipopeptide biosurfactant from Bacillus subtilis C9. J Ferment Bioeng 1997; 84:41-46.
51. Mulligan CN, Gibbs BF. Correlation of nitrogen metabolism with biosurfactant production by Pseudomonas aeruginosa. Appl Environ Microbiol 1989; 55:3016-3019.
52. Ramana KV, Karanth NG. Factors affecting biosurfactants production using Pseudomonas aeruginosa CFTR-6 under submerged conditions. J Chem Technol Biotechnol 1989; 45:249-257.
53. Zhang Y, Miller RM. Enhanced octadecane dispersion and biodegradation by a Pseudomonas rhamnolipid surfactant. Appl Environ Microbiol 1992; 58:3276-3282.
54. Davis DA, Lynch HC, Varley J. The production of surfactin in batch culture by Bacillus subtilis ATCC 21332 is strongly influenced by the conditions of nitrogen metabolism. Enzyme and Microbial Technol 1999; 25:322-329.
55. Syldatk C, Lang S, Matulovic U et al. Production of four interfacial active rhamnolipids from n-alkanes or glycerol by resting cells of Pseudomonas sp. DSM 2874. Z Naturforsch 1985; 40C:61-67.

56. Syldatk C, Wagner F. Production of biosurfactants. In: N. Kosaric, W.L. Cairns, N.C.C. Gray, eds. Biosurfactants and Biotechnology. New York: Marcel Dekker, Inc., 1987:89-120.
57. Ramana KV, Karanth NG. Production of biosurfactants by the resting cells of Pseudomonas aeruginosa CFTR-6. Biotechnol Lett 1989; 11:437-442.
58. Inoue S, Itoh S. Sorphorolipids from Torulopsis bombicola as microbial surfactants in alkane fermentation. Biotechnol Lett 1982; 4:3-8.
59. Kitamoto D, Yanagishita H, Shinbo T et al. Surface active properties and antimicrobial activities of mannosylerythritol lipids as biosurfactants produced by Candida antarctica. J Biotechnol 1993; 29:91-96.
60. Tulloch AP, Spencer JFT, Gorin PAJ. The fermentation of long-chain compounds by Torulopsis magnoliae Structures of the hydroxy fatty acids obtained by fermentation of fatty acids and hydrocarbons. Can J Chem 1962; 40:1326-1338.
61. Cooper DG, Paddock DA. Production of a biosurfactant from Torulopsis bombicola. Appl Environ Microbiol 1984; 47:173-176.
62. Lin SC, Carswell KS, Sharma MM et al. Continuous production of the lipopeptide biosurfactant of Bacillus licheniformis JF-2. Appl Microbiol Biotechnol 1994; 41:281-285.
63. Margaritis A, Kennedy K, Zajic JE. Application of an air-lift fermentor in the production of biosurfactants. Dev Ind Microbiol 1980; 21:285-294.
64. Drouin CM, Cooper DG. Biosurfactants and aqueous two-phase fermentation. Biotechnol Bioeng 1992; 40:86-90.
65. Ohno A, Ano T, Shoda M. Production of lipopeptide antibiotic surfactin with recombinant Bacillus subtilis in solid state fermentation. Biotechnol Bioeng 1995; 47:209-214.
66. Mukherjee S, Das P, Sen R. Towards commercial production of microbial surfactants. Trends Biotechnol 2006; 24:509-515.
67. Hester A. "I.B. Market Forecast". Industrial Bioprocessing 2001; 23(5):3.
68. Deleu M, Paquot M. From renewable vegetables resources to microorganisms: new trends in surfactants. C R Chimie 2004; 7:641-646.
69. Makkar RS, Cameotra SC. Biosurfactant production by microorganisms on unconventional carbon sources. J Surfactants Deterg 1999; 2:237-241.
70. Dubey K, Juwarkar A. Determination of genetic basis for biosurfactant production in distillery and curd whey wastes utilizing Pseudomonas aeruginosa strain BS2. Indian J Biotechnol 2004; 3:74-81.
71. Dubey K, Juwarkar A. Distillery and curd whey wastes as viable alternative sources for biosurfactant production. World J Microbiol Biotechnol 2001; 17:61-69.
72. Joshi S, Bharucha C, Jha S et al. Biosurfactant production using molasses and whey under thermophilic conditions. Bioresour Technol 2008; 99:195-199.
73. Haba E, Espuny MJ, Busquets M et al. Screening and production of Rhamnolipids by Pseudomonas aeruginosa 47T2 NCIB 40044 from waste frying oils. J Appl Microbiol 2000; 88:379-387.
74. Bednarski W, Adamczak M, Tomasik J et al. Application of oil refinery waste in the biosynthesis of glycolipid by Yeast. Bioresource Technol 2004; 95:15-18.
75. Gurye GL, Vipulanandan C, Wilson RC. A practical approach to biosurfactant production using non-aseptic fermentation of mixed cultures. Biotechnol Bioeng 1994; 44:661-666.
76. Makkar RS, Cameotra SC. Utilization of molasses for biosurfactant production by two Bacillus strains at thermophilic conditions. J Am Oil Chem Soc 1997; 74:887-889.
77. Patel RM, Desai AJ. Biosurfactant production by Pseudomonas aeruginosa GS3 from molasses. Lett Appl Microbiol 1997; 25:91-94.
78. Fox SL, Bala GA. Production of surfactant from Bacillus subtilis ATCC 21332 using potato substrates. Bioresource Technol 2000; 75:235-240.
79. Nitchke M, Pastore GM. Production and properties of a surfactant obtained from Bacillus subtilis grown on cassava wastewater. Bioresource Technol 2006; 97:336-341.
80. Wei YH, Wang LF, Chang JS et al. Identification of induced acidification in iron enriched cultures of Bacillus subtilis during biosurfactant fermentation. J Biosci Bioeng 2003; 96:174-178.
81. Vega CA, Cerrato RF, Garcia FE et al. Effect of combined nutrients on biosurfactant produced by Pseudomonas putida. J Environ Sci Health 2004; A39:2983-2991.
82. Joshi S, Yadav S, Nerurkar A et al. Statistical optimization of medium components for the production of biosurfactant by bacillus licheniformis K51. J Microbiol Biotechnol 2007; 17:313-319.
83. Sen R. Response surface optimization of the critical media components for production of surfactin. J Chem Tech Biotechnol 1997; 68:263-270.
84. Sen R, Swaminathan T. Application of response-surface methodology to evaluate the optimum environmental conditions for the enhanced production of surfactin. Appl Microbiol Biotechnol 1997; 47:358-363.
85. Sen R, Swaminathan T. Response surface modeling and optimization to elucidate the effects of inoculum age and size on surfactin production. Biochem Eng J 2004; 21:141-148.

86. Joshi S, Yadav S, Desai AJ. Application of response-surface methodology to evaluate the optimum medium components for the enhanced production of lichenysin by Bacillus licheniformis R2. Biochem Eng J 2008; 41:122-127.
87. Abalos A, Maximo F, Manresa MA et al. Utilization of response surface methodology to optimize the culture media for the production of rhamnolipids by Pseudomonas aeruginosa AT10. J Chem Technol Biotechnol 2002; 77:777-784.
88. Jacques P, Hbid C, Destain J et al. Optimization of biosurfactant lipopeptide production from Bacillus subtilis S499 by Plackett-Burman design. Appl Biochem Biotech 1999; 77-79:223-2330.
89. Rodrigues L, Teixeira J, Oliveira R et al. Response surface optimization of the medium components for production of biosurfactants by probiotic bacteria. Process Biochem 2006; 41:1-10.
90. Wei Y–H, Chin—Chi L, Chang JS. Using Taguchi experimental design methods to optimize trace element composition for enhanced surfactin production by Bacillus subtilis ATCC 21332. Process Biochem 2007; 42:40-45.
91. Yeh MS, Wei YW, Chang JS. Bioreactor design for enhanced carrier-assisted surfactin production with Bacillus subtilis. Process Biochem 2006; 41:1799-1805.
92. Lin SC, Carswell KS, Sharma MM et al. Continuous production of the Iipopeptide biosurfactant of Bacillus licheniformis JF-2. Appl Microbiol Biotechnol 1994; 41:281-285.

CHAPTER 18

Biosurfactants from Yeasts:
Characteristics, Production and Application

Priscilla F.F. Amaral, Maria Alice Z. Coelho, Isabel M.J. Marrucho, and João A.P. Coutinho*

Abstract

B iosurfactants are surface-active compounds from biological sources, usually extracellular, produced by bacteria, yeast or fungi. Research on biological surfactant production has grown significantly due to the advantages they present over synthetic compounds such as biodegradability, low toxicity, diversity of applications and functionality under extreme conditions. Although the majority of microbial surfactants have been reported in bacteria, the pathogenic nature of some producers restricts the wide application of these compounds.

A growing number of aspects related to the production of biosurfactants from yeasts have been the topic of research during the last decade. Given the industrial importance of yeasts and their potential to biosurfactant production, the goal of this chapter is to review the biosurfactants identified up to present, focusing the relevant parameters that influence biosurfactant production by yeasts and its characteristics, revealing the potential of application of such compounds in the industrial field and presenting some directions for the future development of this area, taking into account the production costs.

Introduction

Surfactants are amphiphilic compounds possessing both hydrophilic and hydrophobic moieties. They can reduce surface and interfacial tensions by accumulating at the interface between two immiscible fluids, thus stabilizing emulsions, or increasing the solubility of hydrophobic or insoluble organic compounds in aqueous media. They can be of synthetic or biological origin and the market for these compounds is on expansion.[1]

Due to their interesting properties such as lower toxicity, higher biodegradability, higher foaming capacity and higher activity at extreme temperatures, pH levels and salinity,[2] biosurfactants have been increasingly attracting the attention of the scientific community as promising candidates for the replacement of a number of synthetic surfactants. These compounds are biological molecules with noticeable surfactant properties similar to the well-known synthetic surfactants and they also include microbial compounds with surfactant properties.[3-6]

The majority of microbial biosurfactants described in literature is of bacterial origin and the genders most reported as biosurfactant producers are *Pseudomonas sp.*, *Acinetobacter sp.*, *Bacillus sp.* and *Arthrobacter sp*. However, due to the pathogenic nature of such producing organisms, the application of these compounds is restricted, not being suitable for use in food industry, among others.[7]

*Corresponding Author: João A.P. Coutinho—CICECO, Department of Chemistry, University of Aveiro, Aveiro 3810-193, Portugal. Email: jcoutinho@dq.ua.pt

Biosurfactants, edited by Ramkrishna Sen. ©2010 Landes Bioscience and Springer Science+Business Media.

The study of biosurfactant production by yeasts has been growing in importance, with production being reported mainly by the genders *Candida sp., Pseudozyma sp.* and *Yarrowia sp.* The great advantage of using yeasts in biosurfactant production is the GRAS (generally regarded as safe) status that most of theses species present, for example *Yarrowia lipolytica, Saccharomyces cerevisiae* and *Kluyveromyces lactis.* Organisms with GRAS status are not toxic or pathogenic, allowing the application of their products in the food and pharmaceutical industries.[8]

Biosurfactant Classification and Characteristics

Many microorganisms have the ability to produce molecules with surface activity. Two main types of surface-active compounds are produced by microorganisms: biosurfactants and bioemulsifiers.[9] Biosurfactants significantly reduce the air-water surface tension while bioemulsifiers do not reduce as much the surface tension but stabilize oil-in-water emulsions. During the last decades, there has been a growing interest in isolating microorganisms that produce surface active molecules with good surfactant characteristics such as low CMC and high emulsification activity, simultaneously presenting low toxicity and good biodegradability.[10]

Biosurfactants are categorized mainly by their microbial origin and chemical composition. Most extracellular yeast surfactants characterized and reported in literature have been identified as glycolipids, protein-carbohydrate-lipid or protein-carbohydrate complexes, lipids or fatty acids. Table 1 presents the yeast producing species identified up to present and the type of biosurfactant produced.

Glycolipids biosurfactants are carbohydrates in combination with long-chain aliphatic acids or hydroxyaliphatic acids. Among these the most interesting are the sophorolipids, which have been identified in *Torulopsis bombicola,*[11,12] *T. petrophilum*[13] and *T. apicola*[14,15] and consist of a dimeric carbohydrate sophorose linked to a long-chain hydroxy fatty acid. Although sophorolipids can lower surface and interfacial tension, they are not very effective emulsifying agents.[16] Both lactonic and acidic sophorolipids were reported to lower the interfacial tension between n-hexadecane and water from 40 to 5 mN/m and to display remarkable stability toward pH and temperature changes.[13] Another glycolipid produced by yeasts, mannosylerythritol lipids, was identified from *Candida antarctica*[22] and *Pseudozyma rugulosa*[18] and exhibits excellent surface-active and vesicle forming properties.

Sarrubo et al[19] report the production of a biosurfactant from *Y. lipolytica* in the presence of glucose as carbon source, composed by 47% protein, 45% carbohydrate and 5% lipids. Although produced using the same carbon source but from a different *Y. lipolytica* strain, Yansan, a biosurfactant consisting of a polysaccharide-protein complex with negligible lipid content, shows a much lower protein content (15%).[9] Another *Y. lipolytica* derived surfactant,[20] produced with hexadecane as carbon source, was found to be also a lipid-carbohydrate-protein complex with an even lower protein content, 5% and very high lipid concentration, 75%. Liposan, a biosurfactant produced in the presence of a water-immiscible substrate by yet another *Y. lipolytica* strain, contained no lipid in its constitution, only carbohydrate (83%) and protein (17%) and the yeast seems not to be able to produce surfactants using glucose as carbon source.[21]

In what concerns their ability to produce and stabilize emulsions, Liposan only displays emulsification activity with long chain hydrocarbons[3] while the surfactant produced by *Y. lipolytica* reported by Zinjarde et al[20] was not able to emulsify *n*-alkanes. Yansan was observed to present high emulsification activity with several hydrocarbons tested, including both aliphatics and aromatics.[6]

It has been demonstrated that the protein content of these polymers plays an important role in the emulsification activity. In fact, many mannoproteins extracted from yeasts' wall, have been reported to have high emulsification properties due to the presence of hydrophilic mannose polymers covalently attached to the protein backbone providing the amphiphilic structure common to surface-active agents.[22]

Table 1. Main biosurfactant producing yeast species

Biosurfactant	Producing Microorganisms	References
Sophorolipids	*Candida bombicola*	11
	Candida bombicola	12
	Torulopis petrophilum	13
	Candida (torulopsis) apicola	14
	Torulopsis apicola	15
	Candida bogorienses	65
Mannosylerythritol lipids	*Candida antarctica*	17
	Pseudozyma rugulosa	18
	Candida sp. SY16	44
	Pseudozyma aphidis	55
	Kurtzmanomyces sp. I-11	66
	Pseudozyma fusifornata, P. parantarctica, P. tsukubabaensis	67
Carbohydrate—protein—lipid complex	*Candida lipolytica UCP0988*	5
	Candida lipolytica IA 1055	19
	Yarrowia lipolytica NCIM 3589	20
	Debaryomyces polymorphus	68
	Candida tropicalis	68
Carbohydrate—protein –complex	*Candida lipolytica ATCC 8662*	3,21
	Yarrowia lipolytica IMUFRJ 50682	6
Mannanoprotein	*Saccharomyces cerevisiae*	22
	Kluyveromyces marxianus	27
ND[a]	*Candida utilis*	7
Fatty acids	*Candida ingens*	47
Lipids	*Rhodotorula glutinis*	69

[a]ND not determined.

Production Processes

The Influence of the Culture Medium Composition

Biosurfactants are produced by a number of yeasts, either extracellularly or attached to parts of the cell, predominantly during their growth on water-immiscible substrates. However, some yeasts may produce biosurfactants in the presence of different types of substrates, such as carbohydrates. The use of different carbon sources changes the structure of the biosurfactant produced and, consequently, its properties. These changes may be welcomed when some properties are sought for a particular application.[23] There are a number of studies in biosurfactant production involving the optimization of their physicochemical properties.[6,24,25]

The composition and characteristics of biosurfactants are also reported to be influenced by the nature of the nitrogen source as well as the presence of iron, magnesium, manganese, phosphorus and sulphur. The influence of the culture media on the biosurfactant production is discussed in detail below.

Carbon Source

Several reports in the literature address the influence of the carbon source in biosurfactant production by different yeast strains showing the possibility to use a wide variety of substrates.

Pareilleux[26] isolated surface-active compounds in the growth medium of *Candida lipolytica* using *n*-alkane as carbon source, but when this yeast was cultivated with glucose as carbon source no bioemulsifier was produced. In a similar study, Zinjarde and Pant[4] demonstrated that the surfactant biosynthesis by *Y. lipolytica* NCIM 3589 using soluble substrates such as glucose, glycerol, sodium acetate or alcohol was not viable. The authors identified, however, the presence of a bioemulsifier in culture media containing crude oil and alkanes (C_{10}-C_{18}).

Cirigliano and Carman[3] have also shown that a strain of *Y. lipolytica* produces biosurfactants through different carbon sources such as hexadecane, paraffin, soybean oil, olive oil, corn oil and cottonseed oil, with hexadecane identified as the best one.

Many vegetable oils (corn, soybean, sunflower and safflower) have been used as substrate for biosurfactant production by *T. bombicola*. The biosurfactants yield were similar for all the oils investigated.[16]

In 2001, Sarubbo et al[19] identified for the first time a biosurfactant produced by *Y. lipolytica* IA 1055 using glucose as carbon source. These authors demonstrated that the induction of biosurfactant production is not dependent on the presence of hydrocarbons. Another strain, *Y. lipolytica* IMUFRJ 50682, producing a bioemulsifier from glucose with high emulsification activity for oil-in-water emulsions, was identified by our group.[6]

Lactose has also been used as soluble substrate for the production of compounds with emulsifying activity, such as the production of mannan-proteins by *Kluyveromyces marxianus*.[27]

Although it is also possible to produce biosurfactants in the presence of water soluble carbon sources, several studies show that often higher production yields are obtained when hydrophobic substrates are added.[3,4,26] A number of works describe the importance of combining a water insoluble substrate with a carbohydrate in the culture medium.

Biosurfactant production was identified on a *Candida glabrata* strain isolated from mangrove sediments. The maximum bioemulsifier production was observed when the strain was cultivated on cotton seed oil (7.5%) and glucose (5.0%), reaching values of 10 g l^{-1} after 144 hours. The cell-free culture broth containing the biosurfactant produced presented a surface tension of 31 mN m^{-1}.[25]

Casas and Ochoa[11] studied the medium composition of sophorolipids production by *Candida bombicola*. The carbon sources promoting the best biosurfactant production were glucose (100 g l^{-1}) and sunflower oil (100 g l^{-1}), used simultaneously, resulting in a biosurfactant concentration of 120 g l^{-1} after 144 hours of fermentation.

Sarrubo et al[5] investigated the production of a biosurfactant by *C. lipolytica* in a medium containing canola oil (100 g l^{-1}) and glucose (100 g l^{-1}). The surface-active compound produced was constituted by a protein—lipid—polysaccharide complex and was able to reduce the surface tension of water from 71 mN m^{-1} to 30 mN m^{-1}.

The hydrophilic substrates are initially metabolised by the microorganism for its energetic requirements and afterwards it also uses such substrates in the synthesis of the polar portion of the biosurfactant molecule. On the other hand, hydrophobic substrates are exclusively used for the production of the apolar moiety of the biosurfactant. *Candida* species seem to be capable to incorporate fatty acids directly into the production of biosurfactants.[15]

There are various pathways for the synthesis of the two main parts that constitute a biosurfactant molecule and they are generally accomplished through specific sets of enzymes. In most cases, the first enzymes used in the synthesis of these precursors are regulatory ones; therefore, in spite of their diversity, there are some common features in the synthesis of biosurfactants and regulation.[28] According to Syldatk and Wagner,[29] the synthesis of the different moieties of biosurfactants and their linkage follows one of four possible paths: (i) the hydrophilic and hydrophobic moieties are synthesized de novo by two independent pathways; (ii) the hydrophilic moiety is synthesized de novo while the synthesis of the hydrophobic moiety is induced by substrate; (iii) the hydrophobic moiety is synthesized de novo, while the synthesis of the hydrophilic moiety is substrate dependent; and (iv) the synthesis of both the hydrophobic and hydrophilic moieties are substrate dependent.

One important factor affecting the surfactant synthesis is naturally the alkyl chain length of the compounds used as carbon source. Kitamoto et al[30] studied the production of mannosylerythritol lipids (MEL), a biosurfactant produced by *C. antarctica*, using different *n*-alkanes as carbon source. The authors found that *C. antarctica* T-34 did not grow well on *n*-alkanes (3%, v/v) ranging from C_{10} to C_{18} and no MEL were produced. However, it was possible to successfully produce MEL from *n*-alkanes ranging from C_{12} to C_{18} using 13.6 g resting cells l^{-1}. Only small quantities of MEL were obtained from *n*-alkanes longer than nonadecane (C_{19}), probably due to their high melting points, above the culture temperature of 30°C. The authors observed that the productivity of MEL was markedly affected by the chain-length of the alkane substrates, with the highest productivity obtained from *n*-octadecane. Cavalero and Cooper[12] have shown that the sophorolipid yield from *C. bombicola* ATCC 22214 increases with the *n*-alkane chain length (from C_{12} to C_{15}). However, Zinjard and Pant[4] demonstrated that the production of a biosurfactant by *Y. lipolytica* did not change when using different *n*-alkanes as substrate.

Carbon Source from Renewable Resources

To date, biosurfactants are unable to compete economically with chemically synthesized compounds available in the market, due to their high production costs resulting from the use of expensive substrates. These costs may be significantly reduced by the use of alternative sources of nutrients with lower costs and by reaching high yields of product.[31] A possible solution for the first approach would be the re-utilization of industrial wastes, for instance, the agro-industrial or the oil-containing wastes. This strategy decreases the costs of biosurfactant production, reducing simultaneously, the pollution caused by the waste disposal in landfills.[32]

Many food industries using fats and oils, generate large quantities of wastes, tallow, lard, marine oils or soapstock and free fatty acids from the extraction of seed oils. Waste disposal is a growing problem, which explains the increasing interest in the waste valorisation through microbial transformation.[33]

Oil refinery waste, either with soapstock or postrefinery fatty acids, was used by Bednarski et al[34] to synthesize surfactants in the cultivation medium of *C. antarctica* or *Candida apicola*. The authors showed that the production of glycolipids, in a medium supplemented with soapstock and postrefinery fatty acids, was 7.5 to 8.5-fold greater than in the medium without addition of oil refinery waste.

The soy molasses, a by-product from the production of soybean oil, plus oleic acid were tested as carbon sources for the production of sophorolipids by the yeast *C. bombicola*.[35] The authors reported a production of 21 g l^{-1} after seven days of fermentation, which is a low value when compared to the production in the presence of glucose and oleic acid (79 g l^{-1}).

Used frying oil is produced in large quantities both in the food industry and from domestic uses. Haba et al[36] compared the composition of used olive and sunflower oils with the standard unused oils in their study and found that the most important difference is the presence of 22.52 wt% of fatty acids of low chain length (<C_{14}) in used oil. Thanomsub et al[37] isolated yeast strains from plant material in Thailand and a strain of *Candida ishiwadae* was able to produce glycolipid biosurfactants from used soybean cooking oil. The biosurfactants produced were characterized to be monoacylglycerols and exhibited high surfactant activities.

The production of sophorolipids by *C. bombicola* was stimulated by the addition of animal fat, a residue of the meat processing industry. A high biosurfactant production (120 g l^{-1}) was obtained after 68 hours of fermentation.[38]

Nowadays, a very important renewable origin carbon source is glycerol. The increase in the world production of biodiesel is generating large quantities of raw glycerol, which is a by-product from this bio-fuel production. With the production of 10 kg of bio-diesel from rapeseed oil, 1 kg of glycerol becomes available[39] and its price is decreasing and tends to decrease even more as the traditional glycerol markets become saturated. Morita et al[40] used glycerol for the production of glycolipids by *Pseudozyma antarctica*, obtaining 16.3 g l[-1] of biosurfactant after seven days of fermentation. The biosynthesis of sophorolipids by *C. bombicola* was also studied in the presence of a by-product of bio-diesel production, with 40% of glycerol and 34% of hexadecane soluble compounds (92% of fatty acids and 6% of monoacylglycerol/triacylglycerol) and 26% of water. The fermentation yielded 60 g l[-1] of sophorolipids.[41]

Another good substrate for biosurfactant production is lactic whey. It is composed of high levels of lactose (75% of dry matter), 12-14% protein, organic acids and vitamins. Disposal of whey is a major environmental problem for countries depending on dairy economics.[33] Daniel et al[42] achieved production of high concentrations of sophorolipids (422 g l[-1]) using a two-stage cultivation process: first, deproteinized whey concentrate (DWC) containing 110 g lactose was used for cultivation of *Cryptococcus curvatus* ATCC 20509; cells were then disrupted by passing the cell suspension directly through a high pressure laboratory homogeniser. After autoclaving, the resulting crude cell extract containing the single-cell oil served as a substrate for growth of *C. bombicola* ATCC 22214 and for sophorolipid production in a second stage.

Nitrogen Source

Nitrogen is important in the biosurfactant production medium because it is essential for microbial growth as protein and enzyme syntheses depend on it. Different nitrogen compounds have been used for the production of biosurfactants, such as urea,[43] peptone,[44] yeast extract,[11,45-47] ammonium sulphate,[20] ammonium nitrate,[37] sodium nitrate,[34] meat extract and malt extract,[48] etc. Yeast extract is the most used nitrogen source for biosurfactant production, but its concentration depends on the microorganism and the culture medium.

Cooper and Paddok[16] have studied the effect of the nitrogen source, using sodium nitrate, ammonium chloride, ammonium nitrate, urea or yeast extract in the biosurfactant production by *T. bombicola* in agitated flasks. The authors observed that nitrate was not a good nitrogen source since it affected the biomass growth while 5 g l[-1] of yeast extract promoted a higher surfactant production. When the yeast extract was substituted by peptone, the biosurfactant concentration obtained was reduced to half and a very low concentration was obtained when urea was used.

The production of a bioemulsifier by *Y. lipolytica* was also evaluated using different nitrogen sources: ammonium sulphate, ammonium chloride, ammonium nitrate, urea and sodium nitrate. The results showed that ammonium sulphate and ammonium chloride were the best nitrogen sources for the emulsifier production. The emulsifying activity was reduced to half when ammonium nitrate and urea were used and no emulsifying activity was detected in the culture medium with sodium nitrate.[20]

Casas and Ochoa[11] tested different yeast extract concentrations (1 to 20 g l[-1]) to optimize the formulation of the culture medium of *C. bombicola* and described that the production of sophorolipids is better in the presence of low yeast extract concentration (1 g l[-1]). According to the authors when high yeast extract concentrations are used, the biosurfactant production decreases because the carbon source is used in yeast growth.

Johnson[49] reported the influence of the nitrogen source in the production of a biosurfactant by the yeast *Rhodotorula glutinis* IIP-30. The author revealed that the use of potassium nitrate presented the best result in comparison to other nitrogen sources (ammonium sulphate and urea).

As shown in literature, several researchers choose to use more than one nitrogen source, obtaining good surfactant concentrations. Lukondeh et al[27] investigated the production of a biosurfactant by *K. marxianus* FII 510700, by using yeast extract (2 g l[-1]) and ammonium sulphate (5 g l[-1]) as nitrogen sources. The bioemulsifier produced presented high emulsification activity (around 76% of emulsion phase after 90 days at 4°C).

To optimize the production of a bioemulsifier by *C. lipolytica*, Alburquerque et al[50] used a factorial experimental design to investigate the effect and the interaction between urea, ammonium sulphate, potassium dihydrogen orthophosphate and corn oil in the emulsifying activity of the culture medium. Ammonium sulphate, potassium dihydrogen orthophosphate and corn oil had a positive effect in emulsifying activity while urea presented a negative effect.

The production of surface-active compounds often occurs when the nitrogen source is depleted in the culture medium, during the stationary phase of cell growth.[44] Kitamoto et al[22] studied the cell growth of *C. antarctica* and its biosurfactant production in a culture medium containing the ammonium ion (10 g l^{-1}) and peptone (1 g l^{-1}) as nitrogen sources. The authors noticed that the production of glycolipids starts when the nitrogen source is exhausted after 50 hours of fermentation, reaching a concentration value of 38 g l^{-1} after 200 hours of fermentation.

In the same line of thought, Albrecht et al[51] suggested a mechanism in which the biosurfactant synthesis happens in limiting nitrogen conditions. According to the authors, this condition causes the decline of the specific activity of NAD-NADP-dependent isocitrate dehydrogenase, which catalyses the oxidation of isocitrate to 2-oxoglutarate in the citric acid cycle. With the reduction of the activity of this enzyme, isocitrate accumulates, leading to the accumulation of citrate in mitochondria. Citrate and isocitrate are, then, transported to the cytosol, where the first is cleaved by citrate synthase, forming acetyl-CoA, which is the precursor of fatty acids synthesis and, therefore, biosurfactant production increases.

An important parameter studied by several researchers is the quantitative ratio between carbon and nitrogen sources (C/N) used in biosurfactant production. Different C/N ratios and hydrocarbons were used in biosurfactant production by *C. tropicalis*. The emulsifying activity rose with the increase in C/N ratio for almost all cases, when nitrogen was the limiting factor.[52] Similar results were obtained by Jonhson et al[49] for the production of a biosurfactant from *R. glutinis*.

Table 2 presents a compilation of literature data on biosurfactant production by yeasts, including parameters such as the carbon and nitrogen sources concentration, the yield of the production (Yp/s) and volumetric productivity (Qp).

The Environmental Factors Affecting the Production

Environmental factors are extremely important in the yield and characteristics of the biosurfactant produced.[53] In order to obtain large quantities of biosurfactant it is necessary to optimize the process conditions because the production of a biosurfactant may be induced by changes in pH, temperature, aeration or agitation speed.

pH

The effect of pH in the biosurfactant production by *C. antarctica* was investigated using phosphate buffer with pH values varying from 4 to 8. All conditions used resulted in a reduction of biosurfactant yield when compared to distilled water.[30]

Zinjarde and Pant[4] studied the influence of initial pH in the production of a biosurfactant by *Y. lipolytica*. The authors observed that the best production occurred when the pH was 8.0, which is the natural pH of sea water.

The acidity of the production medium was the parameter studied in the synthesis of glycolipids by *C. antarctica* and *C. apicola*. When pH was maintained at 5.5, the production of glycolipids reached a maximum. Without the pH control, the synthesis of the biosurfactant decreased.[34]

The production of a bioemulsifier by *R. glutinis* during feed batch fermentation was significantly influenced by both pH and temperature, with the optimum conditions at 30°C and pH 4.0.[49]

Temperature

Most biosurfactant productions reported were performed in a temperature range of 25 to 30°C. There are many works in literature reporting the influence of this parameter. Casas and Ochoa[11] showed that the amount of sophorolipids obtained in the culture medium of *C. bombicola* at temperature of 25°C or 30°C was similar. Nevertheles, the fermentation performed at 25°C presented a lower biomass growth and a higher glucose consumption rate in comparison to the

Table 2. Data from biosurfactant production by yeasts reported in literature

Strain	Carbon Source (g l⁻¹)	Nitrogen Source (g l⁻¹)	BPᵃ	Tᵇ (h)	Operation Mode	$Y_{P/S}$ᶜ (g g⁻¹)	Xᵈ (g l⁻¹)	$Y_{P/X}$ᵉ (g g⁻¹)	Qp (g (l h)⁻¹)	Reference
Torulopsis bombicola ATCC22214	Glucose (500) Safflower Oil (1000)	Yeast extract (5)	18 g l⁻¹	48	Batch	0.012	12.4	1.45	0.375	16
Candida bombicola ATCC22214	Glucose (100) Animal fat (100)	CSLᶠ (4) Urea (1.5)	120 g l⁻¹	68	Batch	0.6	30	4	1.76	38
Candida tropicalis ATCC20336	n-hexadecane (10)	Yeast extract (0.3) Peptona (0.5)	0.81 U	72	Batch	NDᴳ	ND	ND	ND	68
Debaryomyces polymorphus ATCC20499	n-hexadecane (10)	Yeast extract (0.3) Peptone (0.5)	0.11 U	72	Batch	ND	ND	ND	ND	68
Candida sp. SY 16	Glucose (15) Soybean oil (15)	Peptone (1)	95 g l⁻¹	200	Feed-batch	0.475	15.0	6.33	0.475	44
Candida bombicola NRRL Y-17069	Glucose (100) Sunflower oil (100)	Yeast extract (1)	120 g l⁻¹	192	Batch— Resting cell	0.6	23.0	5.21	0.625	11
Candida antarctica ATCC20509	Soybean oil (80)	Yeast extract (1)	46 g l⁻¹	144	Batch	0.57	28.4	1.61	0.32	45
Candida antarctica ATCC20509	Soapstock (100)	Yeast extract (1) NaNO₃ (2)	15.9 g l⁻¹	85	Feed-batch	0.636	1.8	8.83	0.1870	34
Candida antarctica T-34	Nut oil (80)	Yeast extract (1)	47 g l⁻¹	144	Batch— Resting cell	0.587	24	1.95	0.326	17

continued on next page

Table 2. *Continued*

Strain	Carbon Source (g l⁻¹)	Nitrogen Source (g l⁻¹)	BP[a]	T[b] (h)	Operation Mode	$Y_{P/S}$[c] (g g⁻¹)	X[d] (g l⁻¹)	$Y_{P/X}$[e] (g g⁻¹)	Qp (g (l h)⁻¹)	Reference
Candida antarctica T-34	n-octadecane (60)	Yeast extract (1) NaNO₃ (2)	40.5 g l⁻¹	144	Batch— Resting cell	0,675	16	2.53	0.281	30
Candida ingens CB-216	Corn oil (20)	Yeast extract (2)	5.6 g l⁻¹	168	Batch	0,28	23.9	0.234	0.033	47
Candida lipolytica ATCC 8662	n-hexadecane (10)	Yeast extract (6)	1.3 U/ mL⁻¹	130	Batch	ND	ND	ND	ND	3
Yarrowia lipolytica NCIM3589	Hexadecano (10)	(NH₄)₂SO₄ (5)	3.0 U/ mL⁻¹	144	Batch	ND	3	ND	ND	4
Candida lipolytica IA 1055	Babassu oil (50)	Urea (0.25)	0.66 U ml⁻¹	60	Feed-batch	ND	6 UFC ml⁻¹	ND	ND	43
Yarrowia lipolytica IMUFRJ 50682	Glucose (20)	Peptone (6,4) Yeast extract (10)	2.0 U ml⁻¹	170	Batch	ND	ND	ND	ND	6
Candida lipolytica UCP0988	Glucose (100) Canola oil (100)	Yeast extract (2)	8 g l⁻¹	48	Batch	0,04	ND	ND	0.166	5
Kluyveromyces marxianus FII 510700	Lactose (40)	Yeast extract (2) (NH₄)₂SO₄ (5)	ND	ND	Batch	ND	ND	ND	ND	27
Candida apicola ATCC 20509	Soapstock (100)	Yeast extract (1) NaNO₃ (2)	10.3 g l⁻¹	144	Batch	0,103	6.5	9.70	0.071	34
Candida. ishiwadae	Soybean frying oil (40)	Yeast extract (0.5) NH₄NO₃ (3)	0.25 µg	168	Batch	ND	ND	ND	ND	37

[a]BP: biosurfactant production; [b]T: biosurfactant production time; [c]$Y_{P/S}$: biosurfactant yield related to substrate consumption; [d]X: cell concentration produced; [e]$Y_{P/X}$: biosurfactant yield related to cell produced; [f]CSL: corn steep liquor; [g]ND: not determined.

fermentation performed at 30°C. In a similar study, Desphande and Daniels[38] observed that the growth of *C. bombicola* reached a maximum at a temperature of 30°C while 27°C was the best temperature for the production of sophorolipids.

In the culture of *C. antarctica*, temperature causes variations in the biosurfactant production. The highest mannosylerythritol lipids production was observed at 25°C for the production with both growing and resting cells. When resting cells were used the production occurred in a large range of temperature. The effect of aeration was also investigated using different volumes of medium (20 to 60 ml) in flasks of 300 ml. The best yield was obtained with 30 ml of medium volume, which implies a medium—flask volume ratio of 0.1, demonstrating the importance of aeration in such systems.[22]

Aeration and Agitation

Aeration and agitation rates are important factors that influence the production of biosurfactants, since they facilitate the oxygen transfer from the gas phase to the aqueous phase and it may also be linked to the physiological function of microbial emulsifiers. It has been suggested that the production of bioemulsifiers can enhance the solubilization of water-insoluble substrates and, consequently, facilitate nutrient transport to microorganisms. Therefore, higher shear stress may induce surfactant secretion as the contact of organic droplets dispersed in water with microorganisms becomes more difficult. Desai and Banat,[28] in their review, reported some opposite results regarding *Norcadia erythropolis* and *Acinetobacter calcoaceticus* which produced less biosurfactant due to the increase of shear stress. They mention, however, that biosurfactant production with yeasts generally increases with stirring and aeration rates.

Adamczak and Bednarsk[45] evaluated the influence of aeration in the biosurfactant synthesis by *C. antarctica* and observed that the best production (45.5 g l^{-1}) was obtained when air flow rate was 1 vvm and the dissolved oxygen concentration was maintained at 50% of saturation. Nevertheless, changing the air flow rate to 2 vvm, there was a high foam formation and the biosurfactant production decreased 84%. The formation of foam is not appropriated for biosurfactant production because it removes biosurfactant, some biomass and lipids from the culture medium.

The effect of aeration rate was also investigated by Guilmanov et al[54] in agitated flasks. The best yield of sophorolipids produced by *C. bombicola* was reached with aeration rate between 50 and 80 mM of O$_2$ l^{-1} h^{-1}.

Kinetics and Operation of Biosurfactant Production Process

It is very difficult to draw general guidelines for optimal biosurfactant production by yeasts because the biosurfactants identified are from a diverse group of compounds produced by a variety of microbial species. The process must, therefore, be optimized on a case by case basis. Most biosurfactants are excreted into the culture medium either during the exponential phase or at the stationary phase.[1] Cirigliano and Carman[3] showed that the emulsifier production by *C. lipolytica* IA 105530 was detected when the microorganism growth rate decreased but Amaral et al[6] described a growth-associated bioemulsifier production by *Y. lipolytica* IMUFRJ 50682 using a different carbon source.

T. bombicola produced most of the surfactant in the late exponential phase of growth. Therefore, Cooper and Paddock[16] proposed to grow the yeast on a single carbon source and then add a second type of substrate after the exponential growth phase, causing a burst of glycolipids production. The maximum yield was 70 g l^{-1} or 35% of the weight of the substrate used. An economic analysis demonstrated that this biosurfactant could be produced at significantly lower cost than any of the previously reported microbial surfactants.

Biosurfactant production by resting or immobilized cells is a type of process in which there is no cell multiplication. Nevertheless, the cells continue to utilize the carbon source for their maintenance and for the synthesis of biosurfactants.[28] Several examples of biosurfactant production by resting cells are known. They include production of sophorolipids by *T. bombicola*[11] and *C. apicola*[14] and mannosylerythritol lipid production by *C. antarctica*.[17] Biosurfactant production by resting cells is important in the reduction of costs associated with product recovery, as the growth and the product formation phases can be separated.

Besides the optimization of the culture medium, considerable attention has been directed towards the different ways to operate the biosurfactant production process. The production of biosurfactant by yeasts is generally carried out in batch or feed-batch fermentation, as can be noticed from Table 2. Batch and feed-batch fermentations are ways to operate bioprocesses which gather some advantages such as simpler equipments and less contamination problems. Some promising results with batch operations for biosurfactant production have been reported. For example, the production of mannosylerythritol lipid by *C. antarctica* achieved a concentration of 95 g l⁻¹ after 200 hours of feed-batch fermentation using glucose and soybean oil as carbon source. The yield obtained by feed-batch fermentation was 2.6 times greater than in batch fermentation.[44] Rau et al[55] reported the production of a biosurfactant by *Pseudozyma aphidis* using soybean oil and glucose in a feed-batch fermentation, obtaining a high production (168 g l⁻¹) after eleven days of fermentation.

Other fermentation techniques include the application of air lift fermentor and continuous operation, which can improve biosurfactant production.[1] However these techniques haven't been used for biosurfactant production by yeasts. Therefore, studies on the optimization of the production operation is still lacking.

Potential Commercial Applications

Biosurfactants find applications in a wide variety of commercial areas and industrial processes such as oil recovery enhancement,[1] bio-remediation of oil-polluted soil and water,[56] replacement of chlorinated solvents used in the cleaning up of oil-contaminated pipes,[57] use in the detergent industry[58] and in the formulation of oil-in-water emulsions in the food, biotechnological, pharmaceutical and cosmetic industries.

Synthetic surfactants are commonly used in oils spills to disperse the oil and accelerate its mineralization, being the limiting steps determined by desorption and/or solubilization rates in soil and water. Surfactants increase the aqueous solubility of hydrophobic contaminants and, consequently, their microbial degradation.[2] The main problem associated to the use of synthetic surfactants is their toxicity, representing an additional source of environmental contamination. Thus, in the bioremediation field, biosurfactants come up as a major candidate for the replacement of synthetic surfactants due to their lower toxicity, high biodegrability and the possibility of in situ production.[1] The effects of biosurfactants on the biodegradation of petroleum compounds were investigated by Hua et al.[59] They reported that the addition of a biosurfactant produced by *Candida antarctica* T-34 could improve the biodegradation rate of some n-alkanes (90.2% for n-decane, 90.2% for n-undecane, 89.0% for dodecane), a mixture of n-alkanes (82.3%) and kerosene (72.5%) and showed that this biosurfactant could substitute with advantage synthetic surfactants.

The application of biodegradable and nontoxic biosurfactants can also be of substantial benefit in the biomedical and biotechnological fields. Perfluorocarbon-based emulsions are being exploited as oxygen injectable carriers, contrast agents, drug delivery systems or as cell culture media supplements and the employment of a nontoxic and biodegradable biosurfactant can lead to further improvements in these areas.[60]

Biosurfactants have also showed several promising applications in the food industry as food additives. Lecithin and its derivatives, fatty acid esters containing glycerol, sorbitan, or ethylene glycol and ethyoxylated derivatives of monoglycerides are currently in use as emulsifiers in the food industries worldwide. A bioemulsifier from *Candida utilis* has shown potential use in salad dressing[7] and good results were obtained with mannoproteins extracted from *S. cerevisiae* cell wall in mayonnaise formulation.[61]

Biosurfactants can also have a very important position in the cosmetic industries. A product containing 1 mol of sophorolipid and 12 mol of propylene glycol has excellent skin compatibility and is used commercially as a skin moisturizer.[62] Sophorolipids are being produced and used by Kao Co. Ltd. as a humectant in cosmetics.[2]

Some other potential commercial applications of biosurfactants currently under study include the pulp and paper industry, textiles, ceramics and uranium ore processing.[28]

Conclusion

In the last few years, there has been an increase in the number of publications in the area of yeast biosurfactant production. This is a clear indication that these compounds are showing to be of interest in several areas and becoming technologically important. Despite the advantages of biosurfactant synthesis, its industrial use is still limited due to the costs involved in the production process.

The optimization of the production process is the key factor to improve yield and to reduce costs. Estimates show that the utilization of renewable source as substrates may reduce up to 30% of the production costs. Factors that influence biosurfactant production, such as nitrogen source, carbon source, pH, temperature, agitation and aeration, are also relevant on the optimization of the production and thus on the production cost.

The current cost of sophorolipids production by the yeast *C. bombicola* varies from 2 to 5 € kg⁻¹, depending on the substrate cost and the production scale,[63] while the market price of synthetic surfactants is around 2 € kg⁻¹. Some specific industrial sectors, such as cosmetic and pharmaceutical, biosurfactants have high application potential and will probably play a major role in short period of time, because of its enhanced characteristics and the high margins and value of the final product.

Nowadays, researches are slowly progressing to the genetic engineering through the use of recombinant DNA techniques for the manipulation of biosurfactant production.[64] These studies open new perspectives to increase production yields and might become the instrument to overcome the limitations for biosurfactants industrial application.

Acknowledgements

The authors wish to acknowledge CNPq and FAPERJ (Brazilian Research Foundations).

References

1. Lin SC. Biosurfactants: Recent advances. J Chem Tech Biotechnol 1996; 66:109-120.
2. Banat IM, Makkar IM, Cameotra SS. Potential commercial applications of microbial surfactants. Appl Microbiol Biotechnol 2000; 53:495-508.
3. Cirigliano MC, Carman GM, Isolation of a bioemulsifier from Candida lipolytica. Appl Environ Microbiol 1984; 48:747-750.
4. Zinjarde SS, Pant A. Emulsifier from a tropical marine yeast, Yarrowia lipolytica NCIM 3589. J Basic Microbiol 2002; 42:67-73.
5. Sarubbo LA, Farias CBB, Campos-Takaki GM. Co-utilization of canola oil and glucose on the production of a surfactant by Candida lipolytica. Current Microbiology 2007; 54:68-73.
6. Amaral PFF, Lehocky M, da Silva JM et al. Production and characterization of a bioemulsifier from Yarrowia lipolytica. Process Biochem 2006; 41:1894-1898.
7. Sheperd R, Rockey J, Sutherland I et al. Novel bioemulsifiers from microorganisms for use in foods. J Biotechnol 1995; 40:207-17.
8. Barth G, Gaillard C. Physiology and genetics of the dimorphic fungus Yarrowia lipolytica. FEMS Microbiol Rev 1997; 19:219-37.
9. Rufino RD, Sarubbo LA, Campos-Takaki GM. Enhancement of stability of biosurfactant produced by Candida lipolytica using industrial residue as substrate. World J Microbiol Biotechnol 2007; 23:729-734.
10. Rosenberg E, Ron EZ. High- and low-molecular-mass microbial surfactants. Appl Microbiol Biotechnol 1999; 52:154-162.
11. Casas J, Ochoa FG. Sophorolipid production by Candida bombicola: medium composition and culture methods. J Biosci Bioeng 1999; 88:488-94.
12. Cavalero DA, Cooper DG. The effect of medium composition on the structure and physical state of sophorolipids produced by Candida bombicola ATCC 22214. J Biotechnol 2003; 103:31-41.
13. Cooper DG, Paddock DA. Torulopsis petrophilum and surface activity. Appl Environ Microbiol 1983; 46:1426-1429.
14. Hommel RK, Weber L, Weiss A et al. Production of sophorose lipid by Candida (Torulopsis) apicola grown on glucose. J Biotechnol 1994; 33:147-55.
15. Weber L, Doge C, Haufe G. Oxygenation of hexadecane in the biosynthesis of cyclic glycolipids in Torulopsis apicola. Biocatal 1992; 5:267-72.

16. Cooper DG, Paddock DA. Production of a biosurfactant from Torulopsis bombicola. Appl Environ Microbiol 1984; 47:173-76.

17. Kitamoto D, Fuzishiro T, Yanagishita H et al. Production of mannosylerythritol lipids as biosurfactants by resting cells of Candida antarctica. Biotechnol Lett 1992; 14:305-310.

18. Morita T, Konish M, Fukuoka T et al. Discovery of Pseudozyma rugulosa NBRC 10877 as a novel producer of the glycolipid biosurfactants, mannosylerythritol lipids, based on rDNA sequence. Appl Microbiol Biotechnol 2006; 73:305-13.

19. Sarubbo LA, Marçal MC, Neves MLC et al. Bioemulsifier production in batch culture using glucose as carbon source by Candida lipolytica. Appl Biochem Biotechnol 2001; 95:59-67.

20. Zinjarde SS, Chinnathambi S, Lachke AH et al. Isolation of an emulsifier from Yarrowia lipolytica NCIM 3589 using a modified mini isoeletric focusing unit. Lett Appl Microbiol 1997; 24:117-121.

21. Cirigliano MC, Carman GM. Purification and characterization of liposan, a bioemulsifier from Candida lipolytica. Appl Environ Microbiol 1985; 50:846-50.

22. Cameron DR, Cooper DG, Neufeld RJ. The mannoprotein of Saccharomyces cerevisiae is an effective bioemulsifier. Appl Environ Microbiol 1988; 54:1420-25.

23. Cooper DG. Biosurfactants. Microbiological Sciences 1986; 3:145-9.

24. Kim HS, Yoon BD, Choung DD et al. Characterization of a biosurfactant, mannosylerythritol lipid produced from Candida sp. SY16. Appl Microbiol Biotechnol 1999; 52:713-21.

25. Sarubbo LA, Luna JM, Campos-Takaki GM. Production and stability studies of the bioemulsifier obtained from a new strain of Candida glabrata UCP 1002. Eletronic Journal of Biotechnology 2006; 9:400-406.

26. Pareilleux A. Hydrocarbon assimilation by Candida lipolytica: formation of a biosurfactant; effects on respiratory activity and growth. Appl Microbiol Biotechnol 1979; 8:91-101.

27. Lukondeh T, Ashbolt NJ, Rogers PL. Evaluation of Kluyveromyces marxianus as a source of yeast autolysates. J Ind Microbiol Biotech 2003; 30:52-56.

28. Desai JD, Banat IN. Microbial production of surfactants and their commercial potential. Microbiol Mol Biol Rev 1997; 61:47-64.

29. Syldatk C, Wagner F. Production of biosurfactant. In: Kosaric N, Cairns WL, Gray NCC, eds. Biosurfactants and Biotechnology, 1st ed. New York: Marcel Dekker 1987:89-120.

30. Kitamoto D, Ikegami T, Suzuki GT et al. Microbial conversion of n-alkanes into glycolipid biosurfactants, mannosylerythritol lipids, by Pseudozyma (Candida antarctica). Biotechnol Lett 2001; 23:1709-14.

31. Gallert C, Winter J. Solid and liquid residues as raw materials for biotechnology. Naturwissenschaften 2002; 89:483-96.

32. Maneerat S. Production of biosurfactants using substrates from renewable-resources. Songklanakarin J Sci Technolol 2005; 27:675-83.

33. Makkar RS, Cameotra SS. An update on the use of unconventional substrates for biosurfactant production and their new applications. Appl Microbiol Biotechnol 2002; 58:428-34.

34. Bednarski W, Adamczak M, Tomasik J et al. Application of oil refinery waste in the biosynthesis of glycolipids by yeast. Bioresour Technol 2004; 95:15-18.

35. Solaiman DKY, Ashby RD, Nunez A et al. Production of sophorolipids by Candida bombicola grown on soy molasses as substrate. Biotechnol Lett 2004; 26:1241-1245.

36. Haba E, Espuny MJ, Busquets M et al. Screening and production of rhamnolipids Pseudomonas aeruginosa 47T2 NCIB 40044 from waste frying oils. J Appl Microbiol 2000; 88:379-387.

37. Thanomsub B, Watcharachaipong T, Chotelersak K et al. Monoacylglycerols: glycolipid biosurfactants produced by a thermotolerant yeast, Candida ishiwadae. J Appl Microbiol 2004; 96:588-92.

38. Deshpande M, Daniels L. Evaluation of sophorolipid biosurfactant production by Candida bombicola using animal fat. Bioresour Technol 1995; 54:143-50.

39. Meesters PAEP, Huijberts GNM, Eggink G. High-cell-density cultivation of the lipid accumulating yeast cryptococcus curvatus using glycerol as a carbon source. Appl Microbiol Biotechnol 1996; 45:575-79.

40. Morita T, Konish M, Fukuoka T et al. Microbial conversion of glycerol into glycolipid biosurfactants, mannosylerythritol lipids, by a basidiomycete yeast, Pseudozyma antarctica JCM 10317. J Biosci Bioeng 2007; 104:78-81.

41. Ashby RD, Nunez A, Solaiman DKY et al. Sophorolipid biosynthesis from a biodiesel coproduct stream. J of the American Oil Chemists' Society 2005; 9:625-30.

42. Daniel HJ, Reuss M, Syldatk C. Production of sophorolipids in high concentration from deproteinized whey and rapeseed oil in a two stage fed batch process using candida bombicola ATCC 22214 and cryptococcus curvatus ATCC 20509. Biotechnol Lett 1998; 20:1153-56.

43. Vance—Harrop MHV, Gusmão NB, Takaki GMC. New bioemulsifiers produced by candida lipolytica using D-glucose and babassu oil as carbon sources. Br J Microbiol 2003; 34:120-23.

44. Kim HS, Jeon JW, Kim BH et al. Extracellular production of a glycolipid biosurfactant, mannosy-lerythritol lipid, by candida sp. SY16 using fed-batch fermentation. Appl Microbiol Biotechnol 2006; 70:391-96.
45. Adamczak M, Bednarski W. Influence of medium composition and aeration on the synthesis of biosur-factants produced by candida antarctica. Biotechnol Lett 2000; 22:313-16.
46. Chen J, Song X, Zhang H et al. Production, structure elucidation and anticancer properties of sophoro-lipid from wickerhamiella domercqiae. Enzyme Microb Technol 2006; 39:501-6.
47. Amézcua—Vega CA, Varaldo PHM, García F et al. Effect of culture conditions on fatty acids composi-tion of a biosurfactant produced by candida ingens and changes of surface tension of culture media. Bioresour Technol 2007; 98:237-40.
48. Mata-sandoval JC, Karns J, Torrens A. Effect of nutritional and environmental conditions on the pro-duction and composition of rhamnolipids by P. aeruginosa UG2. Microbiol Res 2001; 155:249-56.
49. Johnson V, Singh M, Saini VS. Bioemulsifier production by an oleaginous yeast rhodotorulaglutinis IIP-30. Biotechnol Lett 1992; 14:487-90.
50. Albuquerque CDC, Filetti AMF, Campos-Takaki GM. Optimizing the medium components in bioemulsi-fiers production by candida lipolytica with response surface method. Can J Microbiol 2006; 52:575-83.
51. Albrecht A, Rau U, Wagner F. Initial steps of sophoroselipid biosynthesis by candida bombicola ATCC 22214 grown on glucose. Appl Microbiol Biotechnol 1996; 46:67-73.
52. Singh M, Saini VS, Adhikari DK et al. Production of bioemulsifier by a SCP-producing strain of candida tropicalis during hydrocarbon fermentation. Biotechnol Lett 1990; 12:743-46.
53. Banat IM. Biosurfactants production and possible uses in microbial enhanced oil recovery and oil pol-lution remediation: A review. Biosource Technol 1995; 51:1-12.
54. Guilmanov V, Ballistreri A, Impallomeni G et al. Oxygen transfer rate and sophorose lipid production by candida bombicola. Biotechnol Bioeng 2002; 77:489.
55. Rau U, Nguyen LA, Roeper H et al. Fed-batch bioreactor production of mannosylerythritol lipids secreted by pseudozyma aphidis. Appl Microbiol Biotechnol 2005; 68:607-13.
56. Volkering F, Breure A, Rulkens W. Microbiological aspects of surfactant use for biological soil remedia-tion. Biodegradation 1997; 8:401-417.
57. Robinson K, Gosh M, Shu Z. Mineralization enhancement of non-aqueous phase and soil-bound pcb using biosurfactant. Water Sci Technol 1996; 34:303-9.
58. Rosenberg E, Ron EZ. Surface active polymers from the genus acinetobacter. In: Kaplan DL, ed. Bio-polymers from Renewable Resources, 1st ed. New York: Springer 1998:281-291.
59. Hua Z, Chen Y, Du G et al. Effects of biosurfactants produced by candida antarctica on the biodegrada-tion of petroleum compounds. World Journal of Microbiology and Biotechnology 2004; 20:25-29.
60. Freire MG, Dias AMA, Coelho MAZ et al. Aging mechanisms of perfluorocarbon emulsions using image analysis. J Colloid Interface Sci 2005; 286:224-232.
61. Torabizadeh H, Shojaosadati SA, Tehrani HA. Preparation and characterisation of bioemulsifier from saccharomyces cerevisiae and its application in food products. Lebensm-Wiss u-Technol 1996; 29:734–737.
62. Yamane T. Enzyme technology for the lipid industry. An engineering overview. J Am Oil Chem Soc 1987; 64:1657-1662.
63. Van Bogaert INA, Saerens K, De Muynck C et al. Microbial production and application of sophorolipids. Appl Microbiol Biotechnol 2007; 76:23-34.
64. Van Bogaert INA, De Maeseneire SL, De Schamphelaire W et al. Cloning, characterization and func-tionality of the orotidine-5⊠-phosphate decarboxylase gene (URA3) of the glycolipid-producing yeast candida bombicola. Yeast 2007; 24:201-208.
65. Tulloch AP, Spencer JFT, Deinema MH. A new hydroxy fatty acid sophoroside from candida bogoriensis. Can J Chem 1968; 46:345-48.
66. Kakugawa K, Tamai M, Imamura K et al. Isolation of yeast kurtzmanomyces sp. I-11, novel producer of mannosylerythritol lipid. Biosci Biotechnol Biochem 2002; 66:188-91.
67. Morita T, Konish M, Fukuoka T et al. Characterization of the genus pseudozyma by the formation of glycolipid biosurfactants, mannosylerythritol lipids. FEMS Yeast Res 2007; 7:286-92.
68. Singh M, Desai JD. Hydrocarbon emulsification by candida tropicalis and debaryomyces polymorphus. Indian J Experimental Biol 1989; 27:224-26.
69. Yoon SH, Rhee JS. Lipid from yeast fermentation: Effects of cultural conditions on lipid production and its characteristics of rhodotorula glutinis. J American Oil Chemists' Society 1983; 60:1281-6.

CHAPTER 19

Environmentally Friendly Biosurfactants Produced by Yeasts

Galba M. Campos-Takaki,* Leonie Asfora Sarubbo
and Clarissa Daisy C. Albuquerque

Abstract

Some yeasts are preferred to bacteria as sources for biosurfactants, mainly due to their GRAS status for environmental and health safety reasons. This chapter thus focuses on the production of biosurfactants by some yeast cultures using renewable resources like fatty wastes from household and vegetable oil refineries as major substrates. The chapter also emphasizes on the importance of the application of response surface methodology and artificial neural network techniques for the optimization of biosurfactant production by yeasts.

Introduction

Biosurfactants are amphipathic molecules with both hydrophilic and hydrophobic (generally hydrocarbon) moieties, a structurally diverse group of surface active molecules synthesized by a variety of microorganism bacteria, filamentous fungi and yeasts.[27,34] These molecules reduce surface and interfacial tensions in both aqueous solutions and hydrocarbon mixtures, which make them potential candidates for enhancing oil recovery and emulsification processes.[9,18,55] Biosurfactants have several advantages over chemical surfactants, such as lower toxicity; higher biodegradability;[82] better environmental compatibility;[28] higher foaming;[47,50,61] high selectivity and specific activity at extreme temperatures, pH and salinity; and the ability to be synthesized from renewable feedstock.[47,50,81,82]

Information concerning the studies of yeast and the biodegradation of hydrocarbons and oil is described in the literature.[9,10,24-27] Studies on emulsifier production by yeasts have been undertaken by Cirigliano and Carman,[15] Cirigliano and Carman[16] and Singh and Desai.[75] Table 1 shows the biosurfactant produced by different yeast strains, according to the literature.

For the last ten years, our research group has been working on the biosurfactant molecules produced by yeasts, given that the criteria for advantage is the low risk associated with the products obtained from the metabolism of yeast i.e., that all molecules are generally regarded as safe (GRAS). This is a concept used in some countries to identify substances that have been assessed as ingredients in many products and found in all cases to be safe. This simplifies the assessment process by eliminating those substances from extensive and repetitive assessment. Most of the substances that have been classified as GRAS are very common ingredients, such as sodium chloride, but also include substances such as emulsifiers, surfactants and wetting or sticking agents. In addition, the production of biosurfactants has been steadily increasing. This is due to their diversity of action, their environmentally friendly nature, the possibility of their production through fermentation,

*Corresponding Author: Galba M. Campos-Takaki—Nucleus of Research in Environmental Sciences, Center of Sciences and Technology, Catholic University of Pernambuco, 50.050-900 Recife, Pernambuco, Brazil. Email: gmctakaki@pesquisador.cnpq.br

Biosurfactants, edited by Ramkrishna Sen. ©2010 Landes Bioscience
and Springer Science+Business Media.

Table 1. Yeast producers of biosurfactants

Microorganism Producer	Chemical Composition of Biosurfactant	Literature Reference
Kluyveromyces marxianus	Mannan protein	48,49
Saccharomyces cerevisiae	"	11
C. tropicalis	Mannan lipoprotein	40,75,76
Rhodotorula bogorienses	Sophorose lipids	56
C. bombicola	"	12,19,23,31,33,58
Torulopsis petrophilum	"	20
Wickerhamiella domercqiae	"	37
Candida bogorienses	"	22
C. Antarctica	Mannosylerythritol lipids	2,42
Kurtzmanomyces sp 1-11	"	39
Pseudozyma rugulosa	"	52
C. glabrata UCP1002	Carbohydrate-protein-lipid complex	47
C. ishiwadae	"	78
C. sphaerica	"	77
Debaryomyces polymorphus	"	75
Yarrowia lipolytica IMUFRJ	"	7
Y. lipolytica NCIM 3589	"	86
C. lipolytica ATCC 8662	"	15,16
C. lipolytica IA 1055	"	50,81
C. lipolytica UCP 0988	"	64-67
C. ingens	"	8
C. utilis	"	75
C. valida	"	75
C. boleticola	"	53
Rhodotorula glutinis	Polyol-lipids	38
R. graminis	"	82

their potential for higher emulsification activity, their stability, their different applications in the food industry, their use in environmental protection and their lower superficial tension, critical micelle concentration (CMC) and toxicity.[47,64,65,68] In addition, in the northeast of Brazil there are large amounts of fatty waste (1890 tons/year) from vegetable oil refineries that could be used as a source of low cost carbons with commercial potential.[51] This chapter describes the success obtained from biosurfactant production by yeasts, the species most used, substrates, the influence of other factors, the properties of the biosurfactants and the use of neural networks. Our initial studies were based on the use of domestic vegetable oils in order to convert renewable resources into higher value products. Among the vegetable oils tested, babassu, palm kernel and coconut have shown good results. In this chapter we discuss the potential roles and applications of biosurfactants, mainly focusing on areas such as food-related industries and environmental pollution by petrol derivates.[50,66,70,71]

Culture Conditions for the Production of Biosurfactants

First *Candida lipolytica* has been shown to produce bioemulsifiers in batch cultures when growing on a number of water-immiscible carbon substrates. In 1979, Pareilleux[57] first isolated surfactant compounds from *Candida lipolytica* when cultivated in n-alkanes. Later, Cirigliano and Carman[15,16] isolated and characterized a bioemulsifier when the yeast was grown on a variety of water-immiscible carbon substrates. The ability of the *Candida* species to produce biosurfactants in fed batch cultures has also been demonstrated, as described by Sarubbo et al,[67] who showed the ability of *Candida lipolytica* to grow on babassu oil and produce bioemulsifiers under various conditions in batch and fed batch cultures.[69] Singh et al[76] used the fed batch culture technique to obtain high cell concentration with *Candida tropicalis* growing in hexadecane as carbon substrate. Davila, Marchal and Vandecasteele[23] also obtained a high production of sophorose lipids from ethyl esters of rapeseed oil fatty acids and glucose by *Candida bombicola* by using fed-batch fermentation and so did Rau et al,[60] who used glucose and oleic acid as combined substrates in an extended fed-batch cultivation of *Candida bombicola*. Recently, batch and fed-batch processes have been investigated in order to improve the yields of sophorolipid from *C. bombicola* grown in industrial fatty acid residues.[31]

Regarding the influence of cultivation conditions on the production of biosurfactants, the size of inoculums and the substrate concentration have been studied for the yeast *Candida lipolytica* which produced extracellular emulsifying agents when it was grown with three Brazilian vegetal oils as carbon sources namely babassu, palm kernel and coconut that could be applied in the future as food additives. The increase in inoculums size did not influence the emulsification activity and the greatest yield was evidenced with 10^2 CFU/mL. The increase in substrate concentration did not stimulate biopolymer production, although the medium supplemented with coconut oil showed greater emulsification activity for higher substrate concentrations.[50]

Substrates Used for the Production of *Candida* Biosurfactant

Yeasts are known to produce extracellular emulsifier when grown on water-immiscible substrates such as alkenes or oils, in order to facilitate their uptake. Among yeasts, species of *Candida* have been widely used in the production of biosurfactants from soluble,[68,70] insoluble[50,65,66,79] and a combination of both soluble and insoluble carbon sources.[47,64,67]

Regarding the use of food grade vegetal oils, waste frying vegetal oils or residues from vegetal oil refineries, isolated or combined with a soluble substrate, promising results have been obtained in the last ten years for *Candida* species in our laboratories. The use of olive oil was not a suitable substrate for cell growth, although the surface tension of the supernatant fluid decreased with *Candida* sp. 39A2 (35 mNm⁻¹), *C. albicans* (39 mNm⁻¹), *C. rugosa* IFO0750 (39 mN m⁻¹) and *C. tropicalis* CECT 1357 (35 mN m⁻¹). In this case, *C. lipolytica* (43 mNm⁻¹) and *C. torulopsis* (45 mN/m) were poor producers. The use of sunflower oil, on the other hand, supported good cellular growth in most cases and the surface tension decreased as follows: *Candida* sp. 39A2 (35 mNm⁻¹), *C. rugosa* IFO0750 (39 mNm⁻¹), *C. lipolytica* and *C. torulopsis* (40 mNm⁻¹).[23,47,64-67] It is important to consider, however, that the substrates act differently for a specific microorganism, as pointed out by Rau et al.[60]

Emulsifying Activities, Surface Tension and Critical Micellar Concentration (CMC) of *Candida* Biosurfactants

In addition to surface and interfacial tension, stabilisation of an oil and water emulsion is commonly used as a surface activity indicator. Most biosurfactants produced by *Candida* species have been tested for both tenso-active and emulsifying activities. Some microbial surfactants such as the sophorolipid from *Torulopsis bombicola* have been shown to reduce surface tension but not to be good emulsifiers.[19] By contrast, liposan has been shown not to reduce the surface tension of water and yet has been used successfully to emulsify commercial edible oils.[15]

The emulsification activities of the biosurfactant produced by *C. lipolytica* grown on vegetal oil refinery residue had been measured with various water-immiscible substrates. The highest emulsion values were obtained using motor oil. Diesel and hexane were not emulsified effectively.

These findings suggested that the activity of the emulsifier depends on its affinity for hydrocarbon substrates which involves a direct interaction with the hydrocarbon itself rather than an effect on the surface tension of the medium.[63] In another research article, the biosurfactant produced by *C. lipolytica* cultivated in glucose plus canola oil showed both emulsification and surface tension reduction capacity properties.[67] The *C. glabrata* isolated from mangrove sediments also produced a biosurfactant which lowered the surface tension of the medium to 31 mN/m and produced stable and compact emulsions with emulsifying activity of 75% of cotton seed oil.[68]

The emulsification properties of some yeast biosurfactants against synthetic surfactants have been described. The emulsification activity of hexadecane by the surfactant from *C. lipolytica* cultivated in glucose plus canola oil was similar to those of other synthetic commercial surfactants.[67] The biosurfactants produced by the thermo tolerant yeast *Candida ishiwadae* also exhibited higher activities when compared to synthetic surfactants.[81]

The presence of a surfactant reduces the surface tension air/water, this effect being proportional to the concentration of the biosurfactant in solution, until it reaches the CMC.[64] Although most of the potent surfactants extensively studied have been those belonging to the group of rhamnolipids from the *Pseudomonas* species and the lipopeptides from the *Bacillus* species,[35,36,61] due to the low CMC value and surface tension reduction capacity of these compounds, in the last few years the *Candida* species has been shown to produce surfactants with similar properties to the ones found for bacteria surfactants.[66,78]

Recently, the yeast *Candida sphaerica* cultivated in a low cost medium based on distilled water supplemented with vegetal oil refinery residue plus corn steep liquor produced a biosurfactant which exhibited excellent surface tension reducing activity. The surface tension of water decreased from 70 mN m^{-1} to 27.5 mN m^{-1} by increasing the solution concentration up to 0.42%.[80] The biosurfactant from *C. sphaerica* showed a lower minimum surface tension than that of the biosurfactant from *C. bombicola* (39-43.5 mN/m),[58] *C. lipolytica* (32 mNm^{-1}),[64] *C. glabrata* (31 mN m^{-1}),[68] *C. antarctica* (35 mN/m)[2] and from *Yarrowia lipolytica* (50 mNm^{-1}).[7] This biosurfactant also showed a smaller CMC (0.42%) value than those of other biosurfactants from yeasts described in the literature, such as values of 2.5% found for biosurfactants from *C. lipolytica*[64] and *C. glabrata*[47] and of 0.6% for the biosurfactant from *C. antarctica*.[2] We have now produced a new biosurfactant from *C. lipolytica* grown in vegetal oil refinery residue plus glutamic acid which is able to reduce the water surface tension to 25.29 mN/m.[66]

Biosurfactant: Isolation Methodology and Yields

The biosurfactants produced by the *Candida* species have been isolated by liquid-liquid extraction using organic solvents. Chloroform, methanol and ethyl acetate are the most organic solvents cited in the literature. The use of ethyl acetate resulted in greater crude extract yield (8 g l^{-1}) compared with systems based on mixtures of chloroform and methanol (2:1, 1:1 and 1:2) which yielded 4 g l^{-1}, 3.43 g l^{-1} and 2.4 g l^{-1}, respectively, for the biosurfactant produced in batch cultures by *C. lipolytica* cultivated in glucose plus canola oil as substrates. The emulsification index of the partially purified biosurfactant in the ethyl acetate extract was 10% higher than that obtained with the broth-free culture of cells. No remaining emulsification activity was found in the aqueous phase, suggesting that the polymer was completely recovered in the organic phase.[66] The bioemulsifier isolated from the culture filtrate of *Candida glabrata* grown in cotton seed oil plus glucose in the aqueous phase recovered 100% of the emulsification activity of n-hexadecane that was present in the culture filtrate, while the emulsification activity of the cotton seed oil increased 25%. The average yield of precipitate in the aqueous phase was approximately 10.0 g/l.[68] Bioemulsifier production by yeast *Candida utilis* varied from 0.26 to 0.93 g/l and depended on process conditions,[75] while the extracellular emulsifying agent from *Candida lipolytica* grown in the vegetal oil refinery industry was approximately 4.5 g l^{-1}.[56] Several research studies have described the scale up of biosurfactant production in fermentation to increase yields. High yields of a sophorolipid from soybean oil and glucose (67 g/L) have been reported by Cooper and Paddock.[20] Improved concentrations of 150 g/L have been obtained using canola oil and lactose as the substrate.[88]

Biochemical Composition and Application of Biosurfactant

Biosurfactants are polymers, totally or partially extracellular, with an amphipathic configuration, containing distinct polar and no polar moieties, which allow them to form micelles that accumulate at the interface between liquids of different polarities, such as water and oil. In relative terms, this process is based upon the ability of biosurfactants to reduce surface tension, blocking the formation of hydrogen bridges and certain hydrophilic and hydrophobic interactions.[9]

The literature shows that a wide range of carbon sources, including agricultural renewable resources, like insoluble substrates as oils or sugars as hydrophilic substrate are suitable carbon sources that can be used for the production of ecologically safe biosurfactants with good properties.[26-29]

In addition, these unique properties allow the use of biosurfactants and make it possible to replace chemically-synthesized surfactants in a great number of industrial applications. However, among yeasts, *Candida* species have been widely employed for insoluble substrates fermentation and have been reported to produce surface active agents.[64,65,69-71]

Optimal yields of bioemulsifier are usually obtained when carbohydrate and vegetable oil are used as substrate. However, the major success of biosurfactant production depends on the development of cheaper processes and the use of low cost raw materials, which account for 10-30% of the overall cost of the isolation and surfactant production of different species of the genus *Candida*.[35,88]

The surfactants produced by this genus can differ widely from one species to another. It has been reported to produce sophorolipid mainly from *Torulopsis bombicola*, *T. petrophilum* and *T. apicola*.[22,23] The chemical structure consists of dimeric carbohydrate sophorose residue linked to a long-chain hydroxyl fatty acid by the linkage of glycosides, whose glycolipids were incapable of stabilizing emulsions. However, when glucose was used as substrate, the yeast produced a potent emulsifier.[13]

Sophorolipids generally occur as a mixture of macrolactones. The free acid form may be possible; the lactone form is necessary, or at least preferable, for many applications. These biosurfactants are a mixture of at least six to nine different hydrophobic sophorolipids, depending on the growth medium.[20,22,23,31,33,58,74]

Most surfactants produced by *Candida* genus are complexes containing carbohydrate and protein or carbohydrate-protein-lipid, in different proportions, when hydrophic was used as substrate. The important study with polymeric biosurfactants produced by yeasts was on liposan, a polysaccharide—protein complex. Liposan is an extracellular water-souble emulsifier synthesized by *Candida lipolytica* and comprises 83% carbohydrate and 17% protein.[16,17] However, the amount and composition of biosurfactants are influenced by the carbon source and changed to lipid-carbohydrate complexes[25-28] or long-chain fatty acids[40] and protein-carbohydrate-lipid complexes[7,47,52,57,64,65] when grown either on hydrophobic or water-miscible substrates.[66-69,75-77,86]

Bushnell and Hass[11] were the first to demonstrate bacterial production of biosurfactants by isolating *Corynebacterium simplex* and a strain of *Pseudomonas* in a mineral medium containing either kerosene, mineral oil or paraffin.

Biosurfactants are considered chemically and ecologically safe and consequently, can be applied in industrial and bioremediation processes. The environmental applications include: wastewater treatment, environmental control of polluted areas, microbial enhanced oil recovery and hydrocarbon degradation. The mechanism of removal hydrophobic contaminants improve oil drainage into well bores, stimulating the release of oil entrapped by capillaries, the wetting of solid surfaces, the reduction of oil viscosity and oil pour point, the lowering of interfacial tension, dissolving of oil and emulsification of hydrocarbons, lowering of interfacial tension, metal sequestration and interaction with lipids, proteins and carbohydrates, as a protecting agent.[76-79]

The use of *C. antarctica* biosurfactant extracted over 50% of oil adsorbed in the sand.[2] Recently, studies carried out by our research group using *Candida* species have been tested in enhanced motor oil recovery. The authors demonstrated it was effective in the release of car engine waste oil from sand, as described where the biosurfactants obtained from *C. glabrata* and *C. sphaerica* removed 84% of the oil adsorbed in the sand by stable emulsions. In addition those properties of biosurfactants as due the characteristics of polymeric surfactants offer additional advantages because they coat droplets of oil, thereby forming stable emulsions.[47,77]

In general, biosurfactants produced by *Candida* genus are more effective and efficient and their CMC is lower than that of chemical surfactants, i.e., rufsan biosurfactant produced by . *lipolytica* 0988 and the less surfactant is necessary to get a maximum decrease in surface tension $(25, mN/m)$. For this biosurfactant, the surface activities are not affected by environmental conditions such as temperature and pH, nor by NaCl concentrations up to 50 and 25 g/l respectively.[64-66]

The three products were isolated and show low toxicity, with LD_{50} between 1600-1700 mg/Kg corporal weight and absence of direct and indirect mutagenic effects. The characteristics described by the biopolymers produced by *Candida lipolytica* suggest future possibilities for the use of these polymers as emulsifier additives in the food industry.[50,82]

Trends and Future Challenges of Biosurfactants

Computer-Based Tools for Optimization and Cost Reduction

During several decades of the twenty century, biological and computation sciences were dealt with separately. However, in the twenty-first century, the key challenge is to increase the convergence between biotechnology and computation technology through the production of new information resources, in ways that were not previously possible and that today increase the quality, reliability and economic efficiency of bioproducts and the bioprocess. The global surfactant industry is a strong and lucrative business. In the economic market it is necessary to work permanently for quality improvement and total cost competitiveness. The use of new technologies by surfactant companies has incremented the supply of the product, reduced costs through economies of scale and strengthened the world-wide surfactant market.[27,54,77,79,82,83]

Much interest has recently centered on biosurfactants as an alternative source of surfactants. However, biosurfactants are not widely available because of their high production costs, which result primarily from low strain productivities and high recovery expenses. The choice of inexpensive raw materials is important to the overall economics of the process because they account for fifty percent of the final product cost.[34,86] To replace conventional surfactants with biological compounds, inexpensive production is necessary.[44,45]

The reduction of the overall production costs of biosurfactants usually depends on strain improvements; the use of low cost raw materials such as agricultural and industrial wastes as substrates; the use of process scale-up; and the use of advanced computer-based techniques for process control and optimization. The optimization of biosurfactant production processes is especially important if the process is to be implemented on an industrial scale. Traditionally, different statistical and mathematical methods are combined to bioprocess identification, control and optimization. Artificial neural networks, fuzzy logic, genetic algorithms and hybrid approaches are some current, emerging and promising computational technologies with biological inspiration that are contributing significantly toward cultural changes and new advances in the modeling, control and optimization of real-world bioprocess, including some recent applications in the biosurfactant production process.[3,4] Artificial neural networks have been shown to be useful alternatives in applications which include complex, nonlinear and time-varying processes.[4-6,30,41,43-46] In such cases, the use of conventional methods is frequently unsuitable. The ability of neural networks to model the dynamics of a nonlinear process makes them an important tool for the modeling, control and optimization of bioprocesses. The intention of this section is to give a rapid overview of the use of: (i) Experimental Design (ED) associated with Response Surface Methodology (RSM) and (ii) an Artificial Neural Network based Software Sensor (ANNSS)—as effective tools for improving yields and reducing costs in the biosurfactant production process.

Experimental Design and Surface Response Methodology

The association of ED and RSM has been shown to be a rapid and effective technique leading to the optimization of bioprocesses.[18,21,22,31,85] To reduce the production costs of the biosurfactant in relation to synthetic surfactants, process improvements are being continuously implemented through 'one-factor-at-a time' techniques. 'One-factor-at-a time' techniques are time consuming, as they require a large number of experiments to be carried out and they do not consider the effects of interactions between the variables of the process. ED associated with RSM resolves this problem. Optimization using factorial design and RSM usually includes: (i) experimental design (ii) estimation of coefficients in a mathematical model based on data (iii) checking the adequacy of the model (iv) using the mathematical model to determine the levels of the factors that give optimum response, in the range of experimental conditions studied (v) predicting the response variable and (vi) experimental validation of the model.

This statistical approach has been successfully applied to the optimization of different objective functions in biosurfactant production processes. More often, the ED and RSM based optimization procedure has been used in optimizing biosurfactant production media components[1,2,37,59,62,65,81,87] and culture conditions such as age and size of inoculums, temperature, pH, dissolved oxygen level, rate of agitation and aeration etc.[24,32,44,71-74] However, the association of ED and RSM has also been used to ensure effective process scale-up, through the analysis and optimization of the biosurfactant process properties on a small-scale before transfer to medium- and large-scale production.[4,5,13,14] The efficiency of these applications have shown that combined ED and RSM techniques are important tools towards obtaining a high yield and a low cost for biosurfactant production over a short period of time.

Novel Tools in Biosurfactant Production, Control and Optimization Processes: Application of an Artificial Neural Network

Nowadays, the convergence between biotechnology and computation technology is an irreversible trend. Both technologies face problems concerning fundamental questions and are still limited in various aspects. Nevertheless, they have overcome limits in multiple fields and yielded novel and significant data and results.

The successful operational control and optimization of bioprocesses rely heavily on the availability of a fast and accurate evaluation of the performance of the system. This in turn requires reliable real-time information.[41] Supervised neural networks are adaptive computer programs with an ability to learn and are capable of stating estimation and prediction once well-trained. They offer a powerful tool as 'software sensors' for on-line control in cases that have been difficult or impossible to deal with efficiently, using conventional process control.[45,46] To overcome the problem of the lack of reliable sensors for on-line measurements of biomass, substrate and product concentration, enzymatic activity and other nonlinear and time-varying variables, numerous artificial neural network based software sensors have been developed.[6,13,17,20,30] The applications of neural networks in biotechnology are extremely diverse, mainly because the field is interdisciplinary.

In spite of the vast number of successful applications of neural-network-based software sensors in the bioprocess, there is still relatively little information on the applications in biosurfactant production processes. Recent results of on-line estimation and prediction of biomass and emulsification activity have shown that artificial neural network based software sensors may be feasible, efficient and cheap tools for biosurfactant production process control and optimization.[3,4] The biggest challenge in developing neural network based software sensors is to gain the confidence of the researchers and engineers that work on biosurfactant production, bearing in mind that the low cost and high quality of the real-time estimations and predictions carried out by an artificial neural network based software sensor will always be the best indicator of the success of this new technology.

Conclusion

In conclusion, this chapter thus discusses the potential roles and applications of biosurfactants, by mainly focusing on the yeast based lipidic biosurfactants and their potential application areas like food and food-processing industries and environmental biotechnology. The chapter also dwells up on the use of various computer-aided optimization techniques for the enhanced production of biosurfactants.

References

1. Abalos A, Maximo F, Manresa MA et al. Utilization of response surface methodology to optimize the culture media for the production of rhamnolipids by Pseudomonas aeruginosa AT10. J Chem Technol Biotechnol 2002; 77(7):777-784.
2. Adamczak M, Bednarski W. Influence of medium composition and aeration on the synthesis of surfactants produced by Candida Antarctica. Biotechnol Lett 2000; 22:313-316.
3. Albuquerque CDC, Vance-Harrop MH, Sarubbo LA et al. Biosurfactant production by Candida lipolytica—study of the culture medium components using factorial design. Revista Symposium 2005; 1:109-115.
4. Albuquerque CDC. Processo de Produção de Bioemulsificante por Candida lipolytica: Otimização, Ampliação de Escala e Desenvolvimento de Softsensor baseado em Redes Neurais Artificiais. D.Sc. Thesis, State University of Campinas, Brazil: 2006.
5. Albuquerque CDC, Filetti AMF, Campos-Takaki GM. Optimizing the medium components in bioemulsifier production by Candida lipolytica with response surface method. Can J Microbiol 2006; 52:575-583.
6. Albuquerque CDC, Campos-Takaki GM, Fileti AMF. Neural network based software sensors: application to biosurfactant production by Candida lipolytica. In: Antonio Mendez-Vilas. (Org.). Modern Multidisciplinary Applied Microbiology—Exploiting Microbes and their Interactions. 1st ed. Weinheim: Wiley-VCH, 2006:628-632.
7. Amaral PFF, da Silva JM, Lehocky M et al. Production and characterization of a bioemulsifier from Yarrowia lipolytica. Process Biochem 2006; 41:1894-1898.
8. Amézcua-Vega C, Poggi-Varaldo HM, Esparza-García F et al. Effect of culture conditions on fatty acids composition of a biosurfactant produced by Candida ingens and changes of surface tension of culture media. Biores Technol 2007; 98:237-240.
9. Banat IM, Makkar RS, Cameotra SS. Potential commercial applications of microbial surfactants. Appl Microbiol Biotechnol 2000; 53:495-508.
10. Bednarski W, Adamczak M, Tomasik J et al. Application of oil refinery waste in the biosynthesis of glycolipids by yeast. Biores Technol 2004; 95:15-18.
11. Bushnell LD, Haas HF. The utilization of certain hydrocarbons by microorganisms. Journal of Bacteriol 1941; 41:653-673.
12. Cameron DR, Cooper DG, Neufeld RJ. The mannoprotein of Saccharomyces cerevisiae is an effective bioemulsifier. Appl Environ Microbiol 1988; 54:1420-1425.
13. Casas JA, Garcia de Lara S, Garcia-Ochoa F. Optimizing of a synthetic medium for Candida bombicola growth using factorial design of experiments. Enz Microbial Technol 1997; 21:221-29.
14. Chen L.-Z, Nguang S.-K, Chen X.-D. Soft sensors for on-line biomass measurements. Bioprocess Biosys Enginee 2004; 26(3):191-195.
15. Chen S.-Y, Lu W.-B, Wei Y.-H et al. Improved Production of Biosurfactant with Newly Isolated Pseudomonas aeruginosa S2. Biotechnol Progress 2007; 23(3):661-666.
16. Cirigliano MC, Carman GM. Purification and characterization of liposan, a bioemulsifier from Candida lipolytica. Appl Environ Microbiol 1985; 50:846-850.
17. Cirigliano MC, Carman GM. Isolation of a bioemulsifier from Candida lipolytica. Appl Environ Microbiol 1984; 48:747-750.
18. Cladera-Olivera F, Caron GR, Brandeli A. Bacterocin Production by Baccilus licheniformis strain P4 in cheese whey using Response Surface Methodology. Biochem Enginee J 2004; 21:53-58.
19. Cooper DG. Biosurfactants. Microbiol Sci 1986; 3:145-147.
20. Cooper DG, Paddock DA. Production of a biosurfactant from Torulopsis bombicola. Appl Environ Microbiol 1984; 47:173-176.
21. Costa AC, Atala DIP, Maugeri Filho F et al. Factorial design and simulation for the optimization and determination of control structures for an extractive alcoholic fermentation. Process Biochem 2001; 37(2):125-137.
22. Crolla A, Kennedy KJ. Optimization of acid citric production from Candida lipolytica Y-p1095 using n-paraffin. J Biotechnol 2001; 89:27-40.
23. Cutler AJ, Light RJ. Regulation of hydroxydocosanoic acid sophoroside production in Candida bogoriensis by the levels of glucose and yeast extract in the growth medium. J Biol Chem 1979; 254(6):1944-1950.
24. Davila AM, Marchal R, Vandecasteele JP. Kinetics and balance of a fermentation free from product inhibition: sophorose lipid production by Candida bombicola. Appl Microbiol Biotechnol 1992; 39(1):6-11.
25. Deepthi N, Rastogi NK, Manonmani HK. Degradation of DDT by a Defined Microbial Consortium: Optimization of Degradation Conditions by Response Surface Methodology. Res J Microbiol 2007; 2(4):315-326.

26. Desai JD. Microbial surfactants: evaluation, types and future applications. J Sci Ind Res 1987; 46:440-449.
27. Desai JD, Banat IM. Microbial production of surfactants and their commercial potential. Microbiol Mol Biol Reviews 1997; 61(1):47-64.
28. Desai JD, Desai AJ. Production of biosurfactants. In: Kosaric N, ed. Biosurfactants: Production, Properties and Applications. New York: Marcel Dekker, 1993:65-86.
29. Desai AJ, Patel RM, Desai JD. Advances in production of biosurfactant and their commercial application. J Sci Ind Res 1994; 53:619-629.
30. Di Massimo C, Montague GA, Willis MJ et al. Towards improved penicillin fermentation via artificial neural networks. Comp Chem Enginee 1992; 16(4):283-291.
31. Elibol M, Ozer D. Response surface analysis of lipase production by freely suspended Rhizopus arrhizu.s Process Biochem 2002; 38:367-372.
32. Felse PA, Shah V, Chan J et al. Sophorolipid biosynthesis by Candida bombicola from industrial fatty acid residues. Enz Microbial Technol 2007; 40(2):316-323.
33. Garcia-Ochoa F, Casas JA. Unstructured kinetic model for sophorolipid production by Candida bombicola. Enzyme Microb Technol 1999; 25:613-621.
34. Gallert C, Winter J. Solid and liquid residues as raw materials for biotechnology. J Naturwissenschaften 2002; 89(11):483-496.
35. Georgiou G, Lin SC, Sharma MM. Surface active compounds from microorganisms. Bio/Technology 1990; 10:60-65.
36. Hommel RK, Stuwer O, Stubrerd W et al. Production of water soluble surface active exolipids by Torulopsis apicola. Appl Microbiol Biotechnol 1987; 26:199-205.
37. Hu Y, Ju LK. Purification of lactonic sophorolipids by crystallization. J Biotechnol 2001; 87:263-272.
38. Johnson V, Singh M, Saini VS. Bioemulsifier production by an oleaginous yeast Rhodotorula glutinis IIP-30. Biotechnol Lett 1992; 14(6):487-490.
39. Kakugawa K, Tamai M, Imamura K et al. Isolation of Yeast Kurtzmanomyces sp. I-11, Novel producer of mannosylerythritol lipid. Biosci Biotechnol Biochem 2002; 66(1):188-191
40. Kappeli O, Muller M, Fiechter A. Chemical and structural alterations at the cell surface of Candida tropicalis, induced by hydrocarbon substrate. J Bacteriol 1978; 133:952-958.
41. Karim MN, Rivera SL. Artificial neural networks in bioprocess state estimation. Adv Biochem Eng 1992; 46:1-33.
42. Kim HS, Jeon JW, Lee HW et al. Extracellular production of a glycolipid biosurfactant, mannosylerythritol lipid, from Candida antarctica. Biotechnol Letters 2002; 24(3):225-229.
43. Koprinkova-Hristova P, Patarinska T. Neural network modelling of continuous microbial cultivation accounting for the memory effects. Inter J Systems Sci 2006; 37:5/15:271-277.
44. Laith AL-A, Rahman RNZA, Basri M et al. The effects of culture conditions on biosurfactant activity of Pseudomonas aeruginosa 181 using response surface methodology. J Medical Biological Sci 2007; 1(1):1-4
45. Linko S, Luopa J, Zhu Y.-H. Neural network as software sensors in enzyme production. J Biotecnol 1997; 52:257-266.
46. Linko S, Zhu Y.-H, Linko P. Applying neural network as software sensors for enzyme engineering. Tibitech 1999; 17:155-162.
47. Luna JM, Sarubbo LA, Campos-Takaki GM. A new biosurfactant produced by Candida glabrata UCP1002: characteristics of stability and application in oil recovery. Brazilian Arch Biol Technol in press, 2008.
48. Lukondeh T, Ashbolt NJ, Rogers PL. Evaluation of Kluyveromyces marxianus FII 510700 grown on a lactose-based medium as a source of a natural bioemulsifier. Journal of Industrial Microbiology and Biotechnology 2003; 30(2):715-720. ISSN 1367-5435.
49. Lukondeh T, Ashbolt NJ, Rogers PL et al. NMR confirmation of an alkali-insoluble glucan from Kluyveromyces marxianus cultivated on a lactose-based medium. World J Microbiol Biotech 2003; 19(4):349-355. ISSN 0959-3993.
50. Marçal M. do CR. Produção de biopolímeros por Candida lipolytica em meios suplementados por óleos vegetais (babaçu, côco e dendê). Recife 1991:147. Thesis. (in Nutrition). Health Sciences Center, UFPE, 1991.
51. Miranda OA, Salgueiro AA, Pimentel MCB et al. Lipase production by a Brazilian strain of Penicillium citrinum using an industrial residue. Bioresource Technol 1999; 69: 145-147.
52. Morita T, Konishi M, Fukuoka T et al. Discovery of Pseudozyma rugulosa NBRC 10877 as a novel producer of the glycolipid biosurfactants, mannosylerythritol lipids, based on rDNA sequence. Appl Microbiol Biotechnol 2006; 73(2):305-313.
53. Moussa TAA, Ahmed GM, Abdel-hamid SMS. Optimization of cultural conditions for biosurfactant production from Nocardia amarae. J Appl Sci Res 2006; 2(11):844-850.

54. Mukherjee S, Das P, Sen R. Towards commercial production of microbial surfactants. TRENDS Biotechnol 2006; 24(11):509-515.
55. Mulligan CN. Environmental applications for biosurfactants. Environ Pollut 2005; 133:183-198.
56. Nunez A, Ashby RD, Foglia TA et al. LC/MS analysis and lipase modification of the sophorolipids produced by Rhodotorula bogoriensis. Biotechnol Letters 2004; 26:1087-1093.
57. Pareilleux A. Hydrocarbon assimilation by Candida lipolytica: formation of a biossurfactant: effects on respiratory activity and growth. Eur J Appl Microbiol Biotechnol 1979; 8:91-101.
58. Pekin G, Vardar-Sukan F. Production of sophorolipids using the yeast Candida bombicola ATTC 22214 for the applications in the food industry. J Eng Nat Sci 2006; 2:109-116.
59. Ramnani P, Kumar SS, Gupta R. Concomitant production and downstream processing of alkaline protease and biosurfactant from Bacillus licheniformis RG1: Bioformulation as detergent additive. Process Biochem 2005; 40:10:3352-3359.
60. Rau U, Manzke C, Wagner F. Influence of substrate supply on the production of sophorose lipids by Candida bombicola ATCC 22214. Biotechnol Letters 1996; 18:149-154.
61. Razafindralambo H, Paquot M, Baniel A et al. Foaming properties of surfactin, a lipopeptide biosurfactant from Bacillus subtilis. J Am Oil Chem Soc 1996; 73:149-151.
62. Rodrigues LR, Teixeira JA, van der Mei H. Response surface optimization of the medium components for the production of biosurfactants by Probiotic bacteria. Process Biochem 2006; 41(1):1-10.
63. Ron EZ, Rosenberg E. Natural roles of biosurfactants. Environm Microbiol 2001; 3:229-236.
64. Rufino RD. Produção de Biosurfactante por Candida lipolytica. M.Sc. Dissertation. Federal University of Pernambuco, Brazil: 2006;
65. Rufino RD, arubbo LA, Campos-Takaki GM. Enhancement of Stability of Biosurfactant Produced by Candida lipolytica using as Substrate Industrial Residue. World J Microbiol Biotechnol 2007; 23(5):729-734.
66. Rufino RD, Sarubbo LA, Barros Neto B et al. Experimental design for the production of tensio-active agent by Candida lipolytica. Journal of Indus. Microbiol Biotechnol 2008; 35(8):907-914.
67. Sarubbo LA, Farias CBB, Campos-Takaki GM. Co-utilization of canola oil and glucose on the production of a surfactant by Candida lipolytica. Curr Microbiol 2007; 54:68-73.
68. Sarubbo LA, Luna JM, Campos-Takaki GM. Production and stability studies of the bioemulsifier obtained from a new strain of Candida glabrata UCP1002. Eletronic J Biotechnol 2006; 9:400-406.
69. Sarubbo LA, Marçal MCR, Campos-Takaki GM. Comparative study of bioemulsifier production by Candida lipolytica strains. Braz Arch Biol Technol 1997; 40:707-720.
70. Sarubbo LA, Marçal MCR, Neves MLC et al. Bioemulsifier production in batch culture using glucose as carbon source by Candida lipolytica. Appl Biochem Biotechnol 2001; 95:59-67.
71. Sarubbo LA, Porto ALF, Campos-Takaki GM. The use of babassu oil as substrate to produce bioemulsifiers by Candida lipolytica. Can J Microbiol 1999; 45:423-426.
72. Sen R. Response surface optimization of the critical media components for production of surfactin. J Chem Tech Biotechnol 1997; 68:263-270.
73. Sen R, Swaminathan T. Application of response-surface methodology to evaluate the optimum environmental conditions for the enhanced production of surfactin. Appl Microbiol Biotechnol 1997; 47:358-363.
74. Sen R, Swaminathan T. Response surface modeling and optimization to elucidate and analyze the effects of inoculum age and size on surfactin production. Biochem Enginee J 2004; 21(2):141-148.
75. Shepherd R, Rockey J, Sutherland IW et al. Novel bioemulsifiers from microorganisms for use in foods. J Biotechnol 1995; 40:207-217.
76. Singh M, Desai JD. Hydrocarbon emulsification by Candida tropicalis and Debaryomyces polymorphus. Ind J Experimental Biol 1989; 27:224-226.
77. Singh M, Sani VS, Adhikari DK et al. Production of bioemusifier by a SCP-producing strain of Candida tropicalis during hydrocarbon fermentation, Biotechnol letters 1990; 12:743-746.
78. Singh A, Van Hamme JD, Ward OP. Surfactants in microbiology and biotechnology. Biotechnol Adv 2007; 25:99-122.
79. Souza-Sobrinho HB. Utilização de resíduos industriais como substratos de baixo custo para a produção de biossurfactante por Candida sphaerica. Recife 2007:99 Thesis. (Master's in the Development of Environmental Processes). Universidade Católica de Pernambuco.
80. Souza-sobrinho HB, Rufino RD, Luna JM et al. Utilization of two agroindustrial by-products for the production of a surfactant by Candida sphaerica UCP 0995. Process Biochem 2008; 43:912-917.
81. Thanomsub B, Watcharachaipong T, Chotelersak K et al. Monoacylglycerols: glycolipid biosurfactants produced by a thermotolerant yeast, Candida ishiwadae. J Appl Microbiol 2004; 96:588-592.
82. Van Hamme JD, Singh A, Ward OnP. Recent Advances in Petroleum Microbiology Microbiol Mol Biol Rev 2003; 67(4):503-549.

83. Vance-Harrop MH. Potencial Biotecnológico de Candida lipolytica na Produção de Biossurfactantes, nos processos de Remoção e Biossorção de Pireno (Derivado do Petróleo). Dsc. Thesis, Federal University of Pernambuco, Brazil: 2004.
84. Vance-Harrop MH, Gusmão NB, Campos-Takaki GM. New bioemulsifiers produced by Candida lipolytica using D-glucose and babassu oil as carbon sources Braz J Microbiol 2003; 34:120-123.
85. Velikonja J, Kosaric N. Biosurfactant in food applications. In: Kosaric N, ed. Biosurfactants: Production, Properties, Applications. New York: Marcel Dekker Inc., 1993:419-446.
86. Wayman M, Jenkins AD, Kormady AG. Biotechnology for oil and fat industry. J Am Oil Chem Soc 1984; 61:129-131.
87. Yang F.-C, Huang H.-C, Yang M.-J. The influence of environmental conditions on the mycelial growth of Antrodia cinnamomea in submerged cultures. Enz. Microbial Technol 2003; 33(4):395-402.
88. Zhou QH, Kosaric N. Utilization of Canola Oil and lactose to produce biosurfactant with Candida bombicola. J Amer Oil Chem Soc 1995; 72:67-71.
89. Zinjarde S, Chinnathambi S, Lachke AH et al. Isolation of an emulsifier from Yarrowia lipolytica NCIM 3589 using a modified mini isoeletctric focusing unit. Lett Appl Microbiol 1997; 24:117-121.

CHAPTER 20

Synthesis of Biosurfactants and Their Advantages to Microorganisms and Mankind

Swaranjit Singh Cameotra,* Randhir S. Makkar, Jasminder Kaur and S.K. Mehta

Abstract

Biosurfactants are surface-active compounds synthesized by a wide variety of microorganisms. They are molecules that have both hydrophobic and hydrophilic domains and are capable of lowering the surface tension and the interfacial tension of the growth medium. Biosurfactants possess different chemical structures—lipopeptides, glycolipids, neutral lipids and fatty acids. They are nontoxic biomolecules that are biodegradable. Biosurfactants also exhibit strong emulsification of hydrophobic compounds and form stable emulsions. The low water solubility of these hydrophobic compounds limits their availability to microorganisms, which is a potential problem for bioremediation of contaminated sites. Microbially produced surfactants enhance the bioavailability of these hydrophobic compounds for bioremediation. Therefore, biosurfactant-enhanced solubility of pollutants has potential applications in bioremediation. Not only are the biosurfactants useful in a variety of industrial processes, they are also of vital importance to the microbes in adhesion, emulsification, bioavailability, desorption and defense strategy. These interesting facts are discussed in this chapter.

Introduction

Surfactants constitute an important class of industrial chemicals used widely in almost every sector of modern industry (Table 1). The industrial demand for surfactants has grown to about 300% within the US-chemical industry during the last two decades and US market value for specialty surfactants will grow 6.1 percent annually through 2006. Gains will be driven by increasing demand for naturally derived, multifunctional surfactants with enhanced mildness and biodegradability for use in personal care products. Cationic surfactants will remain the largest segment, while amphoterics grow the fastest according to the study by Freedonia group USA. According to other study by consulting firm Colin A. Houston Associates (CAHA; Brewster, NY), North American surfactant consumption in consumer products was 4.375 billion lbs last year, valued at $3.6 billion last year and will grow at 3%/year through 2010. Total surfactants used in 25.5 billion lbs of consumer products, worth $42.5 billion, from which the U.S. accounted for more than 81% of the 25.5-billion North American consumer products market, the firm says. Surfactant consumption in household products will grow faster than the consumer products sector and for body washes, antiaging skin care, men's toiletries and ethnic hair care, the study says.

*Corresponding Author: Swaranjit Singh Cameotra—IMTECH, Sector 39A, Chandigarh—160036, India. Email: ssc@imtech.res.in or swaranjitsingh@yahoo.com

Biosurfactants, edited by Ramkrishna Sen. ©2010 Landes Bioscience and Springer Science+Business Media.

Table 1. Types of modern surfactants used in industries

Surfactant Type	Examples	% of Total Production	Major Uses
Anionic	Carboxylates, sulphonates, sulphuric acid esters	66	Washing powders
Cationic	Amine oxides, monoamines quaternary ammonium salts	9	Fabric softners shampoos
Non-ionic	Carboxylic acids and carbohydrate esters, glycerides and their ethoxylated derivatives	24	Laundry cosurfactants, washing up liquids' Personal care products and foods
Amphoteric	Alkyl betaines, Alkyl dimethylamines, Imidazonilinum derivatives	~1	Speciality uses

Adapted from Banat et al (2000)[5] and Desai and Banat (1997).[3]

Deleu and Paquot[1] have described surfactants as molecules of strong economic and socio-economics impetus and this has been a driving force behind the current active research in exploiting new ways, process, resources and new applications for the surfactants. In addition, the increased global environmental protection concern, has resulted in the use of chemical products in harmony with environment and environmental regulations. The chemical industries anticipate revolutionary transformation in future where biological methods and materials will outgrow some chemical applications and many industries now recognize the potential of biological processes in wide areas e.g., pretreatment of raw materials, processing operations, product modifications, selective waste management, energy recycling and conservation. Recent advances in biological sciences stress on tremendous potential for application of natural products, which involves the use of simple sugars and other renewable substrates as a synthetic feedstock instead of petroleum. Another factor for the interest in biotechnology is the prediction of sales for biotechnology by-products, which is expected to be more than US$500 billion at a rate of 3-5% annually.[2-5] All these concerns have put impetus for more serious consideration of biological surfactants (Biosurfactants, a term derived from biologically active surface active compounds) as possible alternatives to existing products. The new world order and environmental concern have widened the role of biosurfactants with possible applications in agriculture, in detergency and in public health, in waste utilization, in bioremediation and.[5-10]

In this chapter the authors are giving a comprehensive study of biosurfactants: their nature, production and potential applications as bioactive and environmental control agents. Since the applications of biosurfactants are in very diverse area and they are being applied for newer applications the authors have tried to revise the approach to cover the information reported as reviews, articles and added on new findings in this chapter.

Surfactants and Biosurfactants

Surfactants are amphipathic molecules with both hydrophilic and hydrophobic moieties that partition preferentially at the interface between fluid phases that have different degrees of polarity and hydrogen bonding, such as oil and water, or air and water interfaces. Usually the hydrophobic domain is a hydrocarbon whereas the hydrophilic domain can be non-ionic, positively or negatively charged or amphoteric.[3,11] The formation of ordered molecular film at the interface lowers the interfacial energy (interfacial tension, IFT) and surface tension and is responsible for unique properties of the surfactant molecules. The most common non-ionic surfactants are ethoxylates, ethylene and propylene oxide copolymers and sorbitan esters.

Table 2. *Major types of glycolipids produced by microorganisms*

Biosurfactant Type	Producing Microbial Species	Application
Sophorolipids	*Candida bombicola* ATCC 22214	Emulsifier, MEOR
	Candida bombicola	Alkane dissimilation
Trehalose lipid	*Rhodococcus sps.*	Bioremediation
	Tsukamurella sp.	Antimicrobial properties
	Arthrobacter sp. EK 1	
	Rhodococcus ruber	Oxidise the gaseous alkanes
Rhamnolipids	*Pseudomonas aeruginosa* 57SJ	Bioremediation
	Renibacterium salmoninarum 27BN	Bioremediation
	P. putida Z1 BN	Bioremediation
	P. aeruginosa PA1	Bioremediation
	P. chlororaphis	Biocontrol agent
	P. aeruginosa GL1	Hydrocarbon assimilation
	P. aeruginosa GL1	Surface active agent
	Pseudozyma fusiformata VKM Y-2821	Antifungal activity
	Bacillus subtilis 22BN	
Rubiwettins R1 and RG1	*Serratia rubidaea*	Swarming and spreading
Liposan	*Candida lipolytica*	Emulsifier
Schizonellin A and B	*Schizonella melanogramma*	Antimicrobial and Antitumour agent
Mannosylerythritol lipids	*Candida antarctica*	Neuroreceptor antagonist, anti microbial agent
	Kurtzmanomyces sp. I-11	Biomedical applications
Ustilipids	*Ustilago maydis and Geotrichum candidum*	Dopamine D3 receptors antagoist
Cellobiose lipid (microcin)	*Cryptococcus humicola*	Antifungal agent
Flocculosin	*P. flocculosa*	Antifungal, biocontrol agent
Anionic glucose lipid	*Alcanivorax borkumensis*	Biomarkers

Examples of commercially available ionic surfactants include fatty acids, ester sulphonates or sulphates (anionic) and quartenary ammonium salts (cationic). These properties make surfactant suitable for an extremely wide variety of industrial application involving emulsification, foaming, detergency, wetting and phase dispersion or solublization. Table 1 shows the various areas of their applications.

Many biological molecules are amphiphilic and partition preferentially at interphases.[5,12] Microbial compounds, which exhibit particularly high surface activity and emulsifying activity, are classified as biosurfactants.[5,12] The biosurfactants a term derived from the biological surface active agents is a molecule of the future because of the numerous advantages over their chemical counterparts because they are biodegradable and less toxic and are effective at extreme temperatures or pH values and can be produced from several inexpensive waste substrates, thereby decreasing their production cost.[5-10] Different groups of biosurfactants have different natural roles in the growth of the organisms in which they are produced (see Tables 2, 3, 4). These include increasing the surface area and bioavailability of hydrophobic water-insoluble substrates, heavy metal binding, bacterial pathogenesis, quorum sensing and biofilm formation.[2,10,13,14] Although literature is full of the reports with many types of biosurfactants (Fig. 1),

Table 3. Lipopeptides produced by various microorganisms

Name	Producer Organism	Properties and Activities
Amphomycin	*Streptomyces canus*	Antibiotic, inhibitor of cell wall synthesis
Chlamydocin	*Diheterospora chlamydosporia*	Cytostatic and antitumour agent
Cyclosporin A	*Tolypocladium inflatum (Trichoderma polysporum)*	Antifungal agent, immunomodulator
Enduracidin A	*Streptomyces fungicidicus*	Antibiotic
Globomycin	*Streptomyces globocacience*	Antibiotic, inhibitor of cell wall synthesis
HC-Toxin	*Helminthosporium carbonum*	Phytotoxin
Polymyxin E1 (ColistinA)	*B. polymyxa*	Antibiotic
Surfactin	*B. subtilis*	Antifungal, antibacterial and antiviral agent
Bacillomycin L	*B. subtilis*	Antifungal, antibacterial and antiviral agent
Iturin A	*B. subtilis*	Antifungal and antiviral agent
Mycosubtilin	*B. subtilis*	Antimicrobial agent
Putisolvin I and II,	*P. putida*	Biofilm formation inhibitor
BL1193, plipastatin and surfactin	*B. licheniformis* F2.2	Antimicrobial agent
Bacillomycin/Plipastatin/ Surfactin	*B. subtilis* BBK1	Inhibitors of phospholipase A(2)
Plipastins	*B. cereus* BMG 302	Antimicrobial agents
Surfactant Bl-86	*B. lichiniformis*	Antimicrobial agent
Halobacillin	*Bacillus*	Acyl-CoA and cholesterol acyltransferase inhibitor
Lichenysin G	*B. licheniformis* IM 1307	Hemolytic and chelating agent
Arthrofactin	*Arthrobacter*	Oil displacement agent, antimicrobial agent
Fengycin	*B. thuringiensis* CMB26,	Biocontrol agent, fungicidal, bactericidal and insecticidal activity
	B. subtilis F-29-3	Antifungal lipopeptide
Mycobacillin	*B. subtilis*	Antifungal

no single surfactant is suitable for all the potential applications. This makes very important and urgent to develop even more multifunctional biosurfactants to broaden the spectrum of properties available. The losing economics of the biosurfactants production makes it more worthy for better and efficient bioprocesses to make them competitive are unable to compete economically with the chemically synthesized compounds in the market, due to high production costs. This is due to inefficient bioprocessing methodology available; poor strain productivity and need to use expansive substrates.

Table 4. Bioemulsants produced by different microorganisms

Producing Strain	Biochemical Nature	Activity References
A. calcoaceticus RAG-I	Heteropolysaccharide with bound fatty acids	Stabilizes oil-in-water emulsion; lowers oil viscosity
A. calcoaceticus BD413	Complex of hydrophilic polysaccharide and proteins	Stabilizes oil-in-water emulsions; reconstitution from constituents
A. calcoaceticus A2	Polysaccharide	Disperses limestone powders
A. calcoaceticus MM5	Polysaccharide-protein	Emulsifies heating oils
A. radioresistens KA53	Alanine-containing polysaccharide-protein	Forms oil-in-water emulsions; stable to alkali and 100%
M. thermoautotrophium	Protein complex	Forms oil-in-water emulsions; effective at high temperatures
B. stearothermophilus	Protein-polysaccharide-lipid	Emulsifies benzene at high temperature
P. tralucida	Acetylated extracellular polysaccharide	Emulsifies insecticides
Sphingomonas paucimobilis	Acetylated heteropolysaccharide	Suggested use in bioremediation
F! marginalis ST	Lipopolysaccharide-protein	Emulsion stabilizer and antioxidant
Klebsiella sp	Polysaccharide	Excellent emulsifier; yeast has food-grade status
C. ufilis 80%	Polysaccharide	Forms stable emulsions with food oils

Adapted from Rosenberg and Ron.[19]

Significance and Role of Biosurfactants to Microbes

The most ingoing question is why the microbes produce these surfactants and what is the significance and role of biosurfactants to the microorganism, which produce them.[12,15] This question is of fundamental importance for understanding the physiology of these organisms and provides a logical framework for the discovery of new microbial surfactants, improved production and proper choice of commercial application of these surfactants. With new genetic and molecular biology tools new biosurfactants and producing organisms have been discovered and identified, which indicate that microbial surfactants have very different structures, are produced by a wide variety of microorganisms and have very different surface properties and functions.[16,17] The various roles that a biosurfactant will have could be unique to the physiology and ecology of the producing microorganisms and it is impossible to draw any universal generalizations or to identify one or more functions that are clearly common to all microbial surfactants. In this section, we will present the few natural roles for biosurfactants that have been suggested or demonstrated.

Adhesion

The most significant role of microbial surfactants is documented for adhesion of the cells to the interfaces. Adhesion is a physiological mechanism for growth and survival of cells in the natural environments.[18] A special case of adhesion is the growth of bacteria on water insoluble hydrocarbons and is one of the primary processes affecting bacterial transport, which determines the bacterial fate in the subsurface. Bacterial adhesion to abiotic surfaces is attributed to attractive interactions between bacteria and the medium. When surfactants are immersed in water, surfactant molecules cause a distortion of the local tetrahedral structure of water and the hydrogen bonds between water

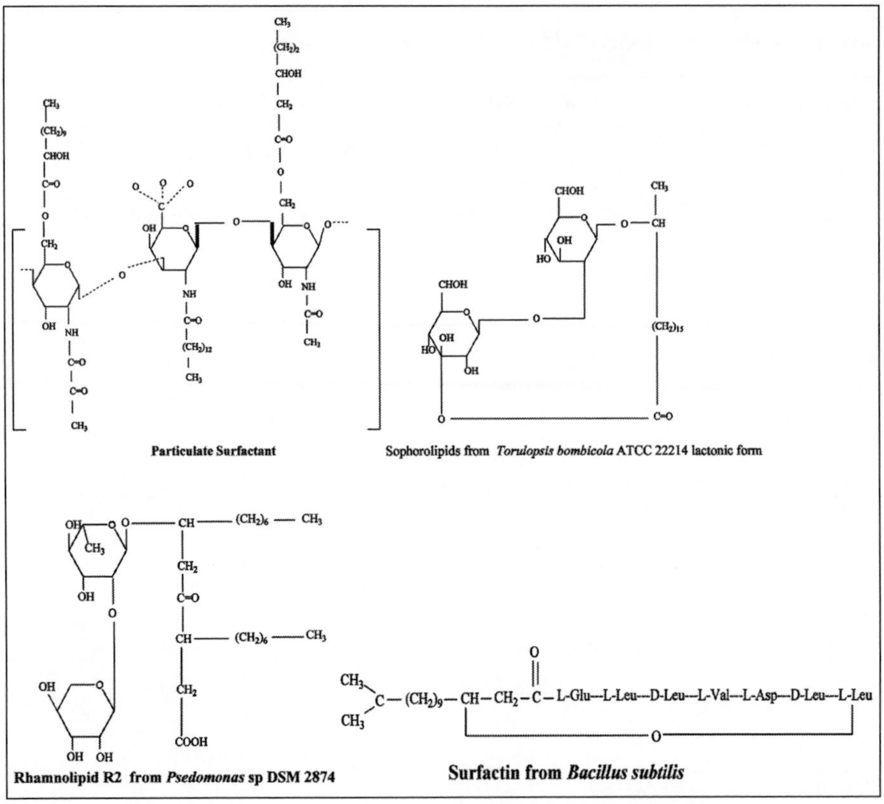

Figure 1. Structures of most common biosurfactants produced by microbes.

molecules are energetically disfavored, resulting in a decrease in interactions between bacteria and the porous medium. The mass of bacteria eligible for desorption varies directly with the magnitude of the interaction reduction. Since the enzymes necessary for hydrocarbon oxidation are on the cell membrane, the microbe must come into contact with its substrate. Adhesion is shown to be a prerequisite for the growth of *A. calcoaceticus* RAG-1 on liquid hydrocarbons under two conditions: low cell density and limited agitation.[19,20] Neu[21] have shown the growth of the microbes on certain surfaces is influenced by the biosurfactant, which forms a conditioning film on an interface, thereby stimulating certain microorganisms to attach to the interface, while inhibiting the attachment of others. In another case the cell surface hydrophobicity of *P. aeruginosa* was greatly increased by the presence of cell-bound rhamnolipid,[22,23] whereas the cell surface hydrophobicity of *Acinetobacter* strains was reduced by the presence of its cell-bound emulsifier.[19,20] These results indicate that the microorganisms can use their biosurfactants to regulate their cell surface properties in order to attach or detach from surfaces according to need.

Emulsification

Many hydrocarbon-degrading microorganisms produce extracellular emulsifying agents, the inference being that emulsification plays a role in growth on water immiscible substrates.[19,20,24] There is correlation between emulsifier production and growth on hydrocarbons. The majority of *Acinetobacter* strains produce high-molecular-mass bioemulsifiers. The best studied are the bioe-mulsans of *Acinetobacter calcoaceticus* RAG-1 and *A. calcoaceticus* BD4.[19,20] Other *Acinetobacter* surfactants that have been reported include biodispersan from *A. calcoaceticus* A2[25] an emulsifier effective on heating oil and whole cells of *A. calcoaceticus* 2CA2.[26] Emulsifier producing organisms were able to on water insoluble substrates while, the mutants, which do not produce emulsifier, grow poorly on hydrocarbons. In similar studies Hua et al[27] applied the emulsification capability of biosurfactant BS-UC produced by *Candida antarctica* from n-undecane as the substrate and found the positive influence of amendment of BS-UC on the emulsification and the biodegradation of a variety of n-alkanes substrates. For the growth of microbe on hydrocarbons, the interfacial surface area between water and oil can be a limiting factor and the evidence that emulsification is a natural process brought about by extracellular agents is indirect and there are certain conceptual difficulties in understanding how emulsification can provide an (evolutionary) advantage for the microorganism producing the emulsifier.

Bioavailability and Desorption

One of the major reasons for the prolonged persistence of high-molecular-weight hydrophobic compounds is their low water solubility, which increases their sorption to surfaces and limits their availability to biodegrading microorganisms. Biosurfactants can enhance growth on bound substrates by desorbing them from surfaces or by increasing their apparent water solubility.[28] Surfactants that lower interfacial tension are particularly effective in mobilizing bound hydrophobic molecules and making them available for biodegradation. Another important characteristic of the biosurfactants is that above the CMC (critical micelle concentration), they form micelles (stable aggregates of 10 to 200 molecules), which, brings about a sudden variation in the relation between the concentration and the surface tension of the solution that can increase the solubility of Hydrophobic Organic Compounds (HOCs).[9,29]

Zhang and Miller[22,23,30] have shown the mechanisms involved in the increased dissociation of hydrocarbon by *Pseudomonas*. Much less is known about how polymeric biosurfactants increase the apparent solubility's of hydrophobic compounds. Recently, it has been demonstrated that Alasan (a polymeric biosurfactant) increases the apparent solubility's of PAHs 5 to 20-fold and thus significantly increases their rate of biodegradation.[20,31]

Makkar and Rockne[9] have evaluated the various mechanisms involved in enhancing of bioavailability of the HOCs specially the polyaromatic hydrocarbons. In addition to adhesion, desorption also plays an important part in the natural growth of the microorganisms. After a certain period of growth, conditions become unfavorable for further development of microorganism e.g., toxin accumulation and impaired transport of necessary nutrients in crowded conditions. Desorption is advantageous at this stage for the cells and need arises for a new habitat. In fact mechanisms for detachment seem to be essential for all attached microorganisms in order to facilitate dispersal and colonization of new surfaces. One of the natural roles of an emulsifier/biosurfactant may be in regulating desorption of the producing strain from hydrophobic surfaces[32] Chen et al 2004 also[33] investigated the effects of transients in elution chemistry on bacterial desorption in water-saturated porous media. They used a rhamnolipid biosurfactant to see the desorption kinetics of *Lactobacillus casei* and *Streptococcus mitis*. It was found with the increase in rhamnolipid biosurfactant concentrations, interactions between bacteria and silica sand decreased and consequently resulted in desorption. This research is of importance for in situ bioremediation applications as rhamnolipid biosurfactant-enhanced bioremediation is effective and economical and is also a nontoxic solution for many subsurface and aquatic sites contaminated with hydrophobic organic chemicals.

Defense Strategy

According to Puchkov[34] apart from two main natural roles suggested for surface-active compounds (increasing availability of hydrophobic substrates and regulating attachment—detachment to and from surfaces) the biosurfactants could be an evolutionary defense strategy of microbe as evidenced by high mycocidal activity of the MC secreted by *C. humicola*. Similar analogy can be made for the lipopeptides biosurfactant producing strains of *B. subtilis*. The lipopeptide (antibiotic) would have strong influence on the survival of *B. subtilis* in its natural habitat, the soil and the rhizosphere.[35,36]

Advantages of Biosurfactants

Special properties of microbial surfactants, which may be useful for their commercialization, are summarized below.

Biodegradability and Controlled Inactivation of Microbial Surfactants

Several chemically synthesized, commercially available surfactants (e.g., perfluorinated anionics) resist biodegradation and accumulate in nature causing ecological problems. Microbial surfactants like all natural products are susceptible to degradation by microorganisms in water and soil.[37,38]

Selectivity for Specific Interfaces

Biological molecules have been found to show more specificity as compared to the chemically synthesized materials. Microbial surfactants show a specificity not seen in presently available commercial surfactants[24,39,40] for example, specificity of emulsan towards a mixture of aliphatic and aromatic hydrocarbons and that of solublizing factor of Pseudomonas PG1 towards pristane.[24,39]

Surface Modification

An emulsifying or dispersing agent not only causes a reduction in the average particle size but also changes the surface properties of the particle in a fundamental manner. Small quantities of a dispersant can dramatically alter the surface properties of a material such as surface charge, hydrophobicity and most interestingly pattern recognition based on the three dimensional structure of the adherent polymer.

Diversity of Microbial Surfactants

Microorganisms produce a wider range of surfactant molecules than are available through chemical synthesis. A broad spectrum of surfactants is required to satisfy the industrial demand. Almost every commercial application has a unique set of growth conditions that dictates the optimum type of surfactant formulation, a single isolate often generates chemical variations of the same surfactant, resulting in the production of a surfactant mixture with an associated characteristic surface.[17,41,42] Even small differences in the structure of a surfactant can have profound effects on its function and its potential industrial applications.[43] Biosurfactants are an example of a class of microbial natural products that has coevolved among many genera and have developed in parallel with respect to genotype and phenotype.[16]

Toxicity

Surfactants are one of the major components (10-18%) of detergent and household cleaning products and are used in high volumes. Most of these ends up in natural waters and consequently, their impact on the environment has been and continues to be, a worldwide concern. Scientific literature is full of the reports, which describe and discuss the toxic effects of surfactants.[44-46] The biological surfactants or biosurfactants have an added advantage of being less toxic or non toxic in comparison to the synthetic surfactants.[47] This property make them a better candidate for taking are of pollutants in environment rather than a menace by itself.

Biosurfactants Types and Producing Organisms

Traditionally it was considered that various types of biosurfactants are synthesized by a number of microbes (bacteria in most of the cases), particularly during their growth on water immiscible substrates (Fig. 1). These biosurfactants have a definite structure, with a lipophilic portion which is usually the hydrocarbon (alkyl) tail of one or more fatty acids that can be saturated, unsaturated, hydroxylated or branched and is linked to the hydrophilic group by a glycosidic ester or amide bond. Most biosurfactants are either neutral or negatively charged and the list includes both ionic and non-ionic surfactants, which range from a short fatty acid to large polymers. Basically there are five major classes of biosurfactants[3,5,48] namely; (i) glycolipids (ii) phospholipids and fatty acids (iii) lipopeptides/lipoproteins (iv) polymeric surfactants and (v) particulate surfactants. Some of the most common types with wider applications will only be discussed in this chapter.

Glycolipids are the most common biosurfactants that have been isolated and studied. Extracellular glycolipids consist of different mono- or disaccharides that are either acylated or glycosidically linked to long-chain fatty acids. These microbial glycolipids have attracted technological interest and some of the best/most studied representative examples of glycolipids are trehalose lipids of *Mycobacterium* and related bacteria,[49] rhamnolipids of *Pseudomonas* sp[8,50] and sophorolipids of yeasts.[51] Major types of glycolipids are tabulated in Table 2.

Lipopeptides represent a class of microbial surfactant which have attained and will be of increasing scientific, therapeutic and biotechnological interest with widespread occurrence over the whole spectra of microorganisms.[3,52] The characteristic structural element of such lipopeptides is a specific fatty acid, which is combined with an amino acid moiety. Such bioactive peptides usually appear as mixtures of closely related compounds which show slight variations in their amino acid composition and/or in their lipid portion. The spectrum of the manifold activities of lipopeptides covers antibiotics, antiviral and antitumor agents, immunomodulators or specific toxins and enzyme inhibitors.[5,10,53] Though mechanism of action of the majority of such compounds has not been clarified in detail so far, it is obvious that their surface- and membrane-active properties play an important role in the expression of their activities. Some of these agents have been listed in Table 3.

Another important class of biosurfactants/bioemulsfiers are bioemulsans.[19,20,25,54] Bioemulsans are amphiphatic proteins and/or polysaccharides which stabilize the oil-in-water emulsion. As other biosurfactants they are also produced by wide diversity of microbes and have potential applications in various bio based industries. Some of the bioemulsans produced from different microbes is listed in Table 4.

Applications of Biosurfactants

Biosurfactants have not been extensively exploited as industrial chemicals as production costs remain uncompetitive compared to synthetic surfactants.[55] The most attractive application of biosurfactants in the near future will be environmental remediation, where they may be used to enhance oil dispersion and biodegradation[22,30,56] and for the solubilisation of heavy metals.[2,14,57,58] The largest market and most applied application of the biosurfactants traditionally had been petroleum industry, where they are used in petroleum production and incorporation into oil formulations. Recent advances in biological sciences and analytical methods has led to expontial increase in the present arsenal of surfactant for applications in medicne, food and cosmetics industries.[10,53] In the forthcoming section we have tried to cover various applications of biosufactants.

Biosurfactant and Environment

Biosurfactant applications in the environmental industries are promising due to the advantages they have over the synthetic surfactants as discussed in review before. As discussed in previous sections the activity of bacterial biosurfactants in bioremediation is due to their ability to increase the surface area of hydrophobic water-insoluble substrates and to increase the solubility and bioavailability of hydrocarbons. They can be added to bioremediation processes as purified materials or in the form of biosurfactant-overproducing bacteria. In either case, they can stimulate the growth of hydrocarbon degrading bacteria and improve their ability to utilize hydrocarbons. There are variable results as to the utility of using biosurfactants especially rhamnolipids in hydrocarbon biodegradation (Mulligan 2005). Role of biosurfactants in particular rhamnolipids, for biodegradation of hydrocarbons has been thoroughly.[3,5,8,46,48,59,60] There is enhanced biodegradation of individual hydrocarbons and hydrocarbon mixtures in soil involving two plausible mechanism for this either because of enhanced solubility of the substrate for the microbial cells or because of increased hydrophobicity of the surface thus increasing the association of hydrophobic substrate.[9,61,62]

Oil is one of the most important resources of energy in the modern industrial world. Contamination of the seas and coasts with hydrocarbons containing crude oils from oil tankers leaks and accidents is worldwide problem and may persist in the marine environment for many years after an oil spill in areas such as salt marshes and mangrove swamps.[63,64] However, in most cases, environmental recovery is relatively swift and is complete within 2-10 years, the effects may be measurable for decades after the event.[65,66] The primary means of hydrocarbon degradation are photo oxidation, evaporation and microbial degradation. The reports which applied biosurfactants for oil removal are numerous and are the contents of many excellent reviews and papers.[67-69] Rhamnolipid surfactants have been used for release of oils from the beaches in Alaska after the Exxon Valdez tanker spill,[70] in a bioslurry for enhancing the solubilization of four-ring PAHs,[71] as an algal-bacterial consortium for degradation of phenanthrene dissolved in silicone oil or tetradecane,[72] to remove the oil from the soil core and subsequent degradation of mobilized oil by soil bacteria.[73]

Heavy crude oil recovery, facilitated by microorganisms, was suggested in the 1920s and received growing interest in the 1980s as microbial enhanced oil recovery (MEOR), although there are not many reports on productive microbial enhanced oil recovery project using biosurfactant and microbial biopolymers.[74] In MEOR processes the microbes are applied for the enhanced recovery of oil from the oil reservoirs and can be considered a applied processes of in situ bioremediation.[74] The process which is fusion of microbiology and engineering technology is dependent on many factors and prevailing conditions of the reservoir such as salinity, pH, temperature, pressure and nutrient availability.[75] Thermophilic and halophilic bacteria capable of thriving at 80 to 110°C under anaerobic conditions hold a promise to be used in the system[76-78] and respective isolates potentially useful for microbial enhanced oil recovery have been described.[75,79-81] Biosurfactants aid MEOR by lowering interfacial tension at the oil-rock interface thus reducing capillary forces that prevent oil from moving through rock pores. Added or in situ-produced biosurfactants, which aid oil emulsification and detachment of oil films from rocks, have considerable potential in MEOR.[75,79,80,82,83] For MEOR, either ex situ (microbial polymers and surfactants can be produced above ground and introduced into the reservoir through wells) or in situ approach (microorganisms within the reservoir can be stimulated to produce these compounds) can be considered, although the ex situ method is expensive due to capital involved surfactant production, purification and introduction into oil containing wells. For in situ approach the biosurfactants producing microorganisms in the wells are amended with a low cost substrates such as molasses and inorganic nutrients which promote growth and surfactant production.[84-87] The effectiveness of MEOR has been reported in field studies carried out in the United States, Czechoslovakia, Romania, USSR, Hungary, Poland and the Netherlands, with significant increase in oil recovery noted in some cases. Some of the biosurfactants applied for environmental bioremediation are listed in Table 5.

Other fields of application of biosurfactants in environment restoration is in aiding the metal and PAH bioremediation which is a persistent threat to environment and human health because of their ubiquitous distribution in the environment. Principal sources for PAH pollution into the environment include emissions from combustion processes or from spillage of petroleum products, coal gasification facilities vehicle emissions, heating and power plants, industrial processes and refuse and open burning.[9,88] The biosurfactants have also been applied bioremediation of PAHs and have been a topic of tremendous interest because of intrinsic properties of biosurfactants to increase the solubility and bioavailability of these pollutants. Some of the recent reports[2,6,9,89] have taken into account the positives of biosurfactant application for PAH bioremediation. Anionic biosurfactants such as rhamnolipids are a better candidate suitable for the application in biosurfactant aided metal remediation as they can remove metal form soil such as cadmium, copper, lead and zinc by making complex with the respective metal ions.[58,90,91] Rhamnolipids have been applied for remediation of cocontaminated soils[58,92,93] or in washing mixtures for the soils contaminated with various metals.[94-96] For details on the biosurfactant aided metal remediation we will suggest reading recent reviews by Mulligan[2] and Singh and Cameotra.[89]

In summary the biosurfactants are effective for remediation of hydrocarbons (and related compounds) and the future success of biosurfactant technology in bioremediation initiatives will require the precise targeting of the biosurfactant system to the physical conditions and chemical nature of the pollution-affected site.[9,97] Although many laboratory studies indicate the potential for use of biosurfactants in field conditions, a lot remains to be demonstrated in cost-effective treatment of marine oil spills and petroleum-contaminated soils compared to chemical surfactants.

Table 5. Studies done in last decade involving the biosurfactants for the environmental bioremediation

Biosurfactant	Source	Remediation Medium	Pollutant	Year of Study
Rhamnolipid	Phenanthrene	Soil slurries	P. aeruginosa UG12	1995
Rhamnolipid	Metals, phenanthrene and PCBs	Soil	P. aeruginosa ATCC 9027	1995
Rhamnolipid and oleophilic fertilizer	Mixture of alkanes and naphthalene	Soil	P. aeruginosa	1995
Rhamnolipid	4,4'-dichlorobiphenyl	Soil	P. aeruginosa	1996
Sodium dodecyl sulfate and rhamnolipid	Phenanthrene, pyrene B(a)P	Soil	P. aeruginosa UG2	1996
Rhamnolipid	Naphthalene	Soil	P. aeruginosa 19SJ	1996
PM-factor	Phenanthrene and other PAHs		P. marginalis PD-14B	1996
Rhamnolipid	Naphthalene and phenanthrene	Soil	P. aeruginosa ATCC 9027	1997
Glycolipid and tween 80	Naphthalene and methyl naphthalene	Liquid	Rhodococcus sp H13A	1997
EKoil	Oil polluted waters	Liquid	Mycobacterium flavescens	1997
Crude surfactin	Hexadecane, kerosene oil	Soil	B. subtilis MTCC2423	1997
Biosurfactant	Crude oil	Liquid	P. aeruginosa	1997
Glycolipids (GL-K12)	Arochlor 1242	Soil	P. cepacia	1997
Rhamnolipid	Phenanthrene, hexadecane	Soil	P. aeruginosa UG2	1998
Monorhamnolipid	Hexadecane	Sand	P. aeruginosa	1998
Biosurfactant	Pyrene	Soil columns	P. aeruginosa UG2	1998
Rhamnolipid	PAHs and Pentachlorophenol (PCP)	Soil	P. aeruginosa # 64	1999
Crude surfactin	Endosulfan	Soil	B. subtilis MTCC2423	1999
Surfactin	Heavy metals	Soil	B. subtilis	1999

continued on next page

Table 5. *Continued*

Biosurfactant	Source	Remediation Medium	Pollutant	Year of Study
Glycolipid	PCB	Soil	*Alcanivorax borkumensis*	1999
Alasan	Phenanthrene, fluoranthene and pyrene	Liquid	*Acinetobacter radioresistens* KA53	1999
Rhamnolipids mixture + triton X100	Trifluralin, coumaphos, atrazine	liquid	*P. aeruginosa UG2*	2000, 2001
Crude surfactin	Aliphatic and aromatic hydrocarbons	Seawater	*B. subtilis O9*	2000
Sophorolipid	Phenanthrene	Soil	*C. bombicola ATCC 22214*	2000
Rhamnolipid	Phenanthrene, cadmium	Soil	*P. aeruginosa ATCC 9027*	2000
Mono-rhamnolipid	Naphthalene, cadmium	Soil	*P. aeruginosa ATCC 9027*	2000
Di-rhamnolipid	Toluene, ethyl benzene, buytl benzene	Liquid	*Pseudomonas sp*	2001
Rhamnolipid + poultry litter + coir pith	gasoline	soil	*Pseudomonas sp DS10-129*	2002
Rhamnolipid	Hexadecane	Silica matrices	*P. aeruginosa UG2*	2002
Rhamnolipids	n-paraffin	Soil	*Nocardioides sp*	2002
Saponin	Metal remediation	Soil	*Plant derived*	2002
Biosurfactant	PAHs	Batch solutions	*P. aeruginosa PCG3*	2003
Biosurfactant + ground rice hulls	PAHs	Soil	*P. aeruginosa strain-64*	2003
Rhamnolipids + bacterial consortium + nutrients	n-alkanes,	Petroleum sludge	*Flavobacterium sp DS5-73, Pseudomonas sp DS10-129*	2003
Rhamnolipids	PCP	soil	Jeneil biosurfactant (saukville, WI, USA)	2003
BOD Balance	Waste water oils and grease	liquid	*Cactus*	2003

continued on next page

Table 5. Continued

Biosurfactant	Source	Remediation Medium	Pollutant	Year of Study
Rhamnolipids	Heavy metals	Soil	Jeneil biosurfactant (saukville, WI, USA)	2003
Rhamnolipid	Hexadecane	Liquid	*Renibacterium salmoninarum* 27BN	2004
Biosurfactant	PAHs	Soil	*P. aeruginosa* PCG3	2004
Rhamnolipid foam	Metals	Soil	Jeneil biosurfactant (saukville, WI, USA)	2004
Rhamnolipid/SDS	Crude oil	Stirred tank Reactor	Jeneil biosurfactants company, USA	2005
Biosurfactant	Oil	Soil	*Rhodococcus ruber*	2005
Biosurfactant	Kerosene and disel	Liquid	*Pseudoxanthomonas kaohsiungensis*	2005
Rhamnolipids	Pyrene	Soil	*P. aeruginosa* 57SJ	2005

Biodegradability and the low toxicity are the two factors which make them suitable for remediation, but more efforts and research is required to understand their behavior in the fate and transport of contaminants and co cocontaminants, their cost of ex situ production and the factors influencing the bioavailability of contaminants.

Biosurfactants and Medicine

Most of the work with applications of biosurfactants has been limited to their use in mainly pollution control where intrinsic properties of biosurfactants are applied but they have applications for therapeutic purposes and in medicine. Some biosurfactants, such as rhamnolipids produced by *P. aeruginosa,* lipopeptides produced by *Bacillus* sps and yeast glycolipid mannosylerythritol lipid (MEL) biosurfactants has numerous applications in medicine and has been shown to exhibit properties of antimicrobial and immunological agents.[8,10,53,59]

Biosurfactants have find applications as a cell differentiation inducers in the human promyelocytic leukemia cell line HL60, as a affinity ligand of human immunoglobin G (IgG) and as a granulocyte colony stimulating molecule.[10,53] There have been reports for their use as transfection agents and are better non viral vector mediated gene transfection and gene therapy procedures.[98,99] The use of biosurfactants as antiviral agents and antibacterial agents have been documented.[8,50,100-103] The discovery of surfactin by Arima et al[104] was a consequence of search for antimicrobial agents and it is one of the most potent biosurfactants known has been applied as antifungal, antibacterial and antimycoplasma agent.[105] Apart from antimicrobial property surfactin has been shown to inhibit the fibrin clot formation, inhibitor of cyclic adenosine monophosphate, platelet and spleen cytosolic phospholipase A2 (possible role on cell signaling). Some of the other lipopeptide biosurfactants with reported antimicrobial activity other than surfactin are iturin,[106] pumilacidin,[107] gramicidin, polymixins,[108] viscosinamide,[36,109] amphisin[110] and Massetolides A-H.[111] Applications of glycolipids as antimicrobial agents is gaining attention in recent years. Some of the glycolipids with antimicrobial activities are rhamnolipids of *P. aeruginosa* AT10,[112] glycolipids of *Borrelia burgdorferi,*[113] glycolipid fungicide from *Psueudozyma fusiformata*[114,115] and MEL lipids *Candida antarctica.*[59]

Apart form these traditional applications, role of biosurfactants as probiotic agents has been gaining interest.[116-118] The term probiotic often used to describe food supplements that contain live bacteria, which can help your health. Use of *Lactobacilli,* as probiotic agents has received greater attention as an alternative, inexpensive and natural remedy to restore and maintain health.[116-118] Two strains, *Lactobacillus* GG (ATCC 53103) and *Lactobacillus rhamnosus* GR-1 appear to be effective at decolonizing and protecting the intestine and urogenital tract against microbial infection.[119] The e probiotic effects of these strains are due to the byproducts (biosurfactants) of *Lactobacillus* metabolism that have an antagonistic effect against urinary and vaginal pathogens. With the increased evidence in term of more research results the concept of treating and preventing urogenital infection by instillating probiotic organisms has great appeal to patients and caregivers.[116,117,120-122]

Biosurfactants have been found to inhibit the adhesion of pathogenic organisms to solid surfaces or to infection sites[123,124] and have been shown to inhibit formation of biofilms on different surfaces, including polyvivyl wells and vinyl urethral catheters.[123,125,126] Precoating the catheters and medical devices by biosurfactant solution can and have potential applications for treating. Opportunistic infections with *Salmonella* species, including urinary tract infections of AIDS patients.[10,53] The prior adhesion of biosurfactants to solid surfaces might constitute a new and effective means of combating colonization by pathogenic microorganisms and a promising strategy for prolonging the prostheses lifespan.[123-127]

Biosurfactants and Miscellaneous Applications

Biosurfactants are products of interest for biotechnological and industrial applications as discussed in previous sections and have application in many diverse areas. Role of biosurfactants as cellular architect has recently been reported for a number of bacteria. They have been shown to play role *B. subtilis* fruiting body formation (surfactin) and role of streptofactin in formation

Streptomyces tendae aerial mycelia.[128,129] They have potential use in modern day agricultural practices as a hyrophilizing and wetting agent for achieving the equal distribution of fertilizers and pesticides in the soils.[130,131]

They have been applied as dewatering agents in pressing peat,[132] as dispersion agent of inorganic minerals in mining and manufacturing processes,[3,5] in cosmetic formulations,[3,5] as an anti algal agents[133,134] and as biocontrol agent.[135-138] In the food industry the biosurfactants are used as emulsifier for the processing of raw materials.[3,5]

Conclusion

The rapid and dramatic advancement in medical and environmental sciences have increased the public interest in natural products such as biosurfactants and propelled these molecules closer to the mainstream of healthcare and consumer products. As explained in the chapter biosurfactants have potent antimicrobial and environmental applications. Their broad range of applications and flexibility of production makes them a suitable alternative synthetic medicines and antimicrobial agents. They could be applied for betterment of environment and health care. For economical penetration of the market the biosurfactants have to overcome the cost of production by better downstream processing and strain improvement for the upscale production. It is just matter of time when some pharmaceutical company will invest in lowering the cost of biosurfactant production and toxicity and other approval tests for specialty uses in medicine and will earn revenues from introducing biosurfactants in market on large scale.

References

1. Deleu M, Paquot M. From renewable vegetables resources to microorganisms: new trends in surfactants. Comptes Rendus Chimie 2004; 7(6-7):641-646.
2. Mulligan CN. Environmental applications for biosurfactants. Environ Pollut 2005; 133(2):183-198.
3. Desai JD, Banat IM. Microbial production of surfactants and their commercial potential. Microbiol Mol Biol Rev 1997; 61(1):47-64.
4. Cameotra S, Makkar R. Synthesis of biosurfactants in extreme conditions. Appl Microbiol Biotechnol 1998; 50(5):520-529.
5. Banat IM, Makkar RS, Cameotra SS. Potential commercial applications of microbial surfactants. Appl Microbiol Biotechnol 2000; 53(5):495-508.
6. Cameotra SS, Bollag J-M. Biosurfactant-Enhanced Bioremediation of Polycyclic Aromatic Hydrocarbons. Critical Reviews in Environmental Science and Technology 2003; 30(2):111-126.
7. Lang S. Biological amphiphiles (microbial biosurfactants). Curr Opin Colloid Interface Sci 2002; 7(1-2):12-20.
8. Maier RM, Soberon-Chavez G. Pseudomonas aeruginosa rhamnolipids: biosynthesis and potential applications. Appl Microbiol Biotechnol 2000; 54(5):625-633.
9. Makkar RS, Rockne KJ. Comparison of synthetic surfactants and biosurfactants in enhancing biodegradation of polycyclic aromatic hydrocarbons. Environ Toxicol Chem 22(10):2280-2292.
10. Singh P, Cameotra SS. Potential applications of microbial surfactants in biomedical sciences. Trends Biotechnol 2004; 22(3):142-146.
11. Georgiou G, Lin SC, Sharma MM. Surface-active compounds from microorganisms. Biotechnology (NY) 1992; 10(1):60-65.
12. Holmberg K. Natural surfactants. Curr Opin Colloid Interface Sci 2001; 6:148-159.
13. Mulligan CN, Eftekhari F. Remediation with surfactant foam of PCP-contaminated soil. Engineering Geology 2003; 70(3-4):269-279.
14. Mulligan CN, Yong RN. Natural attenuation of contaminated soils. Environ Int 2004/6 2004; 30(4):587-601.
15. Ron EZ, Rosenberg E. Natural roles of biosurfactants. Environ Microbiol 2001; 3(4):229-236.
16. Maier RM. Biosurfactants: evolution and diversity in bacteria. Adv Appl Microbiol 2003; 52:101-121.
17. Bodour AA, Drees KP, Maier RM. Distribution of biosurfactant-producing bacteria in undisturbed and contaminated arid Southwestern soils. Appl Environ Microbiol 2003; 69(6):3280-3287.
18. Rosenberg E. CRC Crit Rev Biotechnol 1986; 3:109.
19. Rosenberg E, Ron EZ. Bioemulsans: microbial polymeric emulsifiers. Curr Opin Biotechnol 1997; 8(3):313-316.
20. Rosenberg E, Ron EZ. High- and low-molecular-mass microbial surfactants. Appl Microbiol Biotechnol 1999; 52(2):154-162.

21. Neu TR. Significance of bacterial surface-active compounds in interaction of bacteria with interfaces. Microbiol Rev 1996; 60(1):151-166.
22. Zhang Y, Maier WJ, Miller RM. Effect of rhamnolipids on the dissolution, bioavailability and biodegradation of phenanthrene. Environ Sci Technol 1997; 31(8):2211-2217.
23. Zhang Y, Miller RM. Effect of a Pseudomonas rhamnolipid biosurfactant on cell hydrophobicity and biodegradation of octadecane. Appl Environ Microbiol 1994; 60(6):2101-2106.
24. Rosenberg E. Exploiting microbial growth on hydrocarbons—new markets. Trends Biotechnol 1993; 11(10):419-424.
25. Rosenberg E, Rubinovitz C, Gottlieb A et al. Production of biodispersan by Acinetobacter calcoaceticus A2. Appl Environ Microbiol 1988; 54:317-322.
26. Toren A, Navon-Venezia S, Ron E et al. Emulsifying Activities of Purified Alasan Proteins from Acinetobacter radioresistens KA53. Appl Environ Microbiol 2001; 67(3):1102-1106.
27. Hua Z, Chen J, Lun S et al. Influence of biosurfactants produced by Candida antarctica on surface properties of microorganism and biodegradation of n-alkanes. Water Res 2003; 37(17):4143-4150.
28. Deziel E, Paquette G, Villemur R et al. Biosurfactant Production by a Soil Pseudomonas Strain Growing on Polycyclic Aromatic Hydrocarbons. Appl Environ Microbiol 1996; 62(6):1908-1912.
29. Edwards DA, Luthy RG, Liu Z. Solubilization of polycyclic aromatic hydrocarbons in micellar non-ionic surfactant solutions. Environ Sci Technol 1991; 25(1):127-133.
30. Zhang Y, Miller R. Effect of Rhamnolipid (Biosurfactant) Structure on Solubilization and Biodegradation of n-Alkanes. Appl Environ Microbiol 1995; 61(6):2247-2251.
31. Barkay T, Navon-Venezia S, Ron EZ et al. Enhancement of solubilization and biodegradation of polyaromatic hydrocarbons by the bioemulsifier alasan. Appl Environ Microbiol 1999; 65(6):2697-2702.
32. Jordan RN, Nichols EP, Cunningham AB. The role of (bio) surfactant sorption in promoting the bioavailability of nutrients localized at the solid-water interface. Water Sci Technol 1999; 39(7):91-98.
33. Chen G, Qiao M, Zhang H et al. Bacterial desorption in water-saturated porous media in the presence of rhamnolipid biosurfactant. Res Microbiol 2004; 155(8):655-661.
34. Puchkov EO, Zahringer U, Lindner B et al. The mycocidal, membrane-active complex of Cryptococcus humicola is a new type of cellobiose lipid with detergent features. Biochimica et Biophysica Acta (BBA)—Biomembranes 2002; 1558(2):161-170.
35. de Souza JT, de Boer M, de Waard P et al. Biochemical, Genetic and Zoosporicidal Properties of Cyclic Lipopeptide Surfactants Produced by Pseudomonas fluorescens. Appl Environ Microbiol 2003; 69(12):7161-7172.
36. Nielsen TH, Sorensen J. Production of cyclic lipopeptides by Pseudomonas fluorescens strains in bulk soil and in the sugar beet rhizosphere. Appl Environ Microbiol 2003; 69(2):861-868.
37. Cooper DG. Biosurfactants. Microbiol Sci 1986; 3(5):145-149.
38. Oberbremer A, Muller-Hurtig R, Wagner F. Effect of the addition of microbial surfactants on hydrocarbon degradation in a soil population in a stirred reactor. Appl Microbiol Biotechnol 1990; 32(4):485-489.
39. Chayabutra C, Wu J, Ju LK. Rhamnolipid production by Pseudomonas aeruginosa under denitrification: effects of limiting nutrients and carbon substrates. Biotechnol Bioeng 2001; 72(1):25-33.
40. Wick LY, Ruiz de Munain A, Springael D et al. Responses of Mycobacterium sp. LB501T to the low bioavailability of solid anthracene. Appl Microbiol Biotechnol 2002; 58(3):378-385.
41. Mulligan CN, Mahmourides G, Gibbs BF. The influence of phosphate metabolism on biosurfactant production by Pseudomonas aeruginosa. J Biotechnol 1989; 12(3-4):199-209.
42. Robert M, Mercade M, Bosch M et al. Effect of the carbon source on biosurfactant production by Pseudomonas aeruginosa 44Ti. Biotechnol Lett 1989; 11:871-874.
43. Symmank H, Franke P, Saenger W et al. Modification of biologically active peptides: production of a novel lipohexapeptide after engineering of Bacillus subtilis surfactin synthetase. Protein Eng 2002; 15(11):913-921.
44. Poremba K, Gunkel W, Lang S et al. Marine biosurfactants, III. Toxicity testing with marine microorganisms and comparison with synthetic surfactants. Z Naturforsch (C) 1991; 46(3-4):210-216.
45. Poremba K. Influence of synthetic and biogenic surfactants on the toxicity of water-soluble fractions of hydrocarbons in sea water determined with the bioluminescence inhibition test. Environ Pollut 1993; 80(1):25-29.
46. Kanga SA, Bonner JS, Page CA et al. Solubilization of Naphthalene and Methyl-Substituted Naphthalenes from Crude Oil Using Biosurfactants. Environ Sci Technol 1997; 31(2):556-561.
47. Edwards KR, Lepo JE, Lewis MA. Toxicity comparison of biosurfactants and synthetic surfactants used in oil spill remediation to two estuarine species. Mar Pollut Bull 2003; 46(10):1309-1316.
48. Banat IM. Biosurfactants, more in demand than ever: Les biosurfactants, plus que jamais sollicites. Biofutur 2000; 198:44-47.

49. Lang S, Philp JC. Surface-active lipids in Rhodococci. Antonie Van Leeuwenhoek 1998; 74(1-3):59-70.
50. Lang S, Wullbrandt D. Rhamnose lipids—biosynthesis, microbial production and application potential. Appl Microbiol Biotechnol 1999; 51(1):22-32.
51. Rau U, Hammen S, Heckmann R et al. Sophorolipids: a source for novel compounds. Industrial Crops and Products 2001; 13(2):85-92.
52. Bonmatin JM, Laprevote O, Peypoux F. Diversity among microbial cyclic lipopeptides: iturins and surfactins. Activity-structure relationships to design new bioactive agents. Comb Chem High Throughput Screen 2003; 6(6):541-556.
53. Cameotra SS, Makkar RS. Recent applications of biosurfactants as biological and immunological molecules. Curr Opin Microbiol 2004; 7(3):262-266.
54. Navon-Venezia S, Zosim Z, Gottlieb A et al. Alasan, a new bioemulsifier from Acinetobacter radioresistens. Appl Environ Microbiol 1995; 61(9):3240-3244.
55. Fiechter A. Biosurfactants: moving towards industrial application. Trends Biotechnol 1992; 10:208-217.
56. Zhang Y, Miller RM. Enhanced octadecane dispersion and biodegradation by a Pseudomonas rhamnolipid surfactant (biosurfactant). Appl Environ Microbiol 1992; 58(10):3276-3282.
57. Mulligan C, Yong R, Gibbs B. Heavy metal removal from sediments by biosurfactants. J Hazard Mater 2001; 85(1-2):111-125.
58. Mulligan CN, Yong RN, Gibbs BF. Remediation technologies for metal-contaminated soils and groundwater: an evaluation. Engineering Geology 2001; 60(1-4):193-207.
59. Kitamoto D, Isoda H, Nakahara T. Functions and potential applications of glycolipid biosurfactants—from energy-saving materials to gene delivery carriers. J Biosci Bioeng 2002; 94(3):187-201.
60. Makkar RS, Cameotra SS. Synthesis of Enhanced biosurfactant by Bacillus subtilis MTCC 2423 at 45°C by Foam Fractionation. Journal of Surfactants and Detergents 2001; 4:355-357.
61. Noordman WH, Bruining J-W, Wietzes P et al. Facilitated transport of a PAH mixture by a rhamnolipid biosurfactant in porous silica matrices. J Contam Hydrol 2000; 44(2):119-140.
62. Noordman WH, Janssen DB. Rhamnolipid stimulates uptake of hydrophobic compounds by Pseudomonas aeruginosa. Appl Environ Microbiol 2002; 68(9):4502-4508.
63. Kingston PF. Long-term Environmental Impact of Oil Spills. Spill Science and Technology Bulletin 2002; 7(1-2):53-61.
64. Page DS, Boehm PD, Brown JS et al. Mussels document loss of bioavailable polycyclic aromatic hydrocarbons and the return to baseline conditions for oiled shorelines in Prince William Sound, Alaska. Mar Environ Res 2005; 60(4):422-436.
65. Wiens JA. Recovery of seabirds following the Exxon Valdez oil spill: an overview. Exxon Valdez Oil Spill: Fate and Effects in Alaskan Waters. ASTM Special Technical Publication 1995:854-893.
66. Dauvin J-C. The fine sand Abra alba community of the bay of morlaix twenty years after the Amoco Cadiz oil spill. Mar Pollut Bull 1998; 36(9):669-676.
67. Urum K, Pekdemir T. Evaluation of biosurfactants for crude oil contaminated soil washing. Chemosphere 2004; 57(9):1139-1150.
68. Urum K, Pekdemir T, Ross D et al. Crude oil contaminated soil washing in air sparging assisted stirred tank reactor using biosurfactants. Chemosphere 2005; 60(3):334-343.
69. Wei QF, Mather RR, Fotheringham AF. Oil removal from used sorbents using a biosurfactant. Bioresour Technol 2005; 96(3):331-334.
70. Harvey S, Elashvili I, Valdes JJ et al. Enhanced removal of Exxon Valdez spilled oil from Alaskan gravel by a microbial surfactant. Biotechnology 1990; 8(3):228-230.
71. DeschÂªnes L, Lafrance P, Villeneuve J-P et al. Adding sodium dodecyl sulfate and Pseudomonas aeruginosa UG2 biosurfactants inhibits polycyclic aromatic hydrocarbon biodegradation in a weathered creosote-contaminated soil. Appl Microbiol Biotechnol 1996; 46(5-6):638-646.
72. Munoz R, Guieysse B, Mattiasson B. Phenanthrene biodegradation by an algal-bacterial consortium in two-phase partitioning bioreactors. Appl Microbiol Biotechnol 2003; 61(3):261-267.
73. Kuyukina MS, Ivshina IB, Makarov SO et al. Effect of biosurfactants on crude oil desorption and mobilization in a soil system. Environ Int 2005; 31(2):155-161.
74. Van Hamme JD, Singh A, Ward OP. Recent Advances in Petroleum Microbiology. Microbiol Mol Biol Rev 2003; 67(4):503-549.
75. Khire JM, Khan MI. Microbially enhanced oil recovery (MEOR). Part 2. Microbes and the subsurface environment for MEOR. Enzyme Microb Technol 1994/3 1994; 16(3):258-259.
76. Abu Ruwaida A, Banat I, Hadithirto S et al. Isolation of biosurfactant producing bacteria product characterization and evaluation. Acta Biotechnol 1991; 11:315-324.
77. Banat I. The Isolation of Thermophilic Biosurfactant producing Bacillus sp. Biotechnol Lett 1993; 15:591-594.

78. Margesin R, Schinner F. Potential of halotolerant and halophilic microorganisms for biotechnology. Extremophiles 2001; 5(2):73-83.
79. Banat IM. Biosurfactants production and possible uses in microbial enhanced oil recovery and oil pollution remediation: a review. Fuel and Energy Abstracts 1995; 36(4):290.
80. Khire JM, Khan MI. Microbially enhanced oil recovery (MEOR). Part 1. Importance and mechanism of MEOR. Enzyme Microb Technol 1994; 16(2):170-172.
81. Yakimov MM, Amro MM, Bock M et al. The potential of Bacillus licheniformis strains for in situ enhanced oil recovery. Journal of Petroleum Science and Engineering 1997; 18(1-2):147-160.
82. Madihah MS, Ariff AB, Akmam FH et al. Hyper-thermophilic fermentative bacteria in Malaysian petroleum reservoirs. Asia-Pacific J Mol Biol Biotechnol 1998; 6:29-37.
83. Al-Maghrabi IMA, Bin Aqil AO, Isla MR et al. Use of thermophilic bacteria for bioremediation of petroleum contaminants. Energy Sources 1999; 21:17-29.
84. Rahman KS, Banat IM, Thahira J et al. Bioremediation of gasoline contaminated soil by a bacterial consortium amended with poultry litter, coir pith and rhamnolipid biosurfactant. Bioresour Technol 2002; 81(1):25-32.
85. Rahman KS, Rahman TJ, Kourkoutas Y et al. Enhanced bioremediation of n-alkane in petroleum sludge using bacterial consortium amended with rhamnolipid and micronutrients. Bioresour Technol 2003; 90(2):159-168.
86. Makkar RS, Cameotra SS. Utilization of molasses for biosurfactant production by two Bacillus strains at thermophilic conditions. J Am Oil Chem Soc (JACOS) 1997; 74:887-889.
87. Makkar R, Cameotra S. An update on the use of unconventional substrates for biosurfactant production and their new applications. Appl Microbiol Biotechnol 2002; 58(4):428-434.
88. Harrad S, Laurie L. Concentrations, sources and temporal trends in atmospheric polycyclic aromatic hydrocarbons in a major conurbation. J Environ Monit 2005; 7(7):722-727.
89. Singh P, Cameotra SS. Enhancement of metal bioremediation by use of microbial surfactants. Biochem Biophys Res Commun 2004; 319(2):291-297.
90. Herman DC, Zhang Y, Miller RM. Rhamnolipid (biosurfactant) effects on cell aggregation and bio-degradation of residual hexadecane under saturated flow conditions. Appl Environ Microbiol 1997; 63(9):3622-3627.
91. Ochoa-Loza FJ, Artiola JF, Maier RM. Stability Constants for the Complexation of Various Metals with a Rhamnolipid Biosurfactant. J Environ Qual 2001; 30(2):479-485.
92. Mulligan CN, Kamali M, Gibbs BF. Bioleaching of heavy metals from a low-grade mining ore using Aspergillus niger. J Hazard Mater 2004; 110(1-3):77-84.
93. Maslin P, Maier RM. Rhamnolipid-Enhanced Mineralization of Phenanthrene in Organic-Metal Cocontaminated Soils. Bioremediat J 2000; 4(4):295-308.
94. Mulligan CN, Yong RN, Gibbs BF. Removal of Heavy Metals from Contaminated Soil and Sediments Using the Biosurfactant Surfactin. Journal of Soil Contamination 1999; 8(2):231-254.
95. Mulligan CN, Yong RN, Gibbs BF. Surfactant-enhanced remediation of contaminated soil: a review. Engineering Geology 2001; 60(1-4):371-380.
96. Jeong-Jin H, Seung-Man Y, Choul-Ho L et al. Adsorption of tricarboxylic acid biosurfactant derived from spiculisporic acid on titanium dioxide surface. Colloids Surf B Biointerfaces 1996; 7(5-6):221-233.
97. Finnerty WR. Biosurfactants in environmental biotechnology. Curr Opin Biotechnol 1994; 5(3):291-295.
98. Inoh Y, Kitamoto D, Hirashima N et al. Biosurfactants of MEL-A Increase Gene Transfection Mediated by Cationic Liposomes. Biochem Biophys Res Commun 2001; 289(1):57-61.
99. Inoh Y, Kitamoto D, Hirashima N et al. Biosurfactant MEL-A dramatically increases gene transfection via membrane fusion. J Control Release 2004; 94(2-3):423-431.
100. Vollenbroich D, Ozel M, Vater J et al. Mechanism of Inactivation of Enveloped Viruses by the Biosurfactant Surfactin from Bacillus subtilis. Biologicals 1997; 25(3):289-297.
101. Vollenbroich D, Pauli G, Ozel M et al. Antimycoplasma properties and application in cell culture of surfactin, a lipopeptide antibiotic from Bacillus subtilis. Appl Environ Microbiol 1997; 63(1):44-49.
102. Lang S, Kaiswela E, F W. Antimicrobial effects of biosurfactants. Fat Sci Technol 1989; 91:363-366.
103. Lang S, Wagner F. Biological Activities of Biosurfactants. New York: Marcel Dekker INc; 1993.
104. Arima K, Kakinuma A, Tamuri G. Surfactin, a crystalline peptidolipid surfactant produced by Bacillus subtilis. Isolation, Characterization and its inhibition of fibrin clot formation. Biochem Biophys Res Comm 1968; 31:361-369.
105. Nir-Paz R, Prevost MC, Nicolas P et al. Susceptibilities of Mycoplasma fermentans and Mycoplasma hyorhinis to membrane-active peptides and enrofloxacin in human tissue cell cultures. Antimicrob Agents Chemother 2002; 46(5):1218-1225.
106. Sandrin C, Peypoux F, Michel G. Coproduction of surfactin and iturin A, lipopeptides with surfactant and antifungal properties, by Bacillus subtilis. Biotechnol Appl Biochem 1990; 12(4):370-375.

107. Naruse N, Tenmyo O, Kobaru S et al. Pumilacidin, a complex of new antiviral antibiotics: production, isolation, chemical properties, structure and biological activity. J Antibiot (Tokyo) 1990; 43:267-280.
108. Kitatsuji K, Miyata H, Fukase T. Isolation of microorganisms that lyse filamentous bacteria and characterization of the lytic substance secreted by Bacillus polymyxa. J Ferment Bioeng 1996; 82(4):323-327.
109. Nielsen TH, Sorensen D, Tobiasen C et al. Antibiotic and biosurfactant properties of cyclic lipopeptides produced by fluorescent Pseudomonas spp. from the sugar beet rhizosphere. Appl Environ Microbiol 2002; 68(7):3416-3423.
110. Andersen JB, Koch B, Nielsen TH et al. Surface motility in Pseudomonas sp. DSS73 is required for efficient biological containment of the root-pathogenic microfungi Rhizoctonia solani and Pythium ultimum. Microbiology 2003; 149:37-46.
111. Gerard J, Lloyd R, Barsby T et al. Massetolides A-H, antimycobacterial cyclic depsipeptides produced by two Pseudomonads isolated from marine habitats. J Nat Prod 1997; 60(3):223-229.
112. Abalos A, Pinazo A, Infante MR et al. Physicochemical and Antimicrobial Properties of New Rhamnolipids Produced by Pseudomonas aeruginosa AT10 from Soybean Oil Refinery Wastes. Langmuir 2001; 17(5):1367-1371.
113. Hossain H, Wellensiek H-J, Geyer R et al. Structural analysis of glycolipids from Borrelia burgdorferi. Biochimie 2001; 83(7):683-692.
114. Golubev WI, Kulakovskaya TV, Golubeva EW. The yeast Pseudozyma fusiformata VKM Y-2821 producing an antifungal glycolipid. Microbiol 2001; 70:553-556.
115. Kulakovskaya TV, Kulakovskaya EV, Golubev WI. ATP leakage from yeast cells treated by extracellular glycolipids of Pseudozyma fusiformata. FEMS Yeast Research 2003; 3(4):401-404.
116. Reid G, Bruce AW, Fraser N et al. Oral probiotics can resolve urogenital infections. FEMS Immunol Med Microbiol 2001; 30(1):49-52.
117. Reid G, Heinemann C, Velraeds M et al. Biosurfactants produced by Lactobacillus. Methods Enzymol 1999; 310:426-433.
118. Gan BS, Kim J, Reid G et al. Lactobacillus fermentum RC-14 inhibits Staphylococcus aureus infection of surgical implants in rats. J Infect Dis 2002; 185(9):1369-1372.
119. Reid G, Charbonneau D, Erb J et al. Oral use of Lactobacillus rhamnosus GR-1 and L. fermentum RC-14 significantly alters vaginal flora: randomized, placebo-controlled trial in 64 healthy women. FEMS Immunol Med Microbiol 2003; 35(2):131-134.
120. Rastall RA, Gibson GR, Gill HS et al. Modulation of the microbial ecology of the human colon by probiotics, prebiotics and synbiotics to enhance human health: an overview of enabling science and potential applications. FEMS Microbiol Ecol 2005; 52(2):145-152.
121. Reid G. The Scientific Basis for Probiotic Strains of Lactobacillus. Appl Environ Microbiol 1999; 65(9):3763-3766.
122. Reid G. Probiotic agents to protect the urogenital tract against infection. Am J Clin Nutr 2001; 73(2 Suppl):437S-443S.
123. Velraeds MM, van de Belt-Gritter B, Busscher HJ et al. Inhibition of uropathogenic biofilm growth on silicone rubber in human urine by lactobacilli—a teleologic approach. World J Urol 2000; 18(6):422-426.
124. van Hoogmoed CG, van der Mei HC, Busscher HJ. The influence of biosurfactants released by S. mitis BMS on the adhesion of pioneer strains and cariogenic bacteria. Biofouling 2004; 20(6):261-267.
125. Meylheuc T, van Oss C, Bellon-Fontaine M. Adsorption of biosurfactant on solid surfaces and consequences regarding the bioadhesion of Listeria monocytogenes LO28. J Appl Microbiol 2001; 91(5):822-832.
126. Rodrigues L, Van Der Mei H, Teixeira JA et al. Biosurfactant from Lactococcus lactis 53 inhibits microbial adhesion on silicone rubber. Appl Microbiol Biotechnol 2004.
127. Batrakov SG, Rodionova TA, Esipov SE et al. A novel lipopeptide, an inhibitor of bacterial adhesion, from the thermophilic and halotolerant subsurface Bacillus licheniformis strain 603. Biochimica et Biophysica Acta (BBA)—Molecular and Cell Biology of Lipids 2003; 1634(3):107-115.
128. Branda SS, Gonzalez-Pastor JE, Ben-Yehuda S et al. Fruiting body formation by Bacillus subtilis. Proc Natl Acad Sci USA 2001; 98(20):11621-11626.
129. Richter M, Willey JM, Su(ss)muth R et al. Streptofactin, a novel biosurfactant with aerial mycelium inducing activity from Streptomyces tendae Tu 901/8c. FEMS Microbiol Lett 1998; 163(2):165-171.
130. Mata-Sandoval JC, Karns J, Torrents A. Influence of rhamnolipids and triton X-100 on the desorption of pesticides from soils. Environ Sci Technol 2002; 36(21):4669-4675.
131. Awashti N, Kumar A, Makkar R et al. Enhanced Biodegradation of endosulfan, a chlorinated pesticide in presence of a biosurfactant. J Environ Sci Health 1999; 34:793-803.
132. Cooper DG, Pillon DW, Mulligan CN et al. Biological additives for improved mechanical dewatering of fuel-grade peat. Fuel 1986; 65(2):255-259.

133. Ahn C-Y, Joung S-H, Jeon J-W et al. Selective control of cyanobacteria by surfactin-containing culture broth of Bacillus subtilis C1. Biotechnol Lett 2003; 25(14):1137-1142.

134. Wang X, Gong L, Liang S et al. Algicidal activity of rhamnolipid biosurfactants produced by Pseudomonas aeruginosa. Harmful Algae 2005; 4(2):433-443.

135. Souto GI, Correa OS, Montecchia MS et al. Genetic and functional characterization of a Bacillus sp. strain excreting surfactin and antifungal metabolites partially identified as iturin-like compounds. J Appl Microbiol 2004; 97(6):1247-1256.

136. Assie LK, Deleu M, Arnaud L et al. Insecticide activity of surfactins and iturins from a biopesticide Bacillus subtilis Cohn (S499 strain). Meded Rijksuniv Gent Fak Landbouwkd Toegep Biol Wet 2002; 67(3):647-655.

137. Ongena M, Duby Fl, Jourdan E et al. Bacillus subtilis M4 decreases plant susceptibility towards fungal pathogens by increasing host resistance associated with differential gene expression. Appl Microbiol Biotechnol 2005; 67(5):692-698.

138. Toure Y, Ongena M, Jacques P et al. Role of lipopeptides produced by Bacillus subtilis GA1 in the reduction of grey mould disease caused by Botrytis cinerea on apple. J Appl Microbiol 2004; 96(5):1151-1160.

Enrichment and Purification of Lipopeptide Biosurfactants

Simon C. Baker* and Chien-Yen Chen

Abstract

A great many methods are available for the concentration of biosurfactants from microbiological media. The strongest known biosurfactant, surfactin, serves as a model in many studies, so is used here to illustrate the diversity in approaches to product enrichment. Common physiochemical properties mean that many of these methods can be applied to other systems. Although acid precipitation is the most commonly used form of enrichment, phase separation is both an intrinsic property of surfactants and a useful tool for biotechnology. Direct liquid partitioning, membrane ultrafiltration and foam fractionation can all be regarded as phase separation technologies.

Introduction

In comparison to fossil-fuel-derived surfactants, biologically produced surfactants are still relatively high in price, despite the rising costs of crude oil. The main reasons for their expense are associated with the costs of downstream bioprocessing even when the product is to be used in a relatively impure form. Biosurfactants occur in relatively low concentrations and must be removed from bulk, spent biological media.

This chapter of the current methods used in the separation or purification of biosurfactants from microbiological media will be limited to cyclic lipopeptides, particularly the lipoheptapeptide 'surfactin', since these amply illustrate the principles used. Since surfactants in general have similar physiochemical properties in aqueous solution, the methods discussed here could equally be applied to nonlipopeptide surfactants such as rhamnolipid.

Biosurfactants can be classified as intracellular or extracellular depending on the location of the biosurfactant accumulation. An intracellular biosurfactant is either bound up with the wall surface of the microorganism cell or exists in the cytoplasm, which makes it more difficult to recover. For example, Cameron et al[1] extracted a cell-bound bioemusifier from the cell wall of *Saccharomyces cerevisiae* using a high temperature (121°C) following by protease treatment. Heat-extracted emulsifier was purified by ultrafiltration and precipitation in ethanol-acetic acid. The difficulties associated with the extraction of intracellular surfactants has meant that extracellular biosurfactants (those excreted into the medium by cells) have proved more attractive in commercialisation and provide the focus for this chapter.

Properties of Biosurfactants Useful in Separation

In separating biosurfactants from the medium in which they are produced, the biotechnologist is fortunate that surfactants in general have unique physiochemical properties which distinguish them from the array of other molecules that might be found in solution. Primary

*Corresponding Author: Simon C. Baker—School of Life Sciences, Oxford Brookes University, Gypsy Lane, Oxford OX3 0BP, UK. Email: Simon.baker@brookes.ac.uk

Biosurfactants, edited by Ramkrishna Sen. ©2010 Landes Bioscience and Springer Science+Business Media.

amongst these properties is their amphipathic nature—that some areas of the molecule are hydrophobic, while others are hydrophilic. If the pH and ionic strength are suitable, surfactant molecules will move to phase interfaces where one phase is more hydrophobic than the other. In microbiology, this commonly means water/air, water/organic solvent or more rarely water/solid interfaces. This phase separation property forms the basis on which many of the methods described below are founded.

In common with other biological molecules, biosurfactants tend to function over narrow pH ranges—for example the surfactant activity of surfactin from *Bacillus subtilis* decreases dramatically from pH 7 to 5.5.[2] A similar effect can be observed by changing ionic strength.[3] The ability of many biosurfactants to behave either as hydrophobic molecules or hydrophilic ones and then as a mixture of both gives a separations specialist enormous latitude in designing suitable purification protocols.

When biosurfactants are produced in the fermentation broth, surfactants tend to accumulate at the interface of the medium with air. If this surface layer is separated from the bulk medium, it will be found to contain a higher concentration of some components and a lower concentration of others.[4] Many fractionation processes use some form of separation in which solutes of high surface activity (biosurfactant) are preferentially adsorbed at the interface between a gas phase and bulk liquid phase and are then removed, for example by foaming.[5,4] However, solutes with lower surface activity will tend to remain in the bulk aqueous phase[6] and can be stripped by the use of organic solvents.

Separation by Precipitation

Biosurfactants such as surfactin can be precipitated out of spent media when the pH is several units away from the pI. Most researchers choose to do this at acidic pH, with the addition of hydrochloric acid to pH of 2 commonly used method to achieve this.[7,25,27] The low pH causes the biosurfactant to become positively charged, reducing the effectiveness of the hydrophilic region and possibly causing aggregation. This renders the molecule insoluble and the compound precipitates as a solid.

Although this can under most circumstances yield high-quality surfactant, coprecipitation of other small molecules (e.g., riboflavin[8] in *Bacillus subtilis*, which is also weakly surface active) can occur at such low pH. Altering the pH to 4 reduces yield slightly, but can give a better purity.[9] Acid precipitation has been used to isolate biosurfactants from high-throughput small scale[10] studies to large scale. Most of the methods described in this chapter use preconcentration by acid precipitation before more sophisticated techniques are applied for polishing the product.

Conceptually, ammonium sulphate precipitation could perform the same role as acid in converting the amphipathic biosurfactant into a hydrophobic molecule. However, it is rarely used due to problems with coprecipitation of other small molecules.[11] However, in conjunction with ultrafiltration (see below) to provide enhanced selectivity on the basis of molecular size, concentration from large amounts of media can be achieved.[3]

Liquid Partitioning

Direct from Cell Culture

As an alternative to acid precipitation, some researchers have used phase partitioning as a primary means to enrich for biosurfactant. Few attempts have been made to design systems in which liquid two phase separation is directly coupled to culture growth and production, but Drouin and Cooper[12] used polyethylene glycol or dextran to create a separate aqueous phase above growing cultures of *Bacillus subtilis*. They successfully extracted surfactin and noted that product removal had a stimulatory effect.[12]

Solvent Extraction as a Means of Purification

Acid precipitated biosurfactant (see above) can be separated from contaminating salts by extraction into solvent. Primary alcohols, ethers, hydrocarbons (including chlorinated alkanes), acids, ketones and ethyl acetate have all been used alone or in combination[13] but a detailed study by Chen and Juang[14] suggested that optimisation of the process was essential. Chloroform/methanol in various ratios represents the most flexible method for obtaining the best portioning coefficient of biosurfactant against water,[15] but both of these compounds are deleterious to human health and the environment. As an alternative, it has been found that ethyl acetate extracted surfactin better than *n*-hexadecane,[14] but the best results were obtained with aqueous solutions of biosurfactant against Aliquat 336 (trioctylmethylammonium chloride) dissolved in n-hexane.

Membrane Filtration

The use of filters has the advantage of removing the need for chemical reagents or any phase change during enrichment. As the product remains dissolved in its mother liquor, problems with resuspension are also minimised.[16] Ultrafiltration has been used to purify both surfactin and rhamnolipids using commercially available membranes[17] using various solvents at pressure. Although a pilot-scale study suggested that purification could be achieved for large volumes directly from culture medium,[17] ultrafiltration may not be appropriate under all conditions. Although the molecular weight of most lipopeptides is low (between 1000 and 2000), it is by far unique amongst biological small molecules. An additional consideration is that one step ultrafiltration should be carried out at concentrations below that of the CMC otherwise micelles (and thus the bulk of the biosurfactant) will be removed due to their larger size. Micelle formation has, however, been used as an advantage in a slightly more complex two-step ultrafiltration method.[18] The primary step uses high molecular weight cut-off membranes to isolate micelles from the bulk medium. These are then reduced to component molecules by the addition of methanol and a low molecular weight cut off membrane is then used to separate the biosurfactant from any medium components occluded by the micellar structure.

Cross Flow Ultrafiltration

A major drawback in scaleup of ultrafiltration protocols is membrane clogging[19,20] and the formation of layers of biosurfactant on the membrane itself.[16] To overcome this, the passage of product and solute through the membrane (dead-end filtration) can be changed to flow parallel to the membrane (cross-flow filtration). This limits deposition on the membrane, but does not eliminate it. However, the set up of the cross flow system allows cleaning agents to be better introduced, amongst which pH 11.0 sodium hydroxide solution was found to relieve caking on the membrane.[19] Two-step ultrafiltration, cross flow systems have also been described.[21]

Liquid Membranes

Asymmetrical flow field-flow fractionation (AsFlFFF) has yet to be used on lipopeptides but has been used on uncharacterised biosurfactants from *Pseudomonas*.[22] The stationary phase (i.e., the solid membrane described above) is replaced by an immiscible liquid. If the flow of the two phases is carefully controlled, the partitioning of surfactant, or its movement through a single phase, can give valuable information on the molecular weight and shape of the compound studied. A slightly more complex liquid membrane arrangement has been described very recently, known as pertraction.[23] In this case a three phase system was constructed in which the aqueous medium feed and the product-containing output are separated by a membrane composed of a third liquid which is soluble in neither the feed nor the output. Rotating discs provide mixing in each of the phases, providing mixing without excessive disruption of the interphases between the liquids. Choice of the solvents involved is crucial to a successful extraction and in the case of surfactin a liquid membrane of *n*-heptane was used against two aqueous phases. The pH of the feed and output phases were also found to be important.[23]

Foam Fractionation

Foam fractionation is an unusual process in bioprocessing, since it requires the generation of foam whereas in normal biochemical practice, foam is avoided at all costs. The principle of foam fractionation is straightforward. Bubbles are formed at an aqueous/air interface and these bubbles are guided up a cylinder. While the foam moves up the column, medium drains down the column with gravity. At the top of the column, the draining effect means that the foam is "drier" containing more surfactant than medium. Collapsing the foam by mechanical or chemical means results in a solution ("foamate") which is 50 to 60 times enriched in surfactant compared to the original medium. Many parameters influence the efficacy of the process and include:

- Column height
- Column diameter
- Air flow rate
- Size of bubbles formed within the foam

In addition the physiochemical propertiesof the biosurfactant are important such as the isoelectric point[24] and the portioning coefficient in the medium chosen. It was found that the enrichment ratio of albumin (acting as a biosurfactant) increased with an increase in the height of liquid above the sparger by Uraizzee and Narsimhan (1995, 1996). Additionally, a taller tank results in longer bubble residence times for oxygen supply for microorganism (Bailey and Ollis, 1986).

By manipulating these parameters it is possible to introduce partial selectivity into the process. A tall, wide bore column favours the isolation of biosurfactants with a low CMC value, with the converse being true for weaker compounds. Use of sequential foam fractionation steps can yield enrichments of biosurfactants with successively higher CMC values.[4]

Biosurfactants are very diverse in their chemical composition. It is therefore likely that there are no general guidelines for the isolation of every biosurfactant molecule. As such, a suitable method of product recovery has to be developed and optimised for every newly isolated compound. Some methods are universally applicable, though. In general, recovery techniques include a batch mode consisting of precipitation, solvent extraction and crystallisation; and a continuous mode comprising centrifugation, adsorption, foam separation and ultrafiltration.[13] The choice is dependent on cost and effectiveness. Besides these methods, there are "in situ recovery" methods for biosurfactant recovery where products are continuously removed from the culture broth during cultivation. In situ methods for product recovery can avoid end-product inhibition during fermentation.[25] Some examples of in situ biosurfactant recovery are adsorption of the surfactant onto ion-exchange resins or other suitable adsorbents. As reported by Reiling et al,[26] the rhamnolipids produced by *Pseudomonas* sp. DSM 2874 could be adsorbed onto a support (XAD-2) and recovered by aqueous buffer systems due to their lipophilic ability. However, the use of this method is limited because it is just specific to particular compounds.

Among separation methods, foam separation has drawn the most attention because of its low cost, high effectiveness and the possibility of continuous product removal and in situ recovery. Foam formation is frequently inconvenient because it can fill and clog the reactor during fermentation so that its removal may be advantageous from a practical point of view. In many cases, reactors have to be shut down or antifoam chemicals have to be added to prevent overproduction of bubbles. Foam separation can overcome this problem by continuously removing bubbles. An important reason to remove surfactant by foam fractionation in situ is to overcome product inhibition of catalysis. This can result in much higher yields of desirable product. For example, Cooper et al[27] showed that the yield of surfactin produced by *Bacillus subtilis* ATCC 21332 is enhanced from fermentation by continuously removing the product by foam fractionation. In that study, two types of fermentation were applied to compare production yield. One was carried out without removing the foam and the other was done with the collection of overflowing foam. At the end of these experiments, there was very poor yield in the former reactor. On the other hand, a very good yield of product (0.8 gL^{-1}) was found in the foam from the latter vessel.

In foam fractionation, air is sparged from the bottom of a liquid pool to produce bubbles and these rise to the surface. Whilst the bubbles are travelling, surfactants adsorb at the air-liquid interface. Thereafter, bubbles emerge from the liquid to form a cell in the foam matrix, forming a honeycomb structure. The thin liquid film between air bubbles (lamellae) is stabilised by the adsorbed surfactants.[28] Some of the pool solution will inevitably become entrained (a term coined by Lemlich[29]) in the interstitial spaces of the foam. This interstitial liquid will drain from the foam due to gravity and plateau border suction effects as it rises up the column.[30] Through this mechanism the collapsed foam has much more concentrated surfactant than the bulk liquid solution. Several studies have also been done to investigate recovery of the surfactant itself using foam fractionation and to examine the effects of various parameters on the separation efficiency of surfactants. For example Tharapiwattananon et al[31] applied a continuous foam fractionation column to recover surfactant from water and showed separation to be dependent on airflow rate, foam height, liquid height, surfactant concentration and the size of holes in the porous sparger. The effect of temperature and added salt on surfactant recovery from water using foam fractionation was also discussed by Kumpabooth et al.[32] Recently, a foam fractionation column has also been employed for biosurfactant recovery from a bioreactor by Davis et al,[33] who were able to the concentrate surfactin from *B. subtilis* culture broth. In that study, foam and biosurfactants produced during fermentation were allowed to flow out of the bioreactor using a foam fractionation column and were collected in a separate vessel. Both foam and biosurfactants were effectively removed. The foam separation was integrated with cell culture in a bioreactor to ensure biosurfactant production and recovery were combined. Nevertheless, this system was not closed and so did not provide an aseptic environment. Other species of bacteria might have been able to grow in the system, consume the biosurfactants and affect the biosurfactant activity. Noah et al[34] demonstrated integrated surfactant production in an airlift reactor using an inexpensive low-solids potato process effluent as a medium. In the study, continuous collection of the foam through a tube at the top of the column was used to recover surfactant. They found that 95% of the biosurfactant in *Bacillus subtilis* cultures could be recovered by foam fractionation. Again it was not an aseptic system and indigenous bacteria in the potato process effluent could hamper continuous surfactant production.

A fully aseptic, integrated foam fractionation system for the enrichment of surfactin has been described recently, operating in batch[9] and continuous modes.[35] The yields were comparable to other techniques and the closed system reduced the possibility of contamination. However, while continuous operation was achieved, the system was operating as fed-batch culture and not as a chemostat in steady state. Claims by others to be operating chemostat cultures producing surfactin also turn out to be fed batch cultures rather than true steady state fermentations.[36] True chemostat culture would give valuable information relating to metabolic flux in biosurfactant-producing organisms and such studies are currently under way.[37]

Foam fractionation can give an enrichment of 40 to 50 fold from the bulk medium and can easily be integrated into existing bioprocesses.[35] Coupling foam fractionation to organism culture removes the need to try and control foam during fermentation. Although the method is universally applicable to surface active compounds, some problems still need to be overcome. The primary disadvantage with foam fractionation lies with foam breakage. If bubble size is small, then some biosurfactants with high foam stability (such as surfactin) can form persistent foams. These can resemble shaving foam in consistency and are difficult to collapse either by pH change or mechanically. However, it is straightforward to avoid the formation of such foams during the bubble generation stage.

Surface Skimming

Guez et al[38] have also described an adapted foam fractionation arrangement and have modelled the behaviour of an integrated, continuous fermenter as a variation of Monod-based growth. The design is based on the foam fractionation device of Davies et al[33] but uses a surface agitator to enhance foaming, which then overflows into a collector. A fed-batch strategy to produce yielded mycosubtilin-enriched foam in gram quantities.

Surface Enrichment

The movement of surface-active molecules to an interphase allows the possibility of avoiding foaming altogether if such an interpahse can be collected efficiently. Glazryina et al[39] describe the use of such a device, known as the "flounder". They used it to collect two compounds closely related to surfactin with poorer interfacial properties to demonstrate the efficiency of the method. Cultures of *Bacillus subtilis* DSM 21393 were grown within a combined incubation and extraction vessel, based on apparatus devised by Lunkenheimer et al.[40] Currently the method is only suitable for lab scale volumes, but scale up is not seen as impossible. The apparatus has two modes of action, with growth occurring in a horizontal stage with so that the air/water surface area is maximised. Harvesting occurs at the end of growth and is an iterative process. The vessel is tipped into an upright position so that the biosurfactant moves to a smaller surface area and thus becomes concentrated. The enriched liquid is then removed and the culture returned to the horizontal. After allowing surfactant to move back fro the bulk liquid to the surface, the concentration process can be repeated again, with the authors reporting up to 100 cycles to completely remove surfactant from the bulk medium.[39] As the technique is based on adsorption under defined boundary conditions, it is theoretically possible to isolate compounds with singular surface active properties, devoid of contaminating material.[39]

Adsorption to Solids

Although solid/liquid interfaces are available for binding in many parts of a fermenter, it has been found that surfactin will bind preferentially to some compounds over others. Activated carbon has long been used to clarify acid-precipitated or solvent-extracted surfactin, but was found to be suitable for direct isolation from bacteriological media.[41] Although the process has so far only been modelled,[42] the ultimate goal is to run a fully integrated fixed bed column, with pellets of activated carbon adsorbing surfactin as a means of recovery. Unfortunately the concomitant adsorption of other small molecules found in spent media was not considered.

High Performance Liquid Chromatography

High-performance liquid chromatography (HPLC) has been widely applied to the purification of biosurfactants, as it is a method that is not only an effective separation technique, but also a sensitive tool for biosurfactant analysis. This was shown when[43] proposed a practical approach to separate biosurfactants by incorporating HPLC with ultrafiltration, a technique not requiring any prior structural or physicochemical information about the biosurfactants, but which does need a suitable detector. In addition, rhamnolipids produced by *P. aeruginosa* were purified by HPLC[44] and Mata-Sandoval et al[45] also quantified the biosurfactant mixture using HPLC. These studies show that high-performance liquid chromatography is a rapid and reliable method for purifying biosurfactants for analysis. However, the separation of biosurfactants from large volume cultures by HPLC is a costly and time-consuming process, which cannot be used at an industrial scale. This needs alternative separation strategies as most fermentation products are released into large, dilute, aqueous solutions.

Conclusion

Bulk enrichment or purification of biosurfactants will receive more attention as the price of fossil fuel derived surfactants rises. Although many of the methods for surfactin and related compounds described above could be used in larger scale purifications, the costs have yet to be reduced by a at least two orders of magnitude to allow the use of lipopeptide biosurfactants as household detergents. In the meantime significantly more research is required.

Acknowledgements

The authors thank Professor Richard Darton (University of Oxford, UK) and Dr Peter Martin (University of Manchester, UK) for valuable discussions and the Engineering and Physical Sciences Research Council, UK for providing funding during the preparation of this manuscript.

References

1. Cameron DR, Cooper DG, Neufeld RJ. The mannoprotein of Saccharomyces cerevisiae is an effective bioemulsifier. Appl Environ Microbiol. 1988; 54:1420-1425.
2. Arima K, Kakinuma A, Tamura G. Surfactin, a crystalline peptidelipid surfactant produced by Bacillus subtilis: isolation, characterization and its inhibition of fibrin clot formation. Biochem Biophys Res Commun. 1968; 31:488-494.
3. Chen HL, Chen YS, Juang RS. Recovery of surfactin from fermentation broths by a hybrid salting-out and membrane filtration process. Separation and Purification Technology 2008; 59:244-252.
4. Darton RC, Supino S, Sweeting KJ. Development of a multistaged foam fractionation column. Chemical Engineering and Processing 2004; 43:477-482.
5. Leonard R, Lemlich R. Interstitial liquid flow in foam. I. Theoretical model and application to foam fractionation. II. Experimental verification and observations. AIChE J. 1965; 18-25:25-29.
6. Uraizee F, Narsimhan G. Foam fractionation of proteins and enzymes. II. Performance and modelling. Enzyme and Microbial Technology 1990; 12:315-316.
7. McInerney MJ, Javaheri M, Nagle DP Jr. Properties of the biosurfactant produced by Bacillus licheniformis strain JF-2. J Ind Microbiol. 1990; 5:95-101.
8. Kinnersley HW, Peters RA. The relation of hydrogen ion concentration to the precipitation of purified torulin (yeast vitamin B(1)) by phosphotungstic acid. Biochem J. 1930; 24:1856-1863.
9. Chen C-Y, Baker SC, Darton RC. Batch production of biosurfactant with foam fractionation. J Chem Technol Biotechnol. 2006; 81:1923-1931.
10. Chiocchini C, Linne U, Stachelhaus T. In vivo biocombinatorial synthesis of lipopeptides by COM domain-mediated reprogramming of the surfactin biosynthetic complex. Chem Biol. 2006; 13:899-908.
11. Kim SH, Lim EJ, Lee SO et al. Purification and characterization of biosurfactants from Nocardia sp. L-417. Biotechnol Appl Biochem. 2000; 31:249-253.
12. Drouin CM, Cooper DG. Biosurfactants and aqueous two-phase fermentation. Biotechnol Bioeng. 1992; 40:86-90.
13. Desai JD, Banat IM. Microbial production of surfactants and their commercial potential. Microbiol Mol Biol Rev. 1997; 61:47-64.
14. Chen HL, Juang RS. Recovery and separation of surfactin from pretreated fermentation broths by physical and chemical extraction. Biochem Eng J. 2008; 38:39-46.
15. Kuyukina MS, Ivshina IB, Philp JC et al. Recovery of Rhodococcus biosurfactants using methyl tertia-rybutyl ether extraction. J Microbiol Methods. 2001; 46:149-156.
16. Sen R, Swaminathan T. Characterization of concentration and purification parameters and operating conditions for the small-scale recovery of surfactin. Process Biochemistry 2005; 40:2953-2958.
17. Mulligan CN, Gibbs BF. Recovery of biosurfactants by ultrafiltration. J Chem Technol Biotechnol. 1990; 47:23-29.
18. Hafez M, Isa M, Coraglia DE et al. Recovery and purification of surfactin from fermentation broth by a two-step ultrafiltration process. J Memb Sci. 2007; 296:51-57.
19. Chen HL, Chen YS, Juang RS. Flux decline and membrane cleaning in cross-flow ultrafiltration of treated fermentation broths for surfactinext term recovery. Separation and Purification Technology 2008; 62:47-55.
20. Juang RS, Chen HL, Chen YS. Membrane fouling and resistance analysis in dead-end ultrafiltration of Bacillus subtilis fermentation broths separation and purification technology. In Press doi:10.1016/j.seppur.2008.06.011.
21. Hafez M, Isa M, Frazier RA et al. Recovery and purification of surfactin from fermentation broth by a two-step cross-flow ultrafiltration process Separation and Purification Technology 2008; In Press doi:10.1016/j.seppur.2008.09.008.
22. Cho SK, Shim SH, Park KR et al. Purification and characterization of a biosurfactant produced by Pseudomonas sp. G11 by asymmetrical flow field-flow fractionation (AsFlFFF). Anal Bioanal Chem. 2006; 386:2027-2033.
23. Dimitrov K, Gancel F, Montastruc L et al. Liquid membrane extraction of bio-active amphiphilic substances: Recovery of surfactin. Biochem Eng J. 2008; 42:248-253.
24. Lambert WD, Du L, Ma Y et al. The effect of pH on the foam fractionation of β-glucosidase and cel-lulase. Bioresour Technol. 2003; 87:247-253.
25. Syldatk C, Wagner F. Production of biosurfactants. In: Kosaric N, Cairns WL, Gray NCC eds, Biosurfactants and Biotechnology. New York: Marcel Dekker Inc, 1987:89-120.
26. Reiling HE, Thanei-Wyss U, Guerra-Santos LH et al. Pilot plant production of rhamnolipid biosurfactant by Pseudomonas aeruginosa. Appl Environ Microbiol. 1986; 51:985-989.
27. Cooper DG, MacDonald CR, Duff SJB et al. Enhanced production of surfactin from B. subtilis by continuous product removal and metal cation addition. Appl Environ Microbiol. 1981; 42:408-412.

28. Grieves RB, Wood RK. Continuous foam fractionation: the effect of operating variables on separation. AIChE J. 1964; 10:456-460.
29. Lemlich R. Adsorptive bubble separation methods. Ind Eng Chem Res. 1968; 60:16-29.
30. Scamehorn JF. In: Harwell JH, ed. Surfactant-Based Separation Process, Washington, DC: American Chemical Society, 2000; Chapter 1.
31. Tharapiwattananon N, Scamehorn JF, Osuwan S et al. Surfactant recovery from water using foam fractionation. Separation Science and Technology 1996; 31:1233-1258.
32. Kumpabooth K, Scamehorn JF, Osuwan S et al. Surfactant recovery from water using foam fractionation: Effect of temperature and added salt. Separation Science and Technology 1999; 2:157-72.
33. Davis DA, Lynch HC, Varley J. The application of foaming for the recovery of Surfactin from B. subtilis ATCC 21332 cultures. Enzyme Microb Technol. 2001; 28:346-354.
34. Noah KS, Fox SL, Bruhn DF et al. Development of continuous surfactin production from potato process effluent by Bacillus subtilis in an airlift reactor. Appl Biochem Biotechnol. 2002; 98-100:803-813.
35. Chen C-Y, Baker SC, Darton RC. Continuous production of biosurfactant with foam fractionation. Journal of Chemical Technology and Biotechnology 2006; 81:1915-1922.
36. Noah KS, Bruhn DF, Bala GA. Surfactin production from potato process effluent by Bacillus subtilis in a chemostat. Appl Biochem Biotechnol 2005; 121-124:465-473.
37. Baker SC, Mullins S. Unpublished results Oxford Brookes University, 2008.
38. Gueza JS, Chenikher S, Cassar JP et al. Setting up and modelling of overflowing fed-batch cultures of Bacillus subtilis for the production and continuous removal of lipopeptides. J Biotechnol. 2007; 131:67-75.
39. Glazyrina J, Junne S, Thiesen P et al. In situ removal and purification of biosurfactants by automated surface enrichment. Appl Microbiol Biotechnol. 2008; In Press. doi 10.1007/s00253-008-1620-1.
40. Lunkenheimer K, Wienskol G, Prosser AJ. Automated highperformance purification of surfactant solutions: study of convective-enhanced adsorption. Langmuir 2004; 20:5738-5744.
41. Liu T, Montastruc L, Gancel F et al. Integrated process for production of surfactin: Part 1: Adsorption rate of pure surfactin onto activated carbon. Biochem Eng J. 2007; 35:333-340.
42. Liu T, Montastruc L, Gancel F et al. Integrated process for production of surfactin: Part 2. Equilibrium and kinetic study of surfactin adsorption onto activated carbon. Biochem Eng J. 2008; 38:349-354.
43. Lin SC, Chen YC, Lin YM. General approach for the development of high performance liquid chromatography methods for biosurfactant analysis and purification. J Chromatogr A. 1988; 2:149-59.
44. Schenk T, Schuphan I, Schmidt B. High-performance liquid chromatographic determination of the rhamnolipids produced by pseudomonas aeruginosa. J Chromatogr A. 1995; 693:7-13.
45. Mata-Sandoval JC, Karns J, Torrents A. High-performance liquid chromatography method for the characterization of rhamnolipid mixtures produced by pseudomonas aeruginosa UG2 on corn oil. J Chromatogr A. 1999; 2:211-220.

CHAPTER 22

Production of Surface Active Compounds by Biocatalyst Technology

Smita Sachin Zinjarde* and Mahua Ghosh

Abstract

In the current scenario, there is immense concern regarding the environmental issues. Eco-friendly surfactants are becoming a preferred choice for specific applications in spite of their possibly inferior performance or more expensive nature than conventional ones. This chapter deals with the use of enzymes in non-aqueous media for the synthesis of surfactants such as monoglycerides, sugar fatty acid esters, fatty acid amides, alkyl glycosides and lysophospholipids. The conventional methods of synthesizing these classes of surfactants, the variety of enzymes involved, process parameters, yields, advantages and disadvantages have been discussed in detail.

Introduction

The term surfactant, a surface-active agent, is used rather loosely to designate any substance whose presence in small amount markedly affects the surface behavior of a system. Surfactant molecules have dual nature, a hydrophilic group at one end and a hydrophobic group at the other end; this dual nature is the essential condition for a surface-active agent. These molecules decrease surface tension between the liquid medium and the substrate or interfacial tension between two liquid layers and thereby can act as emulsifying, foaming, defoaming, cleaning, wetting, solubilizing, spreading and dispersing agent.

The 21st century is specially focused on efficient, effective and environmentally friendly surfactants that can deliver high levels of performance in a cost effective manner and on biotechnology. The improvement in technical properties has not been the main reason for this development. The traditional surfactant classes, whether alkyl benzene sulfates, or alcohol ethoxylates, generally perform well, are based on readily available feedstock and have synthesis routes that are under control. Instead, the main driving force behind the development of novel surfactants is the search for products benign to the environment. Today, there are further strong requirements, more than ever, concerning ecological and toxicological aspects. Several of the traditional surfactant types exhibit an insufficient rate of biodegradation and too high aquatic toxicity. With environmental concern becoming a major issue in society, a new "green" surfactant may be preferred choice for a specific application even if it is somewhat inferior in performance or slightly more expensive than the conventional ones. Therefore, identification and characterization of biosurfactants i.e., surfactants directly obtained from microbial origin as well as surfactants produced through biochemical route, have attracted immense research interest. Recent developments in biological services, particularly in molecular biology has a tremendous potential for application. Biosurfactants have become an important product of biotechnology for industrial, cosmetic and medical applications.[17,27]

*Corresponding Author: Smita Sachin Zinjarde—Institute of Bioinformatics and Biotechnology, University of Pune, India. Email: smita@unipune.ernet.in

Biosurfactants, edited by Ramkrishna Sen. ©2010 Landes Bioscience and Springer Science+Business Media.

The term biosurfactant is usually given to a naturally obtained chemical produced by living organism that decreases the surface tension of water. But it could be also given to the surface-active compounds, which are obtained, by involving biocatalyst technology or by bio-catalytic modification of existing surfactants. There is a basic difference between enzymatic and microbial syntheses of surfactants. The former is, essentially, an organic synthesis, where hydrolytic enzymes are used as biological alternatives to conventional catalysts. However, the latter is a biosynthetic process catalyzed by a cascade of enzymes in metabolically active cells.[18]

This chapter will only deal with the biosurfactants, which are produced from various natural compounds through biochemical processes. Hydrolytic enzymes such as lipases and glycosidases, that are available in large quantities and are very robust and inexpensive, can be used for these types of synthesis in non-aqueous media. They also do not require any cofactors to manifest their catalytic activity.[21] Processes like synthesis of monoglycerides, sugar-fatty acid esters, fatty acid amides, lysophospholipids and anomerically pure alkyl glycosides are examples of such biosurfactants.

Biocatalysis

Catalytic synthesis of surfactants, involves the extensive use of lipases. In addition, glucosidases have also been implicated in the synthesis of alkyl glycosides.

Lipases (glycerol ester hydrolases) are enzymes that catalyze the hydrolysis and synthesis of esters of long chain fatty acids and glycerol, triglycerides (Fig. 1).

Triglycerides are insoluble in water and lipases are characterized by the ability to rapidly catalyze the hydrolysis of ester bonds at the interface between the insoluble phase and aqueous phase in which the enzyme is soluble. The ability to catalyze the hydrolysis of insoluble long chain fatty acid esters distinguishes lipases from other esterases that catalyze hydrolysis of soluble esters in preference to insoluble esters. Depending on the positional specificity, lipases may be nonspecific releasing fatty acids from all three positions on the glycerol moiety or may specifically release fatty acids from 1-3 or 1-2 positions.

Lipases are produced by plants, animals and microorganisms. Microbial lipases are cheaper and less subject to batch variation. A reason which may partly account for the trend of lipases being studied extensively is the increased availability of lipases from genetically engineered microbial sources, coupled with their capacity to act as catalysts at the hydrophilic/hydrophobic interface.[32]

Lipases find applications in the following fields:

- In the detergent industry for increasing washing efficiency.
- In the dairy industry they are use in cheese making, in cheese ripening, in taste development and in producing low fat products.
- In the food industry for the production of triglycerides, diglycerides, monoglycerides and free fatty acids.
- In the fine chemical industry as an industrial catalyst.
- For the production of polymers, polyesters, ring opening and polymerization of lactones.

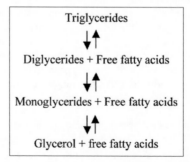

Figure 1. Catalytic activity of lipase displaying hydrolysis and synthesis of triglycerides.

Lipases have conquered a special position in the field of biotechnology since the advent of the enzyme catalyzed reactions in micro aqueous media. The reactions catalyzed by lipases proceed with high regioselectivity and/enantioselectivity making these enzymes as an important group of biocatalysts in organic chemistry.

Their importance is due to the following properties exhibited by them

- Stable in organic solvents.
- Do not require cofactors.
- Have broad substrate specificity.
- Exhibit enantioselectivity.

Several applications of these lipases have been developed for a wide variety of organic synthesis and modification of existing fats and oils. Performing chemical conversions under mild and environmentally benign conditions is currently a topical issue. The ability of enzymes to efficiently catalyze reactions under mild conditions makes them of great interest to the food and chemical industry.[22]

Enzymatic Synthesis of Monoglycerides

Monoacylglycerols (MG) and their numerous derivatives (ethoxylated monoglycerides, acetic, lactic, citric and diacetyl tartaric esters of monoglycerides) are widely used as emulsifiers in the food, cosmetic and pharmaceutical industries. Furthermore, they have generally recognized as safe status, which contributes to their larger applications. Mono- and diglycerides are consumed at an annual level of 85,000,000 kg in the United States, corresponding roughly to 70% of the total emulsifiers used in the food industry. Besides bulk applications in the food and dairy industries, some other applications for special monoacylglycerols have been established in cosmetic and pharmaceutical industries. Recently, the antimicrobial activities of particular types of monoglycerides such as monolaurin, monomyristin, monolinolein and monolinolenin have been reported. It has also been proposed that fatty acids and monoglycerides (lauric acid, monocaprin) may be used as intravaginal microbiocides for protection against sexually transmitted diseases. Moreover, MG of different chain lengths have different properties, e.g., HLB values and therefore possess different biological functions and have various industrial applications.

Normally monoglycerides are produced by alcoholysis of the corresponding triglyceride with two equivalents of glycerol, as is shown in Figure 2.

Monoglycerides are currently produced by the glycerolysis of fats and oils; temperatures of 240-260°C and elevated pressure are required primarily to achieve satisfactory miscibility of the reactants employing inorganic alkaline catalysts.[35] Drawbacks of this process include high-energy consumption and the products are often unusable as obtained, requiring redistillation to remove impurities, degradation products and color. In addition, the highly unsaturated, heat-sensitive oils cannot be processed directly without prior hydrogenation. Thus, energy conservation and minimizing thermal degradation are probably the main advantages of introducing an enzyme-based technology.

Enzymatic glycerolysis of fats and oils has been performed in a nearly stoichiometric solvent-free mixture of substrates at ambient temperatures using a variety of lipases. The equilibrium shift required for the reaction to proceed towards accumulation of the final product was achieved by decreasing the reaction temperature to below the melting point of the

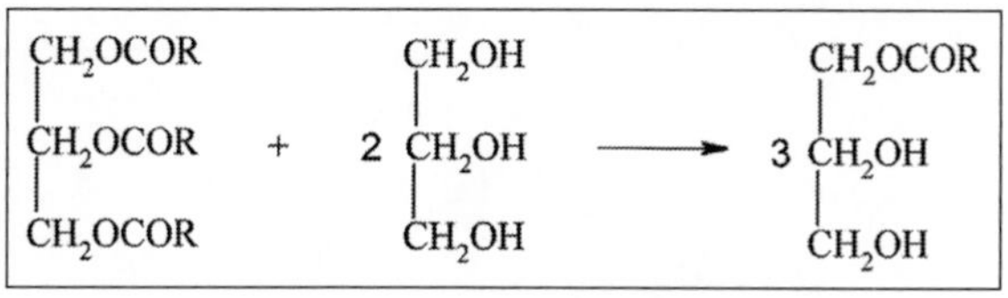

Figure 2. Scheme for the alcoholysis of a triglyceride with glycerol giving 1-monoglyceride (the 2-monoglyceride will also form).

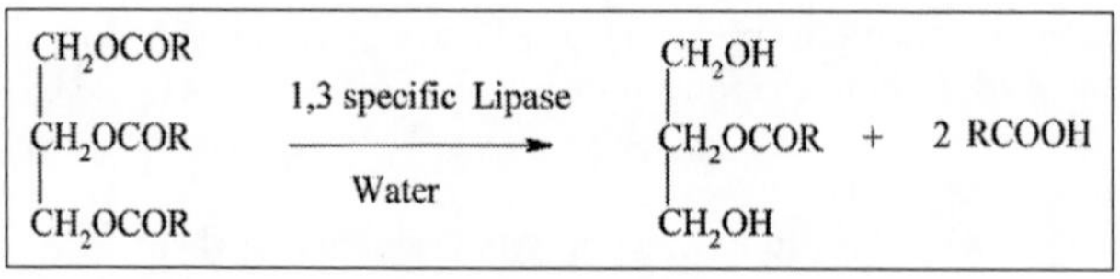

CH$_2$OCOR
|
CH$_2$OCOR   1,3 specific Lipase   CH$_2$OH
| →   CH$_2$OCOR + 2 RCOOH
CH$_2$OCOR   Water   CH$_2$OH

Figure 3. Scheme for the enzymatic hydrolysis of triglyceride to 2-monoglyceride.

monoglycerides. Yields of up to 90% were obtained with a variety of animal and plant lipids, including beef tallow, lard, rapeseed, olive and palm oils.[24,28,46,47,54]

Lipases can be divided into two groups with regard to the regiospecificity exhibited with acylglycerol substrates. Enzymes in the first group show no regiospecificity and catalyze hydrolysis of all ester bonds of the triglyceride and can produce monoglycerides of all variety. Lipases from the second group can release fatty acids regiospecifically from the outer 1- and 3-positions of the glycerol moiety thereby producing 2-mono glycerides only as shown in Figure 3.

The regiospecificity of the enzyme, which normally is almost absolute, results from a poor accessibility of the hindered ester of the secondary alcohol to the active site of the enzyme. However, both 2-monoglycerides and 1,2-diglycerides are chemically unstable species and undergo acyl group migration to give 1-monoglycerides and 1,3-diglycerides, respectively. These, in turn, are good substrates for the regiospecific enzyme and complete hydrolysis to fatty acids and glycerol will eventually take place. It is, therefore, important not to allow the reaction to proceed too long if a specific product is desired, because the rate of acyl group migration is comparable with the rates of di- and monoglyceride hydrolysis.

Monoglycerides have been prepared by enzymatic hydrolysis and alcoholysis of oils catalysed by 1,3-specific lipases. The former method is probably more suitable for the production of mono- and diglyceride mixtures with desirable emulsifying properties. Enzymatic alcoholysis yields very pure monoglyceride products as shown in Figure 4. The alcoholysis of oils, although often carried out in batch, can be run continuously in a packed column reactor to facilitate product separation and recovery.

The production of monoglycerides rich in high-value, polyunsaturated fatty acids are a particularly good example of the successful implementation of enzyme technology. The synthesis of specialty monoglycerides is best achieved by direct condensation of glycerol and a fatty acid. This reaction could be performed continuously in membrane-based hollow-fibre reactor. High conversion was also achieved in batch experiments that were conducted under vacuum to shift the equilibrium towards the final product by evaporation of water produced during the reaction.[25,59]

The lipase-catalyzed production of MG has been shown to be quite successful with long-chain fatty acids. However, it may not be as good as to the synthesis of short-chain MG owing to the relatively high acidity of short chain fatty acids. In that case, *Aspergillus niger* and *Pseudomonas fluorescens* lipase could be used for the alcoholysis of TG with lower alcohols such as ethanol and isopropanol, which could be useful for the production of short-chain MG. The yields of MG are dependent on reaction conditions such as the chain length of TG as well as of the alcohols, the organic solvents and the reaction times.[34,36]

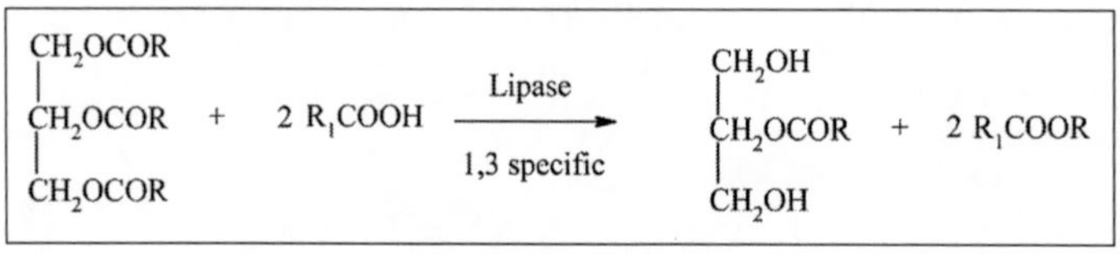

CH$_2$OCOR
|
CH$_2$OCOR + 2 R$_1$COOH   Lipase   CH$_2$OH
| →   CH$_2$OCOR + 2 R$_1$COOR
CH$_2$OCOR   1,3 specific   CH$_2$OH

Figure 4. Scheme for the enzymatic alcoholysis of triglyceride to 2-monoglyceride.

Synthesis of Sugar Esters

Surfactant biodegradability is a crucial factor in determining whether their concentrations in the environment remain below detrimental levels. Surfactants derived from sugar fatty acid esters are attractive because of their ready biodegradability, low toxicity, low irritation to eyes and skin and the renewable nature of the starting materials and novel applications.[29] Sugar fatty acid esters are used as industrial detergents and food emulsifiers in numerous products and processes. They are widely used in food, cosmetic and pharmaceutical formulations. Physicochemical properties of these surfactants can be tailored to suit potential applications by varying the sugar head group size and the length and number of alkyl chains. In addition to the synthesis of non-ionic surfactants, analogous anionic sugar ester surfactants can be produced by incorporation of a sulfonate group. These anionic sugar esters are more water-soluble than their non-ionic counterparts and may more easily replace conventional anionic surfactants in product formulations.[6]

Structural variations of sugar ester surfactants have immense effect on the physicochemical properties, e.g., sucrose fatty acid esters (Fig. 5) are rapidly biodegradable than others.

The presence of side groups on the alkyl chain adjacent to the ester bond has a significant effect on biodegradability. These groups decrease the rate and extent of biodegradation of the sugar esters. This effect is greatest in the presence of an α-sulfonyl group. When α-ethyl or α-methyl groups are attached, the inhibitory effect is weaker, but nonetheless significant. Further studies indicated that these structural changes affect biodegradability of this class of surfactants through their effects on the pathways followed during biodegradation. The biodegradation rate of sulfonated sugar esters is similar to that of the soft anionic standard, linear alkyl benzene sulfonate. Biodegradation of these surfactants is sufficiently rapid and complete to classify them as readily biodegradable, but they do not have the advantage of the very rapid biodegradability as displayed by unsulfonated sugar esters.[50]

Sucrose esters obtained from plants are composed of the lower fatty acids (C_6-C_{12}) and possess very interesting biological properties. The potent insecticidal activities of natural sucrose esters against the persistent and damaging whiteflies have shown that sucrose esters are a new class of "natural" insecticides that should be exploited for commercial use. It was found that C_6-C_{12} sucrose esters had the biological properties and sucrose octanoate the highest insecticidal activity of this group.

Sugar esters have certain advantages over synthetic surfactants as follows:

- Prepared from renewable sources.
- Being tasteless, odorless, stable over a broad pH range and nontoxic, they are the best-suited emulsifiers for foods.
- Being non-irritant to the eyes skin, they are suitable for pharmaceuticals and cosmetics industry.
- Because of the excellent biodegradability, they do not cause environmental pollution.
- Sugar esters offer a full range of HLB values from 1-16 and display good surfactant functionality.

Traditionally, sugar esters are prepared by esterification at 180-260°C in a solvent free mixture of fatty acids and molten sugar molecules. Under these conditions, sugar undergoes rapid dehy-

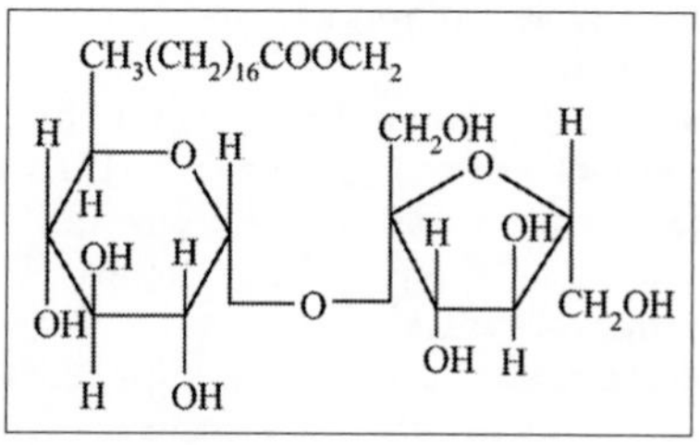

Figure 5. Chemical structure of sucrose monostearate.

dration to yield various regioisomers. To minimize the formation of side products and to prevent browning of sugar it is preferred to do the esterification reaction at a lower temperature. It is also preferred to avoid longer reaction time and harder vacuum, which usually yield more undesirable isomers. Furthermore, a multitude of similar structures is obtained owing to the presence of numerous hydroxyl groups in carbohydrate substrates. Thus, analysis of food-grade sorbitan esters (e.g., SPAN-20) by gas chromatography, showed the presence of at least 65 individual compounds many of which were identified as various isomers of sorbitan, isosorbide and their mono-, di- and tri-esters. There is increasing concern over the allergenicity and carcinogenicity of some of these by-products.[11]

In the current scenario, the enzymatic esterification of sugar ester is gaining importance due to mild reaction conditions and excellent selectivity associated with lipase-catalyzed reactions. They permit the generation of pure materials by more efficient and environmentally friendly processes. Moreover, the enzymatic process can be applied to the regioselective transformations of mono- and disaccharides and does not result in any undue complications. In the enzymatic processes to synthesize sugar esters, several factors can affect both the conversion yield and the rate of glycosylation. These factors include the reaction solvent, reaction temperature, the type and concentration of the acyl donor, enzyme content and initial substrate concentration.[60]

In general, two main approaches have been explored for the lipase-catalyzed preparation of sugar fatty acid esters. The syntheses have been performed either by employing lipases in an organic solvent suitable for solubilization of both substrates or by conducting the reaction in a solvent-free mixture of substrates using sugars that have been modified to improve the miscibility of reactants. The use of highly polar solvents (e.g., dimethyl formamide [DMF], pyridine) is considered to be practically more facile, but the enzyme stability and reaction rates are poor, thus hindering applications on a preparative scale. However, prior acetalization of sugars improves their solubility in or miscibility with molten fatty acids, thus avoiding the use of highly polar solvents in the reaction medium. These solvent-free mixtures allow much higher conversions in a shorter time, even when the reaction is performed in a nearly equimolar mixture of substrates and the high operational stability of the enzyme under these conditions facilitate biocatalyst recycling.[37,49,51,55]

The enzymatic synthesis of sugar esters yields up to 80% conversion within 8 h of incubation and the resulting product contains only 20% of unreacted sugar. The synthesis can be performed in a batch reactor at a temperature as low as 64°C in presence of microbial lipase like *Candida antartica*.

The rate of enzymatic esterification was markedly dependent on the length of the alkyl group. Thus, a yield of only 20% was obtained with glucose and methyl glucoside after 1 and 21 days of incubation, respectively. However, when ethyl-, N- and iso-propyl or butyl-glucosides were used, the reaction was complete in a few hours. Alternatively, sugar acetals have been used as starting materials to facilitate miscibility of the reactants. The final products, mono- and disaccharide fatty acid esters, were obtained in good yields after lipase-catalysed, solvent-free esterification followed by mild acid hydrolysis of the corresponding sugar acetal esters. Although large-scale acetalization and subsequent deprotection do not present serious technological difficulties, the overall production sequence would be somewhat complicated. It remains to be seen, therefore, whether the expected improved quality and superior emulsifying properties of the products will justify these additional steps. At the same time, this methodology provides an efficient route for the synthesis of a variety of (oligo)saccharide fatty acid esters.

It should be noted that the use of isopropylidene groups in these syntheses was designed to improve the miscibility of the reactants and must be distinguished from the conventional protecting strategy employed in regioselective organic synthesis. For example, 6′-0-acyl-lactose was obtained as the sole product after the hydrolysis of isopropylidene groups, even when a crude mixture of partial lactose acetals was enzymatically esterified.

These carbohydrate surfactants made of a hydrophilic sugar head group and a lipophilic fatty acid chain constitute a novel family of non-ionic surfactants that can be used as detergents for washing purposes, as emulsifiers in food products and as active ingredients in personal care products such as shampoos creams and soaps.

Synthesis of Fatty Acid Amides

Fatty acid amides are another class of amphipathic compounds that contain an amino group linked to the hydroxyl portion of the carboxyl group with a general formula of $RCONH_2$. The fatty acid amides thus have a lipophilic hydrocarbon chain derived from a fatty acid that may be straight chain or branched chain. The hydrophilic part of the molecule is based on the amino group. The structure of a typical fatty acid amide is

$$R-CO-NH-CH_2-CH_2-OH$$

Fatty acid amides are conventionally synthesized by reacting a fatty acid or fatty methyl ester with an alkanolamine at 180°C.[15] Alternatively, they are produced by reacting fatty acids with ammonia at high temperature and pressure.

$$150°C \text{ for } 6\text{-}12 \text{ h}$$

$$RCOOH + H_2N-CH_2-CH_2-OH \rightarrow R-CO-NH-CH_2-CH_2-OH$$

Fatty acid amides are economically important and developing novel methods for their synthesis has been an area of extensive research. Biocatalysis has been used as an alternative to the use of traditional methods in the synthesis of fatty acid amides. Enzymes bring about effective and specific catalytic reactions under mild reaction conditions. They have minimal energy requirements and have lesser problems associated with by-product formation. Moreover, the use of enzymes in the synthesis of fatty acid amides is an environmentally benign method. The enzymes that bring about the synthesis are lipases.

Lipases have been used extensively for the synthesis of fatty acid amides. There are several reports on the application of these enzymes as cited below. A majority of the reports have used lipases from the yeast *Candida antarctica*. For example there is an efficient enzymatic procedure for the synthesis of the fatty acid amide, octanamide.[13] The enzyme used in the study was the Lipase SP525 from *C. antarctica* B immobilized on Accurel EP100 using n-butanol in tertiary amyl alcohol as the organic solvent system. The resulting octanamide was isolated in 93% yield. During the synthesis of oleamide, another fatty acid amide, a yield of 90% has been obtained. *C. antarctica* lipase B has also been used as a biocatalyst for the direct amidation of butyric acid 4-methyloctanoic acid with ammonia in organic solvents.[41] The enzymatic amidation reaction proceeded efficiently for various carboxylic acids. There was a very enantioselective amidation of 4-methyloctanoic acid. The enantiomeric excess of the remaining (S)-4-methyloctanoic acid was 95%. An economically viable process using a continuous plug flow reactor has been developed for the synthesis of oleamide using the same lipase from *C. antarctica*, lipase B and 2-methyl-2-butanol as solvent with a yield of 85%.[56] Novozym 435 lipase from *C. antartica* has also been employed as a biocatalyst in the selective preparation of amides from diethanolamine using the direct acylation and transacylation reactions.[16] The choice of the solvents was important and n-hexane, favored the reaction for the formation of the amide by direct acylation. Dioxane, on the other hand, favored the O-acylation reaction. At 60°C, the transacylation route produced both higher conversions (71-77 mol%) and greater selectivities to the amide (74-94%) than the direct acylation reaction (69-74 mol% conversion and 76-86% selectivity).

Selective synthesis of the secondary amide surfactant N-methyl lauroylethanolamide from methyl laurate and N-methylethanol amine using another enzyme Chirazyme L-2 from *C. antarctica* that was carrier-fixed has also been described.[53] In acetonitrile, at 50°C for 16 h the presence of 50 mM of the ester and 150 mM of the amine, a high yield (97.3%) was obtained. With another reaction mixture under a different set of conditions (50 mM ester and 200 mM amine; 60°C for 5 h), a yield of 95.8% was obtained. Lipase B from *C. antarctica* has also been used to catalyze the amidation of the hydroxy fatty acids, ricinoleic acid (RA) and lesquerolic acid (LQA) as well as multihydroxy fatty acids, 7,10-dihydroxy-8(E)-octadecenoic acid (DOD) and 7,10,12-trihydroxy-8(E)-octadecenoic acid (TOD).[38] The optimum temperature for such reactions was 55°C. Transformation percentage at 7 days was better than 95% for all substrates except TOD (93.9%). In another recent report the ammonolysis of erucic acid to erucamide has been described using the lipase Novozym 435 from *C. antartica*.[4] Other optimal conditions for fatty amides synthesis were an incubation period of 48 h shaker speed of 250 rpm, an incubation temperature of 60°C. A molar ratio of erucic acid and urea (1:4) and tert-butyl alcohol (2-methyl-2-propanol) were most suited for the synthetic reaction. In yet another report, lauric acid and monoethanolamine were reacted at 90°C with a lipase from *Candida antarctica* immobilised on a polymeric resin. After 4 h, with the slow addition of the amine and the removal of the water that was formed, high yields were obtained (>90%). The enzyme preparation showed a half-life of 14 days.[57]

Lipase preparations from *Candida rugosa*, *Rhizomucor miehei* and porcine pancreas are other enzymes reported to facilitate the formation of fatty amides at 20°C in hexane. The reactants used were various primary alkylamines and fatty acid methyl esters or triglycerides. Moderate yields of fatty amides were obtained using immobilized *R. miehei* lipase preparation. The lipase preparations tested displayed catalytic activities under these conditions and showed a difference in selectivity for fatty acid and alkylamine chain lengths.[8] Chiral amides have been synthesized from (±)-2-chloropropionate esters and a wide range of amines using a lipase from *Candida cylindracea*. The transamidation reaction was reported to be most effective when N-(trifluoroethyl)-2-chloropropionamide was used as the substrate. Another set of enzymes (Lipozyme and Novozym) has been used to synthesize fatty acid amide surfactants.[45] The amino—sugar derivatives and fatty acids were incubated with lipases in the presence of different organic solvents. Reactions were catalyzed with Lipozyme in hexane or with Novozym in 2-methyl-2-butanol as solvents. 2-methyl-2-butanol was found to be a better solvent that allowed a conversion fatty acid up to 100% when water was removed under reduced pressure.

Although enzymes are important as biocatalysts, processes using microorganisms as catalysts are also suggested as attractive alternatives to chemical synthesis. Microbial transformations producing fatty amides using *Bacillus cereus* are reported.[43] For example *Bacillus cereus* 50 is reported to bring about transformation of 12-hydroxyoctadecanoic acid to 12-hydroxyoctadecanamide when cultivated aerobically in 1% yeast extract medium at 30°C, shaken at 250 rpm for 2 to 5 days. The yields of 12-hydroxyoctadecanamide were reported to be 9.1 and 21.5% after 2 and 5d, respectively.[26] Another isolate of *B. cereus*, Tim-r01 has also been reported to transform the polyaromatic carboxylic acids such as 4-biphenylcarboxylic acid, 4-biphenylacetic acid and 4-phenoxybenzoic acid into corresponding amides. The activity was observed at 37°C (pH 7-8) in the presence of grown cells in nutrients under an aerobic atmosphere.

Alkyl amides display high surface activities and are used as fiber lubricants, detergents, flotation agents, textile softeners, antistatic agents, wax additives and plasticizers.

Enzymatic Synthesis of Alkyl Glycosides

Alkyl glycosides are amphipathic compounds containing a glycosyl moiety (one or several units) linked to the hydroxyl group of a fatty alcohol. The alkyl glycoside structure thus has a hydrophobic (or lipophilic) hydrocarbon chain derived from an alcohol that may be straight chain, branched-chain or phenolic in nature. The hydrophilic part of the molecule is based on glycosides or poly glycosides. The structures of typical alkyl glycoside and alkyl polyglycosides are shown in Figure 6.

Alkyl glycosides are obtained by the condensation of glycosides with a fatty alcohol. During the chemical synthesis of alkyl glycosides such as ethyl glucoside, glucose and anhydrous ethanol are allowed to react in the presence of hydrochloric acid as catalyst. Alkyl glucosides with long alkyl chain (octyl to hexadecyl) have also been synthesized and their surfactant properties have been evaluated. A representative reaction involving the synthesis of alkyl glucosides is shown in Figure 7.

Chemical synthesis reactions have disadvantages and the use of enzymes as alternative sources for such synthetic reactions has been a topic of great interest. The enzymes involved in the synthesis of alkyl glycosides are glucosidases.

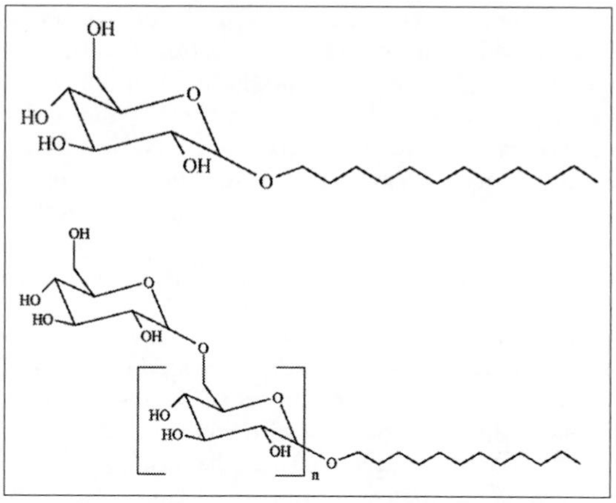

Figure 6. Structures of typical alkyl glycoside and alkyl polyglycosides.

Glucosidases are glycoside hydrolase enzymes categorized under the EC number 3.2.1. The discovery that these enzymes can be active in organic media has greatly expanded their use in synthetic reactions. The nature of the solvents used in such reactions greatly influences enzyme selectivity.[9] Enzymes have a twofold advantage as catalysts for the synthesis of alkyl glycosides. A large number of inexpensive glucosidases are commercially available and they provide stereochemical control at the anomeric center of the newly synthesized glycosydic bond. Consequently, the synthetic potential of glucosidases has been extensively explored. Glucosidases can be used as synthetic catalysts to form glycosidic bonds using two approaches (i) Through reverse hydrolysis where the equilibrium position is reversed. (ii) By transglycosylation whereby retaining glycoside hydrolases can catalyze the transfer of a glycosyl moiety from an activated glycoside to an acceptor alcohol to afford a new glycoside. Several glucosidases derived from plants, fungi and bacteria have been employed for the synthesis of alkyl glycosides. Some representative examples on such studies are as follows:

Yeast and Fungal Glucosidases

α and β-glucosidases from *Saccharomyces cerevisiae* have been applied for the O-glycosylation of different alcohols.[33] The low yields obtained with the native glucosidases were overcome by immobilization of the enzymes on a modified polyacrylamide-type bead support (Acrylex C-100). This increased enzyme stability and resulted in higher yields. The regioselective synthesis of 6-O-phenylbutyryl-1-n-butyl—D-glucopyranose using glucosidase derived from almond and the lipase B obtained from *Candida antarctica* has been described.[48] A yield of 21% yield was obtained when the glucosidase reaction was performed in a biphasic (buffer/n-alcohol) system.

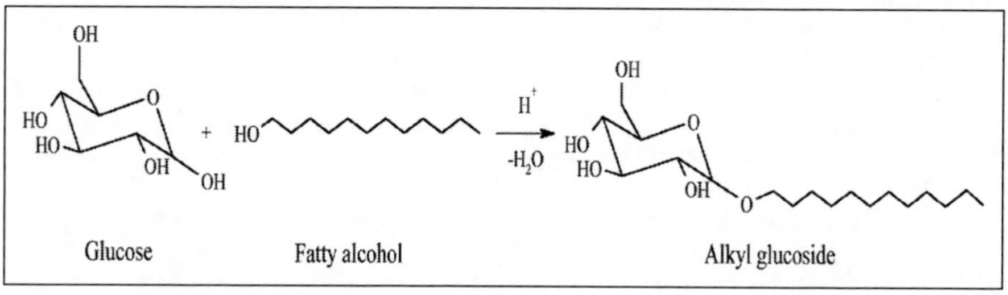

Figure 7. Scheme for the synthesis of alkyl glucoside.

Beta-glucosidase II (BglII) from *Pichia etchellsii* expressed in recombinant *Escherichia coli* has been utilized for synthesis of alkyl glucosides with chain lengths from 6 to 10 carbons as well as for the synthesis of monoterpenyl (nerol, geraniol, citronellol) glucosides.[5] The β-glucosidase from *Fusarium oxysporum* has been employed to catalyze the production of alkyl-β-glucosides from disaccharides, based on the transglucosylation reaction. Although, primary, secondary and tertiary alcohols were as used as glucosyl acceptors, primary alcohols were found to be the best acceptors. The enzyme did not exhibit regiospecificity and was fairly unspecific towards the aglucone part.[42] Enzymatic synthesis of alkyl-D-xylosides by transxylosylation and reverse hydrolysis using the *Trichoderma reesei* xylosidase (EC 3.2.1.37) with primary, secondary and tertiary alcohols as acceptors has been reported.[14]

Plant Derived Glucosidases

There is a report on the synthesis of alkyl glucosides using the β-glucosidase from Thai rosewood (*Dalbergia cochinchinensis Pierre*).[40] The enzyme brought about the catalytic transglucosylation of alcohols to alkyl glucosides. The yields were best with primary alcohols, often approaching 90% in terms of alkyl glucoside. Secondary alcohols on the other hand, gave poorer yields and tertiary alcohols did not react at all. When compared to almond β-glucosidase, the Thai Rosewood glucosidase showed higher transglucosylation yields. The β-glucosidase from apple seed has also been used for the synthesis of O-glucosides synthesis by reverse hydrolysis.[61]

Glucosidases Derived from Bacteria

A novel thermostable beta-glucosidase obtained from *Thermotoga neapolitana* (TnBgl3B) is reported to be an efficient catalyst in alkyl-glucoside forming reactions using transglycosylation with hexanol or octanol as the acceptor molecule. The optimal reaction conditions for the synthesis of the alkyl glycoside, hexyl glucoside from p-nitrophenyl-beta-glucopyranoside were a water/hexanol two-phase system containing 16% (v/v) water, pH 5.8 and a temperature of 60°C.[58] There is another report on the direct coupling of hexanol to glucose by a β-glucosidase derived from the hyperthermophile, *Pyrococcus furiosus*.[44]

Alkyl glucosides are highly effective surfactants in washing and cleansing agents. They are also widely used in the cosmetic products sector, as auxiliaries in crop protection formulations and as surfactants in industrial cleansing agents and today can already be said to be the most important sugar surfactants based on the yearly production amounts.

Enzymatic Synthesis of Phospholipids

Processed phospholipids or 'special lecithin' are used in the manufacturing of paints, leather and numerous foods such as bakery goods, chocolates, margarines, etc. Derivatised phospholipids also have specific applications in pharmaceutical and personal care products. Although several chemical and physical modifications of lecithin have been adopted by industry, there is a clear scope for the application of enzymes to the transformation of phospholipids (PLs) due to the requirement for control over the regioselectivity and/or the degree of modification necessary for obtaining a product with the desired functional properties. Compared to chemical methods, enzymatic modification of PLs has a few advantages.

Selectivity or specificity of enzymes is one of the most important properties of enzymes that make the modification of PLs simple and easy, unlike chemical methods. Enzymatic reactions are often conducted under mild conditions, which help to retain the original properties of those heat- or oxygen-sensitive PLs. The biocatalytic approach greatly reduces the use of toxic and deleterious solvents, which not only simplifies the complicated purification steps and decreases the solvent residue in final products, but also provides a safer alternative for the modified PLs for foods, cosmetics and pharmaceuticals.[2]

The first group of enzymes that could be used for the modification/synthesis of PLs is phospholipases. Phospholipases play crucial roles in cellular regulation, metabolism and biosynthesis of PLs. To act on variable PLs and to serve different functions, phospholipases form a large class of enzymes with wide diversity. The enzymes involved in bond cleavage of ester or ether glycerophospholipids as well as sphingophospholipids and their function sites are Phospholipase A1 (phosphatidylcholine 1-acylhydrolase, PLA1) and A2 (phosphatidylcholine 2-acylhydrolase, PLA2) that belong to acyl hydrolase, which specifically hydrolyze 1- and 2-acyl ester bond of phospholipids, respectively. The phospholipase that can hydrolyze both positional acyl ester bonds is called phospholipase B. Lysophospholipase refers to the enzyme preferable to catalyze monoacylphospholipids to glycerol phospholipids.

Phospholipase C (phosphatidylcholine cholinephosphohydrolase) and D (phosphatidylcholine phosphatidohydrolase,) show similar activity to phosphodiesterases to cleave the phosphorus—oxygen bond between glycerol and phosphate and phosphate and head-group, respectively. Interestingly, phospholipase C can also hydrolyze phosphate ester in sphingomyelin and ether phospholipids at the similar sites. At the same time, phospholipase A2 and lysophospholipase show hydrolytic activity on the acyl ester bond of ether phospholipids.

Besides phospholipases, there are many other enzymes that can be used for the modification of phospholipids. One of the big groups of such enzymes is lipase. Lipases are frequently used for PL modification, which work for the modification of acyl groups in PLs.

Enzymatic Production of Lysophospholipids

Lysophospholipids (lyso-PLs) are the partially hydrolyzed PLs containing fatty acids in only one position. Hydrolysis of PLs with PLA2 yields sn-2 lyso-PLs and hydrolysis with PLA1 or sn-1,3 specific lipases yields sn-1 lyso-PLs. Apart from hydrolysis, other alternative methods include alcoholysis, esterification of glycerophosphorylcholine and thermodynamic transacylation of 2-acyllysophospholipids to 1-acyllysophospholipids. Enzyme-catalyzed production of lyso-PLs has been already implemented in industry. An example of industrial applications of enzyme-catalyzed hydrolysis of lecithin is the egg yolk treatment. With PLA1 or PLA2 treatment, the emulsification properties, heat stability and viscosity of egg yolk products were improved and fortified due to the formation of lyso-PLs, which enhance their applicability, especially in hot food applications. Another process in which enzymatic hydrolysis of PLs to lyso-PLs can be applied is in the oil-degumming step in refining of vegetable oils.[7,12]

Enzyme species, composition of reaction systems, substrate concentration and water activity (aw) were found to play profound roles in the hydrolysis of PLs. Due to the commercial unavailability and thermal instability of PLA1 until recently, lipases and PLA2 had been the often-used biocatalyst for the hydrolysis of PLs (Fig. 8). Amongst the lipases, *Mucor* and *Rhizopus* are found to be the most efficient species.[31,51,52] Up to 80% purity of sn-1 lyso-PC was obtained using Lipozyme IM20 (RML) in water-saturated hexane.[23,30] Solvent polarity had a profound effect on the degree of hydrolysis. Increasing water content stimulated enzyme activity in solvents more polar than hexane; while in less polar solvents, water inhibited activity. Enzymatic alcoholysis of PLs also produce lyso-PLs and along with fatty acid esters.[19,20] The starting alcohol can be glycerol, methanol, or ethanol for example. In general, the reaction rate could be significantly enhanced by the addition of small amounts of water to the reaction mixture. Immobilized RMIM is the best suitable enzyme for this reaction as RMIM had little selectivity with respect to fatty alcohol chain lengths.

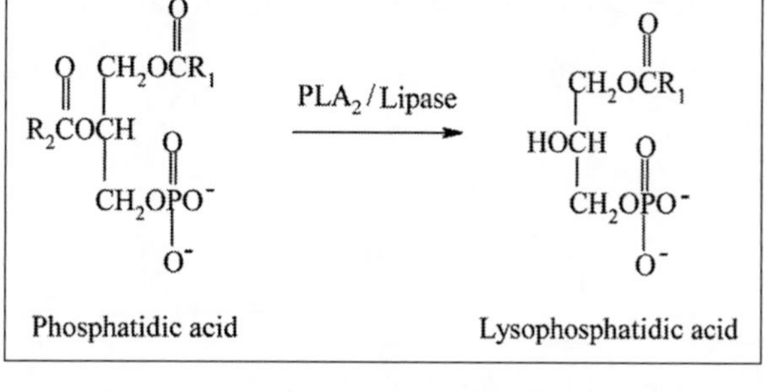

Figure 8. Enzymatic synthesis of lysophosphatidic acid from phosphatidic acid.

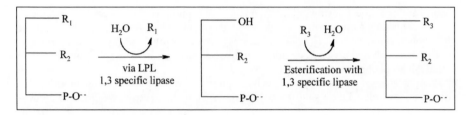

Figure 9. Two step modification of PL by hydrolysis and re-esterification with desired acyl group.

Enzymatic Production of Modified or Structured Phospholipids

Sometimes fatty acid profile of the phospholipid is altered to have some distinct surface properties. Enzymatic modification of PLs is again based on the selective/positional recognition of phospholipase A1, A2 and 1,3-specific lipases. There are two general reaction routes for the modification. The first route is carried out in two steps, i.e., hydrolysis and re-esterification with the acyl group to be incorporated (Fig. 9).

The other route is conducted in one step, i.e., interesterification between PLs and fatty acids or their esters (Fig. 10).

Interesterification reaction is normally simple and easily performed, but the hydrolysis-esterification combination can give products of higher purity. Thus, one can select a proper route according to the requirement of the desired products. Several parameters are considered to be important to influence the esterification and transesterification reactions between acyl donors and PLs. Among them water activity and reaction system design should be paid particular attention.[1,10]

Enzymes phospholipase A1 and A2 or lipases can be used. Increasing enzyme dosage results in higher incorporation but this increase of enzyme may also lead to enhanced hydrolysis. Enzyme can have different reactivity on PLs with different head-groups.[3]

A certain dynamic water environment should be maintained in order to have high enzyme activity. Reaction time to reach equilibrium increases with decreasing water activity. Yield increases when water activity is low. The possibility of using low water activity depends on individual enzymes. For most enzymes the catalytic activity increases with increasing water activity. However many lipases are active at low water activity and this makes it possible to obtain high yields. Water activity influences the molecular organization of phospholipid substrate. The packing density of PL molecules increases with decreasing water activity.

By using a large excess of free fatty acids, hydrolysis reaction is inhibited. Usually it is not a problem to use a high concentration of acyl donors although a slight decrease in reaction rate has been observed for very high concentrations. Generally free fatty acids are more efficient acyl donors than their esters. Reactivity relates to chain length and degree of saturation.

Solvent is not necessarily needed; however, solvent medium reduces viscosity of the substrates and as a consequence the reaction rate is increased through mass transfer increase of substrates. Reaction is solvent type dependent, the rate being inversely proportional to solvent polarity. Polar

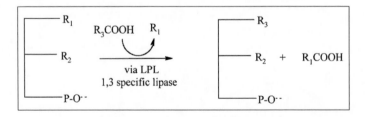

Figure 10. One step modification of PL by intersterification with a desired fatty acid.

solvents compete with enzyme on available water that is required for three-dimensional structure of the enzyme. Such solvents must be avoided as they may disrupt the enzyme activity. The solubility of the substrate depends on solvent types.

The longer the reaction time the higher the incorporation of acyl donors into phospholipids can be expected. Long reaction time however may also result in increased acyl migration.

Optimal temperature changes with enzyme source and type. Increased temperature may result in higher acyl migration. Higher temperature lowers viscosity of reaction medium. Enzyme stability has reverse relationship with temperature.

Most studies on modification of PLs to have better surface properties have been done in laboratory-scale experiments. Only a few process studies have been conducted in order to produce a product. Little effort has been made to upscale the enzymatic modifications of PLs to a practically larger scale. However, results from small-scale operations provide information for the scale-up evaluation and background for the feasibility survey of using enzymes to modify PLs. To make the production of structured PLs feasible, it is essential to develop effective bioreactors and processes.[62]

Conclusion

From the foregoing discussion, it is evident that a variety of novel surfactants benign to the environment can be enzymatically synthesized. Enzymatic approaches lead to processes and products that are less toxic and thus ecologically friendly. Many of the surfactants thus synthesized exhibit properties that make them novel. With environment becoming a major concern, enzymatic synthesis of surfactants provide a "green technology" for the synthesis of "green molecules".

References

1. Adlercreutz D, Budde H, Wehtje E. Synthesis of phosphatidylcholine with defined fatty acid in the sn-1 position by lipase-catalyzed esterification and transesterification reaction. Biotechnol Bioeng 2002; 78:403-11.
2. Adlercreutz P, Virto C, Persson M et al. Enzymatic conversion of polar lipids: principles, problems and solutions. J Mol Catal, B Enzym 1995; 1:173-178.
3. Aura AM, Forssell P, Mustranta A et al. Transesterification of soy lecithin by lipase and phospholipase. J Am Oil Chem Soc 1995; 72:1375-1379.
4. Awasthi NP, Singh RP. Lipase-catalyzed synthesis of fatty acid amide (erucamide) using fatty acid and urea. J Oleo Sci 2007; 56:507-509.
5. Bachhawat P, Mishra S, Bhatia Y et al. Enzymatic synthesis of oligosaccharides, alkyl and terpenyl glucosides, by recombinant Escherichia coli-expressed Pichia etchellsii beta-glucosidase II. Appl Biochem Biotechnol 2004; 118:269-282.
6. Baker IJA, Matthews B, Suares H et al. Sugar ester surfactants: structure and biodegradability. J Surfactants Detergents 2000; 3:29-32.
7. Betzing H. Process for the preparation of a new lysolecithin mixture. 1971; US Patent 3592829.
8. Bistline RG, Bilyk A, Feairheller SH. Lipase catalyzed formation of fatty amides. J Am Oil Chem Soc 1991; 68:95-98.
9. Carrea G, Ottolina G, Riva S. Role of solvents in the control of enzyme selectivity in organic media. Trends Biotechnol 1995; 13:63-70.
10. Chmiel O, Melachouris N, Tritler H. Process for the interesterification of phospholipids. 1999; US Patent 5989599.
11. Chunli G, Whitcombe MJ, Vulfson EN. Enzymatic synthesis of dimeric and trimeric sugar-fatty acid esters. Enzyme Microbial Technol 1999; 25:264-270.
12. Clausen K. Enzymatic oil-degumming by novel microbial phospholipase. Eur J Lipid Sci Technol 2001; 103:333-340.
13. de Zoete MC, Kock-van Dalen AC, van Rantwijk F et al. A new enzymatic one-pot procedure for the synthesis of carboxylic amides from carboxylic acids. J Mol Catal B: Enzymatic 1996; 2:19-25.
14. Drouet P, Zhang M, Legoy MD. Enzymatic synthesis of alkyl-D-xylosides by transxylosylation and reverse hydrolysis. Biotechnol Bioengg 2004; 43:1075-1080.
15. Feairheller SH, Bistline RG, Bilyk A et al. A novel technique for the preparation of secondary fatty amides III. Alkanolamides, diamides and aralkylamides. J Am Oil Chem Soc 1994; 71:863-866.
16. Fernandez-Perez M, Otero C. Selective enzymatic synthesis of amide surfactants from diethanolamine. Enzyme Microbial Technol 2003; 33:650-660.

17. Fiechter A. Biosurfactants: moving towards industrial application. Trends Biotethnol 1992; 10:208-217.
18. Georgiou G, Lin S, Sharma MM. Surface-active compounds from microorganisms. Biotechnol 1992; 10:60-65.
19. Ghosh M, Bhattacharyya DK. Enzymatic alcoholysis reaction of soy phospholipids. J Am Oil Chem Soc 1997; 74:597-599.
20. Ghosh M, Bhattacharyya DK. Lipase-catalyzed glycerolysis reaction of soyphospholipids. J Oil Technol Assoc. India 1995; 27:175-177.
21. Gill I, Vulfson EN. Enzymic catalysis in heterogeneous eutectic mixtures of substrates. Trends Biotechnol 1994; 12:118-122.
22. Greek BF. Sales of detergents growing despite recession. Chem Eng News 1991; 69:25-52.
23. Haas MJ, Cichowicz DJ, Phillips J et al. The hydrolysis of phosphatidylcholine by immobilized lipase: optimization of hydrolysis in organic solvents. J Am Oil Chem Soc 1993; 70:111-117.
24. Holmberg K, Osterberg E. Enzymatic preparation of monoglycerides in microemulsion. J Am Oil Chem Soc 1988; 9:1544-1548.
25. Hoq MM, Yamane T, Shimizu S et al. Continuous synthesis of glycerides by lipase in a microporous membrane bioreactor. J Am Oil Chem Soc 1984; 61:776-781.
26. Huang JK, Keudell KC, Klopfenstein WE et al. Biotransformation of 12-hydroxyoctadecanoic acid to 12-hydroxyoctadecanamide by Bacillus cereus 50. J Am Oil Chem Soc 1997; 74:601-603.
27. Jackson MA, Morton IL. Commercially viable process for high purity of fatty alcohol C to C and its cosmetic application for skin hair and nails; US Patent 1998; 5747305.
28. Kamalngdee N, Yamane T. Monoglyceride formation of fat by immobilized lipases. J Sci Technol 1996; 18:363-370.
29. Kelkar DS, Kumar AR, Zinjarde SS. Hydrocarbon emulsification and enhanced crude oil degradation by lauroyl glucose ester. Bioresour Technol 2007; 98:1505-1508.
30. Kim J, Kim BG. Lipase-catalyzed synthesis of lyosphatidylcholine using organic cosolvent for in situ water activity control. J Am Oil Chem Soc 2001; 77:791-797.
31. Kim J, Kim BG. Lipase-catalyzed synthesis of lysophatidylcholine. Ann NY Acad Sci 1998; 864:341-344.
32. Klibanov AM. Enzymatic catalysis in anhydrous organic solvents. Trends Biochem Sci 1989; 14:141-144.
33. Kosáry J, Stefanovits-Bányai E, Boross L. Reverse hydrolytic process for O-alkylation of glucose catalysed by immobilized α- and β-glucosidases. J Biotechnol 1998; 66:83-86.
34. Langone MAP, De Abreu ME, Rezende MJC et al. Enzymatic synthesis of medium chain monoglycerides in a solvent-free system. Appl Biochem Biotechnol 2002; 98-100:988-1003.
35. Lauridsen JR. A continuous process for the glycerolysis of soybean oil. J Am Oil Chem Soc 1976; 53:400-407.
36. Lee GC, Lin WD, Yi-Fang H et al. Lipase-catalyzed alcoholysis of triglycerides for short-chain mono-glyceride production. J Am Oil Chem Soc 2004; 81:533-536.
37. Lee SH, Ha SH, Dang DT et al. Lipase-catalyzed synthesis of fatty acid sugar ester using supersaturated sugar solution in ionic liquids. J Biotechnol 2007; 131:S88.
38. Levinson WE, Kuo TM, Kurtzman CP. Lipase-catalyzed production of novel hydroxylated fatty amides in organic solvent. Enzyme and Microbial Technol 2005; 37:126-130.
39. Linqiu C, Andreas F, Uwe TB et al. Lipase-catalyzed solid phase synthesis of sugar fatty acid esters. Biocat Biotrans 1996; 14:269-283.
40. Lirdprapamongkol K, Svasti J. Alkyl glucoside synthesis using Thai rosewood β glucosidase. Biotechnol Lett 2000; 22:1889-1894.
41. Litjens MJJ, Straathof AJJ, Jongejan JA et al. Exploration of lipase catalyzed direct amidation of free carboxylic acids with ammonia in organic solvents Tetrahedron 1999; 55:12411-12418.
42. Makropoulou M, Christakopoulos P, Tsitsimpikou C et al. Factors affecting the specificity of β-glucosidase from Fusarium oxysporum in enzymatic synthesis of alkyl-β-glucosides. International J Biol Macromol 1998; 221:97-101.
43. Maruyama R, Kawata A, Ono S et al. Effects of amino acids on the amidation of polyaromatic carboxylic acids by Bacillus cereus. Biosci Biotechnol Biochem 2001; 65:1761-1765.
44. Mattheus de Roode B, van der Meer TD, Kaper T et al. The catalytic potency of β-glucosidase from Pyrococcus furiosus in the direct glucosylation reaction. Enzyme Microbial Technol 2001; 29:621-624.
45. Maugarda T, Remaud-Simeona M, Petre D et al. Enzymatic amidification for the synthesis of biodegradable surfactants: Synthesis of N-acylated hydroxylated amines. J Mol Cat B: Enzymatic 1998; 5:13-17.

46. McNeill GP, Yamane T. Further improvements in the yield of monoglycerides during enzymatic glycerolysis of fats and oils. J Am Oil Chem Soc 1991; 68:6-10.
47. McNeill GP, Shimizu S, Yamane T. High-yield enzymatic glycerolysis of fats and oils. J Am Oil Chem Soc 1991; 68:1-5.
48. Otto RT, Bornscheuer UT, Syldatk C et al. Synthesis of aromatic n-alkyl glucoside esters in a coupled β-glucosidase and lipase reaction. Biotechnol Lett 1998; 20:437-440.
49. Parker KJ, James K, Horford J. Sucrose ester surfactants—A solventless process and the products thereof. In: Hickson JL, ed. Sucrochemistry. Washington DC: ACS Symposium Series 41. American Chemical Society, 1977:97.
50. Ryoto Sugar Ester Technical Information, Non-ionic Surfactant/Sucrose Fatty Acid Ester/Food Additive, Mitsubishi-Kasei Foods Corporation, 1989.
51. Sarney DB, Vulfson EN. Enzymatic synthesis of sugar fatty acid esters in solvent-free media enzymatic synthesis of sugar fatty acid esters In: Vulfson EN, ed. Methods in Biotechnology, Vol. 15. Enzymes in Non-aqueous Solvents: Methods and Protocols. Totowa: Humana Press Inc., 2001:531543.
52. Sarney DB, Fregapane G, Vulfson EN. Lipase-catalyzed synthesis of lyso-PLs in a continuous bioreactor. J Am Oil Chem Soc 2000; 71:93-96.
53. Sharma J, Batovska D, Kuwamori Y et al. Enzymatic chemoselective synthesis of secondary-amide surfactant from N-methylethanol amine. J Biosci Bioengg 2005; 100:662-666.
54. Sonntag NOV. New developments in the fatty acid industry in America. J Am Oil Chem Soc l984; 61:229-232.
55. Stamatis H, Sereti V, Kolisis FN. Lipase-catalyzed synthesis of sugar fatty acid esters in supercritical carbon dioxide. In: Vulfson EN, Halling PJ, Holland HL, eds. Enzymes in Non-aqueous Solvents: Methods and Protocols. Totowa: Humana Press Inc., 2001:517-522.
56. Stoltema WF, Sandoval G, Guieysse D et al. Economically pertinent continuous amide formation by direct lipase catalyzed amidation with ammonia. Biotechnol Bioengg 2003; 82:664-669.
57. Tufvesson P, Annerling A, Kaul RH et al. Solvent-free enzymatic synthesis of fatty alkanolamides. Biotechnol Bioengg 2006; 97:447-453.
58. Turner P, Svensson D, Adlercreutz P et al. A novel variant of Thermotoga neapolitana beta-glucosidase B is an efficient catalyst for the synthesis of alkyl glucosides by transglycosylation. J Biotechnol 2007; 130:67-74.
59. Van der Padt A, Keurentjes JTF, Sewalt JJW et al. Enzymatic synthesis of monoglycerides in a membrane bioreactor with an in-line adsorption column. J Am Oil Chem Soc 1992; 69:748-754.
60. Vulfson EN. Enzymatic synthesis of surfactants. In: Tyman JHP, ed. Surfactants in Lipid Chemistry: Recent Synthetic, Physical and Biodegradative Studies. London: The Royal Society of Chemistry, 1992:17-37.
61. Yua HL, Xua JH, Lub WY et al. Identification, purification and characterization of β-glucosidase from apple seed as a novel catalyst for synthesis of O-glucosides. Enzyme Microbial Technol 2007; 40:354-361.
62. Zheng G, Anders FV, Xuebing X. Enzymatic modification of phospholipids for functional applications and human nutrition. Biotechnol Adv 2005; 23:203-259.

CHAPTER 23

Structural and Molecular Characteristics of Lichenysin and Its Relationship with Surface Activity

Anuradha S. Nerurkar*

Abstract

Lichenysins are most potent anionic cyclic lipoheptapeptide biosurfactants produced by *Bacillus licheniformis* on hydrocarbonless medium with mainly glucose as carbon source. They have the capacity to lower the surface tension of water from 72 to 27 mN/m. Based on species specific variations they are named lichenysin A, B, C, D, G and surfactant BL86. The lowest ever interfacial tension against decane of 0.006 mN/m is obtained with acid precipitated lichenysin B. Surfactant BL86 and lichenysin B have recorded lowest ever CMC of 10 mg/L by any surfactant under optimal conditions. Surface and interfacial tension lowering ability bears significance in the context of oil recovery from oil reservoir. Similarity exists between structure and biosynthesis of surfactin and lichenysin. Surfactin being the most studied of the two, understanding its structure and biosynthesis gives an insight into the structure and biosynthesis of lichenysin. Lichenysin is synthesized by a multienzyme complex, lichenysin synthetase (LchA/Lic) encoded by 32.4 (26.6 kb) lichenysin operon *lch*A (lic). The structure of lichenysin and its operon indicate the nonribosomal biosynthesis with the same multifunctional modular arrangement as seen in surfactin synthetase SrfA. The *lch*A operon consists of *lch*AA-AC (*lic* A-C) and *lch*A TE (*lic*TE) genes encoding the proteins LchAA, LchAB, LchAC and thioesterase LchA-TE. The *lic*A (*lch*AA) gene is 10,746 bp and codes for a 3,582 amino acids protein, *lic*B (*lch*AB) gene is 10,764 bp and codes for a similar sized protein, while *lic*C (*lch*AC) gene is 3,864 bp and codes for protein containing 1,288 amino acid. The biotechnological potential of lichenysin in MEOR has triggered research on structure-activity relationship. Both the nature of peptide and fatty acid dictate the activity of the biosurfactant. Tailormade biosurfactant with desired attributes can be obtained from engineered synthetases. Basic studies are lacking on mechanism of biosynthesis by lichenysin synthetase however, studies on various aspects of lichenysin including regulation are expected to swell in coming years.

Introduction

Surfactants are amphipathic chemicals i.e., they contain both hydrophilic polar head and hydrophobic tail due to which they possess surface and interfacial tension lowering activities. Biosurfactants are structurally diverse surface active molecules of microbial origin that include low molecular weight glycolipids and lipopeptides and high molecular weight biosurfactants that stabilize emulsions like amphipathic polysaccharides, proteins, lipopolysaccharide, lipoproteins and

*Anuradha S. Nerurkar—Department of Microbiology and Biotechnology Centre, Faculty of Science, The Maharaja Sayajirao University of Baroda, Vadodara-390 002, Gujarat, India. Email: anuner@gmail.com

Biosurfactants, edited by Ramkrishna Sen. ©2010 Landes Bioscience and Springer Science+Business Media.

complex biopolymer mixture. Numerous bacteria and fungi esp. yeast of diverse genera produce biosurfactants of varied chemical nature.[1,2] Cyclic lipopeptides class are prominent biosurfactants, produced as secondary metabolites by *Bacillus* spp. having unique structure, exceptional surfactant power and antibiotic activity.[3] Places contaminated with oil or its byproducts commonly yield biosurfactant producers.[4]

The physiological roles of biosurfactants is in solubilisation of hydrophobic substrates, virulence and defense mechanism and regulation of attachment-detachment of microorganisms from surfaces.[5-8] They have advantage over the chemical surfactants due to their high activity, specificity, biodegradability and versatility having varied applications in textile, pharmaceutical, cosmetics, food, detergents and oil industries[9-11] of which MEOR or Microbial Enhanced Oil Recovery is assuming importance in recent years. MEOR is a cost-effective, environment-friendly, alternative tertiary recovery process which uses microorganisms or their metabolites for recovery of oil from the reservoir.[12] *Bacillus mojavensis* JF-2 from oil field injection brine[13] and *Bacillus licheniformis* BAS50 from North German Oil Reservoir[14] are specially isolated for biosurfactant mediated approach and exopolymer producing *Bacillus licheniformis* BNP29 from same reservoir[15] for selective plugging approach of MEOR.

Surfactin

Surfactin of *Bacillus subtilis* and lichenysin of *Bacillus licheniformis* are two important lipopeptide biosurfactants. Surfactin discovered four decades ago[16] and patented in 1972,[17] remains the most studied of the two. *B. subtilis* ATCC 21332 produces a mixture of surfactin with MW between 1007-1035 Da that lowers the surface tension of water from 72 to 27 mN/m and has a CMC of 20-40 mg/L (Table 1). Critical micelle concentration (CMC) is a measure of the efficacy of a surfactant and is the minimum surfactant concentration required to reach the lowest surface/interfacial tension.[18] Large scale continuous production of surfactin on glucose with enhanced yield has been achieved.[19]

Surfactin is an anionic lipopeptide, where 3-hydroxy-1, 3-methyl-tetradecanoic acid is amidated to heptapeptide with LLDLLDL chiral sequence in Glu-Leu-Leu-Val-Asp-Leu-Leu order. In this leucine-rich peptide both D and L isomers are present (Table 2). The residues two and six in surfactin face each other near the first Glu and fifth Asp side chains forming the minor polar domain. On the opposite side, residue four along with the side chains of residues five and seven

Table 1. *Comparison of physical characteristics of lipoheptapeptides of* Bacillus subtilis *and various* Bacillus licheniformis *strains*

Bacillus strain	Biosurfactant	Molecular Weight (Da)	CMC mg/L
B. subtilis ATCC 21332	Surfactin[18]	Mixture 1007-1035	20-40
B. mojavensis JF-2ATCC39307	Lichenysin B[30]	Homogeneous 1035	10
B. licheniformis 86	Surfactant BL86[28]	Mixture 979-1091 (1021,1035 most abundant)	10
B. licheniformis	Lichenysin C[29]	Mixture 1022 and 1036	15
B. licheniformis BAS50	Lichenysin A[14,31]	Mixture 1006-1034	12
B. licheniformis IM1307	Lichenysin G[32]	Mixture 993-1049	
B. licheniformis ATCC10716	Lichenysin D[33]		22
B. licheniformis 603	Novel lipopeptide[37]	1193	
B. licheniformis F2.2	Surfactin (F2.2)[38]	—	
B. licheniformis BC98	Surfactin BC98[39]	1035	—

Table 2. Chemistry of surfactin and lichenysins obtained from B. subtilis *and* B. licheniformis

Biosurfactant	Amino Acid Sequence							Main β-Hydroxy Fatty Acid
	1	2	3	4	5	6	7	
Surfactin	L-Glu	L-Leu	D-Leu	L-Val	L-Asp	D-Leu	L-Leu	i, ai C_{13} n C_{14} (40%) i, ai C_{15}
Lichenysin B	L-Glu	L-Leu	D-Leu	L-Val	L-Asp	D-Leu	L-Leu	n, i, ai branched C_{15}, aiC_{15} (36%)
Surfactant BL86	L-Glx	L-Leu	D-Leu	L-Val	L-Asx	D-Leu	L-Ile (60%) L-Val (40%)	8-9 methyl or more linear and branched mixture
Lichenysin C	L-Glu	L-Leu	D-Leu	L-Val	L-Asp	D-Leu	L-Ile	n, i C_{14}, ai C_{15}
Lichenysin A	L-Gln	L-Leu	D-Leu	L-Val	L-Asp	D-Leu	L-Ile	C_{12} -C_{17}, iC_{15} (39%)
Lichenysin D	L-Gln	L-Leu	D-Leu	L-Val	L-Asp	D-Leu	L-Ile L-Leu L-Val	—
Lichenysin G	L-Gln	L-leu L-Ile	D-Leu	L-Val L-Ile	L-Asp	D-Leu	L-Ile L-Val	i,aiC_{13} n,iC_{14} i,aiC_{15}
Surfactin F2.2	L-Asp	L-Leu	D-Leu	L-Val	L-Val	L-Glu	L-Leu	—
Novel lipopeptide	L-Asp	L-Leu	L-Leu	L-Val	L-Val	L-Glu	L-Leu	
Surfactin BC98	L-Glu	L-Leu	D-Leu	L-Val	L-Asp	D-Leu	L-Leu	3-OH tetradecanic acid

faces the lipid chain constituting a major hydrophobic domain. The fatty acids are branched β hydroxy, in *normal, iso* and/or *anteiso* forms (Fig. 1). The *iso*-methyl branched fatty acids have the branch point on the penultimate carbon (one from the end), while *anteiso*-methyl-branched fatty acids have the branch point on the *ante*-penultimate carbon atom (second from the end). The amino group of N-terminal amino acid is linked via a peptide bond with the carboxylic group of the C_{13}-C_{15} β-hydroxy fatty acid. It exhibits 'horse saddle' conformation that is responsible for

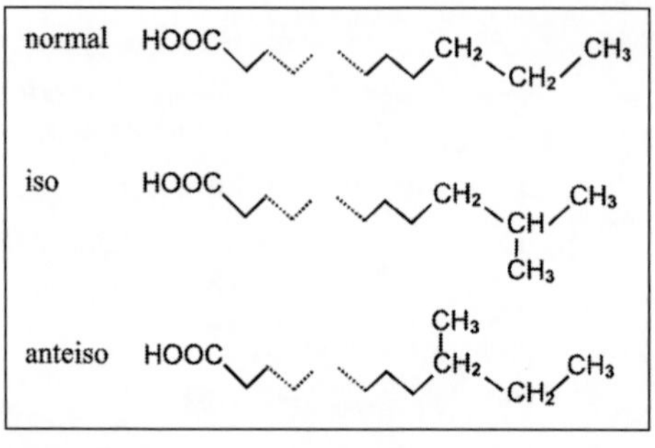

Figure 1. The *normal, iso* and *anteiso* forms of fatty acids found in lipopertide biosurfactant of *Bacillus sp.*

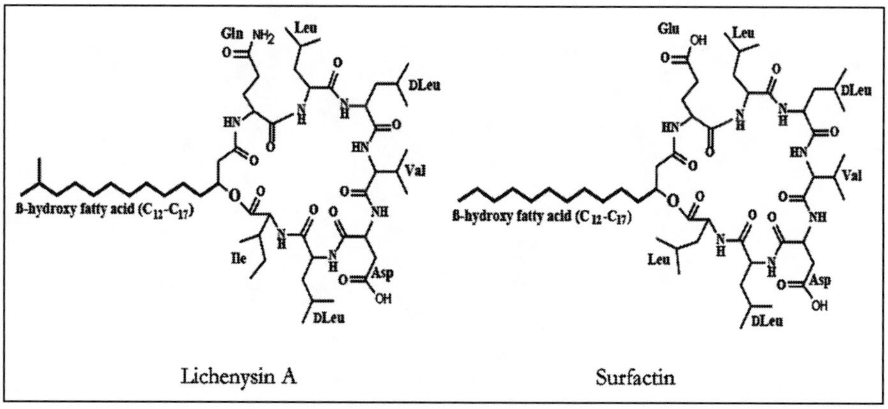

Figure 2. Primary structure of Lichenysin A and Surfactin. Adapted from Yakimov et al[53] 2000, with permission from Horizon Scientific Press.

the broad spectrum of its activities. The β hydroxyl group of fatty acid forms an ester bond with the carboxy group of C-terminal amino acid to form a lactone[18] (Fig. 2).

Nonribosomal Peptide Synthesis

Peptide synthetases of microbial origin act as protein templates for the biosynthesis of the cyclic peptides. They have an adenylation and a thiolation domain that define the sequence and length of the peptide.[20] Sufactin biosynthesis is catalysed by nonribosomal peptide synthetase (NRPS) surfactin synthetase, therefore understanding this reaction would give an idea of the lichenysin synthetase reaction. Surfactin or *srf*A operon encodes three subunits of surfactin synthetase viz. SrfA, SrfB and SrfC. SrfA and SrfB consists of three each and SrfC one amino acid activating module. NRPSs are modular multifunctional enzymes that catalyze the assembly of cyclic peptides possessing biosurfactant, siderophore, immunosuppressant, antibiotic, antitumor, antifungal, antiviral, enzyme inhibitor etc. activity. The cyclic process of chain extension by specific dedicated modules of diverse multifunctional enzymes follows thiotemplate mechanism. A module is a catalytic unit comprising of domains which are necessary for the recognition, activation, covalent binding, occasionally modification of a single monomer and formation of the peptide bond as the chain grows. The three domains of a module are Adenylation (A-domain) that recognizes and activates specific amino acids by adenylation at the expense of an ATP, Thioester forming (T-domain) that catalyzes the covalent binding of the activated amino acid at a specific serine site via a thioester linkage to a 4'-phosphopantetheine cofactor and Condensation (C-domain) that forms peptide bond between two activated amino acids. The terminal domain releases the peptide chain from the enzyme complex in the final step (Fig. 3). The NRP systems according to their biosynthetic mode are categorized as Linear, Iterative and Nonlinear types. A standard NRPS module has a mass of ~110 kDa. Figure 4 illustrates the linear NRPS reaction of surfactin synthetase. The conversion of L to D forms present in the peptide occurs during or after the peptide bond formation. An epimerization (E-domain) that catalyzes the conversion of L-amino acid to D-isomer is associated with the module incorporating D-amino acid. The linear peptide is cyclized and released by C-terminal thioesterase (Te) domain.[21]

Lichenysin Structure

The lichenysins A, B, C, D, G and surfactant BL86 are anionic biosurfactants like surfactin, produced by *B. licheniformis*. Table 1 gives the comparative account of their properties like the producer strain, molecular weight and CMC. Twenty five years after surfactin was first reported by Arima et al.[16] Jenneman et al in 1983 reported a halotolerant, biosurfactant producing *Bacillus* sp. for its application in MEOR.[13] The strain then identified as *B. licheniformis* JF-2 is now

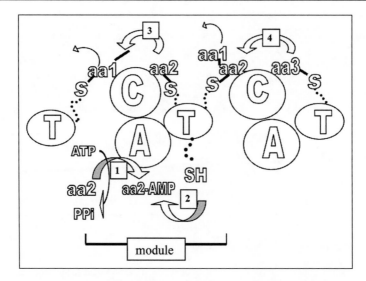

Figure 3. NRPS elongation module—Domain organization and sequence of reaction (1, 2, 3, 4) A-adenylation; T-thiolation/peptidyl carrier domain; C-condensation domain. Modified from Mootz et al[21] 2002 with copyright permission from Wiley-VCH Verlag GmbH & Co. KGaA.

reidentified as *B. mojavensis* JF-2 ATCC 39307.[22] It produced lichenysin in aerobic as well as anaerobic conditions,[23] at temperatures and salinities found in oil reservoirs with very low surface activity which remains unaffected by pH, temperature, calcium or salt concentration.[24]

Lichenysin B is produced by *B. mojavensis* JF2 ATCC 39307,[22] isolated by McInerney's group at Oklahoma University is patented for MEOR[25] and has also been applied in field trials for oil recovery.[26] However, the chemical structure of surfactant BL86 produced by *B. licheniformis* 86 and of lichenysin C were first to be determined by Horowitz et al[27,28] and Jenny et al[29] respectively in 1991. Lin et al elucidated the structure of lichenysin B in 1994.[30] Lichenysin A structure has been worked out in great details by Yakimov's group from Germany[31] in 1999. A petroleum reservoir isolate, *B. licheniformis* BAS50 isolated from a depth of 1500 m produced lichenysin A, when cultured at upto 30% salinities between 35-45°C. Of all the lichenysins the position of lactone ring was determined only in lichenysin A. Grangemarde et al. determined the structure of lichenysin G produced by *B. licheniformis* IM1307[32] in 1999. From sequence analysis of the modules of the lichenysin synthetases of *B. licheniformis* ATCC 10716, the primary structure of lichenysin D was deduced by Konz et al[33] also in 1999.

The lowest CMC of 10 mg/L is exhibited by surfactant BL86 and Lichenysin B under optimal conditions, while Lichenysins A, C and G give 12, 15 and 22 mg/L. This is same or lower

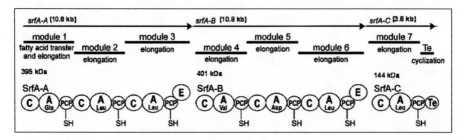

Figure 4. Surfactin synthetase reaction Modified from Mootz et al[21] 2002 with copyright permission from Wiley-VCH Verlag GmbH & Co. KGaA.

than 20-40 mg/L CMC of Surfactin. The whole broth of all the lichenysins reduce the surface tension of water from 72 mN/m to 27(28) mN/m. The Lichenysins A, B and BL86, do so even in presence of NaCl while activity of surfactin is unstable in salt. The whole broth of lichenysin B solution lowers the interfacial tension of octane-5% NaCl mixtures to 0.05 mN/m, while its acid precipitated 50 mg/L solution in 5% NaCl at pH 6, lowers it to 0.006 mN/m, lowest ever recorded. 166 mg/L surfactant BL86 solution in alkaline 4% NaCl lowers the interfacial tension to 0.455 mN/m. It is important indicator for MEOR as it reflects the ability of a surfactant to desorb the oil from rocks using capillary forces. Lichenysin A also has been applied in MEOR field trials with favorable results. Surfactant BL86 is most stable of all retaining the surface activity between pH 4-13, temperatures 25-120°C and 30% NaCl concentration. Comparitively at this concentration lichenysin A and B registered slightly higher ST of 34 and 31 mN/m respectively. Like surfactin and lichenysin B, surfactant BL86 is resistant to 25-120°C for 20 min incubation. Its pH stability is better (pH 4-13) as compared to surfactin (pH 6-12) and lichenysin B (pH 6-10).

Unlike surfactin, lichenysin is synthesized during growth under both aerobic and anaerobic conditions Crude oil is not required for growth or production of lichenysin B. Like surfactin it is produced on mineral-salts medium without hydrocarbon,[34] with glucose or sucrose and has same chemistry and mode of synthesis. The chemistry of lichenysin is dictated by composition of the culture medium e.g., lichenysin G is produced on supplementation of the culture medium with L-Glu or L-Ile as nitrogen source. Lichenysin A exhibits antimicrobial activity against both Gram-positive and negative bacteria but is less potent than surfactin.

The principal techniques used to elucidate the chemical structure of surfactins and lichenysins are TLC, FTIR, HPLC, 2D NMR and Mass spectroscopy (MS). MALDI-TOF provides a sensitive and rapid method for detection and identification of lipopeptides.[35] Variants of lipopeptides from *B. licheniformis* HSN221 when grown in different media are identified by the SCI-MS analysis.[36] Differences exist in chemistry of peptide ring and fatty acid components of surfactin and lichenysins which also give clues about its structure-activity relationship (Table 2). Lichenysins are produced as complex mixtures except Lichenysin B which is a homogenous preparation. The MW of surfactin, lichenysin B, surfactant BL86 (predominant spp.) and lichenysin G (one component) is 1035 Da. The MW of Lichenysin C and A is 1022-1036 and 1066-1034 Da respectively. Different species have MW with an increment of 14 Da units difference due to a methylene group. 1 Da difference in MW is due to the presence of an amide in lichenysin A and surfactant BL86. Lichenysin A structure depicted in Figure 2 represents the general structure of lichenysins.

There are variations at first, fifth and seventh position with respect to surfactin in the heptapeptide of lichenysins. All have D-Leu at the third and sixth position. The peptide portion of lichenysin B is structurally identical to surfactin, only the lipid tail is different. Its biochemical and immunological reactivity is identical to surfactin. The first (N-terminal amino acid) that forms peptide bond with the fatty acid is L-Glu, in lichenysins B, C and surfactant BL86 whereas it is L-Gln in Lichenysin A, G and D while the fifth amino acid is L-Asp in all except in surfactant BL86 which might be Asn. In lichenysin A, C, D and G and surfactant BL86, the C-terminal amino acid is L-Ile instead of L-Leu of surfactin and Lichenysin B. The tentative structure of surfactant BL86 has either Gln/Asp and Glu/Asn in first and fifth positions. It has 40% L-Val and 60% L-Ile as the terminal amino acid. Lichenysin G variants with differences in second, fourth and seventh position, where L-Ile/L-Leu, L-Ile/L-Val and L-Val/L-Ile substitutions respectively are observed.

The β-hydroxy fatty acid in surfactin is i, ai C_{13}; n C_{14}; i, ai C_{15}; n, i, ai C_{15} isoforms in lichenysin B and linear or branched tails with an average 8-9 methylene groups or more with isoforms not known in surfactant BL86. The general structure of lichenysin C is R (1-4) $(CH_2)_8$ CHOH CH_2-CO-NH-heptapeptide with four distinct fatty acid chains viz. R1 = $(CH_3)_2$-CH-, R2 = CH_3-CH_2-CH_2-, R3 = $(CH_3)_2$-CH-CH_2- and R4 = CH_3 – CH_2-CH (CH_3)-. Lichenysin A lipid is a mixture of fourteen linear and branched β hydroxyl fatty acids of C_{12}-C_{17}; the fatty acid chains of C_{13} is 7.3%, n, i C_{14} is 30% and i, ai C_{15} is 59.3% (iC_{15}39%). The fatty acids of Lichenysin G are i, ai C_{13}; i C_{14}, i, ai C_{15}.[14,28-33]

A novel lipopeptide from thermophilic and halotolerant *B. licheniformis* 603 obtained from a mixture of drilling fluid and subsurface thermal water contains same amino acids as surfactin but the sequence is unusual and only L amino acids are present. It inhibits bacterial adhesion and growth of *Corynebacterium variabilis* and *Acinetobacter* sp.[37] The *B. licheniformis* strain F 2.2 isolated from fermented food of Thailand[38] and BC98 isolated from soil,[39] produce surfactin. Surfactin of *B. licheniformis* BC98 exhibits a strong inhibitory activity against the phytopathogenic rice blast fungus *Magnaporthe girsea*, *Curvularia lunata* and *Rhizoctonia bataticola*.

Lichenysin Operon

The structural organization of Lichenysin A and Surfactin operons showing the promoter and location of genes associated within these operons is as in Figure 5. Yakimov et al[40] in 1997 and Konz et al[33] in 1999, cloned and sequenced the 32.4 kb (*lch*A) and 26.6 kb (*lic*) putative lichenysin biosynthesis operon from *B. licheniformis* strains BN29 and ATCC 10716 respectively. The operon consists of *lch*AA-AC (*lic*A-C) and *lch*A TE (*lic*TE) genes encoding the proteins LchAA (LicA), LchAB (LicB), LchAC (LicC) and thioesterase LchA-TE (LicTE). Lichenysin biosynthesis operons for all isoforms of lichenysin have emerged from the same origin. There is one to one similarity between the genes and proteins of *lch*A and *srf*A operons. The *lic*A (*lch*AA) product has approx. 10,746 bp and codes for a 3582 amino acids protein, *lic*B (*lch*AB) gene is 10,764 bp and codes for similar size protein, while *lic*C (*lch*AC) gene is 3864 bp and codes for 1288 amino acid protein. Both have same G+C contents i.e., 50.07 and 49.35% respectively. The genes in *lch*A operon are arranged in modular pattern as required for nonribosomal protein synthesis. This and the 60% similarity between the two suggests same evolutionary origin.

A transcriptional start site upstream of *lch*A operon with 300 bp is identified as against 289 bp of *srf*A operon; however no homology is observed. A *Plch*A corresponding to *Psrf*A promoter with a −10 and −35 consensus sequences is present, again there is a lack of homology. This implies that, *Plch*A must require a help of a positive regulator to initiate transcription. An ABC type transport system operon is predicted to be located upstream of lichenysin A operon which causes the secretion of lichenysin. Several regulatory genes regulate the *srf*A operon. These are components of signal transduction cascade. Environmental signals are sensed by this system, which results in autophosphorylation of comP and subsequent transfer of phosphate group to comA. ComA is a DNA binding activator protein required for transcriptional activation of *srf*A operon needed for genetic competence, sporulation and surfactin production in *B. subtilis*. The ComA-P tetramer binds to regulatory sequences upstream of promoter and activates *srf*A. Similar putative *com*A like

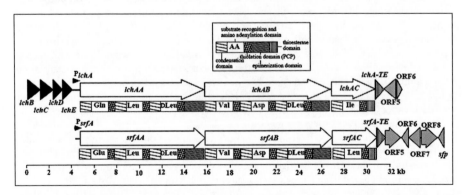

Figure 5. Lichenysin A *lchAA-C* and Surfactin *srfAA-C* operons. Promoters P$_{lchA}$ and P$_{srfA}$, Genes encoding ABC-like transporter systems, *lchB-E*, thioesterase, *lchA-TE*, 4'-PP transferase, *sfp*, genes with unknown functions, ORF5-8. Adapted from Yakimov et al[53] 2000, with permission from Horizon Scientific Press.

box is observed ahead of *lch*A operon. The ComA dependent activation of lichenysin A synthetase promoter is found to be functional in *B. subtilis* and high level production of lichenysin is obtained. A palindromic sequence upstream of cloned *lch*A promoter is the target of ComA. Presence of *com*A operon in *B. licheniformis* indicates similar mechanism.[41]

Lichenysin Synthetase

The *lch*A operon codes for lichenysin synthetase. This like surfactin synthetase multienzymes act as indeependent enzymes whose specific linkage order forms the protein template that decides the primary structure of lichenysin peptide. Yakimov[40] has analyzed several bacterial and fungal peptide synthetase genes and found a high degree of sequence conservation. The similarity suggests that the action of lichenysin synthetase must be similar to that of surfactin synthetase. Very little is known about the lichenysin synthetase molecular nature and biochemistry.

The lichenysin synthetase involves transfer of β hydroxyl fatty acid from acytrasferase to the first module of synthetase followed by hydroxyacylamino acid formation, which is the first intermediate of the sequence of reaction that follows. Like in surfactin synthetase the condensation domain is present in the first module of each protein. The LchAA and LchAB have three modules each namely LchAA1, LchAA2, LchAA3 and LchAB1, LchAB2, LchAB3 respectively while LchAC has one of the total seven modules. First six amino acids are added by LchAA and LchAB and the last one by LchAC. The third and sixth modules of LchAA and LchAB has an epimerization domain each which add the D-amino acids. A putative thioesterase active site is located at the C-terminal end of LchAC product. Its terminal thioesterase is an efficient and versatile enzyme which requires the β-hydroxy fatty acid and side chains of fifth aspartate and seventh isoleucine.[42] The synthetases have specific activating modules that harbor specific pockets for binding of the amino acid substrate on which depends the amino acid sequence of the peptide. As per Yakimov's studies,[40] Lys in Glu recognizing pockets of the SrfAA1 interacts with side chain of Glu, while Gln in the same pocket in LchAA1 interacts with Gln. For Asx the binding pockets were identical in SrfAB2 and LchAB2 as both have Thr and Lys. The binding pocket residues specific for Leu are not highly conserved, while the putative binding pockets for Val are conserved. The putative Ile binding pocket has Phe. In SrfA and LchA modules activating amino acids with neutral side chains have hydrophobic pockets at the bottom due to presence of Phe and Trp. A 100 amino acid peptide between the highly conserved sequences FDXX and NXYGPTE(IV)X within amino acid binding domains of the peptide synthetase is minimal block dictating the substrate specificity of the enzymes.[40]

Konz et al[33] found that the substrate specificity of first, fifth and seventh domain of lichenysin synthetase is Gln, Asp and Ile respectively. As observed in Lichenysin D, LicAA1 and LicAB2 activation of L-Gln and L-Asp respectively occurs with high degree of specificity. LicAC has high side preference for L-Val (30%) and L-Leu (30%) and incorporates them instead of L-Ileu. A single mutation in (His 738→ Glu) Asp-specific A domain of SrfAB2 is sufficient to alter the specificity, which means that the conversion Glu to Gln and Asp to Asn specific domains and vice versa need only slight alteration. Lichenysin operon for the biosynthesis of its isoforms must have such changes due to such strain specific mutations. Different isoforms of lichenysin must be obtained due to such evolution dependent strain specific mutations. In this context, the studies regarding why *lic*A and *lch*AA incorporates Gln and Glu respectively as first amino acid in spite of having 97% identity would be interesting.

Although the A domain recognizes the amino acid and activates it the C domain also is affected by the structure of donor and acceptor amino acids. C domain requires two adjacent amino acid molecules for peptide bond formation. In the NRPS they are clustered into functional groups according to the substrate donor molecules into L-peptidyl, D-peptidyl and *N*-acyl donors as understood by phylogenetic analysis. The C-domain structure is not subject to optical configuration of amino acid acceptor molecule. This indicates that the conversion of L to D form of amino acid must occur after the peptide formation.[43]

Structure-Activity Relationship

Several studies focused on structure-activity relationship with the ultimate goal of rational design of cyclic lipopeptides with enhanced properties have been done. The interest in generation of greater peptide diversity is due to the possibility of creating biotechnologically interesting tailormade products. Several approaches have been adopted based on structural and molecular knowledge of the lipopeptide. Again surfactin has been studied extensively.

The linearization of surfactin by saponification of lactone ring decreases its oil displacement activity which is a function of surface activity. Methylation or amidation of glutamic and aspartic acid residue increases the oil displacement activity however loss of water solubility is observed. The decrease in activity is due to charge repulsion and structural distortion inhibiting micelle formation. pH affects the activity of surfactin in that at alkaline pH higher activity is observed than in acidic pH.[44]

Peypoux[18] has suggested that in surfactin the backbone folding is governed by its chiral sequence, with the requirement of cyclization. The lateral chains favourably interact to stabilize the structure. Accordingly substitutions could be responsible for significant changes in the properties only by modifying the polar/apolar distribution and/or the accessibility of carboxyl groups to cations. Some binding sites of surfactin synthetase are flexible and can bind various hydrophobic amino acids. Surfactin variants were obtained from medium supplemented with isoleucine or valine. On a medium containing L-alanine, *B. subtilis* produced an isoform of surfactin [Ala-4]surfactin containing Ala at fourth position instead of valine.[45] This decreased the surfactant power of surfactin. This implies that replacement of a hydrophobic moiety with longer side chains by the one with shorter chain greatly influences its surface activity. The Ile incorporated in second position improves the hydrophobic and electrostatic interactions and surface properties due to an increase in the hydrophobicity of the apolar domain favouring micellization. Presence of Ile instead of Val in fourth position decreased the CMC two-fold and increased the surface activity. This may be due to the expansion of major domain by the incorporation of more hydrophobic Ile. This Ile in second position also increases the affinity for Ca^{++}, because of the increased accessibility to acidic side chains that bind to Ca^{++}.[46] The 3D topology due to aliphatic chains, side chains of hydrophobic amino acids on one face and the acidic residues of first Glu and fifth Asp on the other, imparts the surface active and chelating properties to surfactin. Ionized surfactin forms surfactin-Ca^{++} in 1:1 ratio, Ca^{++} forming an intramolecular bridge between two acidic residues of cyclic peptide.[47] The monoanionic lichenysin has the same properties but it is more effective than surfactin in surface activity and chelating properties.[18] It forms a complex ratio with divalent cations in 2:1. Its chelating effect is due to its higher association constants with Ca^{++} and Mg^{++} and increase in the accessibility of the carboxyl group to these divalent cations owing to the change in side chain topology.[48]

Surfactin synthetase is used as a model system for the engineering of peptide synthetases with altered amino acid specificities. Symmank et al. have shown a combined in vitro and in vivo recombination approach in which a modified peptide synthetase was constructed by replacing a large internal module of the enzyme by module of different motifs. Such engineered surfactin synthetases produce a novel lipopeptide with reduced toxicity.[49,50]

In *B. licheniformis* too the production of lipopeptides is under the control of culture medium. A relationship involving a minor polar domain also is evident in lichenysin. The fact that the monoanionic lipopeptides are better in binding to divalent cations and lowering surface tension than dianionic ones like surfactin also emphasizes the role of carboxyl group in micellization process. The amidation of one carboxyl group to Gln caused substantial difference in lichenysin G activity. The local variation due to the presence of first Gln bestows higher surfactant power, low CMC and higher hemolytic activity to lichenysin G as compared to surfactin.[32]

The lack of direct correlation between biosurfactant yield and activity points to the fact that structure rather than the change in gene expression dictates the surface activity. The fatty acyl composition too is important for the activity. Addition of exogenous branched chain amino acid to the culture medium brought changes in the fatty acyl moiety. The alteration in the ratio of *n* : *i* even numbered fatty acids has more effect than altering the ratio of *ai* : *i* odd-numbered fatty acid. The branched *iso*-β-hydroxyl myristic acid (C_{14}) was correlated with the surface activity. This in case of lichenysin B gives the optimum HLB for the high surface activity according to Youssef et al.[51] The hydrophile—lipophile balance (HLB) property of the surfactants is a useful guide for choosing a surfactant for appropriate application. It refers to the relative abundance of hydrophilic and lipophilic groups in them. Generally a surfactant that has a low HLB is lipophilic while the one with high HLB is hydrophilic.

The lichenysin A also is less polar than others giving the delicate HLB required for higher surface activity. Supplementation of branched amino acids in the medium caused changes in the lipophilic part of lichenysin A. Addition of L-Glu cause two-fold increase while L-Asn causes a four-fold increase in the production of lichenysin A. The percentage of *n*-β-hydroxy C_{14} acid was correlated with surface activity of Lichenysin A.[52] The surfactant activity varies with both the chain length and branching type of the fatty acid. The order is *normal >iso >anteiso*. The activity of *n* C_{14} was greater than that of *i* or *ai* C_{15}. A hydrophilic domain due to carboxylic group of glutamate and aspartate and the nonpolar residues at second, fourth and seventh position forming the hydrophobic domain with the lipid tail are the major contributions to the activity.[52]

In another approach engineering of NRPS was done. Whole module substitutions were done in *B. subtilis srf*A operon where Glu and Asp incorporating modules were replaced with that of corresponding modules of *lch*A operon. The recombinant lipopeptide ID1 has Gln instead of Glu as the first residue. FAD-MS gave 1 Da difference in the MW which is the difference between Glu and Gln. Also polarity of the ID1 was lower as compared to surfactin due to this substitution. Its yield was 12-14 fold higher than in *B. licheniformis* BNP29. It exhibited high surface activity and achieved a CMC of 13.5 μM, similar to that of native lichenysin A (12 μM) and lower than that of surfactin (20 μM). Structurally the recombinant lipopeptide showed the amino acid composition same as lichenysin A while the fatty acid profile was identical to that of the surfactin. Lipopeptide ID1 has 40% β hydroxymyristic acid (C_{14}) which is responsible for the decrease in the surface tension to 25.5 mN/m. In contrast to surfactin whose activity is progressively inhibited by increasing salt concentrations the recombinant lipopeptide is salt tolerant; upto 250 g/L is tolerated. Glu/Gln difference must be responsible for the observed halotolerance. The lichenysins from *B. licheniformis* BAS50 and *B. mojavensis* JF2 exhibited these properties.[53]

Conclusion

Since the first report of lichenysin, various applied aspects of it has been focus of study. Several strains with lichenysin variants are reported. Knowledge of surfactin has helped to understand lichenysin better. Comparitive structure—activity studies have thrown new insights. While the lichenysin operon is also identified, the biochemistry of the lichenysin synthetase is a grossly neglected field. However, from application viewpoint for its unique properties suitable for oil reservoir conditions the idea of obtaining tailormade lipopeptide by engineering the multienzyme complex has received much attention. The amount of information on lichenysin and its synthetase is expected to swell in the coming years in the wake of its applications. Understanding the relationship of various domains of NRPS with the acceptor and donor molecules is important. It is observed that the culture medium composition to certain extent dictates the production of the lipopeptides. Work on the regulatory mechanisms governing lichenysin synnthesis is warranted.

Acknowledgements

I thank my students Harish Suthar, Sanket Joshi, Nlikanth Faldu and Vipul Gohel for their help in preparation of this chapter.

References

1. Desai JD, Banat IM. Microbial production of surfactants and their commercial potential. Microbiol Mol Biol Rev 1997; 61(1):47-64.
2. Rosenberg E, Ron EZ. High- and low- molecular-mass microbial surfactants. Appl Microbiol Biotechnol 1999; 52:154-162.

3. Vater J. Lipopeptides, an attractive class of microbial surfactants. Prog Colloid Polymer Sci 1986; 72:12-18.
4. Batista SB, Mounteer AH, Amorim FR et al. Isolation and characterization of biosurfactant/bioemulsifier-producing bacteria from petroleum contaminated sites. Biores Technol 2006; 97:868-875.
5. Ron EZ, Rosenberg E. Natural roles of biosurfactants. Env Microbiol 2001; 3(4):229-236.
6. Lin S-C. Biosurfactants: Recent advances. J Chem Tech Biotechnol 1996; 66:109-120.
7. Rodrigues L, Banat IM, Teixeira J et al. Biosurfactants: potential applications in medicine. J Antimicro Chemotherapy 2006; 57:609-618.
8. Neu TR. Significance of bacterial surface active compounds in interaction of bacteria with interfaces. Microbiol Rev 1996; 60(1):151-166.
9. Healy MG, Devine CM, Murphy R. Microbial production of biosurfactants. Resources Conservation Recycling 1996; 18:41-57.
10. Christofi N, Ivshina IB. Microbial surfactants and their use in field studies of soil remediation. 2002; 93:915-929.
11. Mulligan CN. Environmental applications for biosurfactants. Env Pollution 2005; 133:183-198.
12. Banat IM. Biosurfactants production and possible uses in microbial enhanced oil recovery and oil pollution remediation: A review. Biores Technol 1995; 51:1-12.
13. Jeneman GE, McInerney MJ, Knapp RM et al. A halotolerant, biosurfactant—producing Bacillus species potentially useful for enhanced oil recovery. Dev Ind Microbiol 1983; 24:485-492.
14. Yakimov MM, Timmis KN, Wray V. Characterization of new lipopeptide surfactant produced by thermotolerant and halotolerant subsurface Bacillus licheniformis BAS50. Appl Env Microbiol 1995; 61(5):1706-1713.
15. Yakimov MM, Amro MM, Brock M et al. The potential of Bacillus licheniformis strains for in situ enhanced oil recovery. J Pet Sci Engg 1997; 18:147-160.
16. Arima K, Kakinuma A, Tamura G. Surfactin, a crystalline peptidelipid surfactant produced by Bacillus subtilis: isolation, characterization and its inhibition of fibrin clot formation. Biochem Biophys Res' Commun 1968; 31:488-494.
17. Arima K, Tamura G, Kakinuma A. Surfactin 1972; U.S. patent no. 3, 687,926.
18. Peypoux F, Bonmatin JM, Wallach J. Recent trends in biochemistry of surfactin. Appl Microbiol Biotechol 1999; 51:553-563.
19. Cooper DG, MacDonald CR, Duff SJB et al. Enhanced production of surfactin from Bacillus subtilis by continuous product removal and metal cation additions. Appl Env Micro 1981; 42(3):408-412.
20. Marahiel MA, Protein templates for the biosynthesis of peptide antibiotics. Chem Biol 1997; 4(8):561-567.
21. Mootz HD, Schwarzer D, Marahiel MA. Ways of assembling complex natural products on modular nonribosomal peptide synthetases. Chem Biochem 2002; 3:490-504.
22. Folmsbee M, Duncan KH, Nagle D et al. Re-identification of the halotolerant, biosurfactant-producing Bacillus licheniformis strain JF-2 as Bacillus mojavensis strain JF-2. Syst Appl Microbiol 2006:645-649.
23. Javaheri M, Jenneman GE, McInerney MJ et al. Anaerobic production of a biosurfactant by Bacillus licheniformis JF-2. Appl Env Microbiol 1985; 50(3):698-700.
24. McInerney MJ, Javaheri M and Nagle DP Jr. Properties of the biosurfactant produced by Bacillus licheniformis strain JF-2. J Ind Microbiol 1989; 4:1-7.
25. McInerney MJ, Jenneman GE, Knapp RM et al. Biosurfactant and enhanced oil recovery. 1985; U.S. patent no. 482308.
26. McInerney MJ, Knapp RM, Chisholm JL et al. Use of indigenous or injected microorganisms for enhanced oil recovery In microbial Biosystems: New frontiers Proc 8th Int Symp Microbial Ecol Bell CR, Brylinsky M, Johnson-Green P. (eds.) Atlantic Canada Soc Microbial Ecol Halifax, Canada 1999.
27. Horowitz S, Gilbert JN, Griffin WM. Isolation and characterization of a surfactant produced by Bacillus licheniformis 86. J Ind Microbiol 1990; 6:243-248.
28. Horowitz S, Griftin WM. Structural analysis of Bacillus licheniformis 86 Surfactant. J Ind Microbiol 1991; 7:45-52.
29. Jenny K, Kappeli O, Fletcher A. Biosurfactants from Bacillus licheniformis: structural analysis and characterization. Appl Microbiol Biotechnol 1991; 36:5-13.
30. Lin S-C, Minton MA, Sharma MM et al. Structural and immunological characterization of a biosurfactant produced by Bacillus licheniformis JF-2. 1994; 60(1):31-38.
31. Yakimov MM, Abraham W-R, Meyer H et al. Structural characterization of lichenysin A components by fast atom bombardment tandem mass spectrometry. Biochim et Biophys Acta 1999; 1438:273-280.
32. Grangemard I, Bonmatin J-M, Bernillon J et al. Lichemysin G, a novel family of lipopeptide biosurfactants from Bacillus licheniformis IM1307: Production, Isolation and structural evaluation by NMR and mass spectrometry. 1999; 52(4):363-373.
33. Konz D, Doekel S, Marahiel MA. Molecular and Biochemical characterization of the protein template contolling biosynthesis of the lipopeptide lichenysin. J Bac 1999; 181(1):133-140.

34. Mulligan CN, Cooper DG, Neufeld RJ. Selection of microbes producing biosurfactants in media without hydrocarbons. J Ferment Technol 1984; 62(4):311-314.
35. Vater J, Kablitz B, Wilde C et al. Matrix-Assiated Laser desorption Ionisation-Time of Flight mass spectrometry pf lipopeptide biosurfactants in whole cells and culture filtrates of Bacillus subtilis C-1 isolated from petroleum sludge. Appl Env Microbiol 2002; 68(12):6210-6219.
36. Li Y-M, Haddad NIA, Yang S-Z et al. Variants of lipopeptides produced by Bacillus licheniformis HSN221 in different medium components evaluated by a rapid method ESI-MS. Int J Peptide Res and therapeutics 2008:1-7.
37. Batrakov SG, Rodinova TA, Esipov SE. A novel lipopeptide, an inhibitor of bacterial adhesion from the thermophilic and halotolerant subsurface Bacillus licheniformis strain 603. Biochim Et Biophy Acta 2003; 1634:107-115.
38. Thaniyavarn J, Roongsawang N, Kameyama T et al. Production and characterization of biosurfactants from Bacillus licheniformis F2.2. Biosci Biotechnol Biochem 2003; 67(6):1239-1244.
39. Tendulkar SR, Saikumari YK, Patel V et al. Isolation, purification and characterization of an antifungal molecule produced by Bacillus licheniformis BC98 and its effect on phytopathogen Magnaporthe grisea. J App Microbiol 2007; 1-9.
40. Yakimov MM, Kröger A, Slepak TN et al. A putative lichenysin A synthetase operon in Bacillus licheniformis: initial characterization. Biochim et Biophys Acta 1998; 1399:141-153.
41. Yakimov MM, Golyshin PN. Com-A dependent transcriptional activation of lichenycin A synthetase promoter in Bacillus subtilis cells. Biotechnol Prog 1997; 13:757-761.
42. Cao S, Yang Y, Ng NLJ et al. Macrolactonization catalysed by the thioesterase domain of the nonribosomal peptide synthetase responsible for lichenycin biosynthesis. Biorg Medicinal Chem Lett 2005; 15(10):2595-2599.
43. Roongsawang N, Lin SP, Washio K et al. Phylogenetic analysis of condensation domains in the ribosomal peptide synthetases. FEMS Microbiol Lett 2005; 252:143-151.
44. Morikawa M, Hirata Y, Imanaka T. A study of the structure-function relationship of lipopeptide biosurfactants. Biochim et Biophys Acta 2000; 1488:211-218.
45. Peypoux F, Bonmatin J-M, Labbe H et al. [Ala4] Surfactin, a novel isoform from Bacillus subtilis studied by mass and NMR spectroscopies. Eur J Biochem 1994; 224:89-96.
46. Grangemard I, Peypoux F, Wallach J et al. Lipopeptides with improved properties: structure by NMR, purification by HPLC and structure-activity relationships of new isoleucyl-rich surfactins. Biochim Biophys Acta 1999; 1418:307-319.
47. Bonmatin J-M, Laprévote O, Peypoux F, Diversity among microbial cyclic lipopeptides: iturins and surfactins. Activity-structure relationships to design new bioactive agents. Conmbinatorial chemistry and high throughput screening 2003; 6:541-556.
48. Grangemard I, Wallach J, Maget-Dana R et al. Lichenysin: a more efficient cation chelator than surfactin. App Biochem Biotechnol 2001; 90(3):199-210.
49. Symmank H, Franke P, Saenger W et al. Modification of biologically active peptides: production of novel lipohexapeptide after engineering of Bacillus subtilis surfactin synthetase. Protein Engg 2002; 15(11):913-921.
50. Symmank H, Saenger W, Bernhard F. Analysis of engineered multifunctional peptide synthetases: enzymatic characterization of surfactin synthetase domains in hybrid bimodular systems. J Biol Chem 1999; 274(31):21581-21588.
51. Youssef NH, Duncan KE, McInerney MJ. Importance of 3-hydroxy fatty acid composition of lipopeptides for biosurfactant activity. 2005; 71(12):7690-7695.
52. Yakimov MM, Fredrickson HL, Timmis KN. Effect of heterogeneity of hydrophobic moieties on surface activity of lichenysin A a lipopeptide biosurfactant from Bacillus licheniformis BAS50. Biotechnol Appl Biochem 1996; 23(pt 1):13-18.
53. Yakimov MM, Giuliano L, Timmis KN et al. Recombinant acylheptapeptide lichenysin: high level of production of Bacillus subtilis cells. J Mol Microbiol Biotechnol 2000; 2(2):217-24.

CHAPTER 24

Surfactin:
Biosynthesis, Genetics and Potential Applications

Ramkrishna Sen*

Abstract

Even after forty years of its discovery by Arima et al[7], surfactin, a potent lipopeptide biosurfactant, still attracts attention and fancy of the applied microbiologists and bio-technologists worldwide, mainly due to its versatile bioactive properties and potential industrial implications. Starting from its first invented characteristic as an inhibitor of fibrin clot formation coupled with its significant ability to reduce surface tension of water, it has been credited with antifungal, antiviral, antitumor, insecticidal and antimycoplasma activities. These properties of therapeutic and commercial importance and its recent use as an enhanced oil recovery and a bioremediation agent make it a truly versatile biomolecule, the commercial potential of which could not be fully realized, particularly as a therapeutic agent, mainly because of its hemolytic property. This chapter thus addresses the issues related to the versatile nature of the most studied microbial surfactant, surfactin and its potential commercial and health-care applications.

Introduction

Microbial surfactants constitute a class of secondary metabolites, which show the same characteristics as the synthetic surfactants and may have proved to be useful in a broad spectrum of potential industrial applications, which presently utilize synthetic surfactants. Interest and research activities in surfactants produced through microbial routes have increased recently, due mainly to their potential applications in enhanced petroleum recovery and environmental bioremediation.[1,2] These low volume high value products became popular primarily for their specific action, low toxicity, high biodegradability, ease of preparation and potential commercial applications.[3-6] One unique example of such a versatile biosurfactant is surfactin that is produced by various strains of *Bacillus subtilis*. In an attempt to search for an inhibitor of fibrin clot-formation, Arima et al[7] first isolated from *Bacillus subtilis* a crystalline peptide-lipid, which was found to be not only a potent inhibitor of blood clotting, but also a powerful surface active agent. At concentrations as low as 0.005% in distilled water, this surface active compound was found to lower the surfcae tension of water from 72 mN m^{-1} to 27 mN m^{-1} and shown to have surface activity much better than sodium lauryl sulfate, a synthetic surfactant. Arima et al[7] named this powerful bioactive microbial surfactant as Surfactin.

The chemical structure of surfactin, which is a lipopeptide consisting of 3-hydroxy-13-methyl-tetradecanoic acid amidated to the N-terminal amine of a heptapeptid moiety with the carboxy terminal end of the peptide being further esterifeid to the hydroxyl group of the fatty acid, was elucidated and described elsewhere.[8-10] Structural characteristics show the presence of

*Ramkrishna Sen—Department of Biotechnology, Indian Institute of Technology Kharagpur, West Bengal 721302, India. Email: rksen@yahoo.com

Biosurfactants, edited by Ramkrishna Sen. ©2010 Landes Bioscience and Springer Science+Business Media.

a heptapeptide with an LLDLLDL chiral sequence linked, via a lactone bond, to a β-hydroxy fatty acid thereby mimicking a horse-saddle conformation.[11] The cyclic nature of the lipopeptides like surfactin was attributed to the enzyme activity of thioesterases and the corresponding genetic domain SrfTE.[12-13] Further in-depth investigations of surfactin structure using sophisticated techniques provided new insights into the mechanisms of its actions and thus, helped elucidate the structure-function relationship towards designing new bioactive molecules.[14-17] The versatility of surfactin in its action and applications thus lies in its excellent surface and interfacial activities[18] and also in its unique cyclic structure with horse-saddle conformation. Thus the present chapter attempts to address the most pertinent issues related to biosynthesis of surfactin, genetic regulations of its biosynthesis and also its commercial application potentials.

Biosynthesis of Surfactin

Biochemistry and Mechanisms

Although the biosynthetic pathway and the nature of the multienzyme systems involved in the synthesis of surfactin is not well-established, it is generally believed that surfactin and other bioactive lipopeptides are synthesized by their producer organisms nonribosomally, as demonstrated in the presence of inhibitors for protein biosynthesis.[19-20] These lipopeptides contain the rare and modified amino acids, which are not used for ribosomal protein synthesis. Such bioactive lipopeptides usually appear as mixtures of closely related compounds which show little variations in their amino acid composition and/or in their lipid moiety.[19] The enzymatic mechanisms for substrate amino acid activation in nonribosomal biosynthesis of bioactive lipopeptides do not involve the cell's translation machinery but instead utilizes large multienzyme complexes called peptide-synthetases.[21] Many of these enzymes are reported to catalyze peptide synthesis, based on multienzyme thio-template mechanism.[22-23] The growing peptide chain is transferred from one amino acid domain to the next, where a peptide bond is formed. This translocation process is carried out with the aid of a 4'-phosphopantetheine cofactor. Synthesis is then terminated by cyclization of the peptide or its release from the thio-template by a thioesterase.[22]

Biosynthesis of surfactin was studied using growing cells of *Bacillus subtilis* ATCC 21332 and was found to be independent of ribosomal protein synthessis, as was demonstrated by product formation in the presence of the antibiotic chloramphenicol.[20] The results showed that [14]C- labelled precursor amino acids were incorporated directly into the product and a part of the [^{14}C] labelled acetate was found in the fatty acid portion of surfactin. Surfactin biosynthesis was also studied in a cell-free system prepared from *B. subtilis* ATCC 21332 and OKB 105 (mutant) by understanding the mode of substrate activation in biosynthesis and by isolating enzymes, which catalyze ATP-P_i exchange reactions.[20,24] These reactions are mediated specifically by the amino acid components of surfactin.[20,24,25] This mode of activation was reported to be consistent with a peptide-synthesizing multienzyme system, which activates its substrate amino acids simultaneously as reactive aminoacyl phosphates.[20,25] The mechanism involving an amino acid dependent exchange of ATP-P_i has been fully characterized in the case of mycobacillin synthetases.[23,25] Similar studies on in vivo incorporation experiments with ^{14}C-labelled precursor amino acids showed that the biosynthesis of surfactin starts in the exponential phase of growth and continues over a wide range of the cell cycle.[19] Thus, as with other lipopeptides, surfactin is also synthesized by the multienzyme thiotemplate mechanism.[19,20,22,25] Taking cue from the previous studies, a tailor-made strategy for incorporating specific amino acids in target positions in the peptide moiety of the surfactin molecule in a well-controlled biosynthesis process has been reported.[26] In-vitro surfactin production in various fermenter modes and configurations, optimization of media and process parameters for its improved production and recovery were reported.[27-43] However, the scope of this chapter does not allow for a discussion on the production of surfactin in fermenters as it has been critically discussed earlier.[3,5,30,33,36-41]

Role of Genetic Regulations in Surfactin Biosynthesis

The genetic analysis is a prerequisite for understanding the control or regulation mechanisms of the biosynthesis of surfactin. By taking advantage of the easy method of detection of surfactin by studying a zone of lysis on a solid medium containing erythrocytes, Nakano et al (44) identified two genetic loci (*sfp* and *srf*) that are involved in the biosynthesis of surfactin. The genetic locus, *sfp*, which is responsible for surfactin synthesis, was transformed from ATCC 21332 strain into JH642 strain of *Bacillus subtilis* (*sfp⁻*). Molecular genetic studies of the *sfp* locus involved the isolation of a Tn917 insertion mutant that was blocked in surfactin production. The *srf*::Tn917 mutation was found to be closely related to *sfp* and subsequent mapping of both the loci suggested that the transformrd strain JH642 contained at least some of the genes encoding surfactin production. Expression of the *srf* gene(s) was monitored in both *sfp⁺* and *sfp⁻* cells by assaying β-galactosidase activity encoded by a promoterless *lacZ* gene that was fused to the *srf*::Tn917 insertion. Subsequent studies showed that the *sfp* locus altered the transcriptional regulation of *srf* in JH642 cells.[45-47] Studies on the genetic analysis of surfactin biosynthesis involved the isolation of *nul* mutants and subsequent identification of three chromosomal loci responsible for biosynthesis of surfactin in *B. subtilis*.[45] One of the loci, identified as *srf*B, is identical to the *com*A locus responsible for genetic competence in *B. subtilis*.[45,47] The *srf*A locus, which is defined by a transpososn Tn917 insertion required for the synthesis of surfactin, is a large operon of more than 25 kb pairs with four open reading frames that may correspond to sub-units of surfatin synthesis. It was reported that adenylation reaction could be responsible for the activation of the constituent amino acids, which is the same mechanism of activation utilized by the tyrocidine and gramicidine synthetase enzyme complexes. This evidence suggests that *srf*A encodes at least some of the enzymes that catalyze the synthesis of surfactin.[46] *srf*AA contains the amino acid-activating domains for Glu, Leu and D-Leu; *srf*AB contains the amino acid-activating domains for Val, Asp. and D-Leu; and *srf*AC encodes the enzyme that contains the amino acid-activating domain for L-Leu. *srf*AD encodes a product, which resembles in primary structure a family of thioesterases,[48,49] the role of which in the initiation of surfactin biosynthesis has been recently elucidated.[50] In addition to its role in the biosynthesis of surfactin, *srf*A functions in the development of genetic competence in *Bacillus subtilis*,[46,51] a process of cell specialization whereby a fraction of the cell population becomes endowed with the capacity to internalize exogenous DNA in response to conditions encountered in stationary phase cultures of glucose-grown cells.[49] D'Souza et al[49] also studied the effect of Ser-to-Ala substitutions in the amino-acylation site of each domain of *srf*A locus on surfactin production and competence development. This was the first report describing the effects of peptide synthetase active site mutations in vivo on surfactin production and competence development in *Bacillus subtilis*. Further advances on analysis and characterization of surfactin synthetase subunits in srfA mutants of *B. subtilis*, surfactin synthetase C-terminal thioesterase domain as a cyclic depsipeptide synthase and the role of uncoordinated transcription and physical linkage of domains in proper assembly and activity of multienzyme complex system, leading towards the completion of surfcatin synthesis, releasing the assembled lipopeptide chain by hydrolysis and stereospecific macrolactone cyclization have significantly enriched the scientific literature.[50,52-54]

Potential Commercial Applications

Health-Care and Bio-Control Applications

Resurgence in interest in surfactin, which was discovered almost four decades ago, can be a consequence of the increasing number of evidences for its potential efficacy as a therapeutic molecule for health-care applications.[55-58] Surfactin, produced in the culture fluids of various strains of *Bacillus subtilis*, significantly delayed fibrin clot formation process by inhibiting the conversion of fibrin monomer to fibrin polymer.[7] In a similar study, surfactin was reported to enhance the rate of plasminogen activation, which in turn augmentated fibrinolysis both in vitro and in vivo.[59] Interestingly, surfactin, which by acting as a selective inhibitor of platelet cytosolic phospholipase

A2 enzyme, could effectively suppress inflammatory responses.[60] Surfactin, also called subtilysin, showed cytolytic and antibiotic activities.[57,61] It causes lysis of erythrocytes, many bacterial protoplasts and spheroplasts and has some properties in common with two other cytolytic agents of bacterial origin, namely, staphylococcal δ-toxin and streptolysin-S.[61,62] Surfactin was also reported to show very significant antihypercholesterolemic and antifungal properties for potential health-care applications.[63,64] Prominent antimycoplasma and antiviral properties of surfcatin for potential therapeutic applications were also reported.[65-67] This strong antimicrobial and antiviral actions of surfactin could be a consequence of its ability to form ion-conducting channels in bacterial cell membranes by exploiting its detergent-like action on cell membranes, also called membrane active properties.[11,68-71] The membrane active properties which enable it to function as a potent inhibitor of cyclic adenosine 3′,5′-monophosphate phosphodiesterase enzyme.[72] This inhibition is caused by the chelating action of the free carboxyl groups of glutamic acid and aspartic acid residues of surfactin. Unlike conventional antibiotics that penetrate into the target cells to show their actions, antimicrobial membrane active peptides like surfactin are believed to kill target cells by destroying their membrane(s), thereby mimicking the actions of porins.[69-71,73] This mode of action drastically reduces the chance of development of resistance in microbes and hence, offers a promising alternative in the treatment of raging multidrug-resistant infectious diseases.[73] The broad-spectrum antimicrobial activities, even against many multi-drug resistant strains make the lipopeptide biosurfactants, like surfactin, attractive alternatives to conventional antibiotics.[57,74] However, the prominent hemolytic property of surfactin[67,75] has been a major bottleneck in fully realizing its application potential as a novel therapeutic molecule.

Surfactin was also reported to exhibit very significant antitumor activity and antiproliferative actions against many cancer cell lines.[76,77] The mechanisms of its antiproliferative action were attributed to induction of apoptosis, ceasation of cell cycle and suppression of survival signaling.[77] Surfactin has recently been reported to have strong lipopolysaccharide-binding property, which in turn results in its antiendotoxin activity.[78] The ability of surfactin to inhibit biofilm formation on various surfaces may find potential biomedical applications, particularly in surgical devices and implants.[79] Table 1 presents a list of potential therapeutic applications of surfactin with relevant references.

The lipopeptide biosurfactants from *Bacillus* strains were reported to be powerful biocontrol agents, which inhibit or kill phytopathogens and pests causing plant diseases.[80] Application of surfatin as an agent for biological control of plant pathogens showed very good promise. There are several reports on the use and production of surfactin for controlling bacterial,[81] mould[82] and fungal[83,84] pathogens.

Table 1. Potential health-care applications of surfactin

Therapeutic Application Potentials	Reference
Causes hemolysis and inhibits fibrin clot formation	7, 59, 67, 75
Exhibits antifungal, antibacterial and antihypercholesterolemia properties	61-63
Possesses antitumor and antiproliferative activities against cancer cell lines	76-77
Induces formation of ion channels in lipid bi-layer membranes	68-71
Antimycoplasma property	66
Antiviral property—inactivation of herpes and retroviruses	65, 67
Biomedical applications—inhibition of biofilm formation	79
Broad spectrum antimicrobial activity against multi-drug resistant strains	74
Suppression of inflammation by inhibiting platelet cytosolic phospholipase	60
Antiendotoxin property in animal models	78

Table 2. Potential environmental applications of surfactin

Commercial Application Potentials	Reference
Enhanced oil recovery	1, 85
Heavy oil transportation	41
Degradation of hydrocarbons in contaminated sites	86, 87
Promotes metal remediation	2

Environmental Applications

Surfactin has found tremendous potential applications in environmental bioremediation, enhanced oil recovery (MEOR) and heavy oil transportation, due mainly to its very strong surface and emulsification activities.[1,2] Surfactin was characterized as a potentially efficient oil recovery agent.[85] Application of surfactin for enhanced biodegradation of hydrocarbons; particularly diesel present in contaminated soil has been reported.[86,87] Lipopeptides including surfactin from *Bacillus* cultures facilitated transportation of heavy oil.[41] The list of environmental applications of surfcatin is presented in Table 2 with the relevant references.

Conclusion

The world of surfactin, the most studied and potent lipopeptide biosurfactant, was revisited in this chapter. The critical discussion on biosynthesis of surfactin by various strains of *Bacillus subtilis* and the genetic regulations of its biosynthesis would help develop a better understanding of the biosynthesis mechanisms of other lipopeptide biosurfactants and may lead towards developing some hyper-producing recombinant strains for large scale production. The plethora of practical applications in the areas of health-care and environment truly makes surfactin a versatile biomolecule with tremendous commercial application potentials. Discovery of surfactin thus opened up new avenues in biotechnology research for finding, developing and designing bioactive molecules with versatile properties and novel broad-spectrum applications.

Acknowledgement

I do gratefully acknowledge my parents, my wife, Anamika and my son, Yuvraaj for their patience, forbearance and encouragement. I thank Palashpriya Das, my Ph.D student, for helping me with the Tables.

References

1. Sen R. Biotechnology in enhanced petroleum recovery: the MEOR. Prog Energy Combust Sci 2008; 34:714-724.
2. Mulligan CN. Environmental applications for biosurfactants. Environ Pollut 2005; 133:183-198.
3. Desai JD, Banat IM. Microbial production of surfactants and their commercial potential. Microbiol Mol Biol Rev 1997; 61:47-64.
4. Banat IM, Makkar RS, Cameotra SS. Potential commercial applications of microbial surfactants. Appl Microbiol Biotechnol 2000; 53:495-508.
5. Mukherjee S, Das P, Sen R. Towards commercial production of microbial surfactants. Trends Biotechnol 2006; 24:509-515.
6. Nitschke M, Costa SGVAO. Biosurfactants in food industry. Trends Food Sci Tech 2007; 18:252-259.
7. Arima K, Kakinuma A, Tamura G. Surfactin, a crystalline peptidelipid surfactant produced by Bacillus subtilis: Isolation, characterization and its inhibition of fibrin clot formation. Biochem Biophy Res Commun 1968; 31:488-494.
8. Kakinuma A, Hori M, Isono M et al. Determination of amino acid sequence in surfactin, a crystalline peptidolipid surfactant produced by Bacillus subtilis. Agric Biol Chem 1969a; 33:971-997.
9. Kakinuma A, Ouchida A, Shima T et al. Confirmation of the structure of surfactin by mass spectroscopy. Agric Biol Chem 1969b; 33:1669-1671.
10. Itokawa H, Miyashita T, Morita H et al. Structural and conformational studies of [Ile7] and [Leu7] surfactins from B. subtilis. Chem Pharm Bull 1994; 42:604-607.

11. Peypoux F, Bonmatin JM, Wallach J. Recent trends in the biochemistry of surfactin. Appl Microbiol Biotechnol 1999; 51:553-63.
12. Trauger JW, Kohli RM, Mootz HD et al. Peptide cyclization catalyzed by the thioesterase domain of tyrocidine synthetase. Nature 2000; 407:215-218.
13. Bruner SD, Weber T, Kohli RM et al. Structural basis for the cyclization of the lipopeptide antibiotic surfactin by the thioesterase domain SrfTE. Structure 2002; 10:301-310.
14. Morikawa M, Hirata Y, Imanaka T. A study on the structure-function relationship of lipopeptide bio-surfactants. Biochim Biophys Acta 2000; 1488:211-218.
15. Bonmatin J-M, Laprévote O, Peypoux F. Diversity among microbial cyclic lipopeptides: iturins and surfactins. Activity-structure relationships to design new bioactive agents. Comb Chem High Throughput Screen 2003; 6:541-56.
16. Hue N, Serani L, Laprévote O. Structural investigation of cyclic peptidolipids from Bacillus subtilis by high energy tandem mass spectrometry. Rapid Commun Mass Spectrom 2001; 15:203-209.
17. Tsan P, Volpon L, Besson F et al. Structure and dynamics of surfactin studied by NMR in micellar media. J Am Chem Soc 2007; 129:1968-77.
18. Maget-Dana R, Ptak M. Interfacial properties of surfactin. J Colloid Interface Sci 1992; 153:285-291.
19. Vater J. Lipopeptides, an attractive class of microbial surfactants. Progr Colloid Polymer Sci 1986; 72:12-18.
20. Kluge B, Vater J, Salnikow J et al. Studies on the biosynthesis of surfactin, a lipo-peptide antibiotic from B. subtilis ATCC 21332, FEBS Lett 1988; 231:107-110.
21. Zuber P. Nonribosomal peptide synthesis. Curr Opin Cell Biol 1991; 3:1046-50.
22. Lipmann F. Bacterial production of antibiotic polypeptides by thiol-linked synthesis on protein templates. Adv Microb Physiol 1980; 21:227-266.
23. Kleinkauf H, von Döhren H. Nonribosomal biosynthesis of peptide antibiotics. Eur J Biochem 1990; 192:1-15.
24. Ullrich C, Kluge B, Palacz Z et al. Cell-free biosynthesis of surfactin, a cyclic lipopeptide produced by Bacillus subtilis. Biochemistry, 1991; 30:6503-6508.
25. Besson F, Michel G. Biosynthesis of iturin and surfactin by B. subtilis: Evidence for amino acid activating enzymes. Biotechnol Lett 1992; 14:1013-1018.
26. Peypoux F, Michel G. Controlled biosynthesis of (Val7) and (Leu7) surfactins. Appl Microbiol Biotechnol 1992; 36:515-517.
27. Cooper DG, Macdonald CR, Duff SJB et al. Enhanced production of surfactin from Bacillus subtilis by continuous product removal and metal cation additions. Appl Environ Microbiol 1981; 42:408-412.
28. Ohno A, Takashi A, Shoda M. Production of a lipopeptide antibiotic, surfactin, by recombinant B. subtilis in solid state fermentation. Biotech Bioeng 1995; 47:209.
29. Sen R. Response surface optimization of the critical media components for the production of surfactin. J Chem Technol Biotechnol 1997; 68:263-270.
30. Sen R, Swaminathan T. Application of response surface methodology to evaluate the optimum environmental conditions for the enhanced production of surfactin. Appl Microbiol Biotechnol 1997; 47:358-363.
31. Davis DA, Lynch HC, Varley J. The production of surfactin in batch culture by Bacillus subtilis ATCC 21332 is strongly influenced by the conditions of nitrogen metabolism. Enzyme Microb Technol 1999; 25:322-329.
32. Jacques P, Hbid C, Destain J et al. Optimization of biosurfactant lipopeptide production from Bacillus subtilis S499 by plackett-burman design. Appl Biochem Biotech 1999; 77-79:223-233.
33. Sen R, Swaminathan T. Response surface modeling and optimization to elucidate and analyze the effects of inoculum age and size on surfactin reduction. Biochem Eng J 2004; 21:141-148.
34. Noah KS, Bruhn DF, Bala GA. Surfactin production from potato process effluent by Bacillus subtilis in a chemostat. Appl Biochem Biotechnol 2005; 122:465-474.
35. Sen R, Swaminathan T. Characterization of concentration and purification parameters and operating conditions for the small-scale recovery of surfactin. Proc Biochem 2005; 40:2953-2958.
36. Tadashi Y, Yoshiaki M, Kazuo F et al. Production process of surfactin. US Patent No. 7,011,969 (March 2006).
37. Yeh M-S, Wei Y-H, Chang J-S. Bioreactor design for enhanced carrier-assisted surfactin production with Bacillus subtilis. Proc Biochem 2006; 41:1799-1805.
38. Liu Q, Hang Y, Jun W et al. A mutant of Bacillus subtilis with high-producing surfactin by ion beam implantation. Plasma Sci Technol 2006; 8:491-496.
39. Al-Ajlani MM, Sheikh MA, Ahmad Z et al. Production of surfactin from Bacillus subtilis MZ-7 grown on pharmamedia commercial medium. Microbial Cell Factories 2007; 6:17.
40. Wei Y, Lai C, Chang J. Using Taguchi experimental design methods to optimize trace element composition for enhanced surfactin production by Bacillus subtilis ATCC 21332. Proc Biochem 2007; 42:40-45.

41. Ghojavand H, Vahabzadeh F, Roayaei E et al. Production and properties of a biosurfactant obtained from a member of the Bacillus subtilis group (PTCC 1696). J Colloid Interface Sci 2008; 324:172-176.
42. Ponte Rocha M, Gomes Barreto R, Melo V et al. Evaluation of cashew apple juice for surfactin production by Bacillus subtilis LAMI008. Appl Biochem Biotechnol 2009; 155:63-75.
43. Nitschke M, Araújo LV, Costa SGVAO et al. Surfactin reduces the adhesion of food-borne pathogenic bacteria to solid surfaces. Lett Appl Microbiol 2009; Online early view:doi:10.1111/j.1472-765X.2009.02646.x.
44. Nakano MM, Marahiel MA, Zuber P. Identification of a genetic locus required for biosynthesis of the lipopeptide antibiotic surfactin in Bacillus subtilis. J Bacteriol 1988; 170:5662-5668.
45. Nakano MM, Zuber P. Cloning and characterization of srfB, a regulatory gene involved in surfactin production and competence in Bacillus subtilis. J Bateriol 1989; 171:5347-53.
46. Nakano MM, Magnuson R, Myers A et al. srfA is an operon required for surfactin production, competence development and efficient sporulation in Bacillus subtilis. J Bacteriol 1991; 173:1770-78.
47. Nakano MM, Corbell N, Besson J et al. Isolation and characterization of sfp: A gene that functions in the production of the lipopeptide biosurfactant, surfactin, in Bacillus subtilis. Mol Gen Genet 1992; 232:313-321.
48. Fuma S, Fujishima Y, Corbell N et al. Nucleotide sequence of 5' portion of srfA that contains the region required for competence establishment in Bacillus subtilis. Nucleic Acids Res 1993; 21:93-97.
49. C D'Souza C, Nakano MM, Corbell N et al. Amino-acylation site mutations in amino acid-activating domains of surfactin synthetase: effects on surfactin production and competence development in Bacillus subtilis. J Bacteriol 1993; 175:3502-3510.
50. Steller S, Sokoll A, Wilde C et al. Initiation of surfactin biosynthesis and the role of the SrfD-thioesterase protein. Biochemistry 2004; 43:11331-11343.
51. Dubnau D. Genetic competence in Bacillus subtilis. Microbiol Rev 1991; 55:395-424.
52. Vollenbroich D, Mehta N, Zuber P et al. Analysis of surfactin synthetase subunits in srfA mutants of Bacillus subtilis OKB 105. J Bacteriol 1994; 176:395-400.
53. Guenzi E, Galli G, Grgurina I et al. Coordinate transcription and physical linkage of domains in surfactin synthetase are not essential for proper assembly and activity of multienzyme complex. J Biol Chem 1998; 273:14403-14410.
54. Tseng CC, Bruner SD, Kohli RM et al. Characterization of the surfactin synthetase C-terminal thioesterase domain as a cyclic depsipeptide synthase. Biochemistry 2002; 41:13350-13359.
55. Singh P, Cameotra SS. Potential applications of microbial surfactants in biomedical sciences. Trends Biotechnol 2004; 22:142-146.
56. Rodrigues L, Ibrahim MB, Teixeira J et al. Biosurfactants: potential applications in medicine. J Antimicrob Chemother 2006; 57:609-618.
57. Giuliani A, Pirri G, Fabiole Nicoletto S. Antimicrobial peptides: an overview of a promising class of therapeutics, Central Euro J Biol 2007; 2:1-33.
58. Seydlová G, Svobodová J. Review of surfactin chemical properties and the potential biomedical applications. Central Euro J Med 2008; 3:123-133.
59. Kikuchi T, Hasumi K. Enhancement of plasminogen activation by surfactin C: augmentation of fibrinolysis in vitro and in vivo. Biochim Biophys Acta 2002; 1596:234-245.
60. Kim K, Jung SY, Lee DK et al. Suppression of inflammatory responses by surfactin, a selective inhibitor of platelet cytosolic phospholipase A2. Biochem Pharmacol 1998; 55:975-985.
61. Bernheimer AW, Avigad LS. Nature and properties of a cytolytic agent produced by Bacillus subtilis. J Gen Microbiol 1970; 61:361-369.
62. Tsukagoshi N, Tamura G, Arima K. A novel protoplast-bursting factor (surfactin) obtained from Bacillus subtilis IAM 1213. II. The interaction of surfactin with bacterial membranes and lipids. Biochim Biophys Acta 1970; 196:211-214.
63. Arima K, Tamura G, Kakinuma A. Surfactin. US Patent No. 3,687,926; 1972.
64. Thimon L, Peyoux F, Maget-Dana R et al. Surface-active properties of antifungal lipopeptides produced by Bacillus subtilis. JAOCS 1992; 69:92-93.
65. Vollenbroich D, Ozel M, Vater J et al. Mechanism of inactivation of enveloped viruses by the biosurfactant surfactin from Bacillus subtilis. Biologicals 1997a; 25:289-297.
66. Vollenbroich D, Pauli G, Ozel M et al. Antimycoplasma properties and applications in cell culture of surfactin, a lipopeptide antibiotic from Bacillus subtilis. Appl Environ Microbiol 1997b; 63:44-49.
67. Kracht M, Rokos H, Ozel M et al. Antiviral and hemolytic activities of surfactin isoforms and their methyl ester derivatives. J Antibiot 1999; 52:613-619.
68. Sheppard JD, Jumarie C, Cooper DG et al. Ionic channels induced by surfactin in planar lipid bilayer membranes. Biochim Biophys Acta 1991; 1064:13-23.
69. Heerklotz H, Seelig J. Detergent-like action of the antibiotic peptide surfactin on lipid membranes. Biophysical J 2001; 81:1547-54.

70. Carrillo C, Teruel JA, Aranda FA et al. Molecular mechanism of membrane permeabilization by the peptide antibiotic surfactin. Biochem Biophys Acta 2003; 1611:91-97.

71. Heerklotz H, Wieprecht T, Seelig J. Membrane perturbation by the lipopeptide surfactin and detergents as studied by Deuterium NMR. J Phys Chem 2004; 108:4909-4915.

72. Hosono K, Suzuki H. Acylpeptides, the inhibitors of cyclic adenosine 3',5'-monophosphate phosphodiesterase. III. Inhibition of cyclic AMP phosphodiesterase. J Antibiot (Tokyo) 1983; 36:679-683.

73. Amram MOR. Peptide-based antibiotics: a potential answer to raging antimicrobial resistance. Drug Develop Res 2000; 50:440-447.

74. Fernandes PAV, Arruda IRD, Santo AFABD et al. Antimicrobial activity of surfactants produced by Bacillus subtilis R14 against multidrug-resistant bacteria. Braz J Microbiol 2007; 38:704-709.

75. Dufour S, Deleu M, Nott K et al. Hemolytic activity of new linear surfactin analogs in relation to their physicochemical properties. Biochim Biophys Acta 2005; 1726:87-95.

76. Kameda Y, Oira S, Matsui K et al. Antitumor activity of Bacillus natto V. Isolation and characterization of surfactin in the culture medium of Bacillus natto KMD 2311. Chem Pharm Bull (Tokyo) 1974; 22:938-44.

77. Kim S, Kim J, Kim S et al. Surfactin from Bacillus subtilis displays antiproliferative effect via apoptosis induction, cell cycle arrest and survival signaling suppression. FEBS Lett 2007; 581:865-871.

78. Hwang Y-H, Park B-K, Lim J-H et al. Lipopolysaccharide-binding and neutralizing activities of surfactin C in experimental models of septic shock. Euro J Pharmacol 2007; 556:166-171.

79. Mireles II JR, Toguchi A, Harshey RM. Salmonella enterica Serovar Typhimurium swarming mutants with altered biofilm-forming abilities: surfactin inhibits biofilm formation. J Bacteriol 2001; 183:5848-5854.

80. Ongena M, Jacques P. Bacillus lipopeptides: versatile weapons for plant disease biocontrol. Trends Microbiol 2008; 16:115-125.

81. Bais HP, Fall R, Vivanco JM. Biocontrol of Bacillus subtilis against infection of arabidopsis roots by Pseudomonas syringae is facilitated by biofilm formation and surfactin production. Plant Physiology 2004; 134:307-319._

82. Ongena M, Jacques P, Toure Y et al. Role of lipopeptides produced by Bacillus subtilis GA1 in the reduction of grey mould disease caused by Botrytis cinerea on apple. J Appl Microbiol 2004; 96:1151-1160.

83. Snook ME, Mitchell T, Hinton DM et al. Isolation and characterization of Leu⁷-surfactin from the endophytic bacterium B. mojavensis RRC 101, a biocontrol agent for Fusarium verticillioides. J Agric Food Chem 2009; 57:4287-4292.

84. Mohammadipour M, Mousivand M, Salehi Juzani G et al. Molecular and biochemical characterization of Iranian surfactin-producing Bacillus subtilis isolates and evaluation of their biocontrol potential against Aspergillus flavus and Colletotrichum gloeosporioides. Canad J Microbiol 2009; 55:395-404.

85. Schaller K, Fox S, Bruhn D et al. Characterization of surfactin from Bacillus subtilis for application as an agent for enhanced oil recovery. Appl Biochem Biotechnol 115; 2004:827-836.

86. Whang L-M, Liu P-W G, Ma C-C et al. Application of biosurfactants, rhamnolipid and surfactin, for enhanced biodegradation of diesel-contaminated water and soil. J Hazard Mat 2008; 151:155-163.

87. Whang L-M, Liu P-W G, Ma C-C et al. Application of rhamnolipid and surfactin for enhanced diesel biodegradation—Effects of pH and ammonium addition. J Hazard Mat 2009; 164:1045-1050.

Index

X

Y